Modern Hearing Aids

Pre-Fitting Testing and Selection Considerations

Modern Hearing Aids

Pre-Fitting Testing and Selection Considerations

H. Gustav Mueller, PhD
Todd Ricketts, PhD
Ruth Bentler, PhD

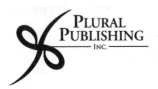

PLURAL
PUBLISHING
INC.

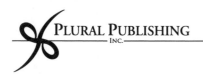

5521 Ruffin Road
San Diego, CA 92123

e-mail: info@pluralpublishing.com
Web site: http://www.pluralpublishing.com

Typeset in 10½/13 Minion Pro by Flanagan's Publishing Services, Inc.
Printed in the United States of America by McNaughton & Gunn, Inc.

Library of Congress Cataloging-in-Publication Data

Mueller, H. Gustav.
  Modern hearing aids. Pre-fitting, testing, and selection considerations / H. Gustav Mueller, Todd Ricketts, and Ruth Bentler. — 1st ed.
      p. ; cm.
  Pre-fitting, testing, and selection considerations
  Includes bibliographical references and index.
  ISBN-13: 978-1-59756-138-9 (alk. paper)
  ISBN-10: 1-59756-138-X (alk. paper)
  I. Ricketts, Todd. II. Bentler, Ruth A. III. Title. IV. Title: Pre-fitting, testing, and selection considerations.
  [DNLM: 1. Hearing Aids. 2. Hearing Tests. 3. Speech Acoustics. WV 274]
  RF300
  617.8'9—dc23
                            2013006758

Contents

Preface

Much of the technical information we need for the practice of audiology can now be accessed electronically, assuming you have enough time and skill with search engines. However, there still are those times when the best solution is to simply reach for a good reliable book. Books about hearing aid function and the fitting of hearing aids have become fairly common in recent years, but that was not always the case. The first book on the topic that we are aware of dates back to 1949, written by LeLand A. Watson and Thomas L. Tolan titled, *Hearing Tests and Hearing Instruments*. As the title suggests, a portion of the book was about hearing testing, but the hearing aid topic made up at least one-half of the 500 pages. The discipline of audiology expanded considerably in the 1950s and 1960s, but books about hearing aids were scarce. This is probably related to the fact that the topic of hearing aids received little attention in academia. It was not uncommon, even as recent as the early 1970s, that graduate training for hearing aids included no more than one-third or one-half of a three-credit hour course—maybe paired with speech audiometry. This all changed, however, in the late 1970s when it no longer was unethical for audiologists to sell hearing aids, and academic interest in the fitting and dispensing of hearing aids increased accordingly.

This increased interest in hearing aids timed nicely with a hearing aid book edited by Michael Pollack, published in 1975, which became the go-to text for many universities for several years. As an aside, an often overlooked aspect of this Pollack book is the 17-page introduction by Raymond Carhart, one of his last writings before his untimely death. Bill Hodgson and Paul Skinner also edited a hearing aid book during this time, which also was well received.

In the 1990s we saw new hearing aid books edited by Michael Valente, a continuing series that has become a useful reference source over the years. Although the trend regarding hearing aid texts has been to have multiauthored contributed books, there have been some notable exceptions. Margo Skinner's book from 1987 is one of our favorites, and of course in recent years, we have seen two hearing aid books authored by Harvey

Dillon. So with all that history, we are ready to throw our hat in the ring. There actually are three books in this series, so technically, that would be three hats!

What were we thinking when we came up with this book idea? First, we immediately decided that we did not want a contributed book, but rather something co-written by the three of us. We are all strong-minded, so we knew for us to reach a consensus may present a challenge on many issues, without having 20 other authors to contend with. Second, we wanted the book to be welcoming to university faculty and their students. Our goal was to include not just reference information, but tools supported by research and clinical experience, presented in a way that was accessible to clinical students with little experience in the field. We also wanted the book to be a handy companion for busy clinicians—a friendly resource where they quickly could find the critical information needed for the next patient. And finally, we wanted enough depth, that even the serious hearing aid researcher would thank us for a few helpful pearls.

As you noticed in the preceding paragraph, we were referencing "the book"; but, as we mentioned, there are three books in this series. Why not just one book, instead of three? That answer is simple. We just have too much to say! When we started this project a few years back, we indeed were going to put everything into one book, but we quickly realized that to include the content that we believed was important, a single text was not practical. We gave considerable thought of how we might break out all the different hearing aid topics—what topic in what book? Although several different approaches probably would have worked, we decided to organize the three books in a time-ordered manner. That is, starting when the patients walk in the door and ending when they complete their post-fitting self-assessment surveys. This tends to be the method used in hearing aid fitting guidelines.

Over the past 20 or more years, there have been several hearing aid fitting guidelines written: Starting back in 1991, we have The Vanderbilt Report, the Independent Hearing Aid Fitting Forum (IHAFF) protocol, and guidelines from both the American Academy of Audiology, and the American Speech-Language-Hearing Association. One or more of the three of us have been involved in the writing of all these documents. Although the various guidelines differ in some of the details, they all lay out the overall process in a fairly similar step-by-step manner: Audiological pre-fitting testing, needs assessment and treatment planning, hearing aid selection, verification, orientation and counseling, post-fitting follow-up, and real-world validation. Using this categorization system, we then have the current book, *Pre-Fitting Testing and Selection Considerations,* the first in the series, and then the two following books, *Function, Features and Advanced Algorithms* and *Verification, Outcome Measures and Follow-up.*

In this first book, we have taken you up to the point of selecting the hearing aid technology. We talk about the initial patient history and counseling, and a wide range of measures that can be used to determine patient needs. We have included numerous pre-fitting tests that can be conducted and given you step-by-step protocols for their administration and scoring. We review the selection of hearing aid styles and fitting arrangements, and take you through the process of obtaining an ear impression and making critical decisions regarding earmolds and hearing aid plumbing. We think you will also like the Appendix, where you can find much of the material needed to facilitate these pre-fitting measures and selection decisions. Because we are discussing the contents of this book, it is important that we acknowledge the tireless efforts of Elizabeth Stangl, AuD, from the Hearing Aid Lab at the University of Iowa. She is responsible for the construction of many of our figures, and she managed all the details regarding references, permissions, and overall organization of the book. Thanks Elizabeth!

Given that a large portion of our target audience is audiology students and busy clinicians, we knew that we had to give the book readability. We wanted to present our material in a manner that was a little unique, but not distracting. To accomplish this (we hope), we introduced callouts, where we could add or emphasize a given point. Throughout the text, you will see short paragraphs that we have identified as Technical Tips, Key Concepts, Things to Remember, and Points to Ponder. Also, every now and then, there was a topic that we felt so strongly about, that we just had to get "On the Soapbox." Finally, while digging through massive amounts of material in writing this book, we sometimes unearthed tidbits that were maybe not quite relevant enough to include in the chapter, yet too good to toss aside. You will find these in the back of the book, which we are calling Endnotes.

We have gone from a time when the topic of hearing aids only occupied a portion of a single class during graduate training, to today, when our AuD programs have three or four classes devoted totally to hearing aids. We have gone from a time when selling hearing aids was unethical, to today, when the majority of hearing aids in the United States are sold and dispensed by audiologists. Fitting hearing aids is what we do. We believe that this area of audiology is fascinating, exciting, rewarding, and sometimes even fun. We hope that you enjoy reading this text as much as we enjoyed writing it.

1

The Audiologist and Hearing Aid Provision

The selection and fitting of hearing aids has been associated with audiology since before audiology was called audiology. In fact, it is probable that the extensive work with hearing aids and aural rehabilitation by several individuals during World War II is what led to the coining of the words audiology and audiologist, but more on that later. In this chapter, we talk about how audiology is associated with the area of hearing aid fitting and dispensing, and discuss many of the overriding principles, guidelines, and regulations that impact on this relationship.

A Little History

Perhaps the first book to provide extensive guidance regarding the fitting of hearing aids was *Hearing Tests and Hearing Instruments* written by Watson and Tolan, published in 1949. Neither Watson nor Tolan were audiologists, or what we would now call audiologists. Thomas Tolan, an MD, was the director of the Department of Otology at the Medical School of the University of Minnesota. Leland A. Watson was the president of the Maico Corporation, a company involved in the manufacture of audiometers and hearing aids.[1] At the time this book was published, many viewed it as simply a promotion of Maico products (one reviewer commented "use-

ful for salesmen"), and to some extent it was, but it also was the first organized publication of many hearing aid fitting concepts, some of which still apply today.

It was around this same time that the terms audiology and audiologist began to be commonly used. When exactly the term audiology was coined is debatable. According to research by Ken Berger, PhD (1976a), the term may have been used by a New York dentist in 1935, by two California hearing aid specialists (approximately 1939), or by individuals working for the Maico company in the late 1930s. Probably unrelated, but well documented, is that a song titled "Audiology" was recorded around 1939.[2] In the academic world, the first use of the term *audiology* usually is credited to either Hallowell Davis, Norton Canfield (prominent military otolaryngologist), or Raymond Carhart, all in the mid-1940s. Relating to what we now know as the profession of audiology, the first use of the word in print was in 1946, in publications in the *Journal of Speech Disorders* (in reference to the U.S. Naval Hospital in Philadelphia) and in the *Volta Review* (in a description of course work offered at Northwestern University; Jerger, 2009).

Military Roots

Regardless of who actually coined the word audiology, there is little question that the advancement of the use of the term was linked directly to the establishment of rehabilitation centers during World War II. These sites were established to handle the large number of returning veterans suffering from hearing loss. Four major military regional sites were established: Hoff General Hospital (Santa Barbara, CA), Borden General Hospital (Chickasha, OK), Philadelphia Naval Hospital, and Deshon General Hospital (Butler, PA). Captain Raymond Carhart (see Figure 1–1), a 1936 PhD graduate of Northwestern University (majoring in speech pathology, experimental phonetics, and psychology), was assigned to Deshon Hospital from 1944 to 1946, and his work there has had a lasting effect on the field of audiology and, specifically, the selection and fitting of hearing aids. In 1946, Carhart published three articles describing the hearing aid selection and fitting procedures developed at Deshon (Carhart, 1946a, 1946b, 1946c). We talk more about the impact that Captain Carhart had on the clinical evaluation of hearing aids in Book Three, which focuses on the verification and validation of hearing aid performance.

Following World War II, there were several additional military audiology facilities established at major hospitals—Walter Reed Army Medical Center in Washington, DC being the most notable. Figure 1–2, is a photo from the 1950s, showing a soldier being fitted with amplification at the Walter Reed audiology clinic, located at the Forest Glen annex. We also saw the emergence of several U.S. Department of Veterans Affairs (VA) audiology clinics. All of these facilities employed audiologists, both military and civilian, who conducted hearing aid evaluations and also dispensed hearing aids to veterans, active duty and retired military personnel. Because of the ethical constraints placed on audiologists

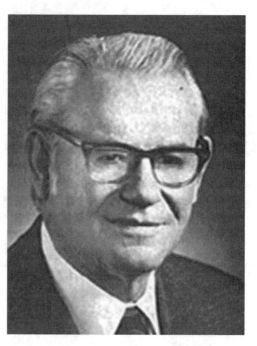

Figure 1–1. Raymond Carhart, PhD, often considered the father of audiology and at least partly responsible for coining the word audiology. Noted professor at Northwestern University until his death in 1975. He conducted pioneering work related to the selection and fitting of hearing aids while serving in the U.S. Army in the 1940s.

fitting hearing aids outside of the government—which we discuss shortly—these military and VA hospital clinics became known as excellent training sites for audiology students wanting to obtain hands-on experience with the selection and fitting of hearing aids.

THINGS TO REMEMBER: WARTIME AUDIOLOGY

If you are interested in audiology history, you will enjoy the monograph written by Moe Bergman titled "American Wartime Military Audiology," a special issue of *Audiology Today* (2002). In it he writes: "It is important for every profession to document its origins. It should be of interest to today's practitioners of audiology to know how the American military 'aural rehabilitation' programs for hearing casualties in the twentieth-century world wars practiced what is now known as 'audiology.'" Even then, professionals were working to help rehabilitate individuals who suffered from hearing loss, many as a result of the unprecedentedly loud equipment and powerful explosives used in World Wars I and II.

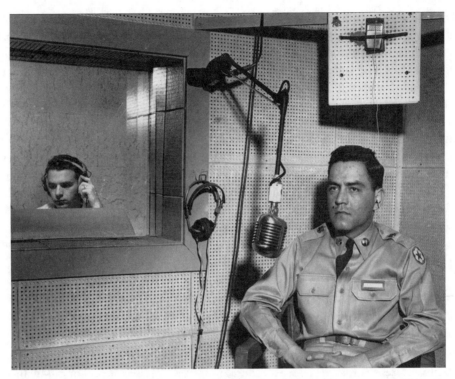

Figure 1–2. Traditional hearing aid evaluation circa 1950 using speech audiometry, a cornerstone of the comparative approach advocated by Raymond Carhart, PhD. Note upper right corner where body-style hearing aid is fixed to loudspeaker, with external receiver to patient.

It was also during this time that audiology training programs began to emerge. These early programs were in the Midwest, at locations such as Northwestern University, the University of Iowa, and Purdue University. The first PhD granted in audiology was from Northwestern in 1946 to John Keys, who went on to establish a noted audiology research and training program at the University of Oklahoma (Jerger, 2009).

Audiologists as the Middle Man

Although audiologists at military facilities enjoyed the benefits of directly dispensing hearing aids to their patients until the 1980s, in the civilian sector, nearly all hearing aids were dispensed by hearing aid dealers, not audiologists. Like today, there were many storefront hearing aid sales facilities, many of them franchises.

Audiologists' clinical activities regarding hearing aid dispensing were influenced greatly by the American Speech and Hearing Association (ASHA), the primary professional organization for audiologists during this time frame. For arguably good reasons, the ASHA had the belief that it could be challenging to professional ethics if an audiologist were to evaluate a patient for a hearing aid, recommend a hearing aid, and then turn around and sell the patient the hearing aid they had just recommended. Selling hearing aids, therefore, was a violation of the ASHA ethical standards.

So it was that during this time frame, audiologists had a somewhat unusual role in the selection and fitting of hearing aids. During this era, although the majority of hearing aids were dispensed by a *dispenser* without the patient first going to an audiologist, there were situations when an audiologist was involved. When this happened, the general fitting process would go something like this:

■ The patient would go to a university or hospital clinic to have his or her hearing tested and be evaluated for hearing aids. We say hearing aids, with an "s," although rarely did audiologists then recommend the use of two hearing aids. In fact, this often caused considerable friction between the hearing aid dealer and the audiologist, as dealers would more frequently fit people bilaterally ("just a way to make more money," audiologists often would say).

■ Audiologists of the time had a large stock selection of behind the ear (BTE) hearing aids on consignment from various manufacturers; it was not unusual to have 20 to 30 consignment aids. A common procedure then was to conduct aided sound field comparative speech testing, usually using monosyllables, with hearing aids from different companies. There usually was only time to test three hearing aids during a typical one-hour appointment, and hence, this selection procedure became known as the *hang three* approach.

■ Following the speech testing, the aided word recognition scores for each instrument were compared, and a *winner* was determined. In some cases, this might mean the patient only scored 2% to 4% higher with one of the instruments—but there had to be a winner! The audiologist would then *prescribe* this fitting (e.g., brand, model, settings of potentiometers, etc.).

TECHNICAL TIP: WHAT IS A POTENTIOMETER?

Audiologists of today are used to easily programming hearing aid gain and output using the manufacturer's software. This procedure, however, only has been common since the early 1990s. Prior to that time, audiologists used a small screwdriver to make adjustments to screw-set controls, called *potentiometers*. Most all BTE models had at least one *tone control* potentiometer (low-frequency cut), and many also had a control for the maximum power output (MPO). Some special models had as many as four potentiometers, with controls for compression kneepoints and even compression time constants.[3] An example of an "older" hearing aid employing potentiometers is shown in Figure 1–3.

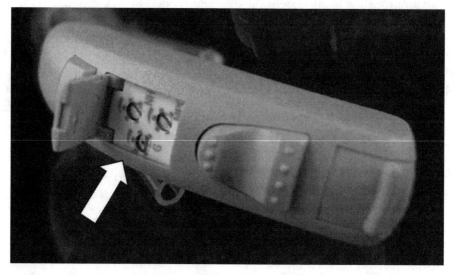

Figure 1–3. Prior to digital programming, hearing aid adjustments were made using screwdriver-controlled potentiometers. This BTE has three: tone control (low-frequency cut), gain, and maximum power output control.

■ The patient was then referred directly to a given hearing aid dealer who sold that brand (most dealers only sold one or two brands), or if the audiologist was concerned about the appearance of a conflict of interest, the patient was simply given a list of several dealers in the area, and the patient would then be on their own to find the product.

■ The protocol for most facilities was that after the patient purchased the new hearing aids, he or she would return to the audiology clinic to obtain aided speech recognition testing with the new product. This was another situation rife with conflict; as in many cases, the patient had purchased a hearing aid different from what the audiologist had recommended. The audiologist and dispenser would disagree regarding what was best, and the patient was caught in the middle.

For a variety of reasons, the fitting and dispensing arrangement just described was less than ideal. Not only was the original comparative selection procedure flawed, but the audiologist was removed from the important post-fitting troubleshooting, tweaking, and counseling. As would be expected, the patients returned to the hearing aid dealer, not the audiologist, for these services. If only audiologists were allowed to sell hearing aids, the process would have been so much more efficient.

Selling Is Not a Bad Word (Anymore)

Regarding the ASHA code of ethics mentioned earlier, it is important to point out that in the 1960s and 1970s state licensure for audiology did not exist for most states. Clinical audiologists, therefore, valued their ASHA certification and did not want to jeopardize their standing as an ASHA member. And, for the most part, audiologists not belonging to the ASHA were considered outsiders. Moreover, most audiologists, especially those in academia, tended to believe that selling hearing aids had a certain sleaze factor associated with it.[4] There of course were audiologists who tested the system, and their expulsion from the ASHA was publicized. James Jerger devotes a couple pages to *The Saga of Barry Elpern* in his book on the history of audiology (Jerger, 2009, pp. 48–49).

As time went on, however, more and more audiologists saw the benefits of providing complete services for their patients, and in the early 1970s, we started to see audiologists going into a dispensing private practice—with or without approval from the ASHA.

The movement to remove the violation for selling hearing aids from the ASHA code of ethics gathered steam in 1977 when a group of ASHA members formed the Academy of Dispensing Audiology (ADA). The name of the organization obviously was selected to make the point that selling hearing aids should be part of the audiologists' scope of practice (the name has since

---

POINTS TO PONDER: WHO KNEW BEST?

As we have mentioned, in the days when audiologists did not dispense, but rather referred their patients to hearing aid dispensers, there tended to be considerable disagreement between the two different disciplines regarding what was the best product for the patient. On one hand, audiologists based their recommendations primarily on the time—honored Carhart comparative speech testing model, testing a large variety of hearing aids from different manufacturers. Dispensers, on the other hand, tended to select a product from their favorite company and relied heavily on what the patient preferred, often taking cosmetics into account (some BTEs of the time were much larger than others). Although the audiologist's more scientific approach would seem to be superior, we need to point out that the different hearing aids tested in the clinic were nearly always adjusted by the audiologist to have very similar frequency responses before testing, and as a result, differential testing usually resulted in small differences in speech recognition—in most cases, differences no larger than the test-retest error. Although speech testing is rarely used today to select the "best" product or fitting arrangement, the role of the patient in determining specific hearing aid gain and output settings is still not well defined, and varies considerably among audiologists.

been changed to the Academy of Doctors of Audiology). Although one might think that this new organization was simply a handful of young maverick audiologists, it actually included several prominent members of the profession, most notably Leo Doerfler, PhD, who was not only the ADA's founding president, but also a former president of the ASHA.

While the internal pressure for change was resulting in many heated discussions at professional meetings, the event that probably triggered the change in ASHA policy was a 1978 U.S. Supreme Court ruling against the National Society of Professional Engineers, saying that their code of ethics could not be used to prohibit price interference for engineers' services. And so it was that selling hearing aids for profit became ethical. By the end of 1979, nearly 1,000 audiologists were selling hearing aids, and that number grew to 5,000 by the end of the 1980s (Harford, 2000).

Audiologists in the Workplace

Things have changed considerably since the days that audiologists only dispensed hearing aids in government facilities. Today, there are approximately 16,000 licensed audiologists in the United States, and 60% to 70% of

these dispense hearing aids. (Note, by comparison, there are approximately 8,000 licensed hearing instrument specialists.) Audiologists dispense from a variety of settings ranging from their own private practice, to an oto-laryngologist's practice, to a university or hospital clinic, to an office owned by a manufacturer, or in more recent years, from a chain department store. Shown in Figure 1–4 are the most recent data from the American Academy of Audiology (AAA) summarizing typical work settings. Observe that the highest percent of audiologists are in privately owned audiology practices. Although this is the most common workplace, data from the AAA suggests that only 15% to 20% of audiology offices are owned and controlled by audiologists, much lower than other similar professions (e.g., optometry 75%, dentistry 93%). Private practice ownership among audiologists also has been decreasing significantly in recent years, as offices are being purchased by manufacturers and other buying groups.

Hearing Aid Distribution Channels

Indirectly and sometimes directly related to the workplace where we find audiologists dispensing hearing aids, is the overall hearing aid distribution system.

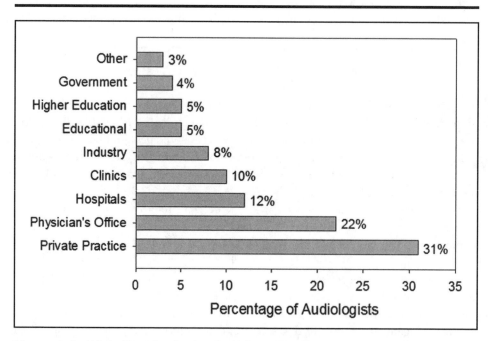

Figure 1–4. Workplace distribution for U.S. audiologists.

Manufacturers

We now have what is referred to as the *Big Six*, composed of Widex, Siemens, Starkey, Great Nordic (GN) ReSound, Sonova (Phonak), and William Demant (Oticon). Among them, these companies own or manage 15 to 20 other brands of hearing aids. In addition, there are probably another 25 to 30 lesser known hearing aid manufacturing companies. Most audiologists have one or two favorite companies, and buy directly from these manufacturers, with over 90% of sales from the Big Six.

Buying Groups

Some audiologists find it advantageous to work with a buying group. That is, because of the increased volume, the groups can demand discounts from the manufacturers and pass these savings on to members of the group. There are several different groups and different types of groups to choose from. Examples are Audigy, AuDNET, EarQ, AHAA, and Sonus. Many of the groups offer a range of practice assistance other than just hearing aid purchases. Some of the buying groups, however, more or less work exclusively with the brands of one or two manufacturers.

Retail Outlets

All of the Big Six have retail outlets, which may consist of established stores such as Beltone (owned by GN ReSound), companies with multicenter clinical sites such as Newport Audiology (Sonova) or HearUSA (Siemens), or the manufacturer may be more subtly involved through corporate-owned, independent practices. In addition to the Big Six, retail offices also are operated by Amplifon (Sonus and Miracle Ear), Costco, and Sam's Club (and probably several more since the writing of this chapter). All the retail outlets employ audiologists,

---

POINTS TO PONDER: TO BUNDLE OR NOT?

Surveys indicate that 80% to 85% of audiologists who sell hearing aids use a *bundled* approach. That is, a single inclusive price that includes the audiologist's cost for the product, fitting fees, counseling, and follow-up visits (either through the life of the hearing aid, or in some cases only during the warranty period). The patient is not informed what percent of the total cost is for the product, or what costs are for services, although our experiences suggest that the average patient believes the bulk of the cost is the product.

Audiologists who use an *unbundled* approach, break out the cost of the product, accessories, fitting fees, consulting, and follow-up services. This has the advantage of clearly showing the value of the fitting and counseling that goes along with dispensing hearing aids. Additionally, it eliminates the patient's concern that the audiologist is upselling when he or she recommends more features, as the fitting fee would likely stay the same (e.g., it does not require more time or counseling to fit a 20-channel product than a 4-channel product). Some audiologists, however, shy away from the unbundled approach because they believe that when the patient sees the true cost of the hearing aid, they will consider the audiologist's fees to be unreasonable (e.g., a $1,000 hearing aid—cost to audiologist—typically is sold for $2,000; in an unbundled scheme, keeping the total cost the same, this would suggest a $1,000 fitting fee). Also, audiologists fear that the patient may not return for the necessary follow-up visits because of the cost involved, and the end result will be dissatisfaction with amplification. Because of this, some audiologists use a partly unbundled approach.

The reason we have included this topic as a "Points to Ponder" is because as Internet sales of hearing aids become more common, audiologists may have to think more about the value of their services, as patients will walk in the door already owning their hearing aids. For a review of the pros and cons of bundling for hearing aid sales, see the *Audiology Today* article by Sjoblad and Warren (2011), and the comments of John Coverstone on page 22.

although the audiologist or hearing instrument specialist mix varies considerably among sites.

Internet Sales

Consumers obtain much of their information about hearing loss and hearing aids from the Internet, so it is not surprising that they buy hearing aids through the Internet too. There are even sites that rate the Internet sales sites. An internet purchase is possible by simply going to eBay, or to Internet sites specializing in Internet sales (conduct an Internet search and you will see that there are several). Although most if not all manufacturers have issued a statement saying that they will not sell hearing aids to retailers who do not conduct an in-person fitting, this is difficult to control. For example, if a regular customer of a hearing aid manufacturer purchases 10 BTE hearing aids, how does the company know how and when they were sold? Internet sales also

may be illegal in some states, but again, enforcement is difficult and as you would expect, something of this nature has a low priority with enforcement officials.

The Ohio Hearing Aid Internet Work Group (September 2011) compiled the chart shown in Table 1–1 regarding state laws related to Internet hearing aid sales.

In most cases, the hearing aid purchased through the Internet will need programming by an audiologist, not to mention that the patient will also need long-term follow-up rehabilitation care. How this is accomplished often becomes a sticky issue for dispensing audiologists. How are these patients handled when they show up for an appointment carrying their newly purchased hearing aids with them? Some Internet hearing aid sales sites such as Hearing Planet (Sonova) have attempted to partner with dispensing audiologists—that is, the patient brings in the Internet-purchased hearing aids and the audiologist conducts the programming. In general, audiologists have not been receptive to this arrange-

Table 1–1. Examples of State Laws that Relate to the Internet Sale of Hearing Aids

State	Citation	Type of Restriction
California	CA BPC Code §3351.5	Catalog/direct mail sellers must be licensed HA dispensers in CA.
Connecticut	CT Public Health Code §20-406-14	Must be licensed by state to fit or dispense HA.
	CT Public Health Code §20-406-1	Reference to "regular place of business" where licensee must be physically available to the public
Florida	FL Statute §484.054	Prohibition on sales or distribution of HA through the mail to the ultimate consumer
Maryland	MD Statute §391-2	Requires MD license for online dispensers; applies general commercial law to HA sales.
Missouri	MO Statute §346.110	Fitting and testing must be done by Mo licensed HAD or AuD prior to mail order sale
Nevada	NV Statute §637A.243	Mail order sales require: proof of otoscopic exam; proof of audiometric exam; earmolds taken by NV licensee; attestation by consumer.
Oregon	OR Statute §694.032	Fitting and sale of HA must be competed in state.
Texas	TX Statue §402.451	Dispensing and fitting must be done by TX licensee.
Washington	WA Statute §18.35.175	Requires face to face contact "to test or otherwise determine needs of purchaser"

ment. However, Internet sales are not going to go away, so we expect that some type of arrangement will evolve so that this group of patients can receive effective benefit from their instruments.

Personal Sound Amplifier Product. We recognize that this is a product and not a distribution channel, but we explain the connection soon. When is a device a personal sound amplifier product (PSAP) and when is it a hearing aid? The distinction becomes more blurred each year. In March 2009, the Food and Drug Administration (FDA) issued guidance describing how hearing aids and PSAPs differ. This guidance defines a hearing aid as a sound-amplifying device intended to compensate for impaired hearing. PSAPs, the guidance states, are not intended to make up for impaired hearing. Instead, they are intended for non-hearing-impaired consumers to amplify sounds in the environment for a number of reasons, such as for recreational activities. You maybe have seen advertisements for such devices as "Game Ear" or "Hunter's Ear." Some PSAPs are more or less novelty items—see Figure 1–5. But today, we also have advanced PSAPs advertised as having 14 bands and channels, digital noise reduction, feedback reduction, and a volume control wheel. Sounds a lot like a hearing aid to us, but such products are being sold over-the-counter at retail outlets. Products like this may have a significant impact on hearing instrument sales and distribution channels.[5]

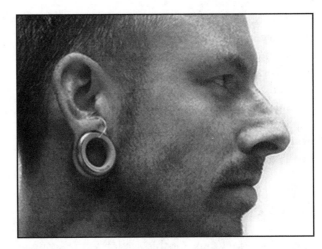

Figure 1–5. An example of a PSAP with a unique ear lobe placement. One of many styles developed to make PSAPs more interesting.

Laws, Regulations, Rules, and Guidelines Related to the Fitting of Hearing Aids

We know that it takes years of education and experience to be successful in the practice of fitting and dispensing hearing aids. The student of this area of audiology must know anatomy and physiology, hearing science, a variety

---

SOAP BOX: WHAT ARE WE SELLING?

We sometimes hear AuD students say in their first or second year, "I'm really not interested in hearing aids, as I don't want to have to *sell* something." Yes, there often is a financial transaction when working with hearing aids, but there are also charges involved for routine diagnostics, balance function testing, auditory processing disorder (APD) evaluations, and most all other audiologic services. Regarding hearing aids, the question really is, what are we selling? We know that properly fitted hearing aids and effective counseling will lead to long-term hearing aid use, benefit, and satisfaction. And, we know that effective hearing aid use is related to not only improved communication, but also increased earning power, emotional stability, improved family relationships, physical health, and increased social participation. So what we really are selling are our skills in addition to a product. Our skills to educate the patient regarding the benefits of hearing aid use, our skills to provide the patient with the optimum fitting through verification and validation, and our counseling skills to handle any bumps in the road that might occur throughout the process. In most cases, a better quality of life for the patient is the result. Not a bad thing to *sell.*

of behavioral test procedures, hearing aid technology, fitting techniques, and a host of other things—superb counseling skills and a good bedside manner also are a must. Fortunately, these areas are all extremely interesting, and some might even say fun to learn. What often is thought of as not so much fun are all the rules and regulations that go along with the practice of dispensing hearing aids. Yet, they are just as critical for success. We briefly discuss some of them here.

Scope of Practice

A good starting point for this section is the scope of practice for audiology. Although we do not usually think of these as regulations or rules, they do serve as a foundation for the development of other documents. All major audiology organizations have a published scope of practice. For example, the AAA scope of practice (last updated January 2004) states as part of its purpose:

> This document outlines those activities that are within the expertise of members of the profession. This Scope of Practice statement is intended for use by audiologists, allied professionals, consumers of audiologic services, and the general public. It serves as a reference for issues of service delivery, third-party reimbursement, legislation, consumer education, regulatory action, state and professional licensure, and interprofessional relations.

> Regarding the fitting of hearing aids, the document states:

> The audiologist is the professional who provides the full range of audiologic treatment services for persons with impairment of hearing and vestibular function. The audiologist is responsible for the evaluation, fitting, and verification of amplification devices, including assistive listening devices. The audiologist determines the appropriateness of amplification systems for persons with hearing impairment, evaluates benefit, and provides counseling and training regarding their use. Audiologists conduct otoscopic examinations, clean ear canals and remove cerumen, take ear canal impressions, select, fit, evaluate, and dispense hearing aids and other amplification systems.

Copies of the scope of practice for audiology from the AAA and the ASHA can be found in Appendix A and B, respectively.

Licensure

Certainly, one of the most important concerns regarding the sale of hearing aids is obtaining appropriate licensure, which is controlled on a state-by-state basis.[6] For audiologists, this could simply mean obtaining your *audiology license* for a given state; however, at this writing, in 13 states, it also is necessary to obtain a second hearing aid dispensing license. For example, in the North Dakota state license for audiologists, it states that the board may refuse to issue or renew a license, or may suspend, revoke, or take other disciplinary action if the licensee has engaged in unprofessional conduct. Such unprofessional conduct includes:

> Receiving remuneration of any kind from the sale of any type of hearing aid, unless licensed under Chapter 43–33. (Note: Chapter 43–33 is the Hearing Aid Dealers license.)

As you might guess, the need for audiologists to hold this second license, and the associated requirements to pass a written and practical examination to obtain this license, has generated considerable angst among audiologists and their professional organizations over the years.[7] In particular, the practical exam that often is required has been criticized; as in some states, points can be deducted for using the wrong color pen! Audiologists argue that after completing the requirements of an AuD degree, the audiologist would have the necessary knowledge and skills needed for the evaluation and fitting of hearing aids. Moreover, to obtain the audiology license, the audiologist already has passed a national examination that includes questions regarding hearing aids and hearing aid dispensing. Not all laws are reasonable, however, and licensure for hearing aid dispensing has a longer history and is more established than that of audiology. These state laws do change fairly frequently, so we suggest that you check with the AAA or the ASHA to obtain the current status for specific states. In some states, even when the hearing aid dispensing license is not necessary, additional requirements to the standard audiology license do apply.

Board Certification

Board certification in audiology is available from both the AAA and the ASHA, although it is not necessary to belong to the organization to obtain and hold the certification. The AAA certification is granted by the American Board of Audiology, and hence it often is referred to by the abbreviation ABA. The ASHA certification is the Clinical Certificate of Competence in Audiology, or CCC-A. Some audiologists have both, so paging through the yellow pages you might see an audiologist listed as AuD, ABA, CCC-A.

Board certification is not required for dispensing hearing aids, and holding such certification, for the most part, is only indirectly related to the services provided. The written test required to obtain either certification often is the same as the test required to obtain state licensure. Board certified individuals have mandatory continuing education unit (CEU) requirements, but mandatory CEUs also are required for licensure. One area, however, where one could argue that board certification leads to enhanced professional services relates to the ABA requirement that CEUs only are granted if the individual passes a written exam on the material, a requirement not in place for state licensure.

Hearing Aid Fitting Guidelines

As with other areas of clinical audiology, over the years various guidelines have been established regarding the selection and fitting of hearing aids. Typically, these guidelines are developed by a group of key experts and reflect what is considered good practice at the time of the writing. Whether these guidelines have had an impact on clinical practice is debatable. Portions of guidelines, however, have found their way into the body of state license documents, and some guidelines have been used by the ASHA when accrediting clinics and training programs. An example of the later is the hearing aid fitting guidelines published in 1967, based on a 1966 Chicago meeting sponsored by the AHSA. The outcome was the 71-page ASHA Reports Number 2 (Castle, 1967). This document included not only recommended test procedures for adults and children, but also minimal requirements for hearing programs.

In more recent years, there have been at least five different sets of guidelines written regarding the selection and fitting of hearing aids:

- 1991: Vanderbilt/VA Hearing Aid Conference 1990 Consensus Statement: Recommended Components of a Hearing Aid Selection Procedure for Adults (Hawkins et al., 1991)
- 1997: The Independent Hearing Aid Fitting Forum (IHAFF) Protocol (Valente & VanVleet, 1997)
- 1998: ASHA Ad Hoc Committee on Hearing Aid Selection and Fitting: Guidelines for Hearing Aid Fitting for Adults (http://www.asha.org)
- 2004: International Society of Audiology: Good Practice Guidance for Adult Hearing Aid Fittings and Services. Prepared by the Good Practice Working Group of the International Collegium of Rehabilitative Audiology (ICRA; http://www.isa-audiology.org)
- 2006: American Academy of Audiology: Guidelines for the Audiologic Management of Adult Hearing Impairment (http://www.audiology.org)

Best Practice

So far, we have talked about *guidelines* and *preferred practice*. The term *best practice* has been a popular buzzword used in industry and management for many years

---

THINGS TO REMEMBER: THIRD-PARTY REIMBURSEMENT

At one time, there was a requirement to hold the ASHA CCC-A to obtain certain types of third-party reimbursement. This was before the presence of audiology licensure in all states. We understand that this requirement has been lifted, or can be successfully contested.

KEY CONCEPT: ASHA PREFERRED PRACTICE PATTERNS

In 2006, the ASHA released a lengthy document titled "Preferred Practice Patterns for the Profession of Audiology," which has a section on the selection and fitting of hearing aids for adults. In the preamble, it was pointed out that the *preferred practice* patterns are neither a yardstick to measure acceptable conduct nor a set of aspirational principles. Rather, they reflect the standard of care relevant to a particular set of circumstances. How do preferred practice statements fit with documents labeled *guidelines*? The ASHA document states that it is useful to regard these practice patterns within the conceptual framework of ASHA policy statements ranging in scope and specificity from broad to narrow, and they are defined as follows:

- Scope of Practice Statement: A list of professional activities that define the range of services offered within the profession of audiology.
- Preferred Practice Patterns: Statements that define generally applicable characteristics of activities directed toward individual patients.
- Position Statements: Statements that specify ASHA's policy and stance on a matter.
- Practice Guidelines: A recommended set of procedures for a specific area of practice, based on research findings and current practice.

American Speech-Language-Hearing Association. (2006). *Preferred Practice Patterns for the Profession of Audiology* [Preferred Practice Patterns]. Retrieved from http://www.asha.org

---

to describe a process of developing a standard way of doing things (a related example is ISO 9001 certification, a standard that has been attained by some hearing aid manufacturers). In more recent years, we have used this term for audiologic practice, with the general definition that best practice is a method or technique that has consistently shown results superior to those achieved with other means, and that this practice can be used as a benchmark. That is, documented outcomes that can be replicated. Regarding the selection and fitting of hearing aids, we sometimes use the term *best practice guidelines* when referring to published hearing aid fitting guidelines. This may or may not be correct, as in some cases, the guidelines were based more on expert opinion than on a critical grading of research evidence. When research evidence is used, the common term is *evidence-based practice*, which often is used interchangeably with best practice.

Because it usually takes considerable time for a given technique or treatment to be researched thoroughly, and for this research to be published in peer-reviewed journals (and therefore qualify for best practice), another term that has been used by the U.S. Department of Health and Human Services is *promising practice*. The definition is as follows:

> Promising Practice: At least preliminary evidence of effectiveness in small-scale interventions or for which there is potential for generating data that will be useful for making decisions about taking the intervention to scale and generalizing the results to diverse populations and settings.

An example of a hearing aid feature that probably would fall into the promising practice category today would be frequency lowering. There appears to be some evidence that when children undergo training using this algorithm, there may be improved performance for the recognition and production of the /s/ and /sh/ sounds. At this point, the available evidence would be weak for best practice, but could be considered promising. A summary of these different terms is shown in Table 1–2.

Table 1–2. Different Levels of Best Practice

Research Validated Best Practice	A program, activity or strategy that has the highest degree of proven effectiveness. Supported by highly rated objective and comprehensive research and evaluation.
Field Tested Best Practice	A program, activity or strategy that has been shown to work effectively and produce successful outcomes and is supported to some degree by subjective and objective data.
Promising Practice	A program, activity or strategy that has worked within one organization and shows promise during its early stages for becoming a best practice with long term sustainable impact. A promising practice must have some objective basis for claiming effectiveness and must have the potential for replication.

Source: Adapted from the U.S. Department of Health and Human Services, Administration for Children and Families Program Announcement. (Federal Register, Vol. 68, No. 131, July 2003)

Evidence-Based Practice

Frank C. Wilson, MD, an authority in *evidence-based practice* once wrote (2009, p. 80):

> Neither unaudited experience nor logical thought can replace controlled clinical trials, so until documentation of a procedure's effectiveness can be demonstrated, it should be considered a false idol and worship withheld.

Although the basic principles date back to the mid-1800s, evidence-based practice is relatively new to medicine, and even newer to audiology. Noted expert David L. Sackett, MD, describes it as "the conscientious, explicit, and judicious use of current best evidence in making decisions about the care of individual patients. The practice of evidence-based medicine [audiology] means integrating individual clinical expertise with the best available external clinical evidence from systematic research" (Sackett, Rosenberg, Gray, Haynes, & Richardson, 1996).

Whereas clinical experience is used in evidence-based treatment decisions, considerable weight is placed on published research. When evaluating a given area of hearing aid selection or fitting, it is therefore useful to provide a rating level of the evidence that is available; certain research designs are viewed more favorably than others. The most commonly used six-point hierarchy rating scale is summarized in Table 1–3. As shown, the strongest evidence would be from Level 1. Unfortunately, there are few decisions regarding the fitting of

Table 1–3. The Hierarchy of Levels of Evidence

Level	Criteria
1	Systematic reviews and meta-analysis of randomized controlled trials (RCT) or other high-quality studies
2	Well designed RCT studies
3	Non-randomized intervention studies
4	Cohort studies, case-control studies, cross-sectional surveys, or uncontrolled experiments
5	Case report
6	Expert opinion

hearing aids where evidence exists in this category. For example, directional microphone technology in hearing aids has been researched for 40 years, and yes, there is one meta-analysis (based on 74 experiments) that concludes that directional technology improves speech recognition in background noise compared with omnidirectional processing (Amlani, 2001). However, the majority of data used in this analysis was collected in listening environments inconsistent with real-world listening (e.g., anechoic chamber, audiometric test booth, etc.), which then limits the strength of the treatment recommendation.

When we design a test protocol or recommend a specific treatment (e.g., hearing aid feature) for our patients, we can examine the levels of the evidence, and

---

THINGS TO REMEMBER: THE IHAFF *JAAA* ISSUE

In 2004, the members of the IHAFF held a special meeting regarding the need for evidence-based practice in the selection and fitting of hearing aids. Following this meeting, a series of systematic review articles were written examining such procedures as the use of speech audiometry, prescriptive fitting approaches, loudness discomfort measures, and the selection of hearing aid special features. These articles were published in a special issue of the *Journal of the Academy of Audiology* (Vol. 16, No. 7, June 2005). The introductory article by Robyn Cox is an excellent review of the use of evidence-based practice in the fitting of hearing aids.

---

then assign a grade. The basis for assigning grades is shown in Table 1–4. The grade then represents the level of confidence we have concerning the recommendation.

The AAA Fitting Guidelines. We mentioned earlier that *fitting guidelines* are only best practice guidelines if they are constructed using the rules of evidence-based practice. The 2006 hearing aid fitting guidelines published by the AAA used this approach. For each recommendation, this guideline provides the level of evidence and a grade. Table 1–5 is an example of six items taken from one of the Tables of Evidence; it includes some items on compression threshold (CT), compression limiting (CL), peak clipping (PC) and threshold of discomfort measures (TD). We selected a section from a table that had mostly Level 1 and Level 2 grades; however, this is not representative of the entire guideline. Michael Valente, chair of the committee who developed these guidelines, provided a review of the recommendations and the procedures used for grading (Valente, 2006). He states that, overall, the combined Tables of Evidence contained 108 statements that were provided to support the 43 recommendations in the guideline. The following is the frequency with which the different levels of evidence were assigned for the 108 recommendations: Level 1: 4.6%, Level 2: 25.9%, Level 3: 14.8%, Level 4: 35.2%, Level 5: 4.6%, and Level 6: 14.8%. Note that less than one-third of the recommendations were judged as Level 1–2.

Efficacy, Effectiveness, and Efficiency

As we have discussed, the treatment of hearing loss using hearing aids falls into the category of a health care

Table 1–4. Grades of Recommendation

Grade	Criteria
A	Level 1–2 studies with consistent conclusions.
B	Level 3–4 studies with consistent findings or extrapolated evidence from Level 1–2 studies.
C	Level 5 studies or extrapolation from Level 3–4 studies.
D	Level 6 evidence; inconsistent or inconclusive studies of any level, any study having a high risk of bias.

intervention, something that epidemiologists have been studying for many years. Simply stated, we need to ask three questions: Can it work? Does it work? And, is it worth it? British epidemiologist Archie Cochrane was one of the first to organize intervention research into three categories:

- Efficacy (Can it work?): This is the extent to which an intervention does more good than harm. This type of testing often is conducted under relatively ideal circumstances.
  Example: The directivity index of a new directional microphone algorithm is evaluated by the manufacturer in an anechoic chamber.
- Effectiveness (Does it work in the real world?): This evaluation assesses if an intervention does more good than harm when used in a typical health care practice.

Table 1–5. Sample Portion of a Table of Evidence Taken From the 2006 AAA Hearing Aid Fitting Guidelines

Treatment Decision	Level	Grade
Hearing aids with low CTs yield better outcomes when compared to linear PC. Patients prefer CL to at least one typical low CT instrument.	2	A
A wide range of CTs and time constants may be appropriate.	1	A
Speech recognition differences can be associated with increased number of compression channels.	1	D
Listeners with greater cognitive ability derive greater benefit from temporal structure in background noise when listening with faster time constants.	2	A
Quantification of a theoretical multichannel compression hearing aid, using intelligibility index And target-gain matching measures, indicate a seven-channel system would suffice for most audiograms in order to meet the strictest root-mean-square (RMS) error criterion evaluated.	2	B
Data support measurement of individual TD and setting of OSPL90 so it does not exceed TD in order to minimize chances of auditory discomfort in the real world.	3	B

Example: Patients are fitted with the new directional algorithm and compare this processing with omnidirectional processing in typical real-world listening situations.

- Efficiency (Is it worth it?): Is the effect of an intervention worth the additional cost that may be related to its use? Is the intervention cost-effective?

    Example: If the new directional algorithm provides an average 2 dB improvement in the SNR (i.e., it is effective), but a pair of hearing aids with this algorithm cost the patient $500 more than other products, is the additional cost to the patient worth the benefit obtained?

In Robyn Cox's 2004 review of evidence-based practice, she offers the following additional explanation to assist us in differentiating efficacy from effectiveness:

- Efficacy: The *efficacy* of a treatment is how well it *can* work given the best possible scenario. This usually means the treatment is administered to highly motivated patients with uncomplicated problems, and the practitioners providing the treatment are extensively trained in the details of the treatment and have plenty of time to get things just right.

- Effectiveness: The *effectiveness* of a treatment is how well it *does* work in the real world where patients may not be very motivated or compliant, and they often lead complicated lives. Also, in the real world, practitioners have limited time and may not understand all the fine points of the treatment.

As an example, Cox (2004) discusses wide dynamic range compression (WDRC), a feature in nearly all hearing aids today, which has been shown in research to improve audibility and speech recognition for soft speech; hence, it is *efficacious*. But, we know that some patients do not adapt well to this amount of gain for soft sounds, they may find it annoying, and they may not want to go through the necessary adjustment period. It may even be that some patients never do adjust to this increased audibility. WDRC processing, therefore, is not always an effective treatment. Although efficacy is important, it is treatment effectiveness that drives our fitting practices.

FDA Regulations

As you might expect, there are government regulations relating to the manufacture, sale, and fitting of hearing aids. These issues are addressed by the U.S. Food and Drug Administration (FDA), Department of Health and Human Services, Medical Devices regulations (Subchapter H, Revised April 1, 2010; see Appendix C). This regulation has definitions for both audiologist and dispenser.

> Audiologist: Audiologist means any person qualified by training and experience to specialize in the evaluation and rehabilitation of individuals whose communication disorders center in whole or in part in the hearing function. In some states, audiologists must satisfy specific requirements for licensure.

> Dispenser: Dispenser means any person, partnership, corporation, or association engaged in the sale, lease, or rental of hearing aids to any member of the consuming public or any employee, agent, sales person, and/or representative of such a person, partnership, corporation, or association.

In general, the term dispenser is used in the regulation, and as shown in the definition above, this term would apply to audiologists involved in selling hearing aids.

FDA Red Flags

One of the things outlined in the FDA regulation are the eight *red flags* for referral (not to be confused with the *Red Flag Rules* issued by the Federal Trade Commission [FTC] in 2010). The regulation states that a dispenser should advise a prospective hearing aid user to consult a licensed physician (preferably an otolaryngologist)

promptly if any of the following is observed through record review, case history, or testing:

1. Visible congenital or traumatic deformity of the ear.
2. History of active drainage from the ear within the previous 90 days.
3. History of sudden or rapidly progressive hearing loss within the previous 90 days.
4. Acute or chronic dizziness.
5. Unilateral hearing loss of sudden or recent onset within the previous 90 days.
6. Audiometric air-bone gap equal to or greater than 15 dB at 500 Hz, 1000 Hz, and 2000 Hz.
7. Visible evidence of significant cerumen accumulation or a foreign body in the ear canal.
8. Pain or discomfort in the ear.

In general, even if these eight conditions were not present in the regulation, the prudent audiologist would probably refer if any of these conditions existed anyway. Depending on your definition of significant, one exception might be cerumen accumulation, which often does not require a medical referral and easily can be handled by most audiologists (assuming it is allowed by the state's licensure law).

FDA Medical Clearance

The FDA also regulates *condition for sale* of certain medical devices. Regarding hearing aids, one condition is the medical clearance, which is summarized as follows (FDA Sec. 801.421 Hearing aid devices; conditions for sale):

- Prospective hearing aid users must obtain a medical clearance from a physician (preferably one who specializes in diseases of the ear) prior to being fit with amplification. The medical clearance must have occurred in the last six months. If the prospective user is over 18 years of age, they may waive this medical clearance and, instead, complete a medical waiver. The medical waiver must be in the language provided by the FDA.
- Prospective hearing aid users under the age of 18 years of age obtain a medical clearance from a physician (preferably one

who specializes in diseases of the ear) prior to being fit with amplification. The medical clearance must have occurred in the last six months. Neither the child or their parent or guardian may waive this medical clearance requirement.

HIPAA

The Health Insurance Portability and Accountability Act (HIPAA) became law in 1996. The part of HIPAA that has the most impact on audiology practice is the Accountability or Administrative Simplification section. Contained in this section are rules regarding transactions and code sets, privacy, and security. There also are rules mandating that that the Employer Identification Number provided to the IRS be utilized when submitting claims to insurers and a rule that mandates the use of the National Provider Identifier (NPI) by audiologists when submitting claims to all insurers including Medicare and Medicaid. Each clinic or facility must also obtain an NPI.

The HIPAA guidelines regarding privacy and confidentially are extensive and complex; some even directly impact the fitting of hearing aids, such as the passwords for fitting software. A thorough description is beyond the scope of this chapter, but an excellent review is provided at the website of the AAA (http://www.audiology.org) and the ADA (http://www.audiologist.org)

Federal Trade Commission

The FTC has issued a set of regulations, effective in June 2010, known as the Red Flag Rules. These rules apply to any audiology practice that accepts and processes third-party payments or insurance, or acts as a creditor for its patients. This rule requires practices to create and implement written identity theft prevention, detection, and management policies and procedures in an attempt to protect their patients from identity theft. The Red Flag Rules can be considered an expansion of the HIPAA privacy rules. As with the HIPAA Privacy Policy, the audiology practice needs to create office policies and procedures that outline how the practice intends to identify, detect, and respond to identity theft red flags.

Laws and Statutes

There are several laws and statutes that have the possibility to directly relate to the sale of hearing aids. In particular, they apply when the audiologist is involved with reimbursement through Medicare or Medicaid.

Antikickback Statute

We are referring to the Medicare and Medicaid Patient Protection Act of 1987, as amended, 42 U.S.C. §1320a-7b. The section of the this statute that relates directly to the sale of hearing aids prohibits the offer or receipt of certain remuneration in return for referrals for or recommending purchase of supplies and services reimbursable under government health care programs. Violation of this statute is a felony, upon conviction the individual could be fined not more than $25,000 or imprisoned for not more than five years, or both. Specially, the statute states:

- Whoever knowingly and willfully solicits or receives any remuneration, including any kickback, bribe, or rebate (directly or indirectly, overtly or covertly, in cash or in-kind) in return for referring an individual to a person for the furnishing or arranging for the furnishing of any item or service for which payment may be made in whole or in part under [Medicare] or a state health care program;
- In return for purchasing, leasing, ordering, or arranging for or recommending purchasing, leasing, or ordering any good, facility, service, or item for which payment may be made in whole or in part under [Medicare] or a state health care program.

The antikickback statute requires intent, but considers that *remuneration* is anything of value, which could include gifts, points, free trips, or equipment that is linked to the purchase of hearing aids from a given manufacturer.

Stark Law

The federal statute dealing with physician self-referral is generally referred to as the *Stark Law*, although there have been modifications. Congress included a provision in the Omnibus Budget Reconciliation Act of 1989, which barred self-referrals for clinical laboratory services under the Medicare program, effective January 1, 1992. This provision is known as *Stark I*. Under this law, if a physician or a member of a physician's immediate family has a financial relationship with a health care entity, the physician may not make referrals to that entity for the furnishing of designated health services under the Medicare program. Generally, to determine whether the Stark statute applies to a particular arrangement, three questions must be answered: Does this arrangement involve a referral of a Medicare or Medicaid patient by a physician or an immediate family member of a physician? Second, is the referral for a *designated health service*? Third, is there a financial relationship of any kind between the referring physician or family member and the entity to which the referral is being made? Violations of Stark can result in civil penalties, denial of payments for the services provided in violation of Stark, and exclusion from participation in Medicare, Medicaid, or any other federal health care program. The Stark statute *does not* require bad intent; a tainted financial relationship violates the Stark law regardless of good intentions.[8]

False Claims Act

The False Claims Act (31 U.S.C. §§ 3729–3733, also called the *Lincoln Law*) is a federal law that imposes liability on persons and companies who defraud governmental programs. As it relates to audiology, the False Claims Act deals with audiologists who submit claims for services that were not done or were not necessary. It applies to any federal health care program. Specifically, violation of this law would include:

- Knowingly submitting a false claim to a federal health care program;
- Submitting claims for services not performed, for medically unnecessary services, and for *upcoding* (i.e., coding at a higher level or for more services than were provided).

Gifts or Inducements to Beneficiaries

Gifts and inducements to beneficiaries is included under section 1128A(a)(5) of the Social Security Act (the Act), enacted as part of HIPAA. Specifically the law states:

It is unlawful to knowingly offer or give remuneration to Medicare or Medicaid beneficiaries to influ-

---

TECHNICAL TIP: CODING

In our discussion of the false claims act, we list *upcoding* as an example of a violation. If you are new to the profession, that term might not have much meaning, so we provide a brief explanation. Current Procedural Terminology, which simply is referred to by the abbreviation CPT, are codes containing a set of five numbers assigned to most tasks and services provided by an audiologist. They are used by insurers to determine the amount of reimbursement. All audiologists use the same set of CPT codes. Within health care, thousands of codes are in use, and they are updated annually. Development and maintenance of these codes is overseen by the American Medical Association. Now, relative to upcoding, if an audiologist only conducted air conduction thresholds for a given patient, that would be CPT Code 92552. If the audiologist entered 92557, which is the Code for *comprehensive audiometry threshold evaluation and speech recognition*, a higher reimbursement rate, that would be considered upcoding. In Appendix E, we have provided a sample audiology superbill, developed by the AAA, which provides a good summary of the different codes that are available. This form is an example only, as these codes change annually—for clinical practice you will need to obtain an updated listing, available from the AAA or the ASHA, as well as other sources.

ence their choice of provider for any item or service covered by Medicare or a state health care program.

You might wonder what this has to do with the sale of hearing aids? Exactly what remuneration would audiologists be giving away? The answer is free hearing testing that usually is termed *free hearing screening*. It is not unusual to see a newspaper ad offering a special "This week only! Come in for your free hearing screening!" (See examples in Figure 1–6). There is some debate

whether screening might be okay and threshold testing is not, but it is no secret that the purpose of the ad is to increase office traffic, and hopefully hearing aid sales. But is it legal? Bryan Liang, who is an MD, PhD, and JD, has spoken on this topic at numerous audiology meetings. Here is the opinion he voiced in 2000:

> This is a very, very difficult and important issue and audiologists are justified in being concerned about it . . . At the outset, let me emphasize that free hearing

---

POINTS TO PONDER: VIOLATION OR NO VIOLATION?

Example #1: A private practice audiologist notes that a new otolaryngologist opened a practice down the street. The otolaryngologist does not employ an audiologist. The audiologist takes the otolaryngologist out to a nice dinner. They discuss the services the audiologist offers, including the dispensing of hearing aids. Violation of Antikickback Law?

Example #2: An otolaryngologist employs an audiologist who dispenses hearing aids. The otolaryngologist refers all patients needing hearing aids to this audiologist. The audiologist earns a handsome salary, which is based almost entirely on commissions from the hearing aids sold. The percent of the commission escalates as a function of the number of units sold each month. Violation of Stark Law?

Example #3: An audiologist sells a large number of hearing aids that are reimbursed through a government agency. The reimbursement rate is very low, and to help him or her out, a manufacturer provides a 25% discount on the Level 1 hearing aids purchased for this population. The invoice sent to the audiologist, however, states the single-unit price, not the discounted price. The audiologist submits this invoice to the government agency for reimbursement, as this is the *true* price of the hearing aid. Violation of False Claims Law?

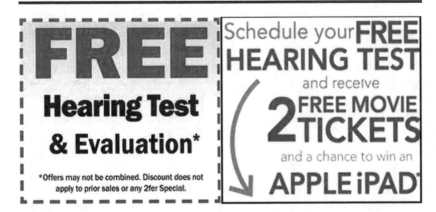

Figure 1–6. Example of two different newspaper ads promoting free hearing tests.

screenings are not *per se* a violation of fraud and abuse laws; it is just that they might be. One thing I think is clear, however: if it is a public health situation where you are not trying to induce referrals to yourself, and if Medicare, Medicaid and other federal health programs are not involved, you are probably okay. If the free screenings become tied to or eventually involve Medicaid or Medicare or the VA program, there may be a problem. (Grayson & Liang, 2000)

Billing and Reimbursement

Although this text focuses mostly on the selection and fitting of hearing aids, we cannot lose sight of the fact that there is a business side to audiology. Any successful practice knows the rules of reimbursement, the specifics of proper coding, and the legalities of billing and financial relationships. To cover all these topics appropriately, we would need several book chapters, or maybe even an entire book (see Glaser & Traynor, 2013). To get you started thinking about some of the key business points associated with dispensing hearing aids, we have asked Paul Pessis, AuD, to help us out. Dr. Pessis, a private practice audiologist in Chicago, has provided numerous workshops for the AAA and other professional organizations. Here is his *Top 20* list of things to remember:

1. First, always determine if a patient has insurance. Patients must present with a current insurance card. Without it, patients should be required to pay out-of-pocket.
2. Most insurance plans only pay for diagnostic services when investigating the etiology of a hearing loss. Testing for the purposes of dispensing a hearing aid may not be reimbursable.
3. More and more, insurance plans are offering a hearing aid benefit. These types of benefits vary widely.
4. Not all hearing aid benefits are created equal. Some examples include:
   - A discount from the provider's fee structure.
   - A fee dictated by the insurance carrier.
   - A dollar amount paid by the insurance company toward a set of hearing aids.
5. Insurance companies may also dictate policies that require:
   - Batteries for the lifetime of the hearing aids.
   - Extended trial periods even beyond what is mandated by state licensure laws.
   - The audiologist to accept the discounted fee structure and not balance bill the patient the difference between third-party payer's allowed amount and the audiologist's customary fee.
   - Discounting or not allowing diagnostic services.
   - Extended free repair warranties.
   - A specific hearing aid type and model has to be fit without any exceptions.
6. Before agreeing to participate in an insurance plan that offers a hearing aid benefit, know the specifics. Can your facility afford to be a provider? High utilization of the benefit does not necessarily yield the desired monetary outcome. In fact, a low differential between cost of goods and the allowable amount paid can be a financial detriment to a practice.
7. Verification of insurance benefits: This is a practice whereby the provider (you) contacts the insurance company to enumerate the patient's hearing and hearing aid benefits. For example, you call the insurance company to see what amount will be paid, what type of hearing aids are covered, etc. Unfortunately, the information given is not always accurate. Also, be aware that the information given is not legally binding. Simply, you can ask, but if wrong information is given, it does not matter. The law does not protect the provider. Many facilities have discontinued the laborious task of verifying benefits because it has no legal weight.
8. All patients should be required to sign an *insurance waiver* stating that services not recognized as a covered benefit by the insurance company are payable by the patient.
9. You must know the proper coding systems to use when billing. These are mandated by HIPAA:
   - CPT: a numeric listing of procedures performed.
   - Health Care Common Procedure Coding System (HCPCS): A numeric listing of medical supplies (such as hearing aids) and services.
   - International Classification of Diseases (ICD-9): The compendium of diagnoses for all medical conditions. The ICD-10 system, with a more comprehensive list, will replace the ICD-9 system in the near future.

10. Not all hearing and hearing aid related procedures have a recognized code. An example is speech-in-noise testing. Without a code, an insurance company cannot be billed. This does not preclude a facility, however, from billing the patient.

11. Your facility must establish a protocol for billing hearing aids and related services:
    - Bundling—a common practice of charging a patient a single amount for all services and supplies. Often, services are included for multiple years without being able to bill the patient for chronic visits.
    - Unbundling—charging a patient for every procedure performed along with a separate charge for supplies (hearings aids, earmolds, batteries, etc.). This specifically differentiates the value of services versus supplies.

12. Do not give diagnostics away for free. Licensure laws define our scope of practice and diagnostic tests are crucial for making a differential diagnosis. Hearing loss is not always a disease. It can often be a symptom of a systemic or serious illness. Maintain your professionalism and bill for these services.

13. It is illegal to bill a Medicare patient more than a non-Medicare patient for an equivalent service. Therefore, if you do not charge for air, bone, and speech audiometry (92557) as part of a free service giveaway when selling hearing aids, it would be illegal to bill other patients for this same service.

14. Credentialing: To be a provider of services for a hearing or hearing aid benefit plan, you must contact the third-party payer provider relations department to become credentialed. It may take in excess of a year to become eligible for participation in some managed care plans. In contrast, Medicare will complete the credentialing process in 60 days or less. Medicare and many managed care payers require providers to have an NPI, which must be used when submitting a claim for reimbursement.

15. Opting out of insurance: Some facilities refuse to accept any type of insurance. Audiologists, however, cannot opt out of Medicare. For managed care, if an audiologist prefers not to become a provider for a plan, then he or she can bill as an out-of-network provider. Out-of-network providers do not have to adhere to the insurance company's fee schedule, and the patient incurs more out-of-pocket expenses than for network providers.

16. Explanation of Benefits (EOB): Every insurance carrier is required to supply both the patient and the provider of service, with an explanation of benefits. The EOB lists the monies paid by the insurance company, the amount to be billed to the patient, the amount to be written off, and co-pay and coinsurance amounts. Effective coding patterns can be learned from the EOB. Simply, the EOB is the *pulse of reimbursement* for a facility.

17. Medicaid: Every state has its own specific Medicaid rules and levels of reimbursement. It is prudent for the provider to learn the rules for participation and provision of services. Be aware if hearing aids are considered durable medical equipment (DME).

18. DME: Falls under the Stark laws that delineate the legal consequences of improper financial relationships between audiologists and other business partnerships. State laws are often more stringent than federal laws.

19. Medicare does not pay for hearing aids. Furthermore, it is illegal to bill Medicare for hearing services when performed for the purpose of a hearing aid. Medicare beneficiaries may have secondary insurance that will pay for hearing aids and/or hearing aid related services. A denial from Medicare is typically needed to bill the secondary. You must bill Medicare using the *GY* modifier in order for the claim to be processed legally. Additionally, line 19 on the CMS 1500 must include a statement indicating that the claim is being submitted to receive a denial for secondary insurance.

20. Cerumen management: If removing cerumen is within the audiologist's scope of practice for your given state, be aware that many insurance companies will not pay for both cerumen removal and a hearing test performed on the same date of service by the same provider/facility. It is illegal to bill Medicare for cerumen removal when performed by an audiologist.

In closing, Dr. Pessis tells us:

View this list as the starting point for the infrastructure necessary for becoming the 'total professional.' The reimbursement/practice management landscape is ever-changing. It is another integral component of our dynamic profession.

More on Bundling and Unbundling

We brought up the topic of bundling and unbundling earlier in this chapter in a "Points to Ponder," and you may have noticed that Dr. Pessis also mentions it in his list. While the majority of audiologists appear to be in favor of bundling, there are a few who speak out in favor of unbundling. One of them is audiologist John Coverstone, and here are what he considers to be the advantages of unbundling, *for the audiologist,* taken from one of his recent articles (2012):

- Unbundling requires conducting a cost analysis. Performing a cost analysis can provide you with a completely different perspective on how your business operates. It can also provide you with a lot more confidence in your fees when you eventually use this information to set them.
- You can ensure that you are paid for the services that you provide. An unbundled model focuses on fees that are appropriate for the time and resources that you dedicate to caring for your patients.
- You have something to promote. There is a good possibility that you will be the first in your area to adopt this fee structure.
- Many audiologists enjoy the intangible benefits of unbundling more than the business ones. Unbundling promotes professionalism, rather than a "sales person."
- There is an additional increase in patient confidence when they know that the recommendations you are making are not tied to how much you will make from the sale. Unbundling removes the burden of tying the income you receive to the product you recommend.
- Unbundling makes it much easier to practice in the modern hearing aid dispensing world:
  - Insurance companies are used to a medical model. Unbundling allows you to fit into that model very easily—and probably bill out more of what you are doing in the process.
  - If you currently bundle and then bill insurance when you can, there is a very good chance that you are in violation of your contract and possibly federal law (if

you accept federal insurance). Medicare in particular does not allow you to bill anyone else less than you bill them. If you include evaluations in the price of a hearing aid, as many people do, you cannot then charge Medicare for the same service.
  - Direct hearing aid sales are not going away. Wherever they purchase the device, unbundling makes it easy for you to provide the services that are so essential for successful hearing aid use.

Ethics

As with all areas of clinical audiology, ethical guidelines relate to several different aspects of dispensing hearing aids. Are the patients treated properly? Do the fitting and verification procedures assure that the patients obtained what is best for them? Are there outside incentives that influence clinical decisions? Ethical guidelines related to hearing aid fitting can also originate from several sources: professional organizations, state licensure documents, hearing aid manufacturers, and health care organizations.

Code of Ethics of Professional Organizations

When we think of a code of ethics, we usually first associate them with professional organizations. You might even know someone who was removed from an audiology organization because of a violation of a given organization's standards. We have included the ethical guidelines for both the AAA (Appendix F) and the ASHA (Appendix G) for your review.

The code of ethics for an organization typically covers a wide range of activities including such areas as: maintaining high standards of professional competence, maintaining patient confidentiality, providing appropriate services and products, making accurate public statements, avoiding commercial interests that could impact patient care, and abstaining from dishonesty or illegal conduct that could adversely affect the profession.

Ethics Related to Hearing Aid Fitting Procedures. One area of the code of ethics that is often overlooked (or simply not remembered) are the statements involving clinical practice. That is, if an audiologist is not performing a given audiologic task appropriately, is that then unethical behavior? For example, we know that preferred practice guidelines say that word recognition testing should be conducted using standardized *recorded* speech material. What if an audiologist used monitored live voice? Is this an ethical violation?

This area of ethics was brought to light in an article by Catherine Palmer, PhD, (2009) in which she related these guidelines specifically to the fitting of hearing aids. Let us say that there are data available that show that certain hearing aid verification and validation methods improve benefit and satisfaction. What if an audiologist does not utilize these measures in the fitting of hearing aids? Is this unethical behavior?

Palmer draws our attention to the following statement from Principle 2 of the AAA *Code of Ethics*, which states: "Members shall maintain high standards of professional competence in rendering services . . . " Principle 4 of the same ethics code states: "Members shall provide only services and products that are in the best interest of those served." She also mentions Principle of Ethics II from the ASHA *Code of Ethics*, which states: "Individuals shall honor their responsibility to achieve and maintain the highest level of professional competence." Palmer adds that all of these statements point to the assumption that an ethical practitioner will follow the best practices supported by evidence and published by their professional organizations.

So is failing to comply with best practice guidelines unethical and justification for removal from an organization? Some might say that this is taking the ethical practice guidelines a bit too far. But the point we are making is that ethical practice is not just about keeping your nose clean and staying out of jail—it is about being a good audiologist, which includes appropriate clinical practice.

Specific Guidelines Regarding Incentives from Manufacturers. In 2003, the AAA added some additional ethical guidelines regarding financial incentives from hearing aid manufacturers. These guidelines are titled, "Ethical Practice Guidelines on Financial Incentives from Hearing Instrument Manufacturers." There did not appear to be a particular event or series of events that prompted this document, although it was about this time that the Office of the Inspector General issued guidelines for gift-giving for the pharmaceutical industry. Perhaps the thought was that a proactive approach would be best, as some of these ethical concerns also could be construed as illegal. These AAA Guidelines are in Appendix D.

Although we encourage you to read the guidelines in detail, here are some examples of what was considered *okay* or *not okay*.

Things that are *probably okay*:

- Gifts that primarily benefit the patient and are related to the audiologist's work, that do not exceed $100 in value.
- The cost of reasonable travel expenses to attend a legitimate educational program.
- Meals and social functions that are part of a legitimate educational program.
- Co-op advertising if there are no strings attached.
- Modest meals from a manufacturer's rep when business related.
- Discount programs as long as they do not compromise professional judgment. (Authors' Note: This becomes less of a problem each year as the array of products from each manufacturer expands.)
- Obtaining a loan from a hearing aid manufacturer is *sort of okay*; see exact wording in Appendix D.
- Consulting for a company, or owning stock, but it must be disclosed to the patient if you fit that product.

Things that are *probably not okay*:

- Accepting invitations to private convention parties or paid tickets for golfing, sporting events, opera, theater, etc.
- Any expenses related to a spouse or significant other attending an educational meeting (e.g., meals, travel, lodging, entertainment).
- Accepting gifts that are over $100 or that do not relate to patient care.
- Incentives or credit toward product purchases (including audiologic or hearing aid related equipment), which are tied to hearing aid purchases.

Hawkins, Hamill, Van Vleet, and Freeman (2002) conducted a survey of audiologists regarding many of the potential conflicts of interest we mention here. Sixteen different scenarios were rated as either *Nothing wrong, May not be in patient's best interest, but comfortable with it, Highly suspect, Borders on unethical,* or

Clearly unethical. In addition, they included the ratings provided by hearing impaired patients for the same items—a reasonable factor to sample, as the *Perception of unethical* can be considered *Unethical.*

Hawkins, Hamill, and Kukula (2006) repeated the survey four years later (for audiologists only) to determine if the increased focus on potential ethical violations by professional organizations had an impact on audiologists' perceptions. We have included a summary of the data from both surveys in Table 1–6. For this

Table 1–6. Summary of possible unethical behavior as rated by audiologists and consumers. (from Hawkins et al., 2006)

Possibly Unethical Behavior	Percent who believe action to be unethical		
	Audiologists (year 2002)	Audiologists (year 2006)	Consumers
Earning credits from companies per hearing aid purchased, redeemable for gifts or cruises	38	70	71
Receiving professional development money from companies for each hearing aid purchased	19	31	85
Receiving equipment from company in exchange for agreeing to purchase a number of aids during the year	30	51	85
Receiving $100 traveler's check for each high-end instrument purchased from company	43	69	85
Receiving visits from sales representatives to discuss company's products	0	1	2
Receiving pens and notebooks with names of company's new products	4	4	7
Sales rep bringing lunch to office while company's new products are discussed	6	8	22
Sales rep taking Audiologist and spouse out to dinner to discuss company's new products	22	48	41
Attending an open party given by manufacturer at a convention regardless of whether they use the company's product	2	3	12
Attending an invitation only party at a convention given by a company	7	16	24
Attending a company sponsored, state approved CEU workshop in town	2	2	10
Attending a company sponsored, state approved CEU workshop in town, with breakfast and lunch provided	3	4	17
Attending CEU workshop in another city; company pays audiologist's expenses to attend	17	32	38
Attending CEU workshop in another city; company pays audiologist's and spouse's expenses to attend	45	74	69
Using Brand X almost exclusively because Aud thinks it is a good product and receives 20% volume discount	7	16	21
Purchasing a franchise and using the product line almost exclusively	9	15	28
Receiving salary plus a commission based on number of instruments sold while working in a clinic	12	19	26

summary, we combined the ratings of *borders on unethical* and *clearly unethical*. Observe that over the four-year interval, audiologists appeared to become more vigilant concerning what activities might be unethical. Also note that for some items there is a considerable gap between the views of audiologists and those of consumers.

So far, we have discussed the ethical guidelines of a professional organization. One might ask, what about all the audiologists who do not belong to a professional organization? It would seem that they would then be exempt from these codes of ethics? Just let your membership in the AAA expire, and then you can take free trips from manufacturers? Well, it is not quite that simple, as state licensure also has ethical guidelines.

Ethics Related to Licensure

In addition to the ethical guidelines of professional organizations, state licensure laws also have ethical guidelines, and failure to comply could result in losing your license—something most audiologists would view as worse than being kicked out of their favorite professional organization. The wording usually is something like this regarding the suspension or revocation of the license: "Engaging in unprofessional conduct, as defined by the rules established by the board, or violating the code of ethics adopted and published by the board."

Most of these licensure ethical violations, of course, involve fairly serious acts such as misrepresentation,

patient confidentiality, discrimination statutes, fraud, deceit, and so forth. However, there are some items that are more in the gray area and do relate to the selling of hearing aids. Here is one example:

> Participating in activities that constitute a conflict of professional interest and adversely affect the licensee's ability to provide appropriate audiology services.

The key here is that it not only must be a conflict of interest, but also must adversely affect audiology services. In most cases, even when a potential conflict of interest exists, hearing aid services are not negatively affected. But how about this example: You work at a dispensing practice owned by one of the Big Six hearing aid manufacturers—a common occurence nowadays. You are audited each month to assure that you are selling a high percentage of their product (e.g., 80%, 90%, or whatever is required). What if you have several patients who require a special feature that is implemented much more effectively by another manufacturer, but you continue to sell the products of your parent company to meet your monthly quota? Is this appropriate audiologic service?

Hearing aid licensure laws also have ethical standards. These ethics tend to be more directly related to the sale of hearing aids. Here are some examples taken from the North Dakota Hearing Aid Dealers license, a license required for all dispensing audiologists in

---

POINTS TO PONDER: OKAY TO HAVE A FAVORITE MANUFACTURER?

Many audiologists purchase 80% or more of their hearing aids from a single manufacturer. (See Johnson, Mueller and Ricketts 2009 for a review of audiologists purchasing trends.) Although some might frown on this, we certainly do not consider this unethical, as long as the amplification needs of each patient are being met. There are many advantages of using a primary manufacturer. The most significant is the greater familiarity with the products and the fitting software. Fine tuning hearing aids quickly on a busy day can be quite challenging for even the seasoned audiologist if several different manufacturers are used. Not only does manufacturer software differ greatly in how changes are made to different hearing aid features, but those features probably will be given different names. In addition, controls with the same name (e.g., gain for soft) may have different effects on compression parameters depending on the specific manufacturer. Another advantage of only using one or two manufacturers is the increased familiarity with the manufacturer's support staff, which can help solve fitting, ordering, repair, and administrative problems. If enough hearing aids are purchased each month, there also will likely be a reduction in the cost of the products, which can be passed along to the patient.

the state. Two of the items listed are fairly straightforward—the patient needs to have been tested properly, and the patient has to have a need for amplification. Ethical violations include:

- Sale of a hearing instrument to a person without adequate and proper audiometric testing.
- Sale of a hearing instrument to a person when the need for a hearing instrument has not been established after adequate and proper audiometric testing.

At this point, we could have a lengthy discussion of what really is *adequate* testing, and how do you really know when hearing aids will *not* benefit a patient? But, we save that discussion for later chapters of this book. Below, we have listed four other ethical violations from the same licensure law. The examples included are from us, not the statute, but do represent actual potential violations that we are aware of from other states:

- Using, or causing or promoting the use of, any advertising matter, promotional literature, testimonial, guarantee, warranty, label, brand, insignia, or any other representation, however disseminated or published, which is misleading, deceptive, or untruthful.

    Example: An audiologist sends out a direct mail piece saying: "Having trouble understanding in background noise? With the advanced NoiseStopper algorithm from MagicTone, you'll notice a remarkable improvement in understanding conversations in background noise."

- Advertising a particular model or type of hearing instrument for sale when purchasers or prospective purchasers responding to the advertisement cannot purchase the advertised model or type, if it is established that the purpose of the advertisement is to obtain prospects for the sale of a different model or type than that advertised.

    Example: Audiologist places a full-page newspaper ad that says: "Thousands of hearing impaired people are now using the totally invisible Phantom II deep-canal hearing aids from MagicTone [very tiny aid shown on the finger tip in the photo].

Stop in today to place your order during a special discount offer." (Note that the audiologist knows that because of the very small size, the fit-rate for the Phantom II is only about 5% of patients; the audiologist nearly always fits the Phantom I, a much larger, more visible completely in-the-canal (CIC) style.

- Advertising a manufacturer's product or using a manufacturer's name or trademark that implies a relationship with the manufacturer that does not exist.

    Example: The dispenser has a newspaper ad that reads: "Be the first to experience the new neural digital technology from MagicTone. Our center has been selected as a MagicTone research site. Enroll in the latest MagicTone research study for new hearing aid users by calling 701-223-XXXX. (Note: This dispenser does sell MagicTone's products, but there is no MagicTone research study.)

- To directly or indirectly give or offer to give, or permit, or cause to be given money or anything of value to any person who advises another in a professional capacity as an inducement to influence them or have them influence others to purchase or contract to purchase products sold or offered for sale by a licensee, or to influence persons to refrain from dealing in the products of competitors.

    Example: A dispenser says to a patient: "What? You're going to go check prices at Bob's Hearing Aids? I've seen some of his patients, and none of them were fit correctly. He doesn't even do probe-mic testing!"

More Ethical Guidelines

It is not just professional organizations and licensure laws that have ethical guidelines. Manufacturers, organizations, medical centers, and other entities sometimes have guidelines that are more rigid than those of the AAA or the ASHA.

Hearing Aid Manufacturers. Although you might think that it is the hearing aid manufacturers that are encouraging audiologists to stray from the straight and narrow (which indeed sometimes has been true in the past), some manufacturers have guidelines more rigid than those of the professional organizations. We know of one company, for example, that has a strict policy regarding issues that are relatively minor, such as who gets a free lunch. If a sales rep takes out an audiology customer for a business lunch, and the audiologist's spouse joins them, the spouse pays for his or her own food. A rep who generously pays the entire bill would most likely receive a letter of reprimand. The same rep takes a group of Chicago audiology customers to a Cubs game? That just might cost the rep his or her job with this company.

Veterans Affairs. The VA employs about 1,000 audiologists; most of these dispense hearing aids and, therefore, work closely with hearing aid manufacturers. About 15%–20% of all hearing aids sold in the United States are to VA clinics. Nearly all major manufacturers have products approved by the VA, and as part of this, the manufacturers provide off-site product training, usually at a major city (e.g., an East Coast VA audiologist might go to Las Vegas for training). Again, the VA has guidelines that are at least as rigid as those of professional organizations. For example, food and lodging can be no more than 150% of the government per diem. This means that if the government per diem for meals for a given city was $56 (e.g., San Antonio, TX), the manufacturer could spend no more than $84/person (150% of $56) for meals and beverages for the day of training. If you consider that the attendees would be served three meals plus snacks, and that a bowl of potato chips or pretzels may cost $25 from hotel catering, you can quickly calculate that the manufacturer will not be serving an expensive wine with dinner (the manufacturer could be removed from the VA contract for noncompliance). The VA guidelines also state:

> Excluded expenses or extras include transportation to and from home/airport, car rental, mileage (gas), baggage fees, entertainment of any kind, cruises, tours, or tickets to any form of entertainment. Contractors will not pay expenses for spouses or partners of government employees.

Medical Centers. And finally, if your dispensing practice is part of a medical center, conflict of inter-

est guidelines may be even more rigid. Recall that the AAA guidelines state that it is okay to accept small gifts (under $100 in value) from manufacturers, as long as the gift relates to your practice or patient care. Certainly a $50 pen would fit into that category—we all need to write something now and then at work, right? Well, that pen had better not have "Starkey" or "Siemens" printed on it, or you could be in trouble. Several medical centers, including our own Vanderbilt, do not allow the use of any gift item that displays the name or logo of a product that we potentially could recommend or sell.

Now, you might be saying, isn't that going a bit too far? Why would the pen I use have any bearing on what brand of hearing aids I sell to my patients? If you are asking that question, especially if you are an audiology student, you might be interested in the intriguing study regarding free pens published by Grande, Frosch, Perkins, Barbara, and Kahn (2009). This was a randomized controlled study of 352 third- and fourth-year medical students at two different medical schools: the University of Miami and the University of Pennsylvania. At the time, these two schools had different policies regarding pharmaceutical marketing items; a more restrictive policy and more negative, school-level attitude toward marketing was in place at the University of Pennsylvania. The medical students were given small marketing items (pens and notepads) promoting Lipitor. There was an exposed and control group at both universities and attitudes were measured pre- and post- for both Lipitor and Zocor using the Implicit Association Test.

What did they find? The small gifts had no effect for the third-year students at either university, but fourth-year students at the University of Miami formed a more favorable attitude toward Lipitor (the drug that was marketed). It is interesting to note that the free gifts had a reverse effect at the University of Pennsylvania, where a more restrictive policy was in place. So free pens do matter! Which leads us to ask, in the marketing world, is a gift ever just a gift?

In Closing

As we have discussed, there is a long history between audiology and the fitting of hearing aids. There is a long and storied history regarding audiology and hearing aid dispensing too. Consider that as recent as the late

---

KEY CONCEPT: IS A GIFT EVER JUST A GIFT?

Most of the data regarding the acceptance of gifts, and how they might impact the behavior of the medical professional, relate to gifts from pharmaceutical companies to physicians. If we assume that the impact would be similar for audiologists, here are some things to remember:

- Companies work harder to influence you than you work to resist their efforts.
- You probably believe that your professional colleagues will be influenced, but that you will not.
- You are probably more influenced than you think.
- Small gifts pack about the same punch as larger ones.

Again, if we use the data from previous studies related to pharmaceuticals and apply the findings to gifts to dispensing audiologists, here are some potentially negative outcomes:

- Dispensing more of a given brand without complete consideration of options.
- Dispensing a higher tier product (more channels, features, etc.) than is needed for certain patients.
- Inability to recognize false claims from favorite brand.
- Developing a close relationship with the manufacturer's rep.

1970s, it was considered unethical for audiologists to sell hearing aids, compared with today, when a large portion of hearing aids sold in the United States are by audiologists who own and operate their own private practice.

Regarding the distribution and manufacturing of hearing aids, we now have the Big Six companies, which includes over 90% of the hearing aids sold. But, as you might expect, the landscape is constantly changing. Two of the Big Six companies have been put up for sale in just the last few years; if one of the sales in particular had gone through, we would now only have a *Big Five*. Nobody is too sure what the impact will be from increased Internet sales or the proliferation of PSAPs.[9] And, what about the increasing number of private practices owned by manufacturers? Are we going back to the days of mostly *franchise offices*?

For the audiologist interested in dispensing hearing aids, we have reviewed many of the related background issues that need to be considered: licensure, certification, guidelines, regulations, laws, reimbursement, and ethics. These topics are maybe not as intriguing as directional polar patterns or new noise reduction algorithms, but important nonetheless. In the following chapters, we focus more on the actual selection and fitting of hearing aids.

2

Understanding the Hearing Aid Candidate

Data from surveys conducted by the National Family Opinion (NFO) panel from over 80,000 households suggest that approximately 32 million, or about 10% of the U.S. population of approximately 305 million, have some degree of hearing loss. It is usually estimated that around 95% of hearing impaired individuals can be helped with hearing aids, at least for some listening conditions. For the current U.S. population, that would be about approximately 30.5 million. Yet, we know from other surveys that only 20% to 25% of those who report having a significant hearing loss use hearing aids, suggesting that there may be 20 million or more individuals in the United States in need of treatment.

As reviewed by Mueller and Johnson (2013), some industry leaders believe that the untapped market is not as large as 20 million, due to an overestimation of the pool of potential hearing aid consumers. This is based on the notion that just because a person has an admitted hearing loss does not mean he believes that he needs hearing aids. Data show that only about ⅓ of the people with admitted hearing loss perceive themselves as having significant need for hearing aids. The real untapped potential market for hearing aids, therefore, may be closer to about 11 million today, considering the latest MarkeTrak VIII estimate of people in the United States who have a hearing impairment.

According to recent data from the Hearing Industry Association (HIA), over 2.7 million hearing aids are sold each year in the United States. However, since about 80% of hearing aids are sold in pairs (for bilateral fittings), only about 1.62 million people actually purchase hearing aids each year; 1,080,000 people purchase two hearing aids and the remaining 540,000 purchase one hearing aid. The unit volume of hearing aid sales has been slow to increase over time, considering that 1 million hearing aids were sold for the first time back in 1983. In 2004, the unit volume of hearing aid sales reached 2 million, indicating only an average of 4.7% increase in sales per year over the 21-year period from 1983. These relatively low sales numbers become even more significant today, given the improvements in hearing aid technology, and when the "aging of America" is considered.

Not surprisingly, the prevalence of hearing loss increases with increasing age: approximately 314 in 1,000 people over age 65 have hearing loss and 40% to 50% of people 75 and older have a hearing loss. Although we know that decreased hearing sensitivity is part of the aging process, the majority (65%) of the 32 million people with hearing loss are under the age of 65, shown in Figure 2–1. Hearing aid use within this younger majority is significantly less than the already disturbing low 20% to 25% figure mentioned earlier—more details on

Percentage of U.S. Citizens with Hearing Loss by Age

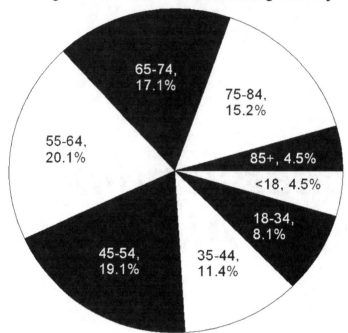

Total number of Americans with hearing loss is about 31.5 million

Figure 2–1. Distribution of U.S. citizens with hearing loss as a function of age.

these demographics shortly. Here are some general summary data from http://www.betterhearing.org regarding the incidence of hearing loss:

- Three in 10 people over age 60 have hearing loss.
- One in six baby boomers (ages 41 to 59), or 14.6%, have a hearing problem.
- One in 14 Generation Xers (ages 29 to 40), or 7.4%, already have hearing loss.
- At least 1.4 million children (18 or younger) have hearing problems.
- It is estimated that 3 in 1,000 infants are born with serious to profound hearing loss.

We of course know that individuals with hearing loss have problems understanding speech. But in addition to this obvious difficulty, we also know that hearing loss is associated with other serious negative consequences such as academic difficulties, various problems in the workplace, and psychosocial problems such as

THINGS TO REMEMBER: UNTREATED HEARING LOSS CAN LEAD TO A VARIETY OF NEGATIVE CONSEQUENCES

- Irritability, negativism, and anger
- Fatigue, tension, stress, and depression
- Avoidance or withdrawal from social situations
- Social rejection and loneliness
- Reduced alertness and increased risk to personal safety
- Impaired memory and ability to learn new tasks
- Reduced job performance and earning power
- Diminished psychological and overall health

Source: Sergei Kochkin, PhD—Better Hearing Institute, Washington, DC

social isolation, depression, anxiety, loneliness, lessened self-efficacy, and mastery (e.g., Abrams & Doyle, 2000; Newman, Jacobson, Hug, & Sandridge, 1997).

MarkeTrak

As mentioned in our introduction, market penetration regarding the use of hearing aids is poor, and the reasons that people do not use hearing aids are complex. This has been a topic of considerable study over the past two decades. In 1984 the Hearing Industry Association (HIA) published a landmark survey of the U.S. hearing aid market. Following an initial large-scale NFO screening survey to identify individuals with hearing loss, a comprehensive 120-question survey was sent to 1,050 hearing aid nonowners and 550 owners of hearing aids. The results provided the first-ever systematic look at the hearing aid market.[10] Given that more than 25 years have passed since this survey was conducted, it is interesting to consider some of the major findings from this landmark survey. How much has really changed?

- Consumers knew where to go for help with their hearing, but 40% of nonowners had never discussed their hearing loss with a physician or an audiologist.
- There was a preference to obtain the hearing aids from the ear, nose, and throat (ENT) doctor and have the hearing aids prescribed.
- Physician recommendations for hearing aids were biased toward the older patients.
- A significant number of nonowners (17%) were told that a hearing aid would not help them (53% by otolaryngologists; 22% by audiologists)
- It is surprising to note that background noise, the price of hearing aids, or cosmetics *was not* considered major problems in converting nonowners.
- And finally, nearly 14% of hearing aid owners did not use their hearing aids.

As you can see, some of the findings from 1984 have not changed significantly today. Unfortunately, one of them is the percentage of *in-the-drawer* (ITD) hearing aids. Throughout all the MarkeTrak surveys over the years, this percentage has remained around 12% to 16%. One area that *has changed* since 1984 is that otolaryngologists are now much more likely to recommend hearing aids—this of course is largely because hearing aids are now sold in most otolaryngologists' offices, usually by audiologists working for the otolaryngologist, although some otolaryngologists are also licensed dispensers.

The results of this HIA (1984) survey led to many initiatives and recommendations; one of which was to launch a family physician education program, based on the importance that survey respondents placed on a family doctor's recommendation. An in-depth review and further analysis of many of the HIA (1984) survey findings was reported in a 1990 *Hearing Instruments* article by Sergei Kochkin titled: "One more time . . . 'What did the 1984 HIA market survey say?'" At the time, Kochkin had been recently hired by Knowles Electronics as Director of Strategic Planning, with the main responsibility of: "developing and market-testing programs to impartially grow the market for hearing instruments." It was in May, 1990, in a *Hearing Journal* publication, that Kochkin introduced MarkeTrak (a consumer-oriented tracking survey of the hearing instrument market), and in this article, he published initial findings from two surveys conducted in 1989. Since this first MarkeTrak report, now referred to as MarkeTrak I, Kochkin and Knowles Electronics teamed to conduct five more surveys of the U.S. hearing loss population, MarkeTrak II through MarkeTrak VI. The two most recent surveys, MarkeTrak VII and MarkeTrak VIII, were conducted and published by the Better Hearing Institute (BHI), with Knowles Electronics sponsorship, and also were reported by Kochkin. Much of the data we report in this chapter originate from one or more of the MarkeTrak surveys.

Willingness to Use Hearing Aids

As we discussed earlier, market penetration regarding hearing aid use is poor. Why is this? As part of MarkeTrak VII, Kochkin examined some of the obstacles to hearing aid use for adults. One area that emerged as significant was the effects of age—that is, there is a perception that the use of hearing aids is probably okay for older people, but not okay for younger people. This is summarized nicely in Figure 2–2. For this analysis, Kochkin (2007) separated degree of hearing loss into 10 hearing loss deciles (#1 = mild, #10 = severe/profound),

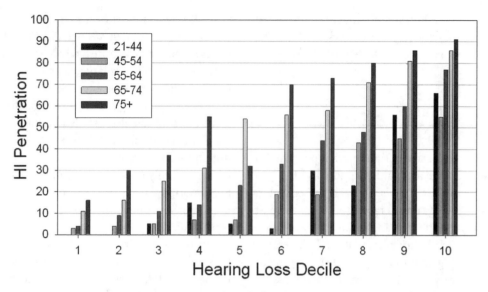

Figure 2–2. Degree of hearing loss categorized into 10 deciles (1 = mild, 10 = severe/profound), showing the percent of hearing aid use for five different hearing loss categories. (Adapted from Kochkin, 2007.)

and then shows hearing aid use as a function for five different hearing loss categories. As expected, the use of hearing aids increases with the degree of loss for all age groups; overall adoption percentages range from 1.9% for decile #1, to 15.5% for decile #5, to 59.9% for decile #10. But, observe that age has a strong influence. For example, for decile #5 (moderate hearing loss), the use rate is over 60% for individuals over 75 years of age, but only around 20% for hearing impaired people in the 55 to 64 age range. The 55 to 64 age range group would have to fall in decile #10 before their hearing aid adoption would exceed 60%.

There are many other interwoven reasons why hearing impaired people are reluctant to use hearing aids. Many of these reasons are summarized in Figure 2–3, which is taken only from deciles #6 through #10 (more significant losses). Note that the leading reason is *type of hearing loss*. Kochkin (2007) explains that this means that the person believes there is something unique about his or her hearing loss suggesting that hearing aids will not be beneficial. In many cases, they believe that their hearing loss is not severe enough to warrant the use of hearing aids. The second leading factor is *financial*. To examine the integrity of this response, Kochkin compared the incomes for this group (controlling for age) with those nonusers who said they *could* afford hearing

aids. For three of the five age groups, there was close to a $40,000 difference in mean household income, suggesting that indeed, the *can't afford* group is probably being truthful. Another significant factor, probably related to age differences shown in Figure 2–2, was the social stigma associated with the use of hearing aids. This is an interesting area, which we discuss in some detail in the next section.

As mentioned, there are several factors that contribute to individuals choosing *not* to use hearing aids. Kochkin (2007) developed a model to illustrate these factors, which is illustrated in Figure 2–4. Notice that there are major factors such as perceived hearing loss, attitude toward obtaining hearing aids, and the intent to solve the hearing loss problem. There are many other drivers, however, which will determine the final choice to proceed with hearing aid use.

Effects of Stigma

Despite considerable marketing effects to the contrary, in most Western cultures like the United States, people with hearing loss are often thought of as old, less able, and maybe even cognitively impaired. This belief is held not only by society in general, but also by the people who have hearing loss (self-stigmatization). This can

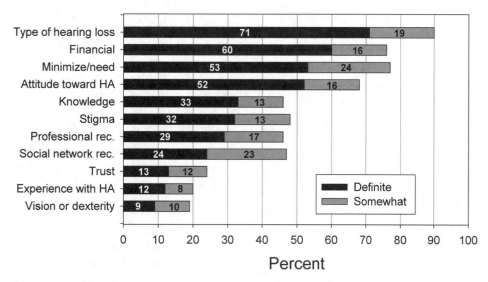

Figure 2–3. Leading reasons for not using hearing aids reported by individuals with hearing loss. (Adapted from Kochkin, 2007.)

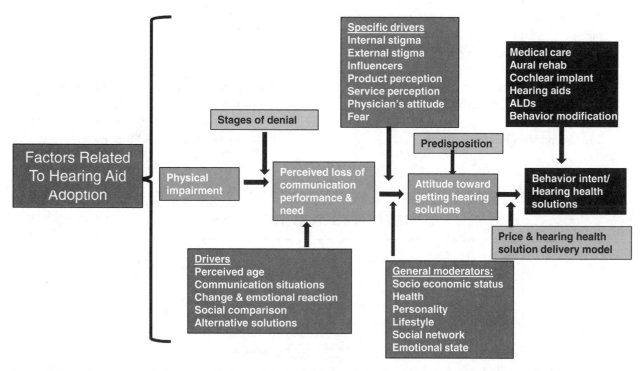

Figure 2–4. Summary of the many factors that interrelate to the use of hearing aids. (Adapted from Kochkin, 2007.)

have a profound effect regarding the initial adoption of amplification as well as the use and acceptance of hearing aids. Because hearing loss is not visible, to avoid stig-

matization, some individuals may try to deny or hide their hearing loss. As described by Gagné, Southall, and Jennings (2009), a variety of strategies might be used.

For example, they will isolate and insulate themselves from the world around them. In this way, they will not need to use communication strategies (e.g., asking someone to repeat) that will reveal that they have a hearing loss. The efforts expended to conceal the hearing require emotional and cognitive resources, which then can lead to an overall decrease in quality of life.

In 1996, Hétu proposed two models related to the stigmatization that occurs for individuals with acquired hearing loss: the *stigmatization process* and the *normalization process*. The work of Hétu (1996) was discussed by Gagné et al. (2009), and the following is a brief summary taken from their review:

Stigmatization Process

- Stigmatization occurs because of *shame* related to their hearing impairment. Shame meaning an emotion that accompanies threats to one's sense of social belonging.
- The shame is related to communication breakdowns that occur when people with hearing loss interact with people who have normal hearing. The person may feel guilt about themselves related to the hearing loss.
- As a result of the feelings of incompetency that might develop, the person's self-esteem and social identity are diminished.

- This may lead the person to attempt to conceal the hearing loss, or withdraw from social activities.

Hétu's model of the Stigmatization Process is shown in Figure 2–5.

Normalization Process (Step 1)

The normalization process is to help the person who is stigmatized by the hearing loss regain a more normal social identity.

- The individual begins by meeting and interacting with other people who have hearing loss. This creates an environment where they can share their feelings and discuss their unsuccessful social interactions.
- They realize that they are not alone, and that many other people have the same feelings of being denigrated or ashamed.
- They begin to realize that the feelings they have are normal.

Normalization Process (Step 2)

- Meeting and interacting with family and friends who do not have hearing loss.
- The hearing impaired person is encouraged to tell family and friends that they have a hearing

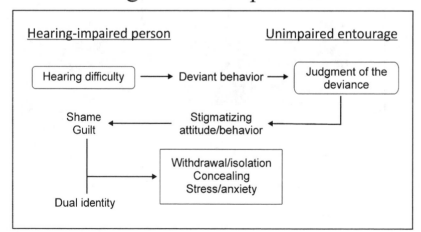

Figure 2–5. Hétu's model of the stigmatization process. (Adapted from Hétu, 1996.)

loss and to solicit the use of communication strategies that will assist in better communication.

■ The use of effective communication strategies will help restore a more factorable social identity; the person with hearing loss will gain more confidence; and as a result, they will be more likely to participate in social situations.

Step 1 and Step 2 of the Normalization Process are shown in Figure 2–6.

Stigma-Induced Identity Threat

Identity threat, often referred to as *stereotype threat*, refers to situations in which individuals feel they might be judged negatively because of a stereotype. The threat refers to being at risk of confirming, as self-characteristic, a negative stereotype about one's group. Identity threat can lead to self-handicapping strategies and a reduced sense of belonging to the stereotyped domain, or their value of the domain in question. Studies in this

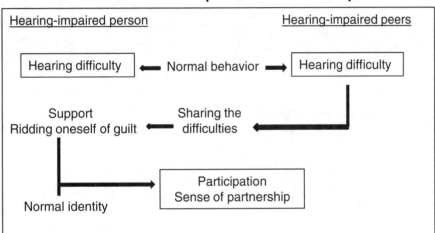

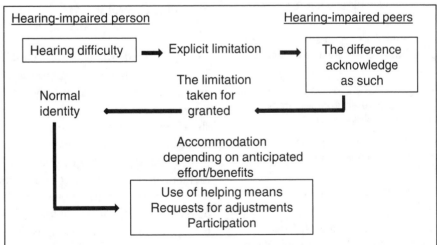

Figure 2–6. Steps 1 and 2 of the normalization process related to stigmatization. (Adapted from Gagné et al., 2009.)

area often have been focused toward minority or gender issues, but identity threat is also something that may need to be considered with hearing aid candidates. We have already discussed one example.

As reviewed by Gagné et al. (2009), stigma related to hearing loss and hearing aid use can put a person at risk for identity threat. This may occur when the patient judges the demands imposed by a stigma-relevant event as potentially harmful to his or her social identity, and when the stress induced exceeds the patient's ability to cope with the demands of the situation. We have already discussed one example. Recall from Figure 2–2, that hearing aid use rate is over 60% for individuals with moderate hearing loss who are over 75 years of age, but the use rate is only 20% for the same hearing loss group in the 55 to 64 age range. It is reasonable to assume that the use of hearing aids is an identity threat to the younger group. In Table 2–1, Gagné et al. (2009) provide

Table 2–1. Components of an Audiologic Counseling Strategy Designed to Address Identity Threat for the Hearing Aid Candidate

---

1. Describe and discuss the stigma-induced identity threat, and explain to the patient the cause, consequences and the potential costs of the stress related to identify threat.

2. Establish a hierarchy of situations in which identity threat occurs.

3. Discuss the effectiveness of the patient's typical coping strategies. Introduce new adaptive strategies when necessary.

4. Implement a problem-solving approach to address a situation of stigma-inducing identity threat identified by the patient.

5. Train and encourage the patient to apply the selected coping strategies in a secure environment (may be practiced during the counseling session).

6. Meet with the patient to discuss the process of implementing and the consequences of applying the strategies discussed.

7. Attempt a similar experience in a slightly more threatening situation.

8. Increase the number of situations in which the patient discloses his or her hearing loss and applies appropriate coping strategies.

Source: Adapted from Gagne et al., 2009.

a set of guidelines to help the audiologist counsel the patient with identity threat.

The Benefits of Hearing Aid Use

As shown in the preceding section, MarkeTrak studies have examined the reasons why people delay their decision to purchase hearing aids. Certainly one reason is that they simply are unaware of the fact that receiving early treatment for hearing loss has the potential to literally transform their lives (e.g., my hearing loss is too mild to benefit from hearing aids). Research by the National Council on the Aging on more than two thousand people with hearing loss, as well as their significant others, demonstrated that hearing aids clearly are associated with substantial improvements in the social, emotional, psychological, and physical well-being of people with hearing loss in all hearing loss categories from mild to severe. Specifically, hearing aid usage is positively related to the following quality of life issues. Hearing loss treatment (use of hearing aids) was shown to improve:

- Earning power
- Communication in relationships
- Intimacy and warmth in family relationships
- Ease in communication
- Emotional stability
- Sense of control over life events
- Perception of mental functioning
- Physical health
- Group social participation

As part of this research, significant others were asked to rate changes they observed in several different areas of their life that they believed were due to the respondent using hearing aids. These findings are shown in Figure 2–7. In general, for nearly all quality of life areas assessed, the observed improvements were positively related to the degree of hearing loss. Family members in nearly every comparison observed greater improvements than the respondent. The top three areas of observed improvement for both respondents and family members were *relationships at home, feelings about self,* and *life overall.* As might be expected, the most substantial improvements were observed for the individuals with more severe hearing loss.

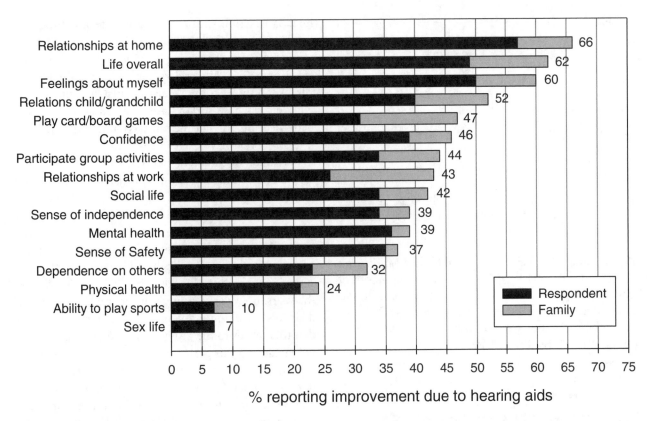

Figure 2–7. Percent of hearing aid owners and their family members reporting improvement in their quality of life in 16 different areas due to the use of hearing aids. Note that in nearly all cases, the family members report that the hearing aid user is experiencing more benefit than the user reports.

Perhaps just as important, this research found that hearing loss treatment was shown to reduce:

- Discrimination toward the person with the hearing loss
- Hearing loss compensation behaviors (i.e., pretending you hear)
- Anger and frustration in relationships
- Depression and depressive symptoms
- Feelings of paranoia
- Anxiety
- Social phobias
- Self-criticism

Given all the factors that can be improved with the use of hearing aids, it is somewhat difficult to explain the large percent of nonusers. Indeed, it could be that they are not aware of the potential advantages. But what about the ITDs—the people who have purchased hearing aids, did not return them during the trial period, but are not using them? Why didn't these patients receive benefit? Why were they not satisfied? This also has been studied, and the reasons are quite variable and include aspects of the patient, the hearing aid, and their environment (see "Things to Remember" on this topic). To combat nonuse, it is important to consider these factors and the potential for them to affect *individual patients* during the process of establishing candidacy, selecting and fitting the hearing aid, and providing counseling. In this way, future nonuse can be reduced. As hearing aids have improved over the years, you might think that the rate of ITDs would have systematically gone down. This is not really true. If we look at MarkeTrak surveys dating back to 1991, we see that the rate of ITDs has ranged from 12% to 18%, with the latest 2008 12% rating no different from that of 1991, shown in Figure 2–8.

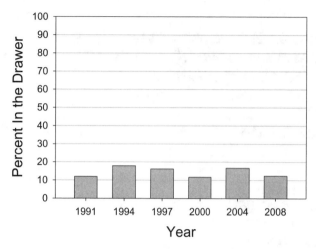

Figure 2–8. Findings from six different MarkeTrak surveys, from 1991 to 2008 regarding the percent of people who own hearing aids but never use them, sometimes referred to as in-the-drawer (ITD) hearing aids. Note that the ITD rate has not improved. (Adapted from Kochkin, 2010.)

Satisfaction with Amplification

We have talked about some reasons why individuals do *not* use their hearing aids, but fortunately most patients do, and most of these individuals are reasonably satis-

fied. Satisfaction with amplification is something that has been tracked by MarkeTrak over the years, with several surveys examining specific aspects of hearing aid fittings (e.g., bilateral versus unilateral, directional versus omnidirectional, custom instruments versus BTE, etc.). These surveys are archived at http://www.betterhearing.org. For the satisfaction ratings, the MarkeTrak surveys have used a five-point Likert scale: very dissatisfied, dissatisfied, neutral, satisfied, and very satisfied. The satisfied and very satisfied categories are then often combined for a single *satisfaction* measure. Figure 2–9 shows the satisfaction levels that have been obtained for surveys dating back to 1989. Fortunately, results from the most recent surveys have revealed satisfaction levels significantly higher than when the first survey was conducted. When observing the levels over the years, however, you might wonder why there was a drop in satisfaction in the mid-1990s. Our best guess is that this relates to the heavy promotion of digital technology during this period, which brought in new users, was significantly more expensive, raised expectations, but may not have delivered *value*. But that's just a guess.

In addition to overall satisfaction, it is important to consider satisfaction for different listening situations. This is shown for MarkeTrak VIII in Figure 2–10. Note that satisfaction is very high for one-on-one communication (92%) and even conversations in small groups (85%). As noise and/or reverberation is added, satis-

---

THINGS-TO-REMEMBER:
OFTEN CITED FACTORS FOR HEARING AID NONUSE

Earlier in this chapter, we examined the reasons why people with hearing loss do not use hearing aids. These data were primarily for individuals who never had tried hearing aids. But what about the people who own hearing aids and do not use them? The main reasons (rank ordered) are listed below. As we read through the different reasons, we can speculate that perhaps some patients simply have unrealistic expectations, but we also have to wonder if some of these factors could have been reduced or eliminated with improved verification, validation and counseling?

- Lack of benefit
- Lack of benefit in noise
- Poor cosmetics
- Disbelief that they need help
- Inability to insert the earmold
- Poor fit and/or comfort

- Negative side effects
- Poor sound quality for own voice
- Poor sound quality for external sounds
- Feedback
- Hearing aid is broken

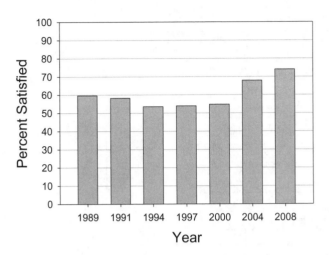

Figure 2–9. Summary of overall hearing aid satisfaction rates for seven different MarkeTrak surveys. Satisfaction has been increasing in recent years following a dip in the 1990s. (Adapted from Kochkin, 2010.)

faction predictably goes down. For common listening situations where background noise is present, such as a restaurant or large group, satisfaction is 68 to 75%. Although these later numbers are not as high as we would like, it is important to point out that as recent as 1995 (e.g., MarkeTrak IV), satisfaction for use in restaurants was only 52% (23% poorer) and the satisfaction for listening in large groups was below 40% (20% poorer). We suspect that the significant increase we have seen in recent years is some combination of today's advanced algorithms, better fitting procedures (more audibility), and probably better counseling.

Another area of satisfaction that can be studied is related to sound quality and the sounds of potentially annoying aspects of hearing aid use (e.g., wind noise, sound of own voice, etc.). These data, from MarkeTrak VIII are shown in Figure 2–11. Again, these values are not as high as we would like, but nearly all of them are

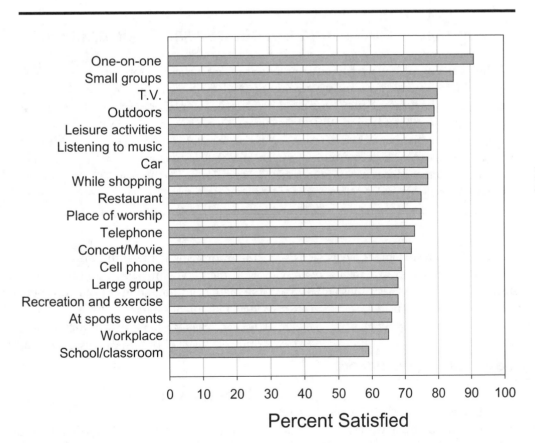

Figure 2–10. Data from MarkeTrak VIII showing satisfaction rates for 18 different listening conditions. (Adapted from Kochkin, 2010.)

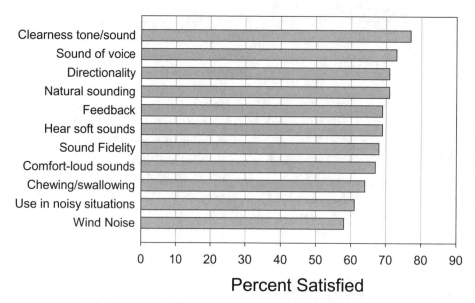

Figure 2–11. Data from MarkeTrak VIII showing satisfaction rates for 11 different conditions related to hearing aid use. (Adapted from Kochkin, 2010.)

POINTS TO PONDER: WHAT IS A GOOD SATISFACTION RATING?

As shown in Figure 2–9, we have seen an upward trend in overall satisfaction with hearing aids in the past 10 years, and we are now at 74%. We do not expect to ever have 100% satisfaction, but what is good? How does 74% compare with other services and products? The good news is that it is about 10% higher than network TV, the IRS, and McDonald's. It is approximately the same as satisfaction for banks, hotels, and waste disposal. Coming in nearly 10% higher are beer and utility companies. BMW owners have an 84% satisfaction rate, and topping the list at 86% is processed food (e.g., Heinz Ketchup) at 86%. At this writing, satisfaction with the U.S. Congress is at 17% and falling!

10% to 15% better than surveys from the 1990s. Consistent with the data shown in Figure 2–9, the *use in noisy situations* satisfaction rating of 62% is a substantial 25% higher than obtained for MarkeTrak IV.

Understanding the Patient

A patient is not defined only by their hearing loss or communication needs, but by a variety of factors. This understanding and respect for individuality must begin the moment a patient walks in the door and continue throughout the entire professional relationship with them. As clinicians, we must also recognize the strengths and limitations of our own personality and how that might interact with the patients. In this way, we can optimize rapport with each patient and maximize our chances at the most positive outcome possible.

Stages of Grief

As reviewed by Taylor and Mueller (2011), it is a commonly held belief that adults with acquired hearing go through Kubler-Ross's five stages of grief: denial, anger, bargaining, depression, and acceptance.[11] It is helpful when initiating the opening counseling and conducting our case history if we have a general understanding of which stage each patient falls into. Whenever possible, it is useful to involve family members and other significant others, as this will help identify the patient's stage. Their assistance also will be helpful as you guide the patient through the first four stages in preparation for using hearing aids—*stage five*. The time it takes a patient to travel through the five stages is extremely variable; for some patients, it seems to happen in a single afternoon, for others it may take years. Not everyone goes through all of the stages or goes through them in linear fashion. Some stages may not be experienced at all. Because hearing loss usually is a slow and gradual process, it is very common to experience a patient in denial. On the other hand, because it is *gradual*, and not life-threatening, the stages of anger and depression are not observed as often as they might be with other pathologies. We do see these stages more commonly in sudden hearing loss, however.

With the typical patient considering the use of hearing aids, the denial stage is so common that it is almost expected. We all have seen a patient in our office who had tried hearing aids four or five years earlier, and returned them for credit because they did not work, and who is now back to try hearing aids again. Our testing reveals that the hearing loss and speech recognition has not really changed in five years, but this time the patient reports that hearing aids provide significant benefit and becomes a satisfied user. Was this because of the changes in hearing aid technology over the years? Maybe, but it is more probable that the fitting is now successful simply because the patient now is accepting of the hearing loss and ready to seek assistance. Insights into how the five stages of grieving can impact patient behavior can be helpful in counseling the new hearing aid user. Examples for each stage are provided in Table 2–2.

Identifying the Hearing Aid Candidate

With all of the problems associated with hearing loss, it is important to discuss what makes someone a hearing aid candidate. Although this question has been debated for decades, it is clear that the answer is much more complex than simply the presence of a certain degree of hearing loss. In fact, success with hearing aids can be more affected by a patient's motivation than the exact degree of hearing loss. Factors such as difficulty hearing sounds, communication difficulty, motivation for improved hearing, financial constraints, expectations related to hearing aids (both positive and negative), and a host of other factors affect candidacy. Before establishing candidacy, the patient must make some effort to be evaluated. Specifically, the patient, some-

Table 2–2. The Elisabeth Kubler Ross Five Psychological Stages of Grieving, Applied to Hearing Loss

Stage	What the patient might say:
Denial	"I don't have a hearing problem, other people mumble." "I hear everything I need to hear."
Anger	To their friends—"Are you purposely talking behind my back?" To the professional: "Are you sure you did the testing correctly?"
Bargaining	"Okay, maybe I just wasn't listening, I'll pay more attention." "Let's see if I'm still having problems next year, maybe my hearing will get better."
Depression	"It seems like my family avoids me because of my hearing loss." "There are things I'll probably never hear again." "I'm getting old."
Acceptance	"Wearing hearing aids is really no big deal." "My quality of life will probably improve with the use of hearing aids." "A lot of people my age have worse health problems than hearing loss."

Source: Adapted from Taylor and Mueller, 2011.

times under the direction (or strong encouragement) of a spouse or significant other, must seek help for their hearing problem.

Making the decision to seek help is obviously a complex one as is shown by the survey data we have discussed. One factor is the magnitude of hearing loss. Specifically, more than 85% of nonusers fall in the range of mild-to-moderate hearing loss and data from Flamme et al. (2005) reveal that fewer than 6% of individuals with mild-to-moderate hearing loss pursue amplification. It is tempting to conclude that these individuals with mild-to-moderate hearing loss may simply not encounter hearing related communication difficulties, although this contradicts everything we know about the importance of audibility and speech understanding. In agreement, Newman et al. (1997) reported that even younger adults with mild hearing loss report a variety of psychosocial problems affecting everyday life.

Concerns about lack of benefit, concerns about how they might look with hearing aids (cosmetics), negative reports from friends and others about hearing aids, and high cost can also keep patients from pursuing amplification. Although it is tempting to think that cosmetic and cost concerns might dominate the worries related to hearing aid use and lead to patient's avoidance of seeking help, they are clearly not the only factors. Surprisingly, one survey reported that only 35% of individuals who have hearing loss, but currently do not have a hearing aid, would wear an instrument even if it was *free* and *invisible* (Kochkin, 2001). Recent data suggests that number has gone up to 55% (Kochkin, 2012)—a sign of the economy perhaps! Obviously, as we discussed earlier, concerns such as expected lack of benefit, negative consequences, and other issues also are being considered by prospective patients.

Once an individual seeks help, it is important to determine if they are an appropriate candidate. At the simplest level, candidacy for adults can be described by a combination of the presence of hearing loss to a degree that obstructs communication (or other reported hearing difficulties) and the motivation to improve hearing. Although these criteria are likely the most important to keep in mind when considering candidacy, a few specific question areas should usually be explored when considering candidacy. Whereas we as clinicians must sometimes gently encourage patients to try amplification, we must also be willing to halt the entire process if the patient is not ready. The answers to a few specific questions can help frame future questions and help us as

clinicians decide how much counseling *needs to be done* prior to thinking about hearing aid selection. Depending on weather there is a red flag or not, the answers to these specific questions might lead to: (1) some counseling during the hearing aid selection stage, (2) the potential need for significant further counseling, or (3) possibly the conclusion that the patient is not an appropriate candidate at this time. Examples of typical and red flag answers are shown in Table 2–3. These are all answers that we actually have heard in the clinic on more than one occasion.

Although it may seem quite surprising on the surface, many adults who seek assessment of their hearing difficulties reject recommendations for remediation of hearing loss. Therefore, in addition to recognizing how the lack of treatment may impact a given individual considering amplification, it is also relevant to determine if and how other nonauditory factors might affect the prognosis for amplification, and whether these factors should be formally assessed. Nonauditory, contextual factors can be internally or externally based.

- Internal (i.e., personal contextual) factors impacting communication include cognitive decline, personality characteristics (expectations, motivation, willingness to take a risk, assertiveness), additional sensory impairments (manual dexterity, visual acuity), prior experience with amplification, general health, and other otologic conditions (tinnitus).
- External (i.e., environmental contextual) factors include environmental characteristics (such as occupational demands and recreational habits) and patient support systems.

Questions asked during the case history should be tailored to address these issues and not just focus on hearing. There is no strong evidence to suggest that any one or a combination of these nonauditory issues can be used to reliably predict success or failure with hearing aids (Valente, 2006). Nevertheless, identifying these factors should be addressed in counseling and in establishing realistic expectations with the patient. In Chapter 6, we review several self-assessment scales that can assist in obtaining important information (often not part of the case history) and categorizing candidacy.

Table 2–3. Questions and Answers That Can Help Frame the Counseling Process

Q1. Why are you here?
- Expected Answer: I have been having some problems hearing (or understanding), especially in background noise.
- Red Flag: **My wife thinks I can't hear.**

Q2. Whose idea was it to come in? (usually indirectly asked)
- Expected Answer: My daughter suggested that I should come in, and I guess she is right. I've been putting if off for years.
- Red Flag: **My husband says he thinks I have a problem, but I really don't.**

Q3. What is your biggest concern?
- Expected Answer: That I won't be able to use a hearing aid correctly.
- Red Flag: **That we really can't afford the hearing aid and my wife will find out we have financial problems.**

Q4. Do you believe you can be helped by the use of hearing aids?
- Typical Answer: I think so. I certainly hope the hearing aids will help me.
- Red Flag: **I really don't have much of hearing problem, so I really don't need help.**

Motivational Interviewing

Based on the patient's answers during the case history, and their personality, a number of different counseling approaches might be necessary when talking to a patient about hearing aid candidacy. It is beyond the scope of this book to address many of these approaches in detail; however, there are many other textbooks that directly address counseling techniques. One counseling philosophy is motivational interviewing, described by Miller and Rollnick (2002; for more information visit motivationalinterview.org). Motivational interviewing is a directive, client-centered counseling style for elicit-ing behavior change by helping clients to explore and resolve ambivalence. This counseling approach, which evolved from treatment of substance abusers, points out the futility of confrontational approaches ("See, you have a hearing loss just like your wife said, now what are you going to do about it?"). Instead, the fact that the patient may experience ambivalence about treatment (a feeling of uncertainty about something due to a mental conflict) that must be explored and resolved is highlighted. Although interested readers are referred elsewhere for detailed techniques, it is worthwhile to at least attempt to capture the spirit of motivational interviewing (see "Technical Tip" on this topic).

TECHNICAL TIP: THE SPIRIT OF MOTIVATIONAL INTERVIEWING

- Motivation to change is elicited from the patient and not imposed from without.
- It is the patient's task, not the audiologist's, to articulate and resolve his or her ambivalence.
- Direct persuasion is not an effective method for resolving ambivalence.
- The counseling style is generally a quiet and eliciting one.
- The audiologist is directive in helping the patient to examine and resolve ambivalence.
- Readiness to change is not a patient trait, but a fluctuating product of interpersonal interaction.
- The therapeutic relationship is more like a partnership or companionship than expert/recipient roles.

(Adapted from motivationalinterview.org.)

In their counseling textbook, Clark and English (2003) describe similar themes that are more directly related to hearing loss, including the importance of getting patients to take ownership of their hearing problem. They describe techniques that can be used for children and adults related to identification of specific problems or difficulties related to hearing and discussing how to best counteract those problems. This type of counseling requires that the clinician switch roles during their time spent with a patient. Specifically, the clinician must relinquish their role as the expert who is determining what is best for the patient until *after* the patient makes the decision they are willing to accept help and pursue amplification.

In addition to the patient, we must also be honest with ourselves as clinicians. This not only includes recognizing when we may be stressed or have external pressures that may affect our performance, but also recognizing our own personality and how it might interact with that of our patients. Some clinicians have naturally warm and friendly styles; others are more businesslike and direct in their approach. Both of these approaches can be successful, although they will likely have the greatest appeal to different patient personalities. Regardless of personality, a caring professional approach and a genuine interest in addressing each individual patient's communication needs is critical for establishing patient trust and building rapport. Without this rapport, many patients will be much less likely to trust your recommendations. The unfortunate consequence of this lack of trust may be reduced satisfaction with hearing aids or even failure to pursue further help for a period of time.

The Patient's Story

Erdman (2009) discusses the importance of an empathetic practitioner-patient relationship, which can facilitate engagement of the patient and which in turn may improve their management of the treatment and their adherence to the treatment regimen. The understanding is based on the accurate perspective of the patient experience and appropriate emotional reactivity. A model illustrating the role of empathic counseling is shown in Figure 2–12 (from Erdman, 2009).

Part of this biopsychosocial counseling approach is the patient's story. Listening to a patient's story will facilitate the counseling process, and the patients are

there to tell their story. It is why they made the appointment. You just need to help them a little. Erdman (2009) provides some guidance in this area:

- Use open-ended statements: "What brought you here today?"
- If at all possible, sit with the patient in a private area face to face. Make eye contact and show that you are sincerely listening.
- Allow the patient to answer. Wait. They may not respond immediately. If the patient does not respond in 10 to 20 seconds, rephrase the question and try again.
- Listen to the story and develop a shared understanding of what the experience of hearing loss means to the patient. This will help you engage the patient and facilitate achieving the treatment goals.

The Four Habits Model

In the final section of this chapter, we take some of the things that we have discussed so far and put them into a model that you can use with your patients. The model that we prefer is from Frankel and Stein (1999) from their article, "Getting the Most Out of the Clinical Encounter: The Four Habits Model." As pointed out by these authors, our bedside manner has a direct influence on the outcome of the treatment; research has shown that patients probably are more concerned about how much we *care*, than how much we *know*. The goals of the Four Habits are:

- To establish rapport and build trust rapidly
- Facilitate the effective exchange of information
- Demonstrate caring and concern
- Increase the likelihood of treatment adherence and positive health outcomes

Habit 1: Invest in the Beginning

It is recommended that three tasks are accomplished at the beginning of the patient encounter (see Table 2–4 for example).

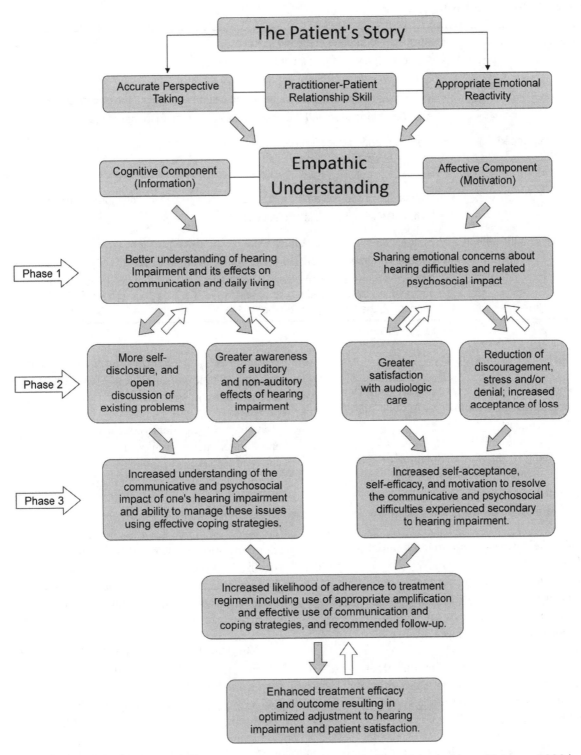

Figure 2–12. A model illustrating the role of empathetic counseling. (Adapted from Erdman, 2009.)

Table 2–4. Habit #1: Invest in the Beginning

Create rapport quickly	• Introduce yourself to everyone in room.
	• Acknowledge wait if patient not seen on time.
	• Convey your knowledge of patient's history.
	• Make social comment or ask a non-medical question to put the patient at ease.
	• Adapt own language and the pace of the conversation to that of the patient.
Elicit patient's concerns	• Use open ended questions:
	"What prompted this visit?"
	"What can I help you with today?"
	"I understand that you are here because of _____, tell me more about that."
	"What else would you like to discuss?"
Plan the visit with the patient	• Repeat patient's concerns back to them to check understanding.
	• Describe course of action. Let the patient know what to expect.
	• Prioritize course of action if necessary. "I know you'd like to talk to someone about your dizziness and the soreness in your right ear, but let's start with conducting the hearing evaluation."

Creating Rapport Quickly

The first few moments of the encounter are important for establishing a trusting relationship. Actions such as the following are suggested:

■ At the initial introduction, to obtain trust and respect, it is helpful if the patient is addressed at the same level of authority. That is, if you are Dr. Smith, then the patient would be Mr. Jones.

■ A handshake during the introduction initiates touch.

■ Assure name of patient and correct pronunciation; names of others if family members or significant others are present.

■ Adapt voice tone and language level to the patient.

■ If possible, review the chart before the initial introduction and inform the patient of this.

■ If the patient is not seen on time, acknowledge this with something like: "I'm sorry for keeping you waiting."

Eliciting Patient Concerns

The second task is to determine the reason(s) for the appointment. Regarding the fitting of hearing aids, this often will help assist in determining if the patient is ready for amplification. Frankel and Stein (1999) recommend two different strategies:

■ Drawing out the patient's concerns with open-ended questions like, "I understand you're having some problems with your hearing?" "Can you tell me about that?"

■ The second strategy is to use *continuers*. Once the patient begins to describe the hearing and communication problems, this then includes vocalizations such as "Uh huh," "Go on," and "Tell me more," and nonverbal behaviors such as silence, head nodding, and an engaged listening posture.

Once you have heard the concerns of the patient, it is time to plan the visit. You could use a summary statement something like: "So it sounds like you're having some trouble understanding speech, especially when background noise is present. What I'd like to do is conduct some testing, so I can tell you what is going on, and then we'll develop a plan together if treatment is needed."

Typically, a patient who is being seen by an audiologist for the potential use of hearing aids has a fairly straightforward problem. It is not like a patient going in to see his or her general practice physician, who may have a list of five or six problems. In some situations, however, the audiology patient might present ear-related issues that need attention that are not directly related to the fitting of hearing aids (e.g., external or middle ear pathology, balance function problems, tinnitus, etc.). Two strategies are suggested for handling this:

Prioritization: Inform the patient of what can be accomplished during the office visit. "In the time we have today, I want to first make sure we obtain a good measure of how you're hearing, and conduct a few tests to identify what might be causing your hearing problems." If time is running short, use *I wish* statements. "I wish I had more time today to talk about the ringing in your ears, but . . . "

Time-framing: Patients usually know the time of their appointment, but are not aware of the time that was allotted for them. It is therefore helpful to provide them information such as: "Mr. Smith, you were scheduled for a 30-minute appointment today. We can take care of your other concerns in a follow-up appointment."

Habit 2: Elicit the Patient's Perspective

The purpose of this habit is to assess the patient's point of view concerning the hearing problem and what treatment he or she is seeking. Eliciting the patient's perspective consists of three skills: assessing patient attribution, identifying patient requests for care, and exploring the impact of symptoms (see Table 2–5 for review).

THINGS TO REMEMBER: TIME MANAGEMENT CAN BE TRICKY

The Four Habits Model discusses the use of prioritization and time-framing when working with patients. This is based on a busy medical practice where patient visits might be scheduled every 15 minutes. Some audiology clinics only allow 30 minutes for a diagnostic appointment, which doesn't leave much time for discussion treatment strategies. When seeing patients who are hearing aid candidates, the audiologist needs to exercise some *clinical judgment* when a time crunch exists. There is something to the old adage "strike while the iron is hot." If after testing and your follow-up counseling a patient appears to be ready to order hearing aids, we suggest that you somehow find time to follow through with this at that patient visit. Often, the patient will be willing to simply wait an hour or so until you have a break, rather than come back on another day—which may not happen for years!

Table 2–5. Habit #2: Elicit the Patient's Perspective

Ask for patient's ideas	• Assess the patient's point of view regarding their hearing problems: "Why do you think that you have a hearing loss?" "What worries you about this problem?" • Ask the patient's friends and family their opinion.
Elicit specific requests	• Determine the patient's goals or desired outcome: "What are you hoping that I can help you with regarding your hearing problems?"
Explore the impact the hearing loss is having on the patient's life	• How has this hearing loss affected your social life? Work? Relations with family members? • Ask the patient's friends and family the same questions.

Assessing Patient Attribution

This consists of determining the patient's perspective about what caused the hearing loss. It is important to ask open-ended questions and to allow the patient to express his or her concerns. This may help you provide reassurance when the testing is finished—a patient who believes that their hearing loss is due to a brain tumor will be relieved to know that the hearing loss is consistent with presbycusis. Because most hearing losses are from similar causes, as audiologists it is tempting to help out the patient with the case history: "Oh, you like to hunt, your hearing loss probably is from noise exposure." Although this may be true, it is important to know what the patient thinks. It has been shown that patients who understand and who are able to explain the problem (e.g., I've worked as a carpenter for the past 20 years, and I'm pretty sure I got my hearing loss from all that saw noise) are able to recall more of the information that we provide them, and are more responsive to treatment (Tuckett, Boulton, Olson, & Williams, 1985).

Identifying Patient Requests

In general, when the patient arrives at your clinic, he or she brings along not only a set of problems, but also expectations regarding the recommendations and treatment that you will provide. This could be related to past experiences, stories from friends, or information acquired from the media. We all have seen the patient who believes that hearing loss could be cured by a simple operation. It is helpful to ask a question such as, "How were you hoping that I could help you with your hearing loss today?" It is interesting to note that Eisenthal and Lazare (1977) found that patients whose requests were fully listened to were more satisfied with their care, regardless of whether the requests were granted.

Exploring the Impact

The final skill in Habit 2 is determining the impact of the patient's hearing loss on their daily activities, work, and family relations. This is best accomplished by using a structured self-assessment scale designed for this purpose. One example is the Hearing Handicap for the Elderly or Adult (HHIE or HHIA). This scale, described in detail in Chapter 6, examines the social and emotional handicap caused by the hearing loss. Another helpful scale, also described in Chapter 6, is the Client Oriented Scale of Improvement, the COSI. Because the COSI relies on communication situations generated by the patient, this often uncovers specific areas regarding work and family where the hearing loss is causing problems.

Habit 3: Demonstrate Empathy

It is of course important to build rapport and show empathy throughout the patient visit, but perhaps the most important time is while you are establishing the patient's concern(s). A review of how this can be accomplished is shown in Table 2–6.

Being Open to the Patient's Emotions

As we have already discussed, clinical practice can be busy, and many times we just want to get down to business—get the patient in the booth, do the testing, order the hearing aids. When do we have time to experience

Table 2–6. Habit #3: Demonstrate Empathy

Be open to patient's emotions	• Assess changes in body language and voice.
	• Look for opportunities to use brief empathic comments or gestures.
Make at least one empathic statement	• Name a probable emotion: "That sounds really upsetting."
	• Compliment the patient on efforts to address the problem.
Convey empathy nonverbally	• Pause; use body language.
Be aware of your own emotions	• Use your feeling as a clue to what the patient might be feeling.
	• Take a break if necessary.

empathy? Frankel and Stein (1999) explain that one strategy is to look for brief windows of opportunity for responding to patients' emotions, a skill noted in *outstanding* clinicians. And, it may not take as long as you think. Research at the University of Western Ontario by Stewart, Brown, and Weston (1989) showed that medical professionals who are sensitive to and explore patients' emotional concerns take on the average only one minute longer to complete a patient visit compared with those who do not. It is also important to identify hints of emotion, which patients might use as a trial balloon. The comment, "I'm thinking about retirement" seems simple enough, unless one considers that communication problems at work could be driving the decision.

Frankel and Stein (1999) suggest that there are two general options available when responding to a potential empathic opportunity:

- The audiologist can avoid the opportunity by changing the topic, ignoring the statement, or by offering premature reassurance. This is the easiest approach and unfortunately often the one employed.
- The audiologist can encourage the expression of the emotion by using open-ended continuers, such as, "Please go on . . . ," "Tell me more," and so forth. Some empathetic responses suggested by Bird and Cohen-Cole (1990) include:
  - Reflection—"I can see that you are . . . "
  - Legitimation—"I can understand why you feel . . . "
  - Support—"I want to help."
  - Partnership—"Let's work together . . . "
  - Respect—"You're doing great."

> ### KEY CONCEPT: ABOUT PATIENT CARE
>
> Dr. Francis Peabody was a well-known pioneer in the area of internal medicine. At the age of 45, he became seriously and incurably ill. His final talk was titled "Care of the Patient," in which he stated the now famous dictum "the secret of the care of the patient is in caring for the patient."[12]

Habit 4: Invest in the End

This habit is more about delivering information than collecting it. It relates to tasks that occur at the end of the patient visit: delivering diagnostic information; encouraging patients to participate in decision making; and negotiating treatment plans (e.g., the fitting of hearing aids). Table 2–7 reviews some of the key skills related to this habit.

Delivering Diagnostic Information

Frankel and Stein (1999) suggest that the most important principle regarding the delivery of diagnostic information is to use the patient's original statement of concerns to frame information to be shared. "Well Bob, you mentioned that you might have a hearing loss because of all that noise exposure during construction work? Well, it looks like you were right." "Well Mrs. Smith, you mentioned that you were having trouble understanding your grandchildren. This testing clearly explains why you have that problem."

Informational Counseling. When we sit down with our patients following the initial audiologic testing, we typically explain the test results. This is something that in general audiologists enjoy doing, almost to a fault. This process is referred to as *informational counseling.* Bob Margolis (2004) has written on this topic, and here are some tips that he provides:

- Present the most important information first. Patients are best at remembering the first thing you tell them.
- Give advice in the form of concrete instructions.
- Use easy-to-understand language; short words and sentences.
- Repeat the most important information.
- Stress the importance of recommendations or other information that you want the patient to remember.
- Ask for questions and confirm the patient understands before moving on to the next category.
- Don't present too much information.
- Present only the information that is important for the patient to remember.

Table 2–7. Habit #4: Invest in the End

Deliver diagnostic information	• Describe the test results in a way that relate back to the patient's concerns: "You were right, you do have problems understanding speech when background noise is present." • Test to determine if patient is understanding your comments.
Provide education	• Explain why you did each test. • Explain prognosis: "This is a permanent hearing loss and it is unlikely it will improve." "Your hearing loss will likely gradually become worse due to the natural aging process." • Provide written materials of support.
Involve patient in making decisions	• Discuss treatment goals: "I believe you will receive significant benefit from the use of hearing aids. We can start the process today if you like." • Listen to the patient's preference. • Set limits respectively. "It's certainly possible that your friend's hearing was helped by surgery, but you don't have that type of hearing loss. The use of hearing aids is the only treatment." • Assess the patient's ability and motivation to carry out the treatment plan.
Complete the visit	• Ask the patient for additional questions? • Assess satisfaction: "Is there anything more about your hearing loss or the use of hearing aids that you would like to know?" • Reassure the patient of follow-up care.

■ Supplement verbal information with written, graphic, and pictorial materials that the patient can take home.

■ Plan on going slower and spending more time with older individuals who may have cognitive problems.

■ Again, repeat the most important information.

Involving Patients in Decision Making

Patient involvement in the decision-making process is important for all types of treatment, including the fitting of hearing aids. As we discussed in the preceding section, it is first important that the patient understands your explanation of the problem. With a typical patient

---

POINTS TO PONDER: WHAT IS REALLY REMEMBERED?

We all have sat down with a patient and provided a detailed description of our test findings, how this relates to ear anatomy and real-world speech communication, and what treatment strategies are needed, such as the use of hearing aids. At the end of our little spiel, we maybe even pat ourselves on the back for doing such a thorough job. Here are a few points to ponder (from Margolis, 2004):

■ About 50% of the information presented to a patient is forgotten immediately.

■ About 50% of the information that the patient *does* remember, is incorrect.

■ One large study reported that 68% of the patients could not remember the diagnoses that were told to them.

■ In another study, the patient and their physician agreed on what needed follow-up only 45% of the time.

with a presbycusic-type hearing loss, it is counterproductive to rush into the ordering of hearing aids, only to have the patient call you the next day to ask about what surgery options are available. Checking comprehension of your informational counseling is important. Once this has been established, proceed with presenting the treatment plan. The model of Frankel and Stein is primarily geared toward medical treatment plans, and we recognize that some modifications may need to be made when the sale of hearing aids is involved; see our earlier discussion regarding the barriers to obtaining hearing aids. However, the basic principles of the model that they outline still apply:

- Provide a clear rationale. Let the patient know why the fitting of hearing aids is the best option. Explain why other treatment options do not apply to them. Use graphics to help explain your plan (see Chapter 4) and take-home, written material to supplement your statements and help them remember.
- Explore potential barriers to implementation. After providing a clear rationale for the plan, check with the patient to determine what barriers might exist? You could ask a question such as: "What might prevent you from purchasing hearing aids?"
- Provide support. Explain to the patient the complete fitting process, pointing out that the two of you will work as a team to assure that optimum benefit is achieved. Acknowledge that this is an important decision, but also remind the patient of the potential benefits of amplification discussed earlier in this chapter. Investing in the end ensures the patient that a partnership exists.

As summarized by Frankel and Stein (1999), the Four Habits Model blends the logic of clinical decision making with the logic of social interaction. With hope, this leads to successful relationships with your patients, which often determines the successfulness of the treat-ment—in our case, obtaining benefit with and satisfaction from the use of hearing aids. It often has been stated that the fitting of hearing aids is both an art and a science. In the following chapters, we focus mostly on the science, but you'll find the science works much better by understanding and implementing the concepts discussed here.

In Closing

As we have reviewed, understanding the hearing aid candidate goes far beyond evaluating his or her pure-tone thresholds and speech recognition scores. We know that the majority of individuals who need hearing aids do not obtain them. And sadly, 12% to 16% of people who own hearing aids never use them. Why is this? Certainly the stigmatization of hearing loss and hearing aid use is one reason. Younger individuals must have a much greater hearing loss than older individuals before they will adopt hearing aid use. And, surveys have shown that even with the new technology available, many of the expected benefits with amplification are not present.

On the positive side, satisfaction with hearing aids continues to increase. Most notably, there has been a 20% increase in the number of patients who are satisfied with their hearing aid's performance while listening in background noise. Recent surveys also have shown that the use of hearing aids significantly improves many quality of life issues, with 50% of wearers reporting improvement for *feelings about myself* and *life overall*.

We must recognize that the patient brings many concerns and feeling to the pre-fitting appointment. How we deal with this can impact the overall fitting process. By listening to the patient's story, using motivational interviewing, and following some of the guidelines of the Four Habits Model, we can better understand our patients and better prepare them for the use of hearing aids. It is then our job to select the right technology, fit it correctly, and conduct appropriate post-fitting follow-up and counseling—all things we address in future chapters.

3

Speech Acoustics

As we discussed in the preceding chapter, there are a large number of factors that are important when assessing and understanding the patient and hearing aid candidacy. As we describe in the following chapters, there also are a series of audiologic tests, both behavioral and self-assessment, that we overview. However, the most common reason patients seek help is because of difficulties in hearing and recognizing speech. There are many variables to consider for speech recognition, but as stated eloquently by Pascoe (1980):

> Although it is true that the mere detection of sound does not insure its recognition, it is even more true that without detection the probabilities of recognition are greatly diminished.

Given the importance of speech recognition to patients and the importance of audibility to speech recognition, it is not surprising that improving speech audibility is a core goal of most hearing aid fittings. One characteristic that is shared by all hearing aids is that they are able to increase sound level. Modern hearing aids affect sound level in sophisticated ways, however. That is, they can provide more amplification for some levels than others, provide less amplification for some types of sounds than others (like noise), and provide this variable amplification differently for different frequency bands. Given the importance of speech recognition and the potential complexity of modern amplification

schemes, it is important to examine how audibility and speech recognition are related. For example, do all parts of the speech signal have to be audible for maximum speech recognition? Are all speech frequencies equally important to speech recognition?

To examine the potential effect hearing aid amplification processing can have, which we do later in this book, we spend considerable space in this chapter defining speech in terms of its level and the frequency regions of importance. Then, the impact of the environments in which speech is produced on speech recognition is discussed. With the information presented in this chapter as a foundation, we can then form a better understanding how hearing aid processing might interact with audibility and room acoustics, giving us a good chance of forming realistic expectations related to hearing aid benefit for current as well as future processing strategies. As you will see in later chapters, we introduce tests to illustrate how individual patients handle speech communication, both in quiet and in background noise.

Long-Term Speech Acoustics

Before considering speech audibility and importance functions, it is first important to quantify speech acoustically. Most often speech is described in static terms (overall level, overall frequency shape, etc.). By static we

---

TECHNICAL TIP:
THREE FACTORS FOR QUANTIFYING SPEECH ACOUSTICS

- Level at each frequency and overall level for various vocal effort levels (e.g., soft, casual, raised, shouted)
- Dynamic range for a single vocal effort level (i.e., range of levels from lowest to highest portions of speech at specified frequencies)
- Level change over time (sometimes described by modulation rate and modulation depth)

---

mean that a single number representing an average value over time is used rather than representing the signal moment by moment. For example, even though the level of speech naturally fluctuates over time, it is common to examine the level across frequency (spectrum of speech) after averaging over some predefined segment (e.g., an entire passage). Graphic plots of these data are referred to as a Long-Term Average Speech Spectrum (LTASS).[13] The LTASS representation is particularly useful because it can be used to quantify the relationship between speech levels and hearing thresholds, giving us a specific indication of audibility for a given patient. By comparing audibility with and without a hearing aid, we can directly demonstrate how much a specific hearing aid changes audibility for an individual listener. An LTASS is usually defined by the vocal effort required for its production rather than being based on the perceived sound level (Pavlovic, 1989; Pearsons, Bennett, & Fidell, 1977).

That is, rather than asking listeners to turn the level of a talker up and down until it is soft; talkers are asked to speak softly, and the level is measured at a predefined distance, typically one meter.

The specific test conditions and instructions matter as well. For example, a talker may be asked to speak at a conversational level, and their vocal output is measured at a distance of one meter. Work that is often referenced in this area is that of Pearsons et al. (1977). Table 3–1 is a summary of their mean speech levels in A-weighed decibels (dBA) for casual, normal, raised, and shouted speech for males, females, and children.

The listener also has an effect on the LTASS, presumably because people talk louder if they know a listener has a hearing loss. For instance, estimates place the overall level of normal conversational speech measured at one meter at 70 dB SPL when the listener has impaired hearing; however when the listener has normal hearing,

---

THINGS TO REMEMBER: SPEECH LEVELS

- Soft vocal effort results in speech that has an overall level of approximately 53 dB SPL
- Conversational vocal effort results in speech that has an overall level of approximately 62 dB SPL
- Shouted vocal effort results in speech that has an overall level of approximately 83 dB SPL
- There is a lot of variability across talkers! Shouted speech might be 72 dB SPL for one talker and 85 dB SPL for another. On average, there are also gender differences; the intensity levels produced by males are about 7 dB higher than those of females.
- More important, these all are *SPL values*. They correspond to approximately 40, 50, and 70 dB HL, for soft, conversational, and shouted levels when played over headphones from an audiometer.

Table 3–1. Mean speech levels in dBA and unweighted sound pressure levels for casual, normal, raised, loud, and shouted speech by males, females, and children in an anechoic chamber. Unweighted sound pressure levels in [ ]. Standard deviations in ( ).

	Casual	Normal	Raised	Loud	Shouted
Females	50[54] (4)	55[58] (4)	63[65] (4)	71[72] (6)	82[82] (7)
Males	52[56] (4)	58[61] (4)	65[68] (5)	76[77] (6)	89[89] (7)
Children	53[56] (5)	58[61] (5)	65[67] (7)	74[75] (9)	82[82] (9)

Note. All values are rounded to the nearest dB.

Source: From Table 1 and Figure 16, 17, and 18 in Pearsons et al. (1977).

KEY CONCEPT: PROBE-MICROPHONE TESTING

Let us go back to the clinic for a moment. The importance of the speech spectrum becomes clear in our probe-microphone verification of hearing aid fittings—a technique often referred to as *speech mapping*, which we discuss in Book Three of this series on verification. This testing approach has increased the awareness of the LTASS and the effects of LTASS amplification among clinicians. Hearing aid verification methods have long used test signals that are intended to mimic some of the properties of speech. Early probe-microphone systems used swept pure tones or noise that was shaped (filtered) to mimic an LTASS. In more recent probe-microphone testing systems, we have seen the introduction of noises that are generated to include both the spectral and temporal modulation properties of speech. Such samples include International Collegium of Rehabilitative Audiology (ICRA) signal, samples of real speech, samples of real speech signals that are shaped to some agreed upon standard LTASS, and a real speech signal that is spliced together from a variety of speech signals that differ in terms of talker, language, and gender such as the International Speech Test Signal (ISTS).

---

the overall level decreased to approximately 63 dB SPL (Stelmachowicz, Mace, Kopun, & Carney, 1993).

As implied, a typical LTASS is an average of many spectra (those that vary across gender, age, and other conditions). Figure 3–1 shows the effect of talker gender and age on the LTASS at a single vocal effort level. Other factors such as the inclusion of one or many languages and the type of speech material are also important when defining an LTASS (Pavlovic, 1989). One choice relates to whether speech material is chosen that is phonemically balanced (uses all phonemes in a language equally) or, more commonly, phonetically balanced (the phonemes in a language are represented using the same pro-

portion for which that occurs in usual speech). There are many common phonetically balanced passages in use. The most commonly referred to being the *Rainbow Passage* and the shortest recognized passage is about a shoe bench! (See related Points-to-Ponder on page 56.)

Differences Across LTASS

Different LTASS will be measured depending on the conditions chosen. That is, there is not just one LTASS, even for the same vocal effort level. On the surface, it might appear that this fact would make it difficult to

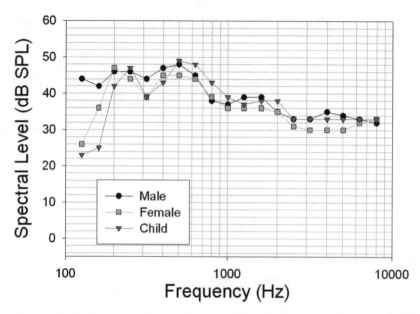

Figure 3–1. Example of LTASS measured for adult male, adult female, and child talkers speaking with casual vocal effort. (Adapted from Pearsons et al., 1977.)

POINTS-TO-PONDER: RAINBOW PASSAGE AND THE SHORTEST PHONETICALLY BALANCED PASSAGE

■ **Rainbow Passage:** When the sunlight strikes raindrops in the air, they act as a prism and form a rainbow. The rainbow is a division of white light into many beautiful colors. These take the shape of a long round arch, with its path high above, and its two ends apparently beyond the horizon. There is, according to legend, a boiling pot of gold at one end. People look, but no one ever finds it. When a man looks for something beyond his reach, his friends say he is looking for the pot of gold at the end of the rainbow. Throughout the centuries, people have explained the rainbow in various ways. Some have accepted it as a miracle without physical explanation. To the Hebrews, it was a token that there would be no more universal floods. The Greeks used to imagine that it was a sign from the gods to foretell war or heavy rain. The Norsemen considered the rainbow as a bridge over which the gods passed from earth to their home in the sky. Others have tried to explain the phenomenon physically. Aristotle thought that the rainbow was caused by reflection of the sun's rays by the rain. Since then, physicists have found that it is not reflection, but refraction by the raindrops which causes the rainbows. Many complicated ideas about the rainbow have been formed. The difference in the rainbow depends considerably on the size of the drops, and the width of the colored band increases as the size of the drops increases. The actual primary rainbow observed is said to be the effect of superimposition of a number of bows. If the red of the second bow falls upon the green of the first, the result is to give a bow with an abnormally wide yellow band, since red and green light, when mixed, form yellow. This is a very common type of bow, one showing mainly red and yellow, with little or no green or blue.[14]

■ **Shortest Balanced Passage:** "Joe took father's shoe bench out; she was waiting at my lawn."[15]

TECHNICAL TIP:
THE LTASS AND PRESCRIPTIVE FITTING APPROACHES

Although similar, there are several different speech spectra used in clinical audiology and the fitting of hearing aids. One example relates to the development and verification of prescriptive fitting algorithms, which we discuss in detail in Book Three of this series on verification. At the time of this writing, there were two primary fitting algorithms in use: the National Acoustic Laboratories Non-Linear version 2 (NAL-NL2) and the Desired Sensation Level version 5.0a (DSL v5.0a).

- NAL-NL2: The development of the NAL-NL1 and NL2 algorithms has been based on the assumed input signal represented by the one-third-octave levels of the International Long-Term Average Speech Spectrum (ILTASS) published by Byrne et al. (1994).
- DSL v5.0a: The evolution of the DSL fitting scheme has focused on placement of third octave speech levels at a desired sensation level for a given hearing loss. The actual values for that speech are an average of male/female/child recordings of speech obtained 30 cm in front of the talker and recordings taken at ear level of the child.

---

measure speech recognition clinically. Fortunately, standards organizations work to reach a consensus on measurement procedures and which measurements will be accepted. Two common such organizations are the American National Standards Institute (ANSI), which was initially formed in 1907, although it was not reorganized into its current form until 1969, and the International Electrotechnical Commission (IEC), which was formed in 1904.

Even though there are many LTASS samples, the spectra across studies and over a wide range of different populations do have some similarities. The characteristic pattern for average vocal effort reveals a peak around 500 Hz and a spectral slope (drop in level across frequency) of about 9 dB per octave (e.g., ANSI S3.5-1997; Dreschler, Verschuure, Ludvigsen, & Westerman, 2001; Pavlovic, 1989; Pavlovic & Studebaker, 1984). It is assumed that the spectral peak corresponds to approximately the frequency of the first formants. The shape is also affected by vocal effort; the spectral slope is slightly steeper for soft speech and becomes flatter as speech level increases as shown in Figure 3–2 (see the Key Concept on this topic for description of why this figure is different from Figure 3–1). The frequency of the spec-

tral peak also is higher for shouted speech than lower vocal effort levels. In fact, if you record shouted speech and play it at the same level as soft speech, one of the most striking (and perhaps surprising) features is that the shouted speech has a higher apparent pitch. Finally, the shape of the LTASS can be affected by the language spoken (Byrne et al., 1994), although those frequency and intensity differences have been deemed fairly insignificant in the fitting of hearing aids.

The spectral levels in Figure 3–2 are based on ANSI S3.5-1997 (average and shouted vocal efforts) and Pearsons et al. (1977; Soft speech).

Dynamics of Speech

Directly related to the LTASS is the dynamic range of speech. The dynamic range of speech at any frequency refers to the difference between the lowest level (speech minima) and highest level (speech maxima). Typically, instead of actually defining the dynamic range with regards to the absolute highest and lowest level segments, some percentage of total energy is often used. For example, the maxima might be defined as the level

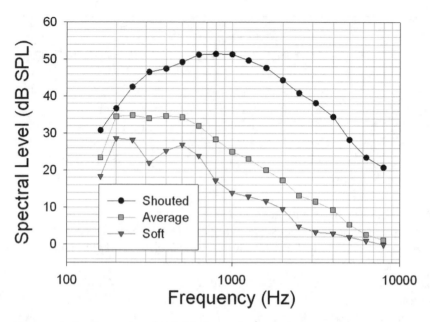

Figure 3–2. Example of LTASS for soft, average, and shouted vocal effort levels. (Adapted from Pearsons et al., 1977 and ANSI S3.5-1997.)

KEY CONCEPT: BAND-LEVEL ACOUSTICS

- You may remember from acoustics that although the level of a signal is most commonly expressed in total level (that is considering all frequencies present and often referred to as *overall* level), we can also describe the sound level of the same signal in a more frequency-specific manner. That is, we can describe the level measured within a particular bandwidth.

- In the specific cases of Figures 3–1 and 3–2, the level in each one-third-octave wide band and one-hertz wide band (spectral level) are given, respectively. This is why the two figures appear at first glance to be so different in level. The relative effect that measurement bandwidth has on level values is demonstrated in Table 3–2.

- The following two formulas can be used to move between the level of relatively narrow and wide measurement bandwidths:

Level of Wider Bandwidth (dB SPL) = Level of Narrower Bandwidth + 10 log
[Wider Bandwidth (Hz)/Narrower Bandwidth (Hz)]

Level of Narrower Bandwidth (dB SPL) = Level of Wider Bandwidth − 10 log
[Wider Bandwidth (Hz)/Narrower Bandwidth (Hz)]

Table 3–2. The LTASS level at octave frequencies for various vocal efforts as measured using spectral, 1/3 octave, and octave measurement bandwidths (adapted from ANSI S3.5, 1997).

Frequency	Bandwidth	Vocal effort				
		Soft	Normal	Raised	Loud	Shouted
	S. Level	—	34.75	38.98	41.55	42.50
250	1/3 octave	48.00	52.38	56.61	59.18	60.13
	Octave	—	57.25	61.48	64.05	65.00
	S. Level	—	34.27	40.15	44.85	49.24
500	1/3 octave	50.00	54.88	60.76	65.46	69.85
	Octave	—	59.77	65.65	70.35	74.74
	S. Level	—	25.01	33.86	42.16	51.31
1000	1/3 octave	42.00	48.65	57.50	65.80	74.95
	Octave	—	53.52	62.37	70.67	79.82
	S. Level	—	17.32	25.32	34.39	44.32
2000	1/3 octave	40.00	43.96	51.96	61.03	70.96
	Octave	—	48.84	56.84	65.91	75.84
	S. Level	—	11.55	20.15	28.21	38.13
3000	1/3 octave	33.00	40.18	48.78	56.84	66.76
	Octave	—	—	—	—	—
	S. Level	—	9.33	16.78	25.41	34.41
4000	1/3 octave	32.50	38.96	46.41	55.04	64.04
	Octave	—	43.86	51.31	59.94	68.94

at which 90% of the speech energy falls below and the minima might be defined as the level for which 10% of energy falls below (i.e., the 10% to 90% dynamic range). Differences between reported values for the dynamic range of speech in the research literature also reflect differences in experimental variables such as frequency range and the length of sampling interval (e.g., Pavlovic, 1987, 1989). Specifically, the shorter the sampling interval, the larger the dynamic range. If we average the intensity level of speech over 500 ms blocks of time, there will be a significantly narrower range than if we average over 1-ms blocks of time. This is because averaging acts to smooth out some of the very short-term peaks and valleys in the speech signal.

Why a 30 dB Dynamic Range?

Choosing the appropriate interval duration is not straightforward because it is of interest to reflect a segment length that is perceptually relevant. That is, the dynamic range of speech is not quantified for purely acoustic reasons; rather, we want to define a range that represents what a listener perceives so that we can estimate audibility.

Most commonly, a dynamic range of 30 dB is advocated for making predictions of speech recognition, although more recent data suggest a dynamic range of greater than 30 dB must be available to optimize speech recognition for all listeners across all conditions. Therefore, we believe that 30 dB should be considered a somewhat conservative estimate of the dynamic range of speech. Data also suggest that the 30 dB dynamic range is not symmetrical around the LTASS; rather, it may be best represented as LTASS +12 and −18 dB for the speech maxima and minima, respectively (Pavlovic, 1989). These issues are primarily still research considerations, however, and it is common to assume a dynamic range of 30 dB that is symmetric around the LTASS. Although perhaps not 100% accurate, this simpler explanation is considered accurate enough for most uses. Clinically however, the 30 dB dynamic range really only encompasses a single vocal effort; if we want to consider the dynamic range across a full range of vocal efforts, the range is much larger as we discuss in the next section.

TECHNICAL TIP: CONSIDERING A *PERCEPTUALLY RELEVANT* DYNAMIC RANGE

■ Let us assume that the acoustic dynamic range of speech for a single talker is measured to be 50 dB using a very small time averaging window.

■ If listeners only require 30 dB of this range (e.g., the 40% to 90% dynamic range) to optimize speech recognition, no matter what the listening condition, one could argue that the remaining 20 dB of this range (which is composed of very short-term maxima and lower level and short-term minima in the speech signal) is not perceptually relevant.

Audibility and Speech Recognition

Although there is a movement to switch to an SPL representation of both hearing loss and the speech spectrum level when discussing hearing aids, it is still common to describe the patient's thresholds in dB HL (decibels hearing level) in the clinic. Because this is so common, the dynamic range of speech for the average vocal effort LTASS shown in Figure 3–2 often has been replotted in dB HL (see Figure 3–3 for example). This dynamic range is shown along with an example hearing loss to demonstrate how hearing loss can impact audibility of speech that was produced at an average vocal effort. When plotted in this way, which is similar to an audiogram, speech that falls below the hearing threshold (*above* the threshold line in this figure) is not audible; speech below the plotted audiogram is audible. In this example, showing speech produced with average vocal effort, no speech sounds above 1500 Hz would be audible to the patient. In Chapter 4, we provide several other examples of using the LTASS and the audiogram, and discuss how this association can be used for patient counseling and illustration of the benefits of amplification.

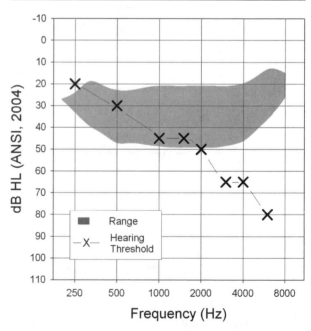

Figure 3–3. An example of speech audibility for the average vocal effort levels in a patient with a sloping hearing loss configuration.

As we mentioned earlier, the commonly used 30 dB dynamic range of speech shown in Figure 3–3 only applies to a single vocal effort level. To provide you with an idea of the *total dynamic range* of speech for a wide range of vocal efforts, the dynamic range from the minima for soft speech to the maxima for shouted speech are shown in Figure 3–4. These data suggest that a reasonable clinical estimate of the total dynamic range of speech is at least 60 dB. When accounting for individual differences in talkers, however, this range is likely more than 70 dB.

The Articulation Index/Audibility Index

Because speech levels and dynamic range have been quantified in so many studies, it is possible to calculate the audibility of speech under conditions of hearing loss and/or masking by a noise signal with a fairly high degree of accuracy.[16] To do this as accurately as possible, we need frequency specific hearing thresholds, thresholds of discomfort, any background noise levels, and the maxima and minima of the exact speech signal of interest. With this information, the audibility of speech at each frequency can be displayed as shown in Figure 3–4; however, rather than just knowing audibility, it is of interest to know how frequency specific audibility translates into importance for speech recognition performance. Calculation of not just audibility, but importance-weighted audibility is the explicit goal of what is referred to as the Articulation Index, or simply AI. These procedures, in one way or another, have been employed since the early 1900s, with the first detailed approach published by Fletcher and Galt (1950). ANSI standards have been developed regarding this measurement, including the current ANSI standard method,

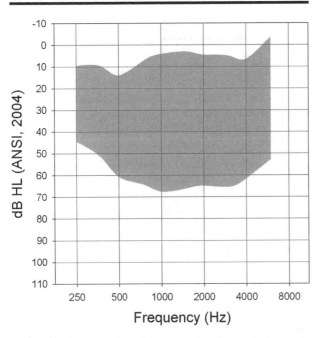

Figure 3–4. Conservative estimate of the full dynamic range of speech across a range of vocal efforts encompassing from the soft speech minima to the shouted speech maxima.

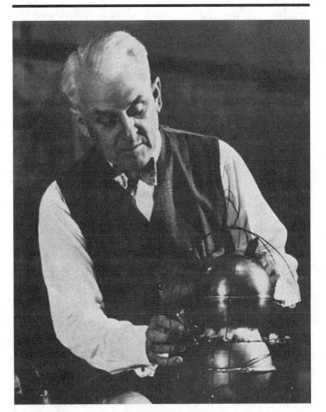

Figure 3–5. The individual most credited with developing the articulation index is Harvey Fletcher, based on his research at Bell Labs conducted over three decades, with the finely tuned version finally published in 1950. Dr. Fletcher is also known for his research relating to loudness scaling, equal loudness contours, loudness summation, and critical band theory. Dr. Fletcher was elected an honorary fellow of the Acoustical Society of America in 1949, the second person to receive this honor after Thomas Edison.[18]

TECHNICAL TIP: AI AND SII—SAME OR DIFFERENT?

One thing you may have noticed is that we have referred to AI as both the Articulation Index and Audibility Index, and referred to the ANSI standard method of the SII. Why are there so many terms? Articulation Index was the original term for these calculations, but as several authors have pointed out, these calculations are really based on audibility, even though they do use audibility importance weighted by frequency. We go into a more detailed explanation of this issue later in this chapter. To make a long story short, AI and SII have both been used to refer to general and specific procedures, whereas the SII is the current standard. Although there is certainly not complete consensus on the issue, we have chosen to use AI as a general term encompassing all procedures of this type and SII to refer to the current specific ANSI standard procedure.

---

which is called the Speech Intelligibility Index (SII; ANSI S3.5-1997 [R2007]).

To examine how AI calculations might be conducted, let us start with an experiment in which we divide the entire dynamic range of speech into blocks. In this experiment, we decide to make the blocks 5 dB high and one-third an octave wide. We could then present different combinations of these blocks by masking out other blocks with background noise and look at the corresponding speech recognition scores. Sounds like a really fun experiment does it not? Although such experiments might prove tedious for participants, they are a way to precisely quantify the relative importance of the speech signal in each frequency band (importance weightings) and can be plotted as Frequency Importance Functions (FIFs) or Band Importance Functions (BIFs). BIFs are usually plotted so that the total importance for all bands adds up to 1.00 (i.e., 100%). An example is shown in Figure 3–6. If we were to add up the frequency importance values on any one line in this figure,

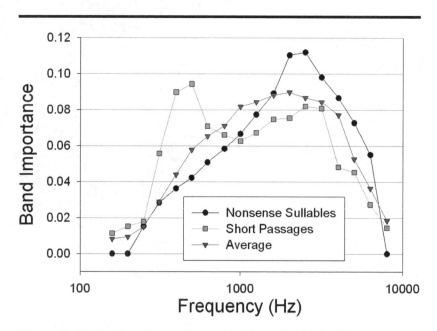

Figure 3–6. The band importance functions (BIFs) for three types of speech, which vary by the amount of contextual information (adapted from ANSI S3.5-1997).

KEY CONCEPT:
CALCULATING BAND IMPORTANCE FUNCTIONS

Let's take a very simple example and just divide speech into two parts or bands, frequencies above 3000 Hz and frequencies below 3000 Hz. That is, we will take a masking noise and cover up all speech energy above 3000 Hz (3000 down) and then cover up all speech energy below 3000 Hz (3000 up) and test speech recognition.

- Depending on the speech material, we would expect that speech recognition scores might be about 100% for the 3000 down condition and about 40% for the 3000 up condition.
- By doing more testing and a little math, we might conclude (in this example) that 80% of speech importance falls below 3000 Hz and about 20% falls above 3000 Hz. This corresponds to BIF weightings of 0.8 and 0.2 for our two tested frequency bands.
- Note that you cannot simply add up the scores from the two conditions because the entire speech signal does not need to be present to obtain 100% correct because of context and redundancy. Listeners with normal hearing only need to have about 40% of the total available weighted important speech energy to obtain 100% correct when listening to sentences.
- This type of work first started in Bell Labs in the 1920s and 1930s (e.g., French & Steinberg, 1947; Fletcher & Galt, 1950). The Bell laboratory work identified the bandwidth of 300 to 3000 Hz as providing enough speech information for listeners to generally understand all words, and this bandwidth is still used today in many telecommunication systems.

---

the total would always be 1.00 (that is, 100% of available speech deemed important).

Band Importance Functions

Band Importance Functions differ in shape depending on the exact speech material evaluated. However, there are some general patterns based on how much contextual information is present. When there is little context, as is the case with nonsense syllables (e.g., /ba/, /da/, and /ga/), the BIF usually peaks in the higher frequencies (around 2000 to 3000 Hz). This is not that surprising when we consider what is needed for correct identification of nonsense syllables. To distinguish /si/ (see) from /ʃi/ (she), a listener must actually hear the difference in the high frequency consonant signals. Increasing the amount of context (i.e., moving from nonsense syllables to running speech) leads to a shift of importance toward the lower frequencies, as shown in Figure 3–6. This shift can be explained by the positive effect that context has on filling in missing information. For example, try reading aloud this target sentence:

"The children _oveled _and on the beach."

Most listeners can fill in the missing two speech sounds and realize the intention was, "The children shoveled sand on the beach." Actually *hearing* the soft high frequency consonants is therefore less important, when you have context to help fill in the blanks.

For calculation of an AI, the audibility of each of the BIFs is examined in order to derive a single number that reflects importance weighted audibility. Specifically, once the importance of various frequency bands for speech (BIFs) is known, the band audibility (BA), or how much of each of these frequency bands is audible, can be calculated based on the 30 dB speech dynamic range. To keep things simple, audibility is also calculated as a portion of the whole. In other words, if 100% of speech is audible in a frequency band (the full 30 dB dynamic range), audibility in that band is 1.00.

If masking noise and/or a hearing loss is present, the full 30 dB dynamic range may not be audible. For example, if only 20 dB of the full 30 dB dynamic range is audible, then the BA would be calculated as: 20/30 = 0.66. Once audibility is measured and band audibility is calculated in each frequency band, the BA is multiplied by that frequency bands BIF, and the resulting product in each band is summed over all the bands. This is described mathematically in the following formula:

$$AI = \sum_{i=0}^{n} (BIF \times BA)$$

Frequency Bands for AI

The number of frequency bands used in the calculation of AI depends on the procedure and the chosen bandwidth (ANSI S3.5-1997; Mueller & Killion, 1990; Pavlovic, 1984; Pavlovic & Studebaker, 1984). Specifically, common procedures currently divide up the frequency range of speech using from 4 to 21 bands. The smaller the bandwidth and larger the number of bands, the greater the calculation accuracy, but obviously the calculation and measurement become more time consuming as more bands are added. For this reason, some procedures have sacrificed precise accuracy (approximately 2% to 3%) to provide a procedure that is easy to use and understand and is clinically friendly (Mueller & Killion, 1990; Pavlovic, 1991). We discuss this clinical application later, and in more detail in Chapter 4.

The narrowest bandwidth used is termed the *critical bandwidth*. The critical bandwidth refers to the assumed bandwidth of the human auditory filters. That is, the total level of any and all signals within the critical bandwidth are integrated over the entire bandwidth and perceived as a single level. Therefore, it is usually assumed that bandwidths smaller than the critical bandwidth are not perceptually relevant because, perceptually, sounds within the critical bandwidth are grouped together. Although a complete description of all of the factors affecting AI calculation are well beyond the scope of this chapter, AI can be of clinical utility provided that we keep several considerations in mind.

KEY CONCEPTS: IMPORTANT AI CONSIDERATIONS

There are many AI derivations that are not perfectly equivalent across test conditions. We explain some of those factors here.

- The AI is not a direct predictor of speech recognition. To improve prediction accuracy, the appropriate band importance function derived specifically for the speech material of interest must be used, and a second formula (specific AI/SII to percent correct transfer function) must also be applied. A commonly used chart for this purpose is based on data from Davis and Silverman (1960) and displayed in Figure 3–7. Even when these steps are taken, prediction of speech recognition performance will only be accurate, on average. AIs are not useful for predicting an individual's speech recognition score. Clinically, however, these measures can be used to predict expected changes in scores due to amplification, noise, or other changes in audibility within an individual listener.
- The AI was developed for listeners with normal hearing. That said, it is often effectively applied to those with hearing loss. To improve accuracy for groups of listeners with hearing impairment, hearing loss desensitization (HLD) and level distortion (LD) factors are sometimes applied.

■ HLDs are applied because of evidence that speech recognition decreases with increasing hearing loss, even when audibility is accounted for. Originally it was called the *Speech Desensitization* factor (Pavlovic, Studebaker, & Sherbecoe, 1986) and was a single multiplier based on averaged thresholds, and applied to the total AI value. Although HLDs assume that performance decrements are directly related to the magnitude of loss, they do not specify what factors are responsible for the deficit (sort of a *catch-all* correction based on degree of loss).There currently is disagreement on how HLDs should be applied and whether frequency specific corrections may be needed (Ching, Dillon, & Byrne, 1998; Ching, Dillon, Katsch, & Byrne, 2001; Hornsby and Ricketts, 2003, 2006; Humes, 2002). Accuracy can also be improved for all AIs by applying corrections for age and for language proficiency.

■ LD factors are applied because data clearly demonstrate that speech recognition performance decreases when speech is presented at very high levels, especially near the threshold of discomfort. In the SII standard, the LD factor is a simple multiplier based on the speech level in each frequency band.

■ Instead of using simple band audibility to estimate audibility when calculating an SII, modulation transfer function techniques (described later in this chapter when discussing the Speech Transmission Index) can be used to estimate signal-to-noise ratio to better account for the effects of room acoustics on speech recognition.

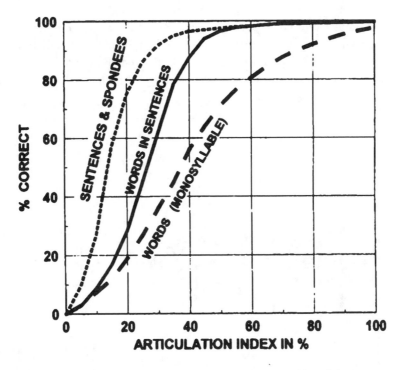

Figure 3–7. The relationship between an *average* AI and the percent correct for a variety of speech materials. (Adapted from data presented by Davis and Silverman, 1960.)

Short-Term Speech Acoustics

Although it is important to discuss the LTASS when considering speech audibility, it is clearly the case that speech level fluctuates over time. We can easily see this by looking at a plot of instantaneous speech amplitude as a function of time as shown in Figure 3–8. In case you are not familiar with this type of display (called a *time waveform*), we provide some background information that will help the interpretation.

Figure 3–8 is the time waveform of one sentence spoken by a male talker. A quick glance at this figure shows that there are segments of speech produced at fairly high levels (at the peak of 0.5 in this example) and other segments produced at much lower levels. Recall

---

TECHNICAL TIP: INTERPRETING TIME WAVEFORMS

- Figure 3–8 shows a common way to display sound using commercially available, computer-based, analysis software; the axis along the bottom (*x*-axis) displays time. In this case, time is shown in seconds, and observe that the entire sample is a little more than 3 seconds long.
- The axis along the side (*y*-axis) is relative amplitude. In this case, the scale is just in relative numbers, but in some software, it is shown in relative dB. Relative amplitude measures like these start in the middle. That is, lower and higher signal levels will appear on the *y*-axis as having smaller and larger excursions, respectively. This is denoted by the brackets marked Lower Level and Higher Level.
- The highest level signal that can be displayed (0.5/–0.5 for a peak-to-peak amplitude of 1 in this example), commonly corresponds to the highest level that can be output by the computers sound card before physical limiting (clipping).
- The dynamic range of the computer sound card, that is the range from the lowest to highest level signals that can be output, will depend on the physical limitations of the sound card and theoretical limitations imposed by the number of bits used when sampling. The theoretical limit is 6 dB per bit, so a 16-bit sample will have a theoretical dynamic range of ($16 \times 6 = 96$ dB).

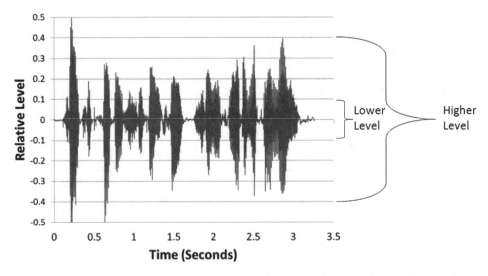

Figure 3–8. The time waveform of an approximately 3.2-second speech sample.

that we described this previously as the dynamic range of speech for a single talker at one vocal effort, which we said was around 30 dB. However, we can see from this figure that the simple explanation of a 30 dB dynamic range of speech is a little misleading because not all levels are present at the same time. This is true even when we examine all frequencies at the same time as we are doing in this figure. If we look at this figure closely, we can see that the amplitude changes occur over different periods of time.

Looking at the Envelope

It is possible to visualize each syllable in Figure 3–8 by highlighting its general outline, commonly referred to as the syllable amplitude *envelope*, by using a bolded black line for the two-second speech sample. This is shown in Figure 3–9. By doing this, we can see a change in the level that corresponds to each syllable that occurs every 125 to 250 ms (0.125 to 0.25 seconds in Figure 3–9). In contrast, we could look as a much smaller time segment of speech. In Figure 3–10, we show a single word *she* that has a total duration of about 275 ms (0.275 seconds). In this case, we can see amplitude changes corresponding to individual phonemes that are much shorter, ranging from approximately 50 to 150 ms.

We can look at a variety of speech segments in this way and see a large range in duration both across and within each type of segment. Figure 3–11, adapted from data presented by Plomp (1986), gives an indication of the range of average durations associated with the amplitude changes within various segments of speech. From this figure, we can see the duration of these amplitude changes ranges from about 33 ms for the shortest phoneme transitions, to more than a few of seconds for sentences.

Instead of discussing the duration associated with amplitude changes within various speech segments, it is more typical to refer to these changes in level over time as amplitude modulations. For example, instead of describing level changes due to the duration of consonants as 50 ms in length; we describe the amplitude modulation associated with these consonant as occurring 20 times a second; or more simply, a modulation rate of 20 Hz (1000 ms [duration of 1 second]/50 ms [duration of level change associated with this consonant]). Using this convention, we can describe speech as having amplitude modulations ranging from about 30 Hz (e.g., 33.3 ms duration) for the shortest phonemes to less than 0.5 Hz (e.g., 2 second duration) for some sentences.

In addition, to the modulation rate, we can also describe speech in terms of its modulation depth; that

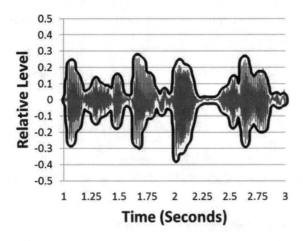

Figure 3–9. The time waveform of a 2-second speech sample. In this example, a bold black line is used to highlight the general amplitude envelope of individual syllables.

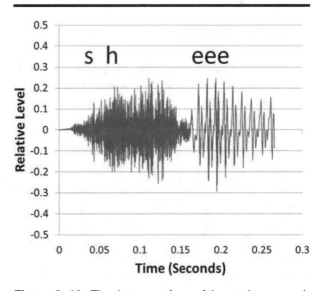

Figure 3–10. The time waveform of the spoken speech sample /shi/, *she.*

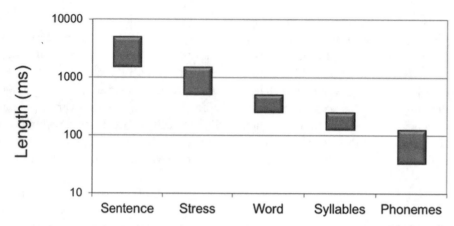

Figure 3–11. The range of average durations of various speech segments. These durations are associated with the amplitude changes within the segments of each type. (Adapted from Plomp, 1986.)

is, how large of a change in amplitude is there from the maxima of the signal to its minima. We have already discussed the assumption that the dynamic range of speech for a single vocal effort level is approximately 30 dB; therefore, this same value can be assigned to the modulation depth of speech. Putting all this information together, we can describe the majority of speech signals as amplitude modulated from approximately 0.5 Hz to more than 20 Hz with a modulation depth at each of those modulation frequencies of about 30 dB.

Practical Applications

You might be wondering why we are spending so much time discussing speech acoustics in a hearing aid textbook. Let us discuss a couple of specific examples of why this information is so important.

First, amplitude modulation information can be useful in hearing aid signal processing when attempting to identify speech. Today's hearing aids utilize a *signal classification system* in which an attempt is made to classify a signal as speech in quiet, speech in noise, broadband noise, music, and so forth. The results of this classification can then be used in controlling features such as digital noise reduction, directional technology, automatic compression learning, and so forth. Specifically, if the incoming signal is not amplitude modulated, or has a modulation rate higher than 30 Hz or so, we can be confident that it is *not* speech. Unfortunately, however,

we are not assured that the signal is speech, just because it has a modulation rate in the range common to speech signals, but usually the classification system is correct if it is speech-in-quiet. We discuss other factors that are used when attempting to differentiate speech from other signals in the signal classification chapter of Book Two.

A second, even more important reason for understanding the speech signal, relates to how the listening environment and hearing aid processing affects acoustics. For example, several factors related to hearing aid processing and the listening environment can affect the modulation depth of speech. What happens to the modulation depth when noise is added? Let us first look at this schematically. In Figure 3–12, an unmodulated noise that has a level that is well below that of the speech has been added to the same speech signal displayed in Figure 3–8. We can see that the noise fills in the modulation valleys, so the lowest level portions of speech are masked by the noise. We can also see that this decrease in modulation depth occurs equally for all modulation rates. That is, there is not greater masking for high modulation rates than for low rates.

Effects of Reverberation

What about environmental factors other than noise? How might reverberation affect the modulation depth of speech? We can examine this question by playing the speech shown in Figure 3–8 in a reverberant room. The

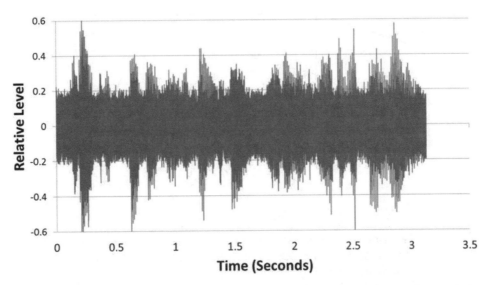

Figure 3–12. The time waveform of an approximately 3.2-second speech sample in background noise. The SNR is +3 dB.

KEY CONCEPT: SOME POINTS ON REVERBERATION

For the most part, we have been talking about speech signals delivered in ideal surroundings. We know, however, that our hearing aid patients will be out in reverberant conditions. In fact, it often is the poor understanding of speech in these difficult conditions that prompt the patient to obtain hearing aids. How does reverberation impact the speech signal?

■ One of the most common measures of a room's effect on sound propagation is reverberation time. Commonly, reverberation time is defined as the time required for a signal to decrease in level by 60 dB after its offset (ANSI S1.1-1994).

■ Reverberation occurs because sound generated from any source inside a room will be reflected (bounce) off room surfaces. Due to these reflections, there will be multiple angles of arrival for sound energy other than the angle of origin. That is, there will be a direct sound pathway (D) and several reflected sound pathways (R), which in combination are referred to as the reflective or reverberant sound field (see Figure 3–13).

■ There are usually many more reflected sound pathways than shown here, and some sound pathways may never reach the listener before they decay away (become so low level they are not heard).

■ As the distance from the sound source increases, the level of the direct sound will decrease. According to the inverse square law, every doubling of distance will halve the intensity. In contrast, the reverberant sound level remains approximately constant (although this changes with proximity to reflective surfaces—for example the reverberant level might go up near a wall). In consequence, as a sound source and a listener are separated in space, there is an increase in the reverberant to direct sound ratio. The distance at which the level of the direct signal is equal to that of the reverberant signal is referred to as the critical distance (Egan, 1988; Peutz, 1971). An example, demonstrating direct sound reverberant sound and a combination of the two as a function of distance, is shown in Figure 3–14.

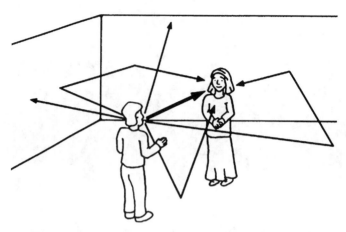

Figure 3–13. A representation of direct (*bold arrow*) and reflected (*thin arrows*) sound pathways, produced by a talker (illustrated by Wilder Boulĕ).

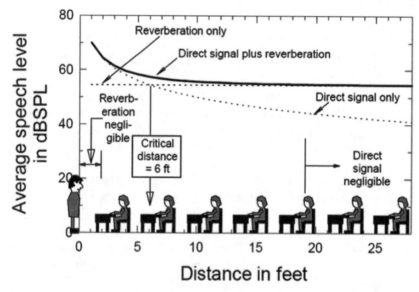

Figure 3–14. Predicted long-term average speech level as a function of the distance from the talker in a room measuring 30 × 20 × 9 feet with a reverberation time of 500 ms.

recording of this signal in a room with a high amount of reverberation (average reverberation time approximately 4 seconds) is shown in Figure 3–15. We can see that reverberation acts to fill-in modulation depth somewhat similarly to noise as was shown in Figure 3–12. Further, the longer the reverberation time, the more the modulation depth is filled in. The effect is a little different from noise, however, because this masking is

occurring because echoes from early portions of speech act to mask later portions (overlap masking) or echoes from a speech segment act to mask that same speech segment (speech self-masking). In consequence, shorter reverberation times or earlier reflections mainly fill in the modulation depth when the modulation rate is high. For lower modulation rates, the echoes may not last long enough to fill in the gaps. Therefore, we must exam-

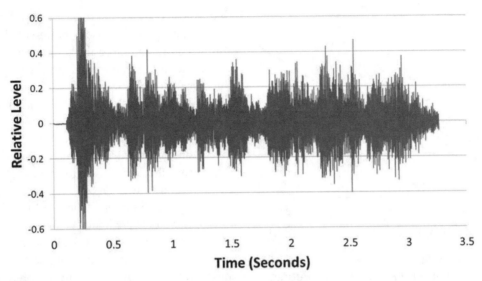

Figure 3–15. The time waveform of an approximately 3.2-second speech sample recorded in a reverberant room.

ine modulation depth over a range of realistic modulation rates for speech to obtain a complete picture of how an environment might affect speech modulations (Houtgast, 1981; Houtgast & Steeneken, 1985; Houtgast, Steeneken, & Plomp, 1980). A graphical representation of how an environment, noise, or any change affects the modulation depth across modulation frequencies of speech is commonly referred to as a modulation transfer function (MTF).

Signal-To-Noise Ratio

Because speech is such a dynamic signal, it might be expected that environmental (e.g., noise, reverberation, distance) and processing factors that affect the MTF might also affect speech recognition. For example, it has been suggested that individuals with normal hearing require a signal-to-noise ratio (SNR) of at least +6 dB for satisfactory communication (e.g., Moore, 1989). SNR refers to the level of the speech in comparison with the level of the noise. Specifically, positive SNR values indicate that on average, the speech is a higher level than the noise, whereas negative SNRs indicate the noise is at a higher level than the speech. Although poor SNR is a problem for all listeners, data overwhelmingly support the contention that individuals with sensorineural hearing

loss generally require a significantly greater SNR to obtain speech recognition performance equivalent to listeners with normal hearing (Carhart & Tillman, 1970; Cooper & Cutts, 1971; Dirks, Morgan, & Dubno, 1982; Groen, 1969; Killion, 1997; Plomp, 1976; Schum, 1996; Sutter, 1985).

From a patient counseling standpoint, it is also important to remember that although we increase our vocal effort as a function of the level of the background noise, there is not a one-to-one relationship. That is, the more intense the background noise, the less favorable the SNR despite the increase in vocal effort. This is illustrated in Figure 3–16 (adapted from Pearson et al., 1977), which shows the level of speech on the y-axis and the level of the background noise on the x-axis. To help your interpretation of this chart, some specific examples are shown in Table 3–3. As you see from Figure 3–16, as noise levels exceed 75 dB SPL, the SNR continues to become more adverse. If you consider that many large group social events and restaurants have background noise levels greater than 75 dB SPL, it is easy to understand the problems faced by the hearing impaired listener.

We discuss different speech-in-noise tests that can be used in the clinic that consider various factors including audibility and the effects of noise in Chapter 5. Some of them apply a fixed SNR for testing, whereas others use an adaptive approach, with either the target speech signal or the background changing in intensity. In addition

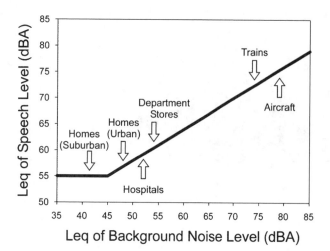

Figure 3–16. The change in SNR as a function of background noise level. (Adapted from Pearsons et al., 1977.)

Table 3–3. SNR as a Function of Background Noise.

If background noise is:	Speech is:	SNR
45 dBA	55 dBA	+10 dB
55 dBA	61 dBA	+6 dB
65 dBA	67 dBA	+2 dB
75 dBA	73 dBA	−2 dB

to the effects of noise and audibility, data also clearly show decreases in speech recognition with increasing reverberation (Bistafa & Bradley, 2000; Bradley, Reich, & Norcross, 1999; Crandell & Smaldino, 2000; Moncur & Dirks, 1967). The negative effect of reverberation is also clearly increased with a greater talker-to-listener distance as described earlier in this chapter during the discussion of reverberation.

The STI

Quantifying the effect of environmental factors such as reverberation on speech recognition is the impetus behind the Speech Transmission Index (STI; Houtgast & Steeneken, 1971, 1973; Steeneken & Houtgast, 1980; IEC 60268-16). The STI shares some general similarities

with AI calculations, but there is a big difference related to how background noise is represented. Both procedures require summing the product of an estimate of speech importance: the band importance function and another factor of importance calculated across several bands. However, instead of calculating simple audibility within each band (BA) as in the case of traditional AI procedures, a type of SNR is estimated in each band by calculating or measuring modulation MTFs for modulation rates that are similar to speech. The typical STI procedure examines or calculates MTFs for modulation frequencies ranging from 0.63 to 12.5 Hz within each of seven octave bands centered at 125; 250; 500; 1000; 2000; 4000; and 8000 Hz. If the modulation depth approaches the case of being completely filled in across modulation frequencies (e.g., by noise and/or due to the effects of reverberation), the SNR function approaches 0. If there is little change in the modulation depth, the SNR function approaches 1:

$$AI = \sum_{i=0}^{n} \left(BIF \times \frac{SNR + 15}{30} \right)$$

The standard STI differs from AI in a few more subtle ways as well. For example, the STI is typically calculated using no more than seven octave bands. In addition, the assumed band importance function is much flatter for the STI than assumed for most AI procedures, although some authors have proposed corrective modifications (e.g., Humes, Dirks, Bell, Ahlstrom, & Kincaid, 1986). However, the flatter band importance function assumed by the STI generally makes it less sensitive to filtering effects than the ANSI standard AI procedure, the SII. That is, noise that drops in level precipitously as a function of frequency provides much less masking than noise that has a more gradual drop in level. These effects are generally not well represented in the standard STI due to the flatter band importance function. However, the STI is much more adept at demonstrating the effect of room acoustics on speech recognition than the original SII. To try to improve accuracy and consider room effects, the SII standard also describes an alternative method for measuring or calculating SNR using procedures similar to those used in the STI.[17]

One way STI has been used is to calculate Percentage Articulation Loss of Consonants (%ALcons). %ALcons is a calculation that is used to estimate how much recognition of consonants is degraded based on STI measures. For example, 2% ALcons would indicate a small degradation, whereas 20% ALcons would indicate a much larger and significant degradation. %ALCONS are often reported by acoustical consultants when describing room effects and are often calculated based on specific measurement equipment. One of the most common formulas used to derive ALcons from STI is: $ALcons = 10^{\frac{1-STI}{0.46}}$; however, empirical formulas such as: $ALcons = 170.5405\ (e-5.419 \times STI)$ are also sometimes used. Because STI is computationally intensive, it presented a challenge for earlier portable test equipment. As a consequence, a simplified STI referred to as the Rapid/Room Acoustics STI (RASTI) is sometimes used. With continued advancements in modern test equipment however, the STI is often advocated over the RASTI due to its greater accuracy.

Mini-Summary

That was a lot of information presented over the last few pages. Before we discuss some clinical applications, here is a mini-summary.

- There are many LTASS. The average shape and overall level of the LTASS depends on factors such as vocal effort, language, and talker characteristics. Speech produced using average vocal effort has an overall level of approximately 62 dB SPL and has a dynamic range of approximately 30 dB. The dynamic range of all speech at all effort levels is greater than 60 dB.
- There are many different AI procedures. In general, these procedures calculate a single value that provides a general indication of the importance-weighted magnitude of speech audibility. AI accuracy can be improved by using actual measured speech and noise levels and the correct band importance function. AI accuracy can further be improved by using hearing loss desensitization, language proficiency, and presentation level factors. Speech can be described as an amplitude modulated signal with a modulation depth

of 30 dB and modulation rates ranging from approximately 0.5 to 20 Hz.
- The STI is a measure that can be used to examine how room acoustics (e.g., reverberation and distance) and noise can affect the transmission of speech information. It is based on measuring or calculating MTFs.
- Room effects such as reverberation can also be accounted for in the SII by using an alternative method for calculating or measuring SNR based on the MTF.

Clinical Use of the AI and the STI

All of the technical aspects of AI and STI may be interesting from a research standpoint, and understanding the effects of audibility and room acoustics on speech recognition performance is clearly important theoretically so that we can really understand how much difficulty a patient might be having and how much benefit a particular hearing aid or processing algorithm may provide. However, as audiologists, we must ask how useful the actual AI and STI measures are in the clinic? We certainly do not have time to measure and calculate the standard SII for all the environments our patients might be in. So, it is of interest to know if there are clinically applicable procedures and (more importantly), are there really opportunities for their use?

With regard to AI/SII, aided and unaided calculations increasingly are showing up on commercial probe microphone equipment and in hearing aid fitting software. Is there a good reason to use these measures clinically? We certainly argue there is; however, there are several potential pitfalls in clinical use.

Despite some apparent clinical limitations, AI can be used clinically as a measure of importance weighted audibility. When used in this way it can help when counseling patients and caregivers of children with hearing impairment regarding what to expect in terms of speech audibility and benefit from a hearing aid. For example, you might use an AI to confirm to a patient, spouse, caregiver, or parent that the hearing loss in question leads to the loss of a significant amount of speech sounds. When using AI procedures for patient counseling, it is sometimes useful to display the findings

---

TECHNICAL TIP: CLINICAL AI CONSIDERATIONS

- AI provides an indication of relative changes in audibility and is not useful for precise prediction of an individual patient's speech recognition score.
- It is important to remember that there is not a one-to-one relationship between the AI and speech understanding—for example, a 70% AI does *not* equal a 70% speech recognition score.
- For an average patient (cochlear hearing loss, no cognitive deficit), the AI can be used to predict speech recognition for different speech material when an appropriate *transfer function* is applied, shown in Figure 3–7.
- It is important to remember that the prediction will be for *average-level speech*, and therefore, their speech recognition might be higher or lower for other input levels.
- The predicted score is based on the AI in quiet and does not consider the masking effects of background noise (although this can be simulated).
- As seen in later chapters (and detailed in the verification section of Book Three), the highest AI does not typically lead to the best hearing aid fitting. (If it did, we could just give 100 dB of gain to everyone!) The goal of a hearing aid fitting is never just to maximize AI without also considering listening comfort, sound quality and loudness perceptioins. Making all speech at all levels audible (maximum AI) will typically lead to most signals being too loud for patient comfort.
- For some patients, increases in audibility in some frequency regions may not lead to increases in speech recognition (see our discussion of effective audibility and cochlear *dead regions* in Chapter 4). In general, use of the AI may lead to an overestimation of the increase in speech recognition expected from an increase in audibility after fitting a hearing aid if cochlear dead regions and/or HLD factors are not considered. However, it is also important to note that the AI is quite accurate for prediction of relative changes in speech recognition performance, even without considering HLDs, for listeners with hearing thresholds better than approximately 65 to 70 dB HL.
- We must also remember to consider *level* effects. As speech peaks approach the listener's threshold of discomfort, the magnitude of speech recognition improvement will be less than predicted from AI, if a level desensitization factor is not considered.

---

graphically (see examples in Chapter 4). We believe that AI calculations are likely not needed for many clinical situations, but they can provide a useful starting point for some patients when talking about the degree of communication deficit, potential hearing aid benefit, or hearing assistive technology (HAT) candidacy and/ or expectations.

Below we provide an introduction to clinical AI procedures that are easy to use and are quick enough for clinical use. There are many clinical procedures available, but rather than overwhelm you, we focus on the detail of only a few of our favorites.

Before we start, let's get a better idea of the expected *average* relationship between speech recognition and AI. To make things simple enough for clinical use, we will assume an average AI procedure that in turn assumes an average band importance function and does not include corrections for hearing loss, level, age, or any other factor. We can obtain a rough idea about this relationship by going back to Figure 3–7. As we mentioned earlier, these data provide a graphical representation of the AI-to-speech-recognition transfer functions. In Figure 3–7, the *x*-axis is the SII, and the *y*-axis is the predicted percent correct score for a given speech material.

Imagine a person who has a downward sloping hearing loss going from 20 dB at 500 Hz to 60 dB at 6000 Hz. Approximately half the speech cues will be available to this listener, and the AI would equal about 0.5. The relationship between AI and intelligibility is not linear, however (see Figure 3–7). We can see that the most linear function between AI and the percent correct scores is for nonsense syllables. This is important because it suggests that higher AI values are especially important when there are less speech context cues available.

The effect of context can be demonstrated clearly by our example listener with hearing loss and an AI of 0.5. Even though this listener misses 50% of the speech cues, he or she will miss only about 30% of the words in a NU-6 monosyllabic word list and only 5% of sentences. The dramatic difference is a result of the brain's remarkable ability to use context to fill in missing information.

One important example of limited context occurs in children who are first learning speech. In this case, the context might be available in the speech source, but the child may not yet know how to use it. As a result, they may not be as able to fill in the blanks as well as an adult when they miss certain words or sounds. As we pointed out previously, another surprising thing we can see from Figure 3–7 is that for sentence materials, the AI only needs to be about 0.4 for adult listeners with normal hearing to approach 100% correct identification. This of course is for sentences in quiet—performance may be much different in background noise.

Clinical AI Procedures

As we have discussed, formal AI procedures can involve considerable mathematical calculations. Even with the computer scoring methods that are available today, use of these procedures has been overwhelming or too time consuming for most clinicians. Recognizing this, Chas Pavlovic designed a simplified method referred to as A_0 (pronounced A-zero), which was published in 1989. One of the advantages for the A_0 was that no form was required and the procedure could be applied to any audiogram. The calculation is based on only four frequencies (500, 1000, 2000, and 4000 Hz), each having the potential of 30 audible dB. Consider the speech box or *speech block* shown in Figure 3–17 that represents a rough estimate of the dynamic range of speech

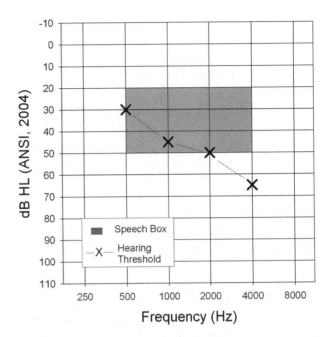

Figure 3–17. An example of the A_0 procedure applied to an audiogram.

from the minima at 20 dB HL to the maxima at 50 dB HL. The procedure is equally weighted, so we have four frequencies with 30 dB at each frequency for a total of 120 potential audible dB. To illustrate how this might be used, let us take an individual with a downward sloping hearing loss of 30 dB at 500 Hz, 45 dB at 1000 Hz, 50 dB at 2000 Hz, and 65 dB at 4000 Hz. Applying this to the speech block shown in Figure 3–17, we see that this patient would have 20 audible dB at 500 Hz, 5 dB at 1000 Hz, 0 dB at 2000 Hz, and 0 dB at 4000 Hz. If we add the audible dB together (20 + 5 + 0 + 0) we find that 25 of the possible 120 dB are audible, for an AI of 0.21 (25 / 120). Pretty simple, huh?

Well, not simple enough for some because dividing anything by 120 in a speedy manner might require a calculator or scratch paper. As a consequence, the 1988 publication of Pavlovic led to several other simplified AI procedures:

- Mueller and Killion (1990) develop a procedure that has 100 dots representing the speech spectrum, commonly called the *count-the-dots audiogram*.

- Humes (1991) develops a similar count-the-dots audiogram, although he only uses 33 dots (and they are bigger).
- Pavolic (1991) develops a *count-the-squares* procedure, using 100 squares with a somewhat different speech spectrum than Mueller and Killion, or Humes.
- Lundeen (1996) publishes a 100-dot version modeled after the 100-square work of Pavlovic.
- Kringlebotn (1999) develops an audiogram form with 100 points for SII calculation.
- In 2010, Killion and Mueller revise their 100-dot audiogram to more closely align it to the SII (more high frequency dots).

Although these approaches are all slightly different, the similarities are such that any of them could be applied routine clinical use. That is, it is unlikely that your clinical decision making will be changed based on an AI difference of 5% or less, which is probably the biggest difference you will see among methods. In addition, when fitting hearing aids, you will more likely use the automatic calculations of the probe-microphone equipment, which may also be different, depending on what speech spectrum or AI method is being used by a given manufacturer. The popular Audioscan Verifit, for example, uses a speech spectrum slightly raised from the 20 to 50 dB HL range of Killion and Mueller (2010) and, therefore, a higher (better) unaided AI will result.

In the next chapter, we illustrate how these count-the-dot audiograms can be used in patient counseling, and for making decisions relating to hearing aid candidacy. In Book Three of this series on verification, we illustrate how AI calculation can be used to compare aided versus unaided performance.

Situational Hearing Aid Response Profile

Another, and somewhat different, clinically useful AI-based procedure that we want to mention is the Situational Hearing Aid Response Profile (SHARP), which was developed by Patricia Stelmachowicz and colleagues (1993). The SHARP is a computer program that provides a graphical representation of speech audibility for 13 typical listening conditions commonly experienced by children. This program also calculates an aided AI (AAI) for each of the listening conditions it includes. Because this tool was developed for pediatric hearing aid fittings, it is not surprising that long-term average speech spectra representations include important situations for children. These include a teacher speaking at various distances, the hearing aid wearer's own voice, a child in a cradle position, and a number of other situations. An example of the SHARP graphical output for two conditions is shown in Figure 3–18. The shaded areas in these figures give a clear indication of the area of audible speech. Similar figures are now available on many probe-microphone systems; however, they usually only include average speech spectrum shapes, even when multiple signal levels are possible. The SHARP is a nice tool for those fitting hearing aids on children and can be used with any hearing aid prescription. In addition to the school setting application, the inclusion of long-term average speech spectra corresponding to the very close listening positions that are experienced by infants and toddlers are especially helpful for coun-

---

POINTS TO PONDER: "A" IS FOR ARTICULATION OR AUDIBILITY?

As we have discussed, the abbreviation AI is commonly used for the *Articulation Index*, but the word articulation makes it sound like the calculation has more to do with how we speak, than how we hear. For the most part, what we are measuring is the audibility of speech cues, so wouldn't *Audibility Index* be a better term? We could still keep the "A." In 1993, Mead Killion, Gus Mueller, Chas Pavlovic, and Larry Humes, who all had independently designed a simplified AI procedure, published the article "A Is for Audibility," supporting the switch from the word articulation. Twenty years have passed and "articulation" still seems to be the word of choice. Perhaps this is only fitting, as this is the term that Harvey Fletcher used over 80 years ago, and his work has certainly withstood the test of time.

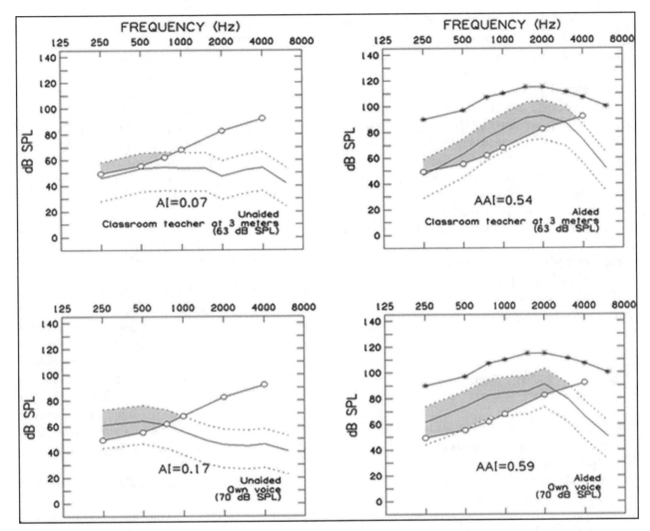

Figure 3–18. An example of aided and unaided audibility for a theoretical child calculated using the SHARP.

seling purposes. At the time of this writing, Boys Town was in the process of updating SHARP to incorporate recent advances in hearing aid signal processing, such as nonlinear frequency compression. A newer version with updated features should be available at the Boys Town website by the time you are reading this (search the web for Situational Hearing Aid Response Profile).

Clinical STI Procedures

Given that estimation of the STI requires measurements in a room and/or complex calculations, rather than just the readily available clinical information, it is reasonable to question whether there are clinical applications for the STI. Although perhaps not in routine clinical hearing aid practice, the STI can be useful when considering the impact of room acoustics, acoustic room treatments, or hearing assistive technology. A complete discussion of this topic is well beyond the scope of this textbook; however, clinicians who routinely do this type of work often choose to obtain a sound level meter and/or computer program that is able to measure and calculate STI or one of its simplified versions such as the Rapid Speech Transmission Index, or RASTI. More recently rough measurements and calculations of the STI for public address systems have even been introduced as smartphone applications.

We should mention that it is also possible to obtain free STI software that can be used in conjunction with an existing personal computer, loudspeaker, and microphone. For example, Harry Levitt has developed a program that can be used to make such measures and is available free-of-charge from Gallaudet University (search the Internet for http://www.hearingresearch .org and LexSTI). This small, easy-to-use program can be quite useful (for example) for clinicians in a school setting arguing for acoustic treatment of a room or hearing assistive technology. A note of caution is also warranted, however. The STI should generally not be used after measuring the modulation transfer function at the output of modern hearing aids. This limitation is due to the fact that some types of commonly used signal processing, such as amplitude compression, are known to affect STI values without producing a concomitant effect on speech recognition.

Mini-Summary

- The calculation of the AI can be helpful for patient counseling and making decisions regarding amplification.
- Maximizing the AI is clearly not the only consideration when assigning hearing aid gain and is expected to lead to excessive and undesirable loudness in many cases. In addition, hearing loss desensitization and level effects must also be considered when interpreting clinical AI values.
- There are several *clinically friendly* AI approaches available. In general, they produce similar and comparable clinical AI values. Clinical application of aided audibility for a variety of different long-term average speech spectra, as is possible with the SHARP instrument, can be useful for examining speech audibility across a range of environments in children

In Closing

Understanding the acoustics of the speech signal is paramount to managing the most common desire of potential hearing aid candidates: understanding speech better. Without a basic understanding of the factors that impact the LTASS (such as vocal effort, talker variables, and measurement techniques), it is not possible to alter or adjust the hearing aid processing in a meaningful or effective manner. Knowing the interactions between speech dynamics and the hearing aid's classification system leads to a better understanding of the function of automatic hearing aid algorithms. Quantifying the resultant audibility after a hearing aid fitting allows both the clinician and patient to better understand the potential success of the effort. Adding the effect of noise and reverberation to that audibility calculation provides a better real-world indication of the potential for success.

4

Pre-Fitting Tests Using Frequency-Specific Measures

In the next few chapters, we discuss some of the pre-fitting tools that we use to assess the patient, the patient's hearing handicap, and their communication needs to begin making decisions regarding hearing aid candidacy and selection. Assessing communication needs for the purpose of hearing aid selection requires knowledge in several areas. Given the time limitations in a typical clinic setting, it is necessary that an appropriately small number of measures are selected that provide the most important information for each specific patient in an efficient manner. Because every patient is different and there is not time to gather exhaustive clinical data, this handful of assessment tools must be selected individually for each patient's situation out of the large group of possible assessment measures available. This is often an iterative process during which the clinician uses information gathered earlier (e.g., general case history, type and degree of hearing loss, general patient goals, and problems) to determine what additional information is most critical to gather for the individual patient via additional assessments. We provide you with a variety of tools in the next three chapters, ranging from tests using pure-tone stimuli, speech recognition in quiet, speech in background noise, and several self-assessment measures.

To select the best assessment measures and interpret their results to assist in selecting the optimal hearing aid model, style, and processing for a given patient, it is important to know how hearing aids work and the various features available. For example, loudness discomfort measures go hand-in-hand with setting the maximum output of the hearing aid; the patient's QuickSIN score might influence the recommendation of directional microphone and wireless streaming technologies, and so forth. Because the hearing aid selection process requires knowledge in so many areas, we sometimes describe assessment tools and techniques without first providing a clear indication of exactly when and how the test results should be applied and interpreted. We do this so that we can provide background information about a variety of techniques. However, it is our philosophy that the cookbook method of learning hearing aids is of little use in the long run, so subsequent chapters provide information about the philosophy underlying the use of these techniques so that future techniques can also be appropriately applied.

Although it is easy to get caught up in learning how to conduct and score all the test procedures and then trying to understand when and how to best implement them, we must remember that each patient is an individual. One of the most challenging and interesting aspects of hearing aid selection and fitting is recognizing this individuality and appropriately modifying the process for each patient. Protocols are a wonderful starting place and an excellent mechanism for helping ensure quality control in our practice. However, a protocol should only serve as a point of reference, and the personality, desire, and needs of the individual patient must drive clinical decision making from beginning to end.

Using the Audiogram for Counseling and Predicting Audibility

In the previous chapter, we provided a detailed description of the speech signal and explained the importance of understanding the components of this signal as they relate to the fitting of hearing aids. As we described, a big part of the success of the overall fitting relates to making speech audible, with the caveat that it also must have the appropriate loudness, minimal distortion, and a reasonable sound quality. It is helpful during the pre-fitting appointment to assure that the patient understands the fitting goals. For the new hearing aid user, who still might be questioning the need for hearing aids, it might be necessary to illustrate how much of the average speech signal is *not* audible. For the experienced hearing aid user obtaining a new pair of hearing aids, it might be helpful to explain why the new hearing aids will sound different from the old ones. For example, if more high frequency gain is being added, an explanation of the importance of these speech cues might encourage the user to be more accepting to this new amplification strategy. These visual demonstrations also can be very helpful for family members, who might be wondering why Mom can "hear but not understand."

The history of audiology is linked to the audiogram. (See Appendix H for an interesting timeline dating back to 377 BC!) There are several methods of using the patient's pure-tone audiogram for pre-fitting counseling. Some are more detailed than others, and the method selected often relates to the sophistication of the patient, the level of interest in learning about hearing loss, and how the loss might impact speech understanding.

Using the Speech Banana with Symbols

As was discussed in the previous chapter, when we plot the LTASS of average speech on the HL scale, it more or less resembles a banana—so much so, that even many lay people know what the *speech banana* is. This is commonly used for counseling patients regarding their hearing loss. Some audiologists only have the banana shaded on the audiogram, other forms have symbols for common environmental sounds, or have the various speech consonants or vowels printed on the audiogram. Usually this is not the audiogram placed in the patient's records or sent out to referral sources, but rather simply something unofficial that can be used for counseling and that the patient can take home for review.

What is displayed in Figure 4–1 is an audiogram that has a shaded banana. Many audiologists have the banana on their standard clinical audiogram, as it provides an immediate reference of the speech range. Figure 4–2 is an audiogram that does not have a banana per se, but shows the individual speech sounds that are contained within the banana. Several environmental sounds also are displayed. This is not an audiogram

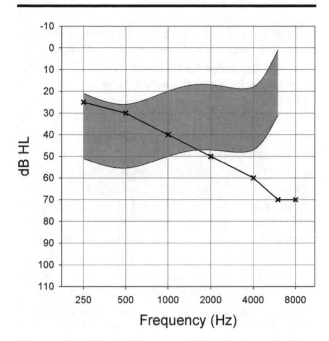

Figure 4–1. Typical downward sloping hearing loss plotted on an audiogram displaying the average speech spectrum.

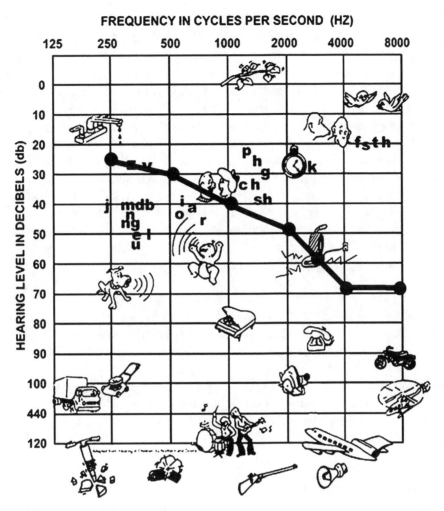

Figure 4–2. Typical downward sloping hearing loss plotted on an audiogram displaying common speech and environmental sounds.

that you would use in a medical record, but it is helpful for patient counseling. After plotting the hearing thresholds, you could then talk about the portion of the banana that was not audible, the speech sounds that are not audible, and also point out specific environmental sounds that might not be heard or not perceived as readily as for people with normal hearing. This later form is a bit extreme, as most audiologists would not want all these symbols for environmental sounds—personally, we probably wouldn't include the whispering chimpanzees on our form. The point is, many forms of this type are available and can serve as useful counseling tools.

Using the Speech Banana with Dots

In the previous chapter, we introduced you to the AI and the SII, and discussed some simplified clinical methods for making these calculations. Of the several methods we reviewed we like the count-the-dots procedure for busy clinicians because frequencies often important in hearing aid fittings, 1500 and 3000 Hz are now also included, and the calculation of AI only involves counting dots—no addition, subtraction, or division required. In case it is not obvious, you would count the dots *below* the hearing thresholds. If you want to venture into the world of math and it is a mild hearing loss, you might

---

SOAPBOX: PICK YOUR BANANA CAREFULLY!

As we have mentioned, it is common to place the speech banana (average LTASS) on the audiogram and use this for counseling. There have been several studies of average speech over the years, and LTASS findings do vary somewhat from study to study, but they are more or less in pretty good general agreement. So why is it then, that if we would do a Google image search on *Speech Banana* today, we find audiograms (apparently used in offices and clinics somewhere) with the 1000 to 2000 Hz frequency region of the LTASS ranging anywhere from 15 to 45 dB for the upper boundary and 40 to 70 dB for the lower boundary, with everything in between also used. A 25 dB difference! This is a pretty fundamental concept of audiology—wouldn't it be nice if we all could get it right? Imagine if you took your three-year-old son in for testing, and the audiometric results revealed that he had a 35 dB loss (or is it really a loss?). If he was tested at Clinic A, where they use the 15 to 45 dB banana, you would be told that your son was missing about two-thirds of the important sounds of average speech. On the other hand, if he were tested at Clinic B, where the audiologists use the 40 to 70 dB speech banana, you would be told that all is well—he is hearing 100% of average speech! In our opinion, this borders on malpractice, as a child suffering from middle ear effusion (which often results in a hearing loss of 30 to 35 dB) might go untreated for months or years, simply because the parents were given the wrong counseling based on the wrong banana.

Refer back to Chapter 3 for more details on the correct LTASS. In general, we recommend using a spectrum that has the soft components for the mid-frequencies around 20 to 25 dB, with the loud components of the LTASS at 50 to 55 dB (see Figure 4–1).

---

want to count the dots above the hearing thresholds and subtract this number from 100.

The 1990 Mueller-Killion audiogram is shown in Figure 4–3. In part, the design was based on a 200-dot SPL chart that was used in industrial acoustics in the 1960s (Cavanaugh, Farrell, Hirtle, & Waters, 1962). Observe that the density of the dots changes as a function of frequency, to represent the importance function of speech. We have used the same hearing loss as before, and note that for this patient, about 20% of the dots are audible.

We have found the count-the-dot audiogram to be particularly helpful when counseling patients who are in denial regarding the degree of handicap that they might have. Using a percentage to make the point is something that everyone can relate to. Showing someone graphically that they are missing 60% of average speech, when they have just said they hear everything, can be a convincing message. As we discussed in Chapter 2, patients often forget much of what we tell them during the prefitting counseling process, but they usually remember the percent of dots they could hear.[19]

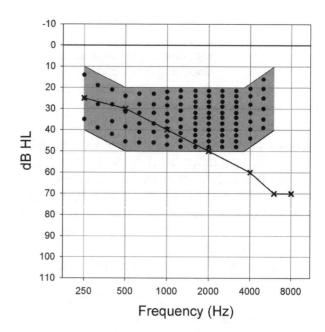

Figure 4–3. Typical downward sloping hearing loss plotted on an audiogram displaying the 1990 Mueller and Killion count-the-dots speech spectrum.

KEY CONCEPT: HEARING, NOT UNDERSTANDING

Although we believe that using *percent audibility* of average speech can be effective for patient counseling, we do need to mention a fine point that often needs to be clarified. It is important to clearly state that this is the percent of speech that the patient *hears*, not the percent of speech that he or she *understands*. Patients sometimes want to think of it as percent understanding, or even percent hearing loss. As we discussed in Chapter 3, it is possible to make a rough conversion from the audibility index to speech recognition using the chart shown in Figure 3–7. As illustrated in this chart, a person who is only hearing 50% of average speech could be understanding nearly 100% of sentence material if listening in quiet.

The dots also can be useful in educating referral sources, as it soon becomes clear that an individual with a high frequency, noise-induced hearing loss really does not have normal hearing for the *speech range*, as this patient often is missing over 40% of average speech. Or, the dots also work effectively for illustrating the audibility deficit a child with middle ear effusion might suffer.

New SII Dots

In 2010, Mueller and Killion modified their 1990 count-the-dot procedure (Killion & Mueller, 2010). The authors state that the form was changed to reflect the research behind the new ANSI standard S3.5-1997(R2007), "Methods for Calculation of Speech Intelligibility Index," which produced a new SII importance function that gives more weight to higher frequencies. The new version, therefore, slightly redistributes the 100 dots and includes weightings for 6000 and 8000 Hz. The revised 2010 audiogram is shown in Figure 4–4 (and also Appendix I), with the same audiogram from Figure 4–3 plotted. Note that the audible dots are now roughly 20%, the same as from the previous calculation. This is because the speech region where the differences between forms exists were not audible for this patient for both versions. The biggest differences would be noted for the patients with more or less normal hearing through 3000 or 4000 Hz. Killion and Mueller (2010) review the basic differences between the two forms:

■ The new audiogram has 11 dots above 4000 Hz, whereas only 6 dots were above 4000 Hz in the older version. There is also an additional dot at 4000 Hz in the new version. Because there are only 100 dots to work with, these extra high-frequency dots were carefully lifted from the frequencies below 4000 Hz.

■ Because a few dots from the mid-frequencies were removed, the typical patient with a gradually downward sloping hearing loss might have an AI score 2% to 3% lower with the new SII version than with the older one.

One thing that did not change in the new Killion-Mueller count-the-dot audiogram is the overall speech spectrum, which is based on a 60 dB SPL equivalence. As we have discussed earlier, there are several different

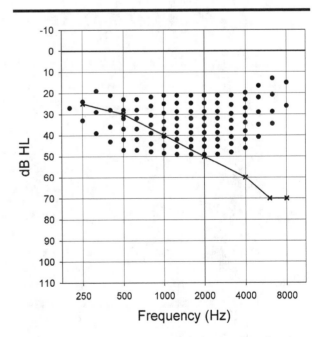

Figure 4–4. Typical downward sloping hearing loss plotted on an audiogram displaying the 2010 Killion and Mueller count-the-dots SII speech spectrum.

speech bananas in clinical use. Killion and Mueller (2010) state that their selection of this spectrum was based on the work of Margo Skinner, who recommended that all conversational speech tests be conducted at 60 dB SPL, 5 dB softer than the generally accepted average for conversational speech, as this level is a better measure of the listener's ability in everyday life (Skinner, Holden, Holden, Demorest, & Fourakis, 1997).[20]

Although the audibility calculations that we have been discussing easily can be computerized (and they have been), there is something to be said about using the paper-and-pencil version. Sitting at a desk with a patient, plotting the audiogram, having the patient help you count the audible dots, showing what happens when the low-frequency dots are covered up because they are masked by noise, all tends to have a memorable counseling impact. The patient takes the sheets home with them, and in general, they seem to get it. But, computer automation is a good thing too, so we discuss how the illustration of audibility also can be used with your fitting software and probe-microphone equipment.

Using Fitting Software or Probe-Microphone Equipment

Most hearing aid fitting software also provides a counseling module, which often includes a method to relate the hearing loss to average speech. An example of this from one manufacturer is shown in Figure 4–5. This form has

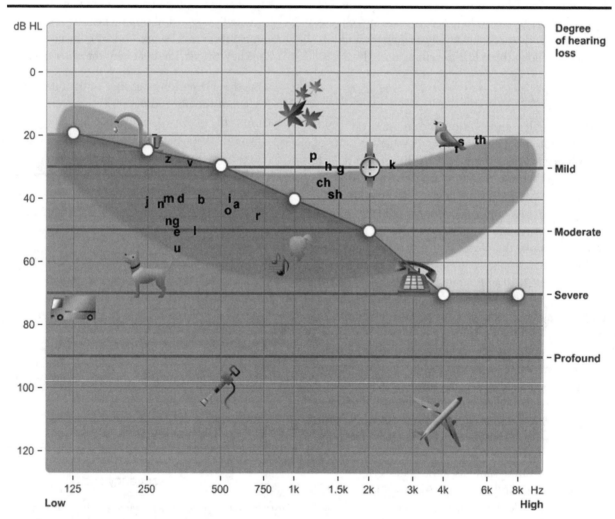

Figure 4–5. Typical downward sloping hearing loss plotted on an audiogram displaying the average speech spectrum in a manufacturer's fitting software. Note that this is the same audiogram as shown in Figures 4–1 to 4–4, except it now appears as if more speech is audible as the overall spectrum is approximately 10 dB louder.

the shaded banana, the important speech sounds, and a few environmental sounds. We specifically included this form to illustrate our earlier point about displaying the LTASS—note that this speech banana is 10 to 15 dB lower (louder) than the one shown in Figures 4–1, 4–3, and 4–4. We have plotted the same hearing loss as before, and good news—now our patient seems to be doing better! The patient previously was only hearing about one-third of average speech in the 1000 Hz range, and now the patient is hearing about three-fourths of the speech signal for this frequency range. But the hearing loss did not change. It is interesting to observe that a hearing aid manufacturer would use a spectrum that makes it appear the patient is doing *better* than most other speech spectrums would indicate. You'd think

that if they'd error, it would be in the other direction. But most importantly, you see how something as simple as the speech banana can cause confusion for both the audiologist and the patient when not used correctly.

Another way to illustrate how the patient's hearing loss relates to the average speech signal is to use your probe-microphone equipment. The advantage of this is that we now have converted everything to ear canal SPL, and we are using an SPL-O-gram, a display method where loud sounds actually fall appropriately above soft sounds, unlike the standard audiogram. One way to use this display is to plot the patient's hearing threshold and use the average speech spectrum that is stored for screen display. This is shown in Figure 4–6. In general, this is more intuitive for patient counseling than the standard

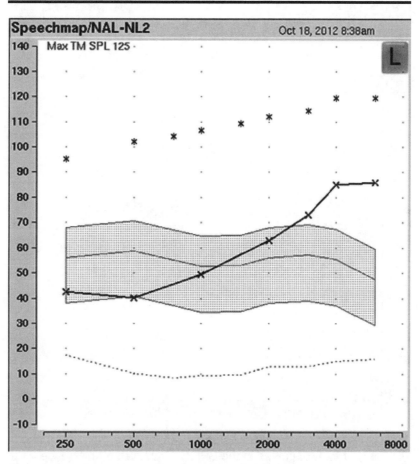

Figure 4–6. Typical downward sloping hearing loss (same as used in Figures 4–1 to 4–5) plotted in the SPL-O-Gram format (reference = ear canal SPL) with the average speech spectrum. Asterisks at the top of the audiogram represent the patient's LDLs; the dotted line near the bottom of the audiogram represents thresholds for normal hearing.

audiogram, as we see that what is *not audible* falls below the patient's thresholds, and what is audible falls above. This display does not involve any extra testing; the probe-microphone equipment monitor is simply used to facilitate the counseling.

It is possible to add a bit more face validity into the pre-fitting counseling and actually measure an average speech spectrum in the patient's ear canal, while comparing the speech levels to hearing thresholds. This is displayed in Figure 4–7. What you see here are the same hearing thresholds as before, compared with the measured real-ear output of the calibrated LTASS (*carrot passage—male talker*) of the Audioscan Verifit probe-microphone equipment (i.e., the measurement is conducted with the test probe at the patient's eardrum). This equipment automatically calculates the SII, which in this case was 41%. This is considerably higher than the 20% that we calculated for Figure 4–4, but recall that the Killion-Mueller spectrum was based on a 60 dB SPL overall level, rather than the approximately 62 dB SPL level used by the SII. The patient's free-field-to-eardrum transfer function also will impact these measures (see the probe-microphone section of Book Three for details). Depending on the time that is available, this counseling and demonstration can be expanded by presenting speech of different input levels (soft, average, loud), or even using live speech of family members to illustrate to the patient what he or she is missing.

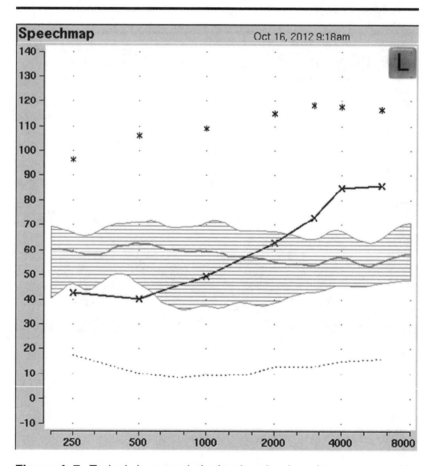

Figure 4–7. Typical downward sloping hearing loss (same as used in Figures 4–1 to 4–5) plotted in the SPL-O-Gram format (reference = ear canal SPL). Rather than displaying the average speech spectrum, the spectrum shown was obtained from a real-speech signal (65 dB SPL) delivered to the patient's open ear with the probe-microphone tip at the patient's eardrum.

What Does It All Mean?

What we have shown in this section is that there are many ways that the pure-tone audiogram can be used to help patients understand their hearing handicap and how it relates to speech understanding. For the most part, it is pretty simple. But, We need to focus on the fact that the goal in this case is not perfect scientific accuracy—we don't care if one SII estimate is 2% different from another. The overall purpose is simply to show patients the impact that hearing loss potentially could have for understanding speech, so that they can make informed decisions regarding the use of hearing aids.

Loudness Discomfort Level Testing

The most critical aspect of the hearing aid verification process is ensuring that the gain and the maximum output are adjusted correctly for a given patient. Although these two adjustments are not totally independent (one could not achieve high gain levels for average inputs without a moderately high output setting), for the average patient, it is usually possible to vary the gain by 40 to 50 dB and the MPO (for maximum power output) by at least 20 dB. Gain prescriptions are typically based on audiometric thresholds, but how do we determine the best MPO setting? The logical approach, which also has been specified in best practice guidelines for the past 25 years, is to conduct frequency-specific loudness

discomfort level (LDL) measures, and use these values to set the hearing aid MPO (often by manipulating the output compression limiting kneepoint) so that loud sounds are loud, but not too loud. These LDL measures are a routine part of the pre-fitting hearing aid battery.

Background

The loudness growth function for both normal hearing and hearing impaired individuals, at some point, reaches a level where the sound is uncomfortable. This is referred to as the uncomfortable loudness level, threshold of discomfort, or the term we use in this chapter, the loudness discomfort level (LDL). A long-standing component of the fitting process is to assure that the MPO of the hearing is appropriate for the patient. Carhart's procedure from the 1940s (1946a) included a "determination of instrument efficiency," which included "transmitting loud sounds without undue discomfort."

Although intuitively it seems likely that the maximum output of the hearing aid could influence use, benefit, and satisfaction, one might question if there are data to suggest that this is a problem? There are. In 2003, in a large survey of audiologists, Jenstad, Van Tasell, and Ewert (2003) reported that "aids too loud" was the most common complaint audiologists received from patients fitted with hearing aids. "Satisfaction with loudness" also has been a common question on the MarkeTrak surveys. Although overall satisfaction with hearing aids has gone from a low of 53% (1994) to a high of 74%

POINTS TO PONDER: DOES THE TERMINOLOGY REALLY MATTER?

As we explain in Table 4–1, there are many terms used to denote the point at which loud sounds become uncomfortable—UL, UCL, ULL, TD, LDL, etc. Does it matter what term we use? This topic has been discussed several times over the years in the Mueller and Bentler "How Loud Is Allowed" trilogy (Mueller & Bentler, 1994, 2002, 2008). Dr. Bentler points out (supported by research; Warner & Bentler, 2001) that TD is the most appropriate term, as dimensions other than the *loudness* of a perceptually abusive sound play a part in what is considered uncomfortable—it is not determined by the RMS level of the signal alone. Factors that tend to cause LDLs to be rated lower include annoyance, peakiness, high-frequency content, and the subjective perception of tinniness. These factors are particularly important during the aided verification process, which we describe in Book Three. For this chapter, however, despite Dr. Bentler's fondness for the TD descriptor, we use LDL to describe this loudness perception.

Table 4–1. Terminology Associated with the Measurement of Loudness Discomfort

- Uncomfortable Loudness (UCL). This is perhaps the most commonly used term among clinicians to describe the point at which loud sounds become uncomfortable. The common use of the letter "C" in the abbreviation is somewhat puzzling, and indeed, some simply use the abbreviation UL. The abbreviation ULL also is used, with the final "L" referring to *level*.

- Loudness Discomfort Level (LDL). The term that we prefer and what we will use throughout this chapter. It is used interchangeably with UCL/ULL.

- Threshold of Discomfort (TD). Another term for the same measure. For the most part (see Point to Ponder on this topic), it can be used interchangeably with LDL, UCL and ULL.

- Upper Level of Comfort (ULC). The category of loudness falling just below the LDL. When using the 7-point Cox Contour Anchors we discuss later, this is the #6 Loud, But Okay rating. In general, we want the output of the hearing aid to fall at this level; the DSL prescriptive software has used ULC values for this purpose.

- Highest Comfortable Level (HCL). The same as the ULC.

- OSPL90: The broadest most powerful output of a hearing aid with the gain control "full on" measured in a 2-cc coupler using 90 dB swept pure tones. A component of ANSI standard S3.22 and used for hearing aid specification, documentation, and quality control.

- Maximum Power Output (MPO). In some cases, the term MPO is used synonymously with OSPL90. More commonly, however, in the clinic, MPO refers to the maximum output of the hearing aid when specific settings have been made (e.g., settings of gain, input and output compression), and not the *potential* maximum output of the instrument (the OSPL90). The MPO, therefore, cannot be higher than the OSPL90, and often it is significantly lower. For example, lowering the AGCo compression kneepoint for a given patient would lower the hearing aid's MPO.

- Real-ear saturation response (RESR). This is an MPO measure obtained with the hearing aid fitted to the patient's ear rather than in a 2-cc coupler. Typically, this measure is made with the hearing aid's gain and compression parameters set to approximate use conditions using an 85-90 dB swept pure tone.

- Real-ear coupler difference (RECD). This is a measure which compares the output of a hearing aid in the real ear to the output in a 2-cc coupler with identical settings. If the RECD is known, it can be added to the hearing aid coupler MPO (*not* the OSPL90) to predict the maximum output in the ear canal.

- Reference equivalent thresholds in SPL (RETSPL). Difference between HL dial setting and output in a 2-cc or 6-cc coupler. Because insert earphones (which are calibrated in a 2-cc coupler), are typically used for HL LDL testing, RETSPL values can be used to convert HL LDLs to 2-cc coupler values (so you can speak the same language as your fitting software).

- Real-ear dial difference (REDD). This is the addition of the RETSPL and the RECD (or it can be measured directly); using this you can convert from HL LDL to ear canal SPL. This provides the RESR output targets you see on the probe-mic fitting screen.

- Automatic Gain Control-input (AGCi): Input compression, typically having a low activation kneepoint (in which case it is referred to as WDRC). It can be used to control the hearing aids' MPO if kneepoints are low enough and the ratios are big enough. Note: Amplitude compression processing will be discussed in much greater detail in Book Two and is purposefully oversimplified here.

- Automatic Gain Control-output (AGCo): Output compression, typically having a high activation kneepoint and high compression ratios (in which case it is referred to as compression limiting)—the most common method to control the MPO.

(2008), the MarkeTrak VIII 2008 survey revealed that satisfaction for "comfort with loud sounds" was only 67%, which had a .60 correlation with overall satisfaction (Kochkin, 2010). It is important to mention, however, that the comfort for loud sounds category only had 42% satisfaction as recent as 2002 (Kochkin, 2002).

In a related finding from MarkeTrak VIII, Kochkin et al. (2010) reported that highly satisfied users from the sample were more apt to have received loudness testing during the fitting process than individuals who were not satisfied. For the weighted protocol, these differences were substantial: For the bottom 15% of satisfaction (*n* = 275), only 40% received the testing versus 98% for the top 15% of satisfied hearing aid users (*n* = 276). The study did not differentiate if the loudness testing had been conducted pre-fitting or during the fitting process.

The research surrounding the clinical measure of LDLs was addressed in an evidence-based review by Mueller and Bentler (2005). Because of the limited number of studies that met their criteria ($n = 3$), the level of evidence, and the statistical power of the studies, they were unable to make a strong recommendation concerning the clinical use of LDL measures. One prospective study published since the Mueller and Bentler (2005) review compared two different fitting protocols; one included LDL measures and the other did not (Shi, Doherty, Kordas, & Pellegrino, 2007). The aided Abbreviated Profile of Hearing Aid Benefit (APHAB) and Satisfaction of Amplification in Daily Life (SADL) findings for the two groups were not significantly different following hearing aid use. However, when the authors examined patient-driven adjustments in the first 45 days following the fittings, there were nearly twice as many adjustments made to the group who were fitted without the LDL measures (mean = 2.7 versus 1.5 adjustments). The authors speculate this was because of the alterations of the output based on the LDL values.

Measures of LDL Variability

An important question regarding the pre-fitting measurement of LDLs relates to the variability of loudness discomfort among individuals. Are the LDLs of the hearing impaired about the same as people with normal hearing? Do individuals with the same hearing loss more or less have the same LDLs? If for example, most all patients with a 50 dB cochlear hearing loss have LDLs within a 10 dB window, then it probably would not be worth the time investment to conduct LDL testing during the pre-fitting process. We would simply predict it from the audiogram.

Perhaps the most extensive study of LDLs was reported by Bentler and Cooley (2001). They determined LDLs for a total of 433 subjects (710 ears) with presumed cochlear pathologies, using an ascending method of limits similar to our recommendations in the next section. Their data (averaged for five test frequencies) is displayed in Figure 4–8. Several important teaching points are evident:

1. From 20 to 60 dB hearing loss, there is no average change in LDLs.
2. Above 60 dB, average LDLs go up roughly 5 dB for each 10 dB increase in hearing loss.
3. The range of LDLs for different individuals with the same hearing loss is 40 to 50 dB or greater for most hearing loss levels.

Other findings from the Bentler and Cooley (2001) study that have clinical importance (multiple regression analysis using almost 2,000 LDLs; subjects ranging in age from 11 to 97 years):

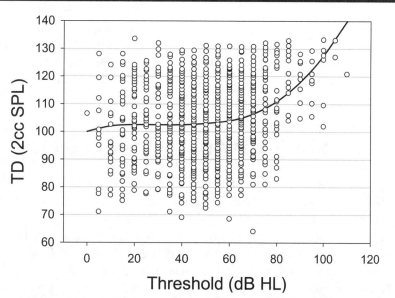

Figure 4–8. Display of LDLs (TDs) referenced to a 2-cc coupler as a function of hearing loss obtained from 710 individual ears. Data points averaged for frequencies 500 to 4000 Hz. (Adapted from Bentler and Cooley, 2001.)

1. LDLs did not vary as a function of the frequency tested (when hearing loss was matched).
2. There were no gender differences.
3. There were no age differences.

As mentioned above and readily observed in Figure 4–8, the variability of LDLs for individuals with the same degree of hearing loss is very large. For example, if we take a common 50 dB hearing loss, we see that values ranged from the mid-70s to over 130 dB—nearly a 60 dB range. Perhaps more important than the range per se, is that there were not just one or two outliers but a fairly even distribution between the lower and upper values. If we were to use average values to predict the correct MPO setting, in this example, the value would be around 102 dB (re: 2-cc coupler; see regression line). Bentler and Cooley (2001), however, report that only 32% of measured LDLs fell within ± 5 dB of this average. Assuming that we would not want an MPO mistake of greater than 5 dB, this clearly points out the problems that can exist when average values are used.

Dillon and Storey (1998) also reported LDL findings for a large group of subjects, showing average values similar to that of Bentler and Cooley (2001). The range of variability for their subject group was smaller, however, around 40 dB, primarily because they did not observe LDLs less than approximately 90 dB once the hearing loss was 50 dB or greater. But even with this somewhat smaller range, predicting from the audiogram could be risky.

If It Is Not Right?

So what happens if we fit a hearing aid and the MPO is not right? Perhaps the biggest problem would be to select an output that is too high, exceeding the patient's LDL. Some probable adverse outcomes are as follows:

■ Because there is not a control for MPO, the patient will turn down gain (and will then not have appropriate audibility for soft and average inputs).
■ The patient will only use the hearing aids when knowing that no loud sounds will be present (missing out on appropriate amplification for the majority of listening situations).
■ The patient will have some initial negative experiences and will simply stop using the hearing aids.

So what if the MPO is set unnecessarily lower than it needs to be? Unlike setting the output too high, this probably will not result in rejection of amplification, but there are several potential negative consequences:

■ Speech may sound somewhat distorted, as the peaks often will be limited by the MPO of the hearing aid (typically an AGCo algorithm).
■ Speech may not have the necessary amplitude dynamics, as the peaks will be limited or clipped. Music may sound dull.
■ The range of loudness perceptions will be limited—average and loud inputs may only differ by a few decibels following processing.
■ For some speech-in-noise listening situations (those with a slightly positive SNR), unnecessary MPO limiting could make the SNR more adverse.

POINTS TO PONDER: *BEST* PRACTICE VERSUS *REAL* PRACTICE

Starting with the Vanderbilt Report of 1991, all subsequent best practice guidelines have included the recommendation of conducting frequency-specific LDL as part of the pre-fitting of hearing aids. So is this a common practice? Mueller (2003a) conducted a survey of over 500 audiologists and Hearing Instrument Specialists who were actively fitting hearing aids and found that 61% routinely conducted pre-fitting LDL measures. However, only 27% of these respondents used frequency-specific test signals (speech stimuli was by far the most popular). If we do the math (27% of 61%), we find that only 16% of audiologists or dispensers were conducting pre-fitting LDL testing according to established protocols. That of course was 2003. Maybe things are different today?

Let the Fitting Software Do the Work?

In the next few pages, we present a clinical protocol that easily can be used to measure the frequency-specific LDL, and then these values can be used to set the MPO of the hearing aid for individual patients. Before we do that, however, it is relevant to discuss what is the *most common* pre-fitting clinical method of deciding the hearing aid's MPO: it is using the decision making of the manufacturer's software. Depending on the audiologist and the manufacturer, there are several options regarding how this could be handled:

- No LDLs entered into the software; the software selects MPO values based on the average for the patient's hearing thresholds using algorithms from validated prescriptive fitting methods. The two most popular methods are the NAL-NL2 (for National Acoustics Laboratory–Nonlinear 2) and the Desired Sensation Level Version 5 (DSL5.0)—see the hearing aid selection section of Book Three for complete review.
- No LDLs entered into the software; the software selects MPO values based on the average for patient's hearing thresholds using the *manufacturer's* correction values.
- LDLs entered into the software; the software selects MPO values based on HL to 2-cc corrections using data from validated fitting methods (e.g., DSL5.0). Note: The NAL-NL2 does not use measured LDLs for MPO calculations, although it is possible that a given manufacturer could use their own correction factors for setting the MPO in conjunction with the NAL-NL2 algorithm.
- LDLs entered into the software; the software selects MPO values based on the *manufacturer's* HL to 2-cc coupler corrections.

Could these different approaches result in different MPO settings? Most certainly. When LDLs are not entered, the DSL prescribes different output values than the NAL-NL2. Moreover, it is reported that some manufacturers use the 1988 data of Pascoe, which are nearly 10 dB higher than the average values from Bentler and Cooley (2001) for common hearing losses in the 50 to 60 dB range. Even when LDLs are entered, not all manufacturers have the same philosophy regarding how the MPO should relate to the measured LDL. Should MPO be set exactly at the LDL? Above? Below?

A Comparative Study of MPO. To examine some of these differences, Mueller, Bentler, and Wu (2008) conducted electroacoustic measures (MPO for a 90 dB SPL swept tone) for the premier hearing aid of each of the top six manufacturers. The hearing aids were programmed based on the manufacturers default settings for a flat 50 dB HL hearing loss. The authors first conducted the fitting without entering LDLs. The resulting MPO for the six different instruments are shown in Figure 4–9, top panel. Observe that at 2000 Hz, there is an approximate 20 dB difference in the MPO among instruments (HA1 versus HA5), with the other four instruments spaced fairly evenly in between the lowest and the highest. Clearly, different manufacturers use different prediction models.

The authors then entered a 90 dB HL LDL for all test frequencies and reprogrammed the instruments. These MPOs are shown in Figure 4–9, bottom panel. Again we see a range of about 20 dB, although the ordering among manufacturers has changed. Note that the output of HA1 and HA2 dropped approximately 10 dB—a somewhat reasonable change, given that the 90 dB LDL that was entered is about 10 dB below the common average of 100 dB for this degree of hearing loss. But also note that the MPO for HA6 did not change, and this hearing aid now has the highest output. The output for HA5 also stayed about the same.

Given the variability of the MPO selected by the different manufacturers, even when LDLs are entered, it seems reasonable that the prudent audiologist would want to select the MPO themselves—that is what we discuss in the next section.

Administration and Scoring

Although measuring LDLs is usually considered a fairly simple task and can be conducted effectively by a technician, there are two important procedural conditions that if not followed correctly, will significantly reduce the validity and reliability of the task: the use of loudness anchors and appropriate instructions. In fact, we suspect that when audiologists state, "I don't do LDL testing because the results are just too unreliable," it is probably

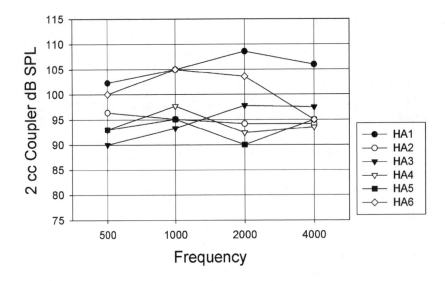

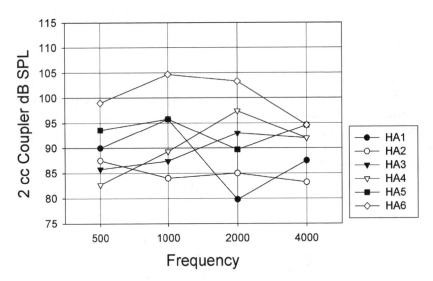

Figure 4–9. Maximum power output (re: 2-cc coupler) for the premier hearing aids from the six major manufacturers when programmed for a flat 50 dB HL hearing loss using default settings. **Top Panel:** Output levels when no LDLs were entered. **Bottom Panel:** Output levels when an LDL of 90 dB HL was entered into the fitting software for all key frequencies.

because these critical components have not been implemented into the test protocol.

Loudness Anchors

Loudness anchors are used to give the patient a reference for the loudness perceptions that he or she will be experiencing. It indicates boundaries and intermediate

steps, which facilitates the understanding of the task and improves reliability; the patient has words to attach to a perception. The loudness anchors that we recommend, shown in Figure 4–10 (and also Appendix K), are from Robyn Cox (1995) and were used in the development of the Cox Contour Test, which became part of the hearing aid fitting protocol of the IHAFF (for Independent Hearing Aid Fitting Forum; Cox, 1995; Mueller, 1994b).

These anchors are an abbreviated form of those used by David Hawkins in much of his LDL research (e.g., Hawkins, Walden, Montgomery, & Prosek, 1987).[21]

Loudness Anchors

#7.   Uncomfortably Loud

#6.   Loud, But Okay

#5.   Comfortable, But Slightly Loud

#4.   Comfortable

#3.   Comfortable, But Slightly Soft

#2.   Soft

#1.   Very Soft

Figure 4–10. Loudness anchors used for LDL testing. Anchors adapted from those used for the Cox Contour Test (Cox, 1995).

Prior to the testing, the patients are familiarized with the loudness anchors, and they are provided the chart to use during testing. They can respond either by stating the loudness category or by simply giving the number. We prefer to have the chart quite large (e.g., 2' × 3'), mounted on cardboard, which patients can hold in their lap during testing, shown in Figure 4–11. They then have the option of pointing to the category rather than calling out the term or the number. (Savvy clinicians have learned to associate the certainty of the judgment with different pointing techniques—a true #7 hits the board with a little more force than an uncertain one!) The pointing technique of course only works if you have the patient positioned in the booth so that you can observe the response. Many audiologists simply have the chart printed on standard size paper and hand it to the patient, or have the chart mounted on the test booth wall. The main point—use the anchors!

Instructions

Going hand-in-hand with the anchors are the instructions. The measured LDL can vary by 15 to 20 dB simply based on the instructions that are used.[22] Given that we

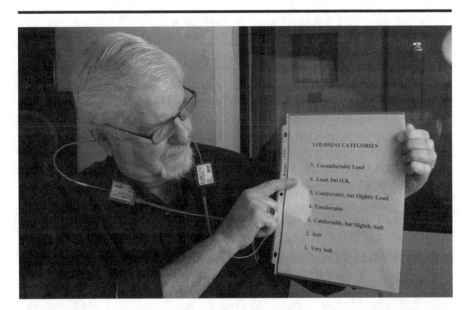

Figure 4–11. Clinical measurement of loudness perception using the Cox Loudness Anchors. The patient can respond by pointing to the correct perception or by calling out the corresponding number. A chart this size may not allow for a font large enough for all patients to easily read—for best results, we recommend putting the anchors on a 2' × 3' board.

are using the loudness anchors of Cox (1995), it is appropriate to also use the instructions that were developed in association with these anchors. They are provided in Figure 4–12 (and also Appendix J). We have modified Cox's instructions slightly, by adding the sentence "It is okay to repeat a loudness category, and it is okay to skip a category," as we've found that patients sometimes have problems regarding these issues. For example, they give a #6 rating when it really is a #7 because they think they have to say #6 at least once, or they immediately go from #4 to #5 because the tone got louder, and they already had said #4 once. Perhaps the most important statement of the instructions is at the end, " . . . louder than you would ever choose on your radio no matter what mood you are in." What we are looking for is when the sound is *first* uncomfortable. Audiologists who are somewhat haphazard in delivering LDL instructions often say something like, "we want to see what you can tolerate." The difference between *uncomfortable* and *tolerate* can be 10 to 20 dB for some patients. We can assure you that when new hearing aid users experience an environmental noise that exceeds their LDL, they do not sit back and say, "Gee, I wonder if I could tolerate that?" Rather, they turn down gain as quickly as possible, which often makes soft speech inaudible. Alternatively, in cases where there is no volume control, the patient may reject the hearing aids completely.

We find it convenient to paste the written instructions on the back of the board that has the loudness anchors on the front. This way you can be reading (yes, *reading*) the instructions while the patient is looking at the anchors. We cannot overstate the importance of using precise and consistent instructions when the goal is a reliable and valid measure.

Test Procedures

Typically, LDL testing is conducted in the test booth, as that is where the equipment is located, and the patient is already seated and hooked up to earphones for the diagnostic testing. If the equipment is available in a hearing aid fitting room, there is no reason that earphone LDL testing could not be conducted there instead, as ambient room noise is not an issue. Once the patient is seated, the earphones have been inserted properly (deep fit of foam tip), the patient has the loudness anchors and the instructions have been given, we recommend the following protocol:

- Use pulsed pure tones as test signal and select frequency.
- First, conduct practice run.
- Begin testing at or near the patient's MCL (e.g., 60 to 70 dB HL).

LDL Instructions

THE PURPOSE OF THIS TEST IS TO FIND YOUR JUDGMENTS OF THE LOUDNESS OF DIFFERENT SOUNDS.

YOU WILL HEAR SOUNDS THAT INCREASE AND DECREASE IN VOLUME. YOU MUST MAKE A JUDGMENT ABOUT HOW LOUD THE SOUNDS ARE. PRETEND YOU ARE LISTENING TO THE RADIO AT THAT VOLUME. HOW LOUD WOULD IT BE?

AFTER EACH SOUND, TELL ME WHICH OF THESE CATEGORIES BEST DESCRIBES THE LOUDNESS. IT IS OKAY TO REPEAT A LOUDNESS CATEGORY, AND IT IS OKAY TO SKIP A CATEGORY.

KEEP IN MIND THAT AN UNCOMFORTABLY LOUD SOUND IS LOUDER THAN YOU WOULD EVER CHOOSE ON YOUR RADIO NO MATTER WHAT MOOD YOU ARE IN.

Figure 4–12. Instructions that are read to the patient prior to administering LDL measures (modified from Cox, 1995).

- Present signal and obtain rating (probably #4).
- Use ascending approach in 5 dB steps and obtain loudness rating for each subsequent level.
- Stop run at the level that results in the first #7 rating.
- Following the practice run, repeat procedure.
- After again establishing the #7 rating, conduct a second run.
- If the #7 rating of the second run is within 5 dB of the first, average the two and record this as the LDL. If the difference is larger than 5 dB, conduct a third run and average the last two.
- Repeat the procedure for other selected frequencies (practice run no longer necessary).
- Repeat the procedure for the other ear.

An example of calculating LDL is shown in Figure 4–13. In this case, we are using the worksheet from Robyn Cox, which is available at her website (http://www.memphis.edu/csd/harl/index.htm). For this patient, testing started at 500 Hz in the right ear. The first run produced a #7 rating of 90 dB HL. Notice that the #7 rating for the second run was 100 dB, 10 dB above the first, so a third run was conducted. The average of the second and third runs resulted in an average LDL of 98 dB (100 + 95 / 2, and rounded up). For 3000 Hz, the first and second runs resulted in the same value, so it was not necessary to conduct a third run. For the left ear, observe that the lower frequency selected was 1000 Hz rather than 500 Hz—this was because the patient had normal hearing for 500 Hz. (No hearing loss, no gain, no MPO problem!) For both frequencies tested in this ear, the #7 values fell within 5 dB for the two runs.

Notice that on the form shown in Figure 4-13, we have the loudness rating for each presentation level. Although it is interesting to see the loudness growth pattern, you really do not have to record the ratings for anything but #7. Most of us can remember the #7 value of the first run, so all you have to record is the average of the two. If that is all you are going to record, the worksheet is a bit of overkill—you could just record the #7 values on the audiogram, scratch paper, or even a bar napkin if you like.

So, now that the LDLs are measured and recorded, what happens next? Will this extra effort and time (five minutes or so) result in a better fitting? That comes next.

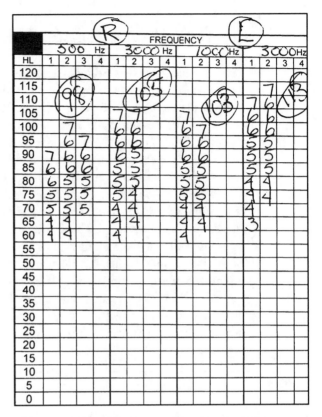

Figure 4–13. Sample score sheet completed by an audiologist while administering LDL measures for 500 and 3000 Hz for the right, and 1000 and 3000 Hz for the left. The numbers that are circled at the top represent average values for the different runs. These average values are then used for setting the hearing aid MPO. The score sheet itself is from the Cox Contour Test.

Clinical Applications

As we discussed earlier, when programming the hearing aids, one option is to enter the measured LDLs into the fitting software. And, as we also discussed (see Figure 4-9, Panels A and B), the impact this has on the setting of the hearing aid MPO varies considerably among manufacturers. If you fit most of your patients with hearing aids from a single manufacturer (85% of audiologists do), then it might be worth taking some time and entering different LDLs into the software (e.g., all 80s, all 90s, all 100s, etc.) and observe how this influences the MPO settings. Do they change? Do the settings agree with your beliefs? It is possible that the manufacturer(s)

TECHNICAL TIP: BILATERAL LDLS FOR BILATERAL FITTINGS?

A common question regarding LDL measures is if it is necessary to conduct bilateral LDLs for a bilateral fitting. On the surface, it would seem that this might be necessary, as we know that usually there are binaural summation effects that can be 6 dB or more at suprathreshold levels. But, it is not that simple. First, the binaural loudness summation that can impact listening through hearing aids may not be the same as experienced with earphone testing or unaided soundfield measures. A partial explanation is that full summation can occur only when the inputs are the same at both ears (and eardrums). That rarely occurs, especially across the frequency range. Second, it seems that summation may be present when the task is a loudness matching paradigm, but when it is couched in loudness discomfort terms, the summation is not observed. This could be related to the improved sound quality of bilateral listening, which may counteract the summation effects that are present (see Mueller and Bright [1994] and Mueller and Hornsby [2002], for review). The fact that bilateral LDLs are essentially the same as unilateral ones is a good thing for both the patient and the audiologist. For the patient, it means that the ceiling of their dynamic range was not reduced, so with bilateral summation effects, the overall dynamic range should be expanded. For audiologists, it means that each ear can be treated independently without making alterations when and if the patient uses bilateral amplification.

---

that you use will do these calculations correctly. If not, we recommend the procedure outlined below.

Converting to 2-cc Coupler

A continual disconnect in the fitting of hearing aids is that we conduct testing in HL; manufacturers commonly provide hearing aid software referenced to 2-cc coupler levels in SPL, and we verify hearing aids in ear canal SPL. As a result, we are continually converting among the three references. If that makes you feel like you are going in a circle, you might enjoy Larry Revit's article, "Circle of Decibels" (Revit, 1997), which nicely illustrates these relationships. So for our task at hand, we

have LDLs in HL, but we want to program hearing aid MPO for specific frequencies, which are defined in 2-cc coupler SPL. How do we get from HL to the 2-cc coupler levels? Fortunately, this is more common of a correction than you might think, and we have an ANSI standard (S3.6-2004) for making these corrections. These values are referred to as *RETSPLs*. This is an acronym for the Reference Equivalent Threshold in SPL and is pronounced *Rhet-Spull*, in case you are curious. It is the difference between HL and the output in a 2-cc or 6-cc coupler. The reason that this is commonly used is that audiometers are calibrated using RETSPL values. For our discussion here, things work out conveniently, as insert earphones, which you used for conducting

---

TECHNICAL TIP: THINKING ABOUT THE RETSPL

One of our favorite quiz questions for audiology students or interns is to ask them to describe the expected differences in the RETSPL for infants versus adults. We have had some interesting answers over the years. The point of course, is that RETSPLs are *device* specific, not *people* specific. You use the same RETSPL corrections for big ears and tiny ears. In contrast, Real-Ear Coupler Differences (RECDs) are *ear* specific.

the LDL measures, are calibrated in a 2-cc coupler, just like hearing aids. If we convert HL values using the RETSPL, it makes it easy to talk to the fitting software, which also is in the language of 2-cc SPL, when adjustments are needed.

As mentioned, RETSPL values for insert earphones are contained in ANSI Standard S3.6-2010, and these values are shown in Table 4–2. Note that the values are somewhat different for the two types of 2-cc couplers commonly used with hearing aids (HA1 and HA2); although except for 4000 and 6000 Hz, these differences are small. For our example here, we will use the HA1 coupler values (the coupler type commonly used with custom hearing aids such as ITEs). These are mostly positive numbers, which means that they are *added* to the HL values to convert to 2-cc. Refer back to our LDL testing shown in Figure 4–13. Note that the LDL for 500 Hz was 98 dB, and the LDL for 3000 Hz was 105. Using the corresponding RETSPLs from Table 4–2, we would then do the following corrections:

For 500 Hz: 98 + 6.0 = 104 dB (re: 2-cc coupler)

For 3000 Hz: 105 + 2.5 = 107.5 (108) dB (re: 2-cc coupler)

This little bit of simple math gives us the values that we need to go into the fitting software and make the necessary adjustments for this patient.

Software Adjustments

All manufacturers have methods to adjust the MPO in their fitting software, and in most cases, this can be accomplished relatively independently of gain for soft, average, and loud(er) input levels. As a consequence, it is preferable to adjust the gain and low threshold compression parameters so that loud speech is loud but okay, and then use the MPO adjustment to assure that loud environmental noises do not exceed the LDL. Rather than having default controls for gain and compression parameters, most modern hearing aids have separate handles (sometimes within each compression channel) to control gain for soft, average, and loud input levels in addition to MPO control and sometimes control of gain for even more input levels. That is, there are different controls for different purposes. In modern hearing aids, these controls attempt to directly affect gain and output as a function of input, but the exact gain, compression, and limiting algorithms manipulated to do this are often kept out of view. When AGCo compression is used to limit the hearing aid output, the compression ratios are usually 10:1 or greater, so the AGCo kneepoint and the MPO value tend to be essentially the same. It is also possible to implement lower threshold compression using smaller compression ratios and then use peak clipping to limit the output, but that approach is much less common in modern hearing aids.

We encourage you to work through this MPO adjustment process with the software from your favorite manufacturer, but we have given you two examples here. One thing that has changed in recent years is that we now have the capability of setting the MPO independently for many different channels. It was not too long ago that the MPO was adjusted in hearing aids using a single-channel output limiter, commonly implemented using AGCo, meaning that you had to pick one value, which usually was driven by the real-ear peak of the response, set the MPO to this value, and then let the MPOs at all the other frequencies fall where they may. This still is seen in a few hearing aids including some entry level models. Single channel limiting, in an effort to set the MPO low enough for one specific frequency, often meant unnecessarily reducing headroom for many others. By comparison, in the two examples that we have here, one product has 16 adjustment possibilities for 16 channels of AGCo; the other product has 10 "handles," which control 64 channels of AGCo—enough MPO software adjustment capability to satisfy even the most fastidious audiologist.

Table 4–2. Reference Equivalent Threshold values in SPL (RETSPL) for Insert Earphones from ANSI S3.6-2004

	250	500	1K	1.5K	2K	3K	4K	6K
3A/5A insert (HA-1)	14.5	6.0	0.0	0.0	2.5	2.5	0.0	−2.5
3A/5A insert (HA-2)	14.0	5.5	0.0	2.0	3.0	3.5	5.5	2.0

Figure 4–14 illustrates the MPO adjustment screen from one manufacturer. Note that there are 16 channels, and the lower values in the chart represent the MPO settings for the average patient with this degree of hearing loss. In the software, this display is accompanied by a graph of the output, which we are not showing due to space limitations. Going back to our earlier calculations, we would simply go to the 500 Hz tab and set the MPO, currently set at 105 dB, to 104 dB—for 1 dB it may not be worth the effort. In some low power instruments, the output at 500 Hz might not go to 104 dB, which in this case we would simply set it as high as it goes. We would then go to 3000 Hz and set this MPO (currently set at 116 dB) to 108 dB. Then, using basic interpolation, we would set all the other intermediate channels to correspond to these values accordingly (e.g., increasing gradually from 104 to 113 dB).

Figure 4–15 shows the MPO adjustment screen from a different manufacturer, which uses a somewhat different approach. Again, these tabs are accompanied by a graphic display of the 2-cc coupler output, which can be used as a visual reference, displayed in Figure 4–16. This manufacturer allows you to control the MPO for 64 channels by using 1, 2, 4, or 10 handles; we are showing the 10-handle option. Note that the values displayed are not absolute SPL, but rather negative numbers (e.g., –9,

200	500	1K	1.5	2K	2.5	3K	3.5	4K	4.5	5K	5.5	6K	6.5	7K	7.5	ALL
-7	-7	2	2	7	12	14	12	10	8	8	2	-1	-3	-4	-6	Loud
3	3	12	12	17	21	23	22	20	18	16	10	7	4	0	-4	Moderate
13	13	20	20	24	30	32	30	27	24	22	16	13	9	5	1	Soft
98	105	111	111	114	114	116	116	112	109	107	103	101	100	99	98	MPO

Figure 4–14. Screenshot from the software of a major manufacturer illustrating the selection of frequency-specific MPO across several channels. MPO values are displayed in the bottom row.

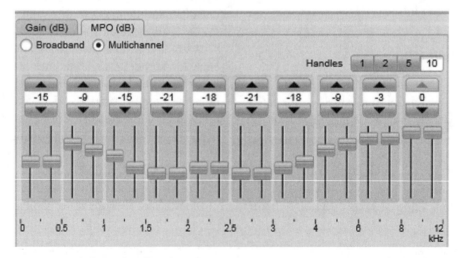

Figure 4–15. Screenshot from the software of a major manufacturer illustrating the selection of frequency-specific MPO across several channels. The values shown across the top row represent what has been subtracted from maximum MPO for each channel (e.g., if the maximum power output available for this instrument was 118 dB SPL, the programmed MPO of this patient for the 2000 to 2500 region would be 100 dB (118 − 18 = 100 dB).

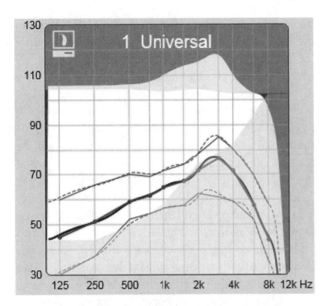

Figure 4–16. Graphic display of the OPSP90 for a given instrument (corresponding to Figure 4–15).

−15, etc.). This represents the dB value that the maximum MPO has been reduced. (The max values are displayed on the graphic display in Figure 4–16 that we mentioned.) So if we again take our desired setting of 104 dB at 500 Hz, we see that the max MPO for 500 Hz is 108 dB (see Figure 4–16), so we would set the tab to −4 dB to obtain our desired MPO. For 3000 Hz, the max output is 118 dB, and our desired setting is 108, so we would set this tab to −10 dB. Like before, we would then interpolate and set the intermediate MPOs accordingly. For patients like this, where the LDL configuration is pretty flat across frequencies, we would probably only use 4 handles instead of 10, as that would speed up the process, with no reduction in accuracy.

Although these type of adjustments might seem a little confusing the first few times, they quickly become routine. And we have to believe that you and your patient will be in a better place than if you had randomly picked a value within a range of 50 to 60 dB (shown in Figure 4–8).

FAQs about LDL Measures

Once audiologists begin conducting LDLs routinely, there tends to be a lot of clinical questions, so we thought we'd end this section with some FAQs.

How Many Frequencies to Test?

Although the *more is better* adage usually applies, we do need to be practical—how much information is really needed to make a good clinical judgment? There is no reason to waste time in a busy clinic conducting LDLs at unnecessary frequencies when that time could be spent conducting other pre-fitting measures or patient counseling. Two frequencies/ear usually are enough, although for some configurations, three probably works a little better. Fortunately, most hearing aids today have multichannel MPO control, but if you are fitting a hearing aid with single-channel, then one frequency is probably enough—it is hoped you pick the right one—as you will not be able to shape the output signal anyway. The overall MPO simply will be moved up or down as a whole based on the lowest LDL, which will determine the setting.

What Are the Best Frequencies to Test?

It would be nice if we could simply give you two frequencies to test and that was all you had to remember. It is not that simple, as the *best* LDL frequencies change from patient to patient. Here are some general rules to remember:

- If the patient has a relatively flat or gradually downward sloping hearing loss across all frequencies, we recommend conducting LDL measures at 500 or 1000 Hz and 3000 Hz. If the hearing loss is not changing significantly frequency to frequency, we certainly would not expect that the LDLs would either. Hence, if you have a value at 500 Hz and one at 3000 Hz, you could set the MPO at the intermediate frequencies by interpolation.

- Many patients have normal hearing in the lower frequencies. If it is obvious that you will not be applying gain for 500 Hz, or very little gain, then there is no reason to conduct LDLs for this frequency, as the MPO setting will not impact the fitting. The patient has normal hearing at 1000 Hz? Then the same logic applies for this frequency.

- As we discuss in a later section of this chapter relating to cochlear dead regions, some patients have downward sloping hearing losses where the extent of the loss makes it very unlikely that we can obtain aided audibility using traditional amplification (e.g., loss of approximately 90 dB or greater). In this case, we might decide to give up on chasing this frequency and even roll-off gain to help prevent feedback. So again, if we are not planning on applying gain, then there is no reason to conduct LDLs at this frequency.

■ To summarize our points, although we often will conduct LDLs for the two frequencies of 500 and 3000 Hz to obtain loudness anchors for the corners of the fitting range, let's take a patient with normal hearing through 1000 Hz, dropping to a 30 dB loss at 1500, down to 60 dB at 2000 Hz, and then 90 dB thresholds at 3000 and 4000 Hz. Although not a common audiogram for a hearing aid fitting (fortunately), we do see audiograms like this. So what are the LDL testing rules for this patient? Well, if the lows are normal, and we are not going to chase the highs, then in this case we would do LDL testing at 1500 and 2000 Hz, as this is the frequency region where a correct setting of the MPO will most probably determine the success of the fitting.

Several Audiologists Use Speech Signals, Such as Spondee Words to Obtain LDLs: Is This an Acceptable Substitute for Pulsed Tones?

In a word, no. The reason for conducting earphone LDLs is to determine the values for setting *frequency-specific* MPO values —the level at which output is limited. Consider this example—your Monday morning patient being fitted for hearing aids has a gradually downward sloping hearing loss ranging from 30 dB in the lows to 75 dB at 4000 Hz. You do speech LDLs and obtain values of 95 dB bilaterally? How do you convert this HL value to 2-cc coupler, so you can talk to the software? How do you use this number to set the AGCo kneepoint at 1000 Hz? At 3000 Hz? At any frequency? We are aware that there are some state dispensing laws that specify that speech material be used for LDL measures. We are not sure why this would ever be the case.

For Patient Flow Purposes, When Is the Best Time to Conduct LDLs?

If you have worked in a busy clinic, you know that what is time-consuming for most audiometric testing is often not the test itself, it is things like finding a booth that is free, getting the patient back to the booth, listening to the patient's stories about their grandchildren, getting the inserts to fit deep enough, and so on. For this reason, we recommend conducting LDL testing the same time that the routine audiogram is conducted. The patient is already seated, they just had some practice listening to pulsed tones, and now all you have to do is go in the room, hand them the loudness chart, and explain the test procedure. Granted, at this point you do not know if the patient will decide to purchase hearing aids, and you indeed will end up conducting testing for many patients who do not, but it still will increase your efficiency in the long run. Moreover, even if the patient does not return for hearing aids for a year or so, if a check of audiometric thresholds at that time reveals that thresholds have not changed, there is a good chance LDLs are the same too, and your testing will already be completed.

Why Use Pure Tones for Testing? The Patients Do Not Hear Pure Tones in the Real World

We partially already answered this earlier when we explained that we somehow have to talk the language of the fitting software, which are values based on 2-cc coupler, pure-tone measures. It is true that listeners do not normally hear pure tones in their daily environment, but they do hear narrowband signals that drive the output of the hearing to a level nearly as high (shrill dog bark, baby crying, clattering of dishes). Our goal is to prepare the patient for a worse-case situation. Moreover, recall that we recommend setting the hearing aid to the #7 rating, which in fact is uncomfortable. We could use #6, which is typically 3 to 5 dB lower, but because the hearing aid is seldom driven to the output produced by a pure tone, we have a cushion of a few dB, and the #7 rating from pure-tone testing seems to work pretty well in the real world. This was supported by the work of Bratt et al. (2002) and Munro and Patel (1998). And, of course, before the patient ever leaves the clinic, we will conduct aided LDL testing using loud speech and obnoxious environmental noises (see the loudness verification section of Book Three), so we should always be okay.

Is It Okay to Use a Warble Tone or Narrowband Noise as the Stimulus?

This is a common question and the short answer is that it probably does not matter. But, we wonder, why you would want to use these stimuli? Given that pulsed pure tones work well for audiometric thresholds and that the patient has just had practice listening to these signals during the audiometric threshold measurements, it seems logical to use these signals for LDL testing too. Why introduce a new signal that could possibly confuse the patient?

Are the Results of LDL Testing Reliable?

The reliability certainly is adequate for clinical measures. This has been studied quite extensively with similar findings among researchers—test/retest variability is around 3 to 4 dB, not much worse than for pure-tone thresholds (Hawkins et al., 1987; Ricketts & Bentler, 1996). The variability will be somewhat influenced by the test procedure employed. Palmer and Lindley (1998) used a LDL test protocol very similar to what we recommended earlier (an ascending method using the Cox Seven-Point Contour Anchors and Cox instructions). They reported a mean test-retest difference of 2.6 dB across five test frequencies for the #7 (uncomfortably loud) anchor rating; 94% of the test-retest differences were less than 10 dB. Related to this question, we might mention that there also does not appear to be a learning effect for the task—repeat measures days or weeks after the initial testing have not shown large differences (Cox, Alexander, Taylor, & Gray, 1997; Palmer & Lindley, 1998).

What If the Patient's LDLs Are Above the Limits of the Audiometer?

With TDH earphones the upper limit of most audiometers is 120 dB HL, which is probably loud enough (although Bentler and Cooley, 2001, appear to have gone to 130 dB in their data collection!) But with insert earphones, the maximum output usually drops to 110 dB, or even lower. Assuming that most audiologists are using insert phones, this can be somewhat of a problem. First, however, if the patient's LDL is greater than 110 dB HL, then you already know that this is not a "sound sensitive" individual, so the exact hearing aid MPO setting is probably not as critical as for someone who is. If you are getting #6 ratings (Cox Anchors) for 110 dB, then it's fairly safe to assume that the LDL is around 115 dB or so—usually, we see a 5 dB or so difference between the #6 rating and the patient's LDL(#7 rating). Or, as an alternative, for these patients you could use the predic-

tive algorithm for MPO from your prescriptive fitting method (e.g. the NAL-NL2). And of course, you'll still have your aided verification ahead of you to do the final tweaking of the AGCo kneepoints.

Does the Patient's LDL Go Up After Hearing Aid Use?

A reasonable question, because if it did, it would be necessary to reassess LDLs periodically after the hearing aid fitting and then readjust the MPO settings accordingly. At one time (e.g., 1940s), researchers actually suggested *tolerance training* to expand the useable dynamic range.[23] Tolerance training is not part of our fitting practices today—at least it is not conducted intentionally.

Research that has examined LDLs after hearing aid use has sometimes noted a slight increase, but there does not seem to be a significant change in loudness perceptions (e.g., Bentler, Niebuhr, Getta, & Anderson, 1993; Hamilton & Munro, 2010; Lindley, Palmer, Durrant, & Pratt, 2000). These studies, however, did not purposely expose patients to outputs above their LDLs, but rather initially fit the hearing aids with output corresponding with the patient's unaided loudness ratings. Similarly, Bratt et al. (2002) followed potential changes in LDLs over a nine-month period following the fitting of hearing aids for 360 patients and noted an average increase of the LDL of only 1 to 3 dB across the five frequencies observed (500, 1000, 2000, 3000, and 4000 Hz).

An interesting exception to all this regarding plasticity for loudness discomfort was reported by Hamilton and Munro (2010). They compared LDLs for individuals fitted bilaterally with those of patients who were fitted unilaterally; both groups had similar symmetric hearing losses. The LDLs for the group aided bilaterally were symmetrical. They found that for the patients fitted unilaterally, there was a significant interaural asymmetry of 3 to 5 dB, with higher LDLs in the fitted ear and lower LDLs in the not-fitted ear. They suggest that changes in the LDL may be a feature of asymmetric sensory input and are consistent with a central gain mechanism.

If the Patient Has a Conductive Loss, or a Large Air-Bone Gap, Is It Still Necessary to Conduct LDL Testing?

In general, we would expect that LDLs would be elevated at about a 1:1 factor of the conductive component. Known to be precise, Harvey Dillon suggests it is actually 87.5% of the conductive component. This means that if the patient has a 60 dB loss, with a 30 dB conductive component, if we use average LDL values for cochlear pathology, it is probable that the LDL is 125 dB or greater—beyond the limits of the earphones. So in many cases, testing probably is not necessary. However, (see Figure 4–8) note that some patients with a 60 dB cochlear loss have LDLs around 90 dB. If again we add the effects of the conductive component (90 + [.875 × 30]), we will have a desired MPO of around 117 dB. For this patient, you will want to adjust the hearing aid output accordingly. So, given the minimal time it takes to conduct a quick LDL check, it might be worthwhile even when a conductive loss or conductive component is present.

For Open-Canal Fittings, Do the Same Rules Apply for Setting the MPO?

Good question. We talk about that in the probe-microphone verification section of Book Three, but it is good to discuss it here too. It gets a little complicated, but stick with us (see Mueller & Ricketts, 2006, for detailed review). The technique we provided earlier for converting LDLs to 2-cc coupler, and then adjusting the MPO, is based on the assumption that the patient has an average real-ear coupler difference (RECD). If your patient truly has an open fitting, the RECD is much smaller (remember Boyles Law), which will *reduce* the ear canal SPL. But, on the other hand, the patient may retain all or most of the open ear resonances, which will *increase* the ear canal SPL. For patients who have average, or larger-than-average resonances, this will outweigh the RECD reduction, and the net effect is that the real-ear MPO will be greater with an open fitting (in the 2000 to 4000 Hz range) than with a closed fitting. You may have to set the hearing aid MPO *lower* for this frequency range for an open fitting. This of course is why we also check aided loudness during the verification process.

Why Is It Necessary to Conduct Pre-Fitting LDLs if Aided LDLs Are Assessed at the Time of the Fitting?

We certainly recommended aided loudness verification, and we discuss a protocol for this in Book Three. And, it's true that a good verification protocol could take care of many fitting mistakes that would result when pre-fitting LDL testing is not conducted. There is one factor, however, that must be considered. With some fitting algorithms, such as the DSL 5.0, the LDL that is entered into the software is not just used for selecting the maximum output. It also is used in the calculations of desired gain for soft, average and loud speech inputs. Here is a simple example to make this point. Consider a patient with a 50 dB loss who has LDLs of 110 dB—a fairly common finding. This patient has a 60 dB dynamic range. Now, what if this patient with a 50 dB hearing loss had LDLs of 90 dB—also a common finding? A 40 dB dynamic range. In general, for patients with the same hearing loss, when the dynamic range becomes smaller, the patient's preferred listening level for average speech falls at a less intense level. Some fitting algorithms, therefore, provide different fitting targets for the same hearing loss for a 40 dB versus a 60 dB dynamic range. If you wait until the verification stage, and then find out that the patient's LDLs are not what you had predicted, you may not only have to change the maximum output, but also may need to go back and change the gain for soft and average. This is why it makes sense to us to include the patient's LDLs up front, so that these values can be used in the initial programming prior to verification.

It Seems That Older People Are More Bothered by Loud Noise; Isn't This Related to Lower LDLs for This Group?

First, we already mentioned earlier that Bentler and Cooley (2001) found no effect of age in their large sample of nearly 2000 LDLs. However, *bothered by loud noise* is somewhat different than the perception of uncomfortably loud. We can, however, look at the aversiveness scale of the APHAB (described in detail in Chapter 6). The norms for this scale include aversiveness results for both young normal hearing and elderly with few or no hearing problems. If we examine the percent of problems for the two groups, the percentile distributions are very similar. If anything, the elderly are less bothered by loud noises—the 50th percentile for the young listeners is 20% problems, for elderly the 50th percentile is 10%. These were people, however, with normal or near-normal hearing. But in general, data to date does not support setting the hearing aid MPO any differently for the elderly than for younger adults when both groups have the same LDLs.

What If Some Patients Simply Don't Understand the Task?

This does happen on occasion. The tip-off usually is when you raise the intensity of the tone by 5 dB, and the patient calls out a number lower than what they had rated the previous softer signal. We usually try reinstructing, and give it one more shot. If problems still occur, we then just predict the MPO from the pure tones using an approach such as that used by the NAL-NL2. In a typical clinic, we'd estimate that 90 to 95% of the patients understand the LDL task well enough to provide valid and reliable responses.

At What Point Do Low LDLs Mean the Patient Has Hyperacusis?

There has been a lot of talk about *hyperacusis* in recent years, and indeed individuals suffering from this under-researched condition do have lower-than-average LDLs. You've probably also heard terms related to hyperacusis such as as phonophobia, misophonia, and selective sound sensitivity syndrome, known as 4S (see Hall, 2013 for review). Given that it's sometimes difficult to differentiate these disorders, we'll refer to the general condition as "decreased sound tolerance" (DST).

For the most part, the patient with DST is a different type of patient than we have been talking about here. DST is not related to cochlear disorders, and in fact, the typical patient with this disorder has normal hearing. In some instances, the term hyperacusis has been inappropriately applied; a patient who simply has LDLs somewhat lower than average is labeled hyperacusic. A comprehensive review of this pathology was provided by Baguley (2003), and in this review, he gives the following definition for hyperacusis:

> *Hyperacusis* has been defined as "unusual tolerance to ordinary environmental sounds" and, more pejoratively, as "consistently exaggerated or inappropriate responses to sounds that are neither threatening nor uncomfortably loud to a typical person." (p. 582)

These are patients that often will not leave the house because of the fear that a loud sound may occur. These are not the typical patients you see for hearing aid fittings who happen to have LDLs 10 to 20 dB or so below average.

In Closing

At some point in the fitting process, we have to get the MPO set correctly. You probably have heard the old adage:

> There's never enough time to do it right, but there is always enough time to do it again.

We believe that taking a few minutes to conduct earphone LDLs will pay off in streamlining the adjustments on the day of the fitting. True, we also recommend aided loudness verification, and yes, one could wait until then to set the MPO, but the process will be much simpler if the hearing aids already are at or near the desired levels. Moreover, for some fitting algorithms, the patient's LDL impacts gain for soft, average, and loud, so if you do not have it right from the beginning, you are more or less starting over with all the hearing aid programming. But more on the complete verification process in Book Three.

Real-Ear Coupler Difference (RECD)

Many of you already have heard of how the RECD applies to the fitting of hearing aids for children, and certainly that is the primary application. There are some compelling reasons, however, why we might want to consider greater use of the RECD when fitting hearing aids to adults.

1662: It Was a Very Good Year

We start this section with a word about Robert Boyle (1627–1691), a 17th-century philosopher, chemist, and physicist. In the world of audiology, he is best known for describing what is now referred to as Boyle's Law, which was published in 1662.

> Boyle's Law: This principle states that the absolute pressure and volume of a given mass of confined gas (air) are inversely proportional, if the temperature remains unchanged within a closed system. That is, if the volume of the closed space becomes smaller, the

pressure (i.e., SPL) becomes proportionally greater; if the volume becomes larger, the pressure becomes smaller. If we now relate this to the residual volume of the ear canal when an earphone tip, earmold, or hearing aid is in place, consider that if we reduce the volume by one-half —the tip is placed deeper in the ear canal, or the patient's ear canal is only one-half as large as average—then the sound pressure within this volume will double. A doubling of sound pressure corresponds to an increase of 6 dB.

Here is one example of the application: A couple in their seventies went to the audiology clinic to have their hearing tested. Bob was a big burly guy with large ear canals. His wife Mary was petite, with small ear canals. When the testing was completed, it showed that they both had bilateral downward sloping losses, and the audiologist observed that both Bob and Mary had a 50 dB loss at 2000 Hz in their right ear. Because Bob had a large ear canal residual volume following the placement of the insert earphone tip, when the audiometer dial read 50 dB HL, the output at his eardrum (what he *heard*) was 55 dB SPL. Because Mary had a small ear canal and a small ear canal residual volume, the output at her eardrum when the dial was set to 50 dB was 65 dB SPL. So Mary's hearing really was 10 dB worse than Bob's at 2000 Hz. But when Bob and Mary are fitted with hearing aids, will this 10 dB be taken into account, or will the audiologist simply enter 50 dB into the fitting software for both of them? Should it be taken into account?

Background

Not all clinicians measure an adult patient's RECD in clinical practice. But, it actually could improve the fitting. As the name suggests, the RECD is the difference between the output of a signal in the real ear versus the output of the same signal in a 2-cc coupler. Because the residual volume of the real ear with an insert earphone or hearing aid/earmold in place is nearly always less than 2 cc, the RECD value is usually a positive number (i.e., output in the ear canal exceeds the output in the coupler). As would then be expected, infants and children have larger RECDs than adults, as the residual volume is even more different than 2 cc. Because the RECDs for infants and children are less predictable, reliable Real-Ear Aided Response (REAR) measures used in hearing aid fittings are more difficult to obtain in children, and because these patients are not able to provide extensive subjective reports regarding the hearing aid fitting, RECDs are an important part of the fitting process with this population. There is no "standard" RECD per se, but several studies have collected RECD data from individuals of different ages, and provided average findings. Table 4–3 is one example, taken from the DSL5.0 (based on foam-tip inserts and the HA2 coupler).

The primary clinical application of the RECD is to use this value to predict ear canal output, which may be difficult to measure, based on the hearing aid's 2-cc coupler output, which is easy to measure. For example, if we know that a hearing aid has a maximum output of 112 dB SPL in the 2-cc coupler at 2000 Hz, and the

Table 4–3. A sampling of age-related foam-tip **HA-2 RECD** values (adapted from Audioscan Verifit User Manual).

Age/Freq	250	500	750	1000	1500	2000	3000	4000	6000
1 month	3	8	9	12	15	15	16	20	23
12 months	3	6	8	10	10	11	11	15	17
24 months	3	5	7	9	9	10	10	14	15
36 months	3	5	7	9	8	9	9	13	14
60 months	3	5	7	9	7	8	8	13	13
8 yrs–Adult	3	4	6	8	7	7	8	13	13

Values are from DSL 5.0 but differ from DSL in that values from 119 months have been used for ages>119 months. DSL 5.0 RECDs differ from DSL 4.1 RECDs.

patient's RECD is 8 dB at 2000 Hz, then we would predict that the MPO in the ear canal would be 120 dB SPL (112 dB + 8 dB). Or, if you knew you wanted the output in the ear canal to be any given value, then the RECD can be applied (in this case, subtracted from the 2-cc coupler), so that the hearing aid is programmed to the corresponding desired values. This application can be used for setting both the input level- specific gain and the maximum power output (e.g., AGCo kneepoints). In other words, if RECD values are known, the hearing aid can be accurately fitted to real-ear target values in the 2-cc coupler test box.

RECD Applications for Adults

As we have mentioned, the RECD is commonly used with infants and toddlers to predict real-ear SPL when conventional probe-microphone measures for verification are not feasible. But why have we included the RECD as a pre-fitting test for adults? We talked about the RETSPL in the previous LDL section, but to help explain why the *individual* (rather than average) RECD might be useful for fitting adult patients, it is necessary to introduce another term, the REDD.

> REDD: This acronym is the Real-Ear Dial Difference. As the name indicates, it is the difference between the intensity setting in HL on the audiometer dial, and the output in the ear canal. It is composed of the RETSPL, which takes us from the audiometer HL to the 2-cc coupler, and the RECD, which takes us from the 2-cc coupler to the real ear. If you like formulas: REDD = RECD + RETSPL. The REDD also can be assessed directly, by using probe-microphone equipment to measure the ear canal SPL when a pure tone is presented from the audiometer. The primary use of this correction factor is related to the probe-microphone verification of hearing aid performance. For example, if we know a patient's HL threshold is 50 dB at 3000 Hz, the RETSPL for 3000 Hz is 3 dB, and the patient's RECD is 8 dB at 3000 Hz (which would then give us an REDD of 11 dB), then we would calculate that the patient's threshold in ear canal SPL would be 61 dB for 3000 Hz (50 + 11 dB).

When we conduct REAR measures such as *speech mapping* with our probe microphone equipment, the patient's thresholds and the LDLs are converted to ear canal SPL from the HL values using the REDD. It is common to use the average REDD for this conversion, which includes the average RECD—recall that RETSPLs are not patient specific. The converted thresholds shown on the screen are then often used to determine if soft sounds have been made audible, and if average speech is matching prescriptive targets, which have been derived from these average values. The converted LDLs are used to determine if the MPO of the hearing aid falls into the appropriate region. Consider, however, that if the patient's RECD differs significantly from average, the on-screen ear canal SPL plots will not be correct, and potentially, what might appear as a good fitting, might not be as good as it looks.

RECD Variability

It is important, therefore, to consider what variability might exist in adult RECDs and how this variability might affect hearing aid fittings. One of the first studies on this topic was published by Valente, Potts, Valente, Vass, and Goebel (1994). Part of the design of the study was to compare supra-aural (TDH39) earphones with insert earphones (ER3A). Given that today, insert earphones are routinely used, we only refer to these results, and they are displayed in Table 4–4. These data are from 50 adult ears; a 90 dB HL pure-tone signal at the frequencies shown was the input stimulus. The mean values are the resulting output ear canal SPLs that were measured (top line on Table 4-4)—the difference between these values and 90 dB would be the mean REDD. For the present discussion, however, our interest is not so much with the absolute REDD, but rather in the variability, shown by the standard deviations and the range for each frequency. Notice that for the key frequencies of 2000 to 4000 Hz, standard deviations are 4.0 to 5.6 dB, with ranges of 20 to 29 dB. If we look at 3000 Hz, where the range is the largest at 29 dB, in practical terms this means that for two different patients with the same hearing loss expressed in HL, their true hearing loss may differ by this amount. Obviously, this could affect prescribed gain and output. Also, consider that this was a research study where the earphone foam tip was carefully placed at a controlled depth. Everyday clinical differences could be even larger.

The largest database for adult RECDs was reported by Saunders and Morgan (2003). Their work included 1,814 ears of 904 subjects; 69% were male. They report

Table 4–4. Mean and Output Range of 90 dB HL Input Signal Measured in the Ear Canal of 50 Adults

ER-3A Earphones						
Frequency	500 Hz	1000 Hz	1500 Hz	2000 Hz	3000 Hz	4000 Hz
Mean	88.9	92.9	96.3	99.5	92.6	88.7
SD	5.8	2.9	4.3	5.6	4.0	5.6
Range	23.0	12.0	21.0	29.0	20.0	25.0

Real-ear SPL values shown were obtained using 90 db HL input signal. Mean REDDs can be calculated by subtracting 90 dB from the mean output values shown in the top line (Adapted from Valente et al., 1994).

KEY CONCEPT: AUDIOGRAM INTERPRETATION FOR YOUNG CHILDREN

Our discussion here has centered on the effects that ear canal acoustics can have on interpreting the standard audiogram with adults. It is also important to remember this concept when viewing serial audiograms for young children that have been obtained over several years. As the young child's ear canal becomes larger when they grow, the residual ear canal cavity for the insert earphone also will become larger. This means that it will require more SPL to reach the child's threshold. This in turn will result in a higher HL value, which when recorded on the audiogram will give the appearance that hearing thresholds have become worse, when in fact they have not.

RECD standard deviations of 3.1 dB for 1000 Hz, 3.5 dB for 2000 Hz, and 5.4 dB for 4000 Hz. The range between the 5th and 95th percentiles was roughly 10 to 17 dB between 1000 Hz and 4000 Hz, increasing as a function of the frequency tested.

To illustrate how RECD variability could impact hearing aid fittings, the authors used five sample patients from their database and calculated desired NAL-NL1 fitting targets based on the individual RECDs, all for the same audiogram. These results are shown in Figure 4–17, Panel A; the NAL-NL1 fitting target for average RECDs used by this algorithm also is included. Notice that the prescribed target output varies by over 10 dB when the individual's RECDs are applied.

Saunders and Morgan (2003) mention that in clinical practice, the differences might not be as great as shown here, as if the patients had a volume control (VC), they would be able to adjust gain. The authors, therefore, arbitrarily matched gain for all prescriptive targets for 500 Hz, and the results of this are shown in Figure 4–17,

Panel B. Note that this did reduce some of the variance, but there is still a 3 to 5 dB range for most key frequencies. And, of course, many patients today are fitted with hearing aids without a VC, which would then take us back to the variability shown in Figure 4–17, Panel A.

Methods to Measure the RECD

As we have stated, calculating the RECD involves two measurements: the output of a test signal in a 2-cc coupler and in the real ear. Although this sounds rather straightforward, there are many variations possible for this measurement, which can lead to different RECDs. These differences could be as large as 10 dB or more between certain test protocols. The following summarizes some of these issues:

- Not only is the RECD dependent on the individual ear residual volume, it also is

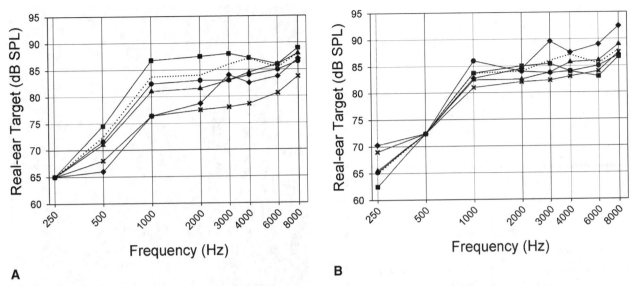

Figure 4–17. Display of how the individual RECDs can influence the calculation (and subsequent hearing aid programming) of prescribed gain. **Panel A:** Distribution of the prescribed gain for five individuals assuming the same hearing loss; the dotted line indicates the values obtained of the NAL average RECDs used. **Panel B:** Differences between the five individuals if we match the prescribed gain at 500 Hz. (Adapted from Saunders and Morgan, 2003.)

dependent on the acoustic impedance of the sound source, the coupling system, and the coupler that is used.

- The transducer for the RECD can be an insert earphone attached to an audiometer or a probe-microphone system, or a special-purpose transducer developed for RECD measures.
- Some have suggested that a hearing aid be used for the transducer (e.g., Munro & Millward, 2006)—the settings of compression and other algorithms of this hearing aid then introduce a new set of variables.
- The transducer used for the RECD measurement can be coupled to the ear using a special-purpose eartip, a foam eartip, or the patient's own custom earmold.
- Both the HA1 and the HA2 coupler have been used as the 2-cc reference, which also introduces differences.
- Although traditionally the real-ear output is measured using conventional probe-microphone measures, in recent years, two hearing aid manufacturers have introduced a

hearing aid equipped with a probe tube, that can then generate the test signal *and* measure it in the real ear, eliminating the need for probe-microphone equipment (assuming these measures are reliable and valid). This *in situ* testing is discussed in more detail later in this chapter.

As illustrated from the above review, the measurement of the RECD is not a simple straightforward matter, and this is why you will see different RECD values published, and it has been difficult to settle on a standard for RECD measures.

Clinical Applications

As we have discussed, RECDs often are used to predict real-ear hearing aid output when traditional probe-microphone measures are not feasible. When this is the purpose of the RECD, all the measurement variables we just mentioned must be carefully considered. We discuss this thoroughly in the probe-microphone verification section of Book Three.

Presently, however, we only are concerned with using the RECD for making appropriate corrections of the audiogram and the LDLs when going from HL to ear canal SPL. For this measurement, the processing and coupling of the hearing aid is not a factor, which simplifies our selection of a measurement procedure. We recommend using an insert earphone with a foam tip as the transducer. (Note: At least one probe-microphone manufacturer has a special *RECD transducer*, which is equivalent to the standard insert earphone.) Munro and Davis (2003) reported that this RECD procedure is reliable, and that when RECDs obtained in this manner were used to predict real-ear SPL and compared with measured real-ear SPL, differences usually were small (approximately 1 dB) and rarely exceeded 3 dB for any subject. That's good enough for our clinical application.

The measurement of the RECD requires probe-microphone equipment, and each manufacturer has some equipment-specific procedures. We suggest you follow their user's manual—each manufacturer provides an easy-to-follow, step-by-step protocol. In general, the protocol will be similar to the following:

- Plug the insert earphone into the earphone jack of the probe-microphone equipment (or use the special RECD transducer if available).
- Remove the foam tip and attach the insert earphone tubing to the 2-cc coupler.
- Conduct the measure and save. (This should not change significantly from day to day; it would not have to be conducted for each patient and may be stored in the equipment.)
- Place the probe tube apparatus on the ear and insert the probe tube to the appropriate depth (3 to 5 mm from eardrum).
- Place the foam tip on the earphone and insert it in the ear. Attempt to place it at the same depth that was used for audiometric threshold testing—shown in Figure 4–18.
- Conduct the measure. Depending on the equipment used, the display may show the absolute ear canal SPL output and/or the calculated RECD.

An example of the probe-microphone RECD measure using an insert earphone is displayed in Figure 4–19. What we see at the top of the screen is the real-ear output with the coupler response below it. This particular equipment then automatically subtracts these two values and

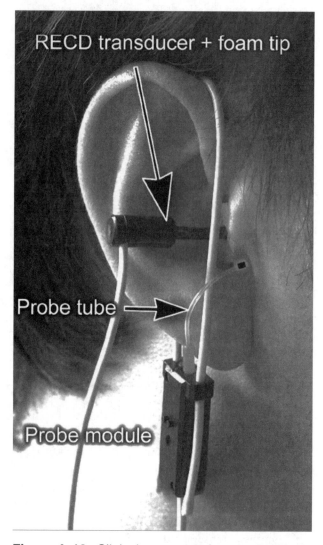

Figure 4–18. Clinical apparatus for measuring the RECD using an earphone and foam tip. (Photo courtesy of Audioscan.)

what you see on the bottom of the screen is the resulting RECD. The average RECD also is displayed, indicating that this patient's RECD is 3 to 5 dB larger than average. The RECD shown here has the general appearance of what you would expect to see, but they don't always look this "predictable." A couple things to troubleshoot when things don't look quite right:

- A negative RECD in the lower frequencies often means a poor seal.
- A negative RECD in the higher frequency suggests a plugged or poorly placed probe tip.

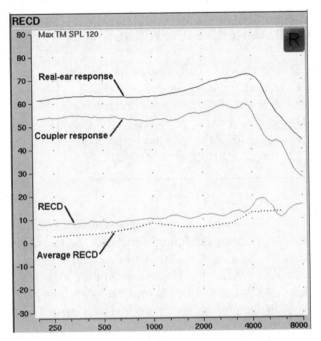

Figure 4–19. Upper portion of the chart shows the absolute values for the input signal measured in a 2-cc coupler compared with the real ear. The lower part of the chart shows the calculated difference between the two upper curves—the patient's RECD—compared with the average RECD.

■ Eardrum or middle ear pathology also might cause an unusual RECD

Applying the Measured RECD

Once the RECD has been measured, it now can be applied as a correction in fitting software, and in your probe-mic equipment. To illustrate specifically how this can impact a fitting, we conducted probe-mic speech mapping with a hearing aid programmed to provide appropriate audibility for soft speech. Shown in Figure 4–20, Panel A, is the aided soft speech output (55 dB SPL input; LTASS for the male talker of Audioscan Verifit). This display is based on average RECD values for this patient. Observe that the average of soft speech (the dark line in the speech spectrum) falls about 5 dB above the patient's threshold. This patient, however, had an RECD somewhat larger than average, fairly similar to that shown in Figure 4–19, so we entered these values into the probe-microphone software to recalculate the REDD, which in turn changes the ear canal SPL plotting of the audiogram and the LDLs. The results of this adjustment are displayed in Figure 4–20, Panel B. We need to emphasize that the output of the hearing aid is the same, but now the average of the soft speech signal is barely above the hearing thresholds.

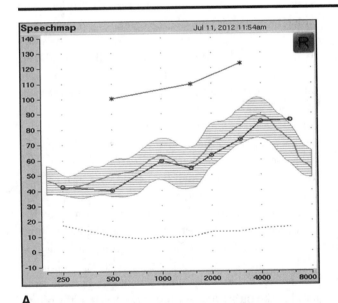

A

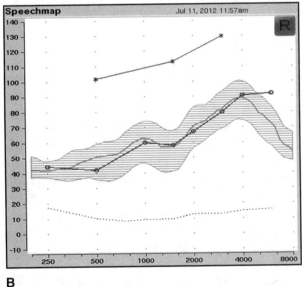

B

Figure 4–20. SPL-O-Gram plot of the patient's thresholds (dark line, connected circles) converted to ear canal SPL. Hatched area represents the amplified real speech signal from the hearing aid. *Panel A:* Hearing thresholds plotted using average corrections—note that the majority of the amplified signal appears audible (above the threshold plot) for the 2000 to 3000 Hz region. *Panel B:* Hearing thresholds plotted using the patient's measured RECD—note that now only about 50% of the speech signal is audible for the 2000 to 3000 Hz region.

> ### TECHNICAL TIP: USE OF THE INDIVIDUAL RECD FOR FITTINGS
>
> As we discuss in this section, the measured RECD can be used to individualize the fitting process, such as the example shown in Figure 4-20 regarding the assessment of audibility. But, as we mentioned, it is also possible to enter an individual RECD into some prescriptive algorithms and manufacturers' fitting software. One potential problem, however, is to use the individual RECD with an algorithm where the average RECD already has been added. Care should be taken to assure that only one RECD is used, or significant errors will result.

In Closing

The data shown in Figure 4–20 provide just one illustration of how these RECD measures can improve the accuracy of the fitting. This is a pretest that probably is best accomplished on the day of the fitting, just before probe-microphone verification begins. Recall that the objective here is to provide a more precise evaluation regarding the patient's thresholds and the ear canal SPL generated by the hearing aid. Most of the published methods recommend using the HA2 coupler as it allows for the most convenient method of attaching a BTE instrument to the coupler. In Book Three, we discuss the use of different couplers to obtain this measure, how these measures can be used for verification, and various sources of error that can impact those values.

In Situ Testing

Another pre-fitting measure that can be conducted to potentially enhance the fitting process is in situ testing. What we are referring to is audiometric thresholds or loudness judgments that are conducted using the hearing aid to transmit the test signal. In situ is a Latin term meaning in place. In this case, meaning that testing is conducted at the ear, without any external device. Related to audiology, there is sometimes confusion regarding what is meant by in situ testing, as historically, probe-microphone measures also have been referred to as in situ—that is, testing conducted in place at the ear rather than in a 2-cc coupler. There doesn't seem to be a better term to use, however, than in situ when the hearing aid is used to deliver signals, so that's what we'll use here.

When in situ testing is implemented, the testing itself is driven by the fitting software of the manufacturer. The hearing aid is fitted to the ear, and the signals are then delivered. The response from the patient (e.g., threshold, MCL, or LDL) is recorded in the software, much the same as with computerized audiomety. These digital values can then be converted to traditional HL values, or used internally by the software to alter the hearing aid fitting.

Background

In the previous section, we discussed how the RECD can be used to account for individual ear canal differences, which has the potential of improving the preciseness of the fitting. In situ audiometry can play much the same role. With the hearing aid serving as the transducer, pure tones, continuous or pulsed, are played directly into the ear for threshold testing. By doing so, many of the same ear canal acoustic properties are taken into consideration as we discussed with RECD measures. It has been suggested that determining an unaided threshold response with the hearing aid/earmold in situ is able to increase the precision of the hearing aid fitting (Kuk, 2003). With the hearing aid coupled to the ear in the same manner as the user would wear it in everyday listening situations, considerations such as residual volume of the ear canal or the effects of venting—intended or slit-leak—are accounted for in the initial stages of fitting the device. Other purported advantages include time saved in the fitting process and space saved in the office.

One possible source of concern involves the reliability of threshold measurements taken in situ. There seems to be little evidence, however, that hearing aid in situ measures are less reliable than those obtained using

> ## KEY CONCEPT:
> ## POTENTIAL USES OF HEARING AID IN SITU MEASURES
>
> Most of the major manufacturers offer the capability of using the hearing aid to conduct in situ measures. In general, we see three major areas of utilization:
>
> - Conduct audiometric testing when standard audiometry is not available, to allow for a "first fit" of a hearing aid.
> - To make corrections to standard audiometry for alteration of the fitting algorithm; this can involve changes relative to the residual ear canal volume with the hearing aid in place (as we discussed with RECD measures) or the effects of venting—applications need to be considered for open canal fittings (Keidser, Yeend, O'Brien, & Hartley, 2011).
> - For hearing aid verification of gain and output when traditional probe-microphone measures are not available.

standard TDH or insert earphones (Smith-Olinde, Nicholson, Chivers, Highley, & Williams, 2006; O'Brien, Keidser, Yeend, Hartley, & Dillon, 2010), although this has not been examined with all devices currently available.

Administration

Obtaining in situ thresholds is similar to obtaining thresholds in a more traditional manner. The patient is seated near the computer used for programming of the hearing aid. The patient's earmold or an appropriate dome tip (depending on the manufacturer and the model of hearing aid chosen) are inserted into the ear. Several of the systems also allow for an evaluation of the environment to determine if the ambient noise level is acceptable. A screen shot of one of those systems is shown in Figure 4–21. The patient is instructed to indicate (by raising of the hand or finger) when he or she hears the tone in the test ear. Depending upon the hearing in the non-test ear, it is advisable to plug that ear to avoid any false positive responses. The thresholds are obtained in the manner of choice (e.g., down 10, up 5) by the examiner with the computer functioning very much like current computer-based audiometers, with the keyboard or the mouse tracking the frequencies and intensities.

Examples of two of the screens used for in situ testing are shown in Figures 4–21 and 4–22. Currently, there

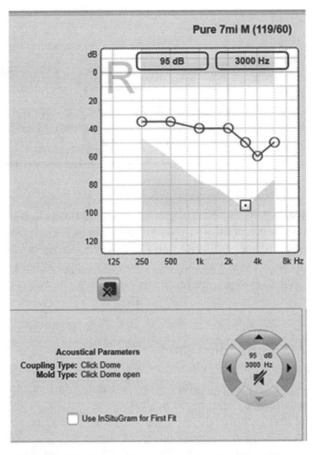

Figure 4–21. Example of screenshot from in situ testing. (Results for the same patient tested with an instrument and software from a different manufacturer is shown in Figure 4–22.)

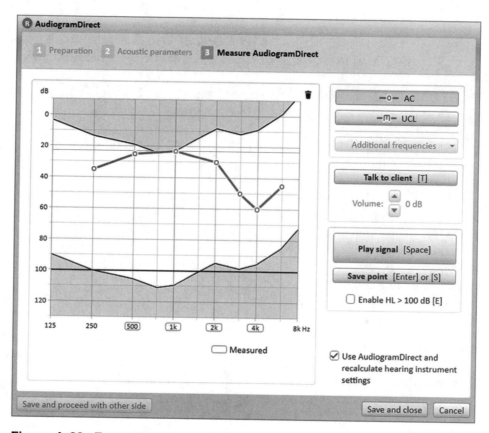

Figure 4–22. Example of screenshot from in situ testing. (Results for the same patient tested with an instrument and software from a different manufacturer is shown in Figure 4–21.)

are six manufacturers of hearing aids that provide in situ testing capabilities in their software. Table 4–5 shows some of the similarities and differences across these options. It is obvious that the frequency ranges, intensities, and even graphic presentation can vary. The manner in which the collected data are used, also will vary.

A Comparative Study

As we mentioned earlier, research has shown that the reliability of hearing aid in situ-testing is good. Many audiologists use this as a replacement or addition to conventional pure-tone thresholds when hearing aids are fitted. This seems to be particularly true when a manufacturers' proprietary fitting algorithm is utilized.

Given that there are now a number of manufacturers who have in situ testing available, we questioned

if the same thresholds would be obtained for a given patient with the different systems. This of course is a different question than test reliability. To do this, we used the right ear of a 64-year-old male patient with a confirmed cochlear hearing loss. For each manufacturer, we used their premier mini-BTE RIC product, and the manufacturer's "closed" fitting tip In general, the tightness of the different domes was similar among manufacturers. Testing was conducted in a quiet hearing aid fitting room.

In Figure 4–23, the results of in situ testing are shown for the hearing aid patient. The circles indicate the measures obtained using a calibrated audiometer and insert earphones. Each of the other symbols represents the thresholds obtained using the six in situ options. There is a noticeable difference observed in the low frequencies, with all in situ thresholds lower than earphone, some as much as 20 to 30 dB. This is no doubt a

Table 4–5. Comparison of In Situ Audiometry Measurement Parameters

Manufacturer	Frequency Range	Intensity Range	Overlays	Measurement of TDs	Mouse or Keyboard Control	Stimuli
Oticon	250–8000 Hz	20/40 to 65/110 dB HL*	None	Can be measured, but not stored	Keyboard	Continuous or Pulsed Pure Tone
Phonak	250–6000 Hz	20/25 to 80/100 dB HL*	None	Yes	Keyboard	Continuous Pure Tone
ReSound	250–6000 Hz	20 to 80/100 dB HL*	Speech Banana, Phonemes, and Familiar Sounds	Can be measured, but not stored	Keyboard	Continuous or Pulsed Pure Tone
Siemens	250–6000 Hz	10 to 40/95 dB HL*	None	Yes	Both	Continuous Pure Tone
Starkey	250–4000 Hz	30 to 100/120 dB HL*	Speech Spectrum and Familiar Sounds	Yes	Both	Continuous or Pulsed Pure Tone
Widex	125–8000 Hz	0 to 80/120 dB HL*	None	No	Mouse	Pulsed Chirp

*Intensity range depends on frequency and instrument model.

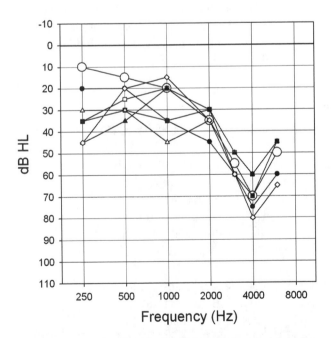

Figure 4–23. In situ thresholds obtained using the software and hearing aids (mini-BTEs) from six major manufacturers, using the manufacturers' stock closed fitting tips. Earphone thresholds are shown for comparison (*larger open circles*).

reflection of the leakage from the fitting tip, when compared to the tight fitting foam of the insert earphone. Even in the high frequencies, we see some relatively large differences among manufactures—20 dB at 4000 and 6000 Hz. Interestingly, at 3000 Hz, all thresholds were remarkably similar.

The purpose of this testing was not to determine what method or device was best. While the earphone threshold is included as a reference, it's certainly possible that any one of the in situ thresholds might be "best" for the fitting of this product—depending on how these data are used in the software. Perhaps a more interesting question would be what real-ear gain is present for each instrument when these in situ data are applied? We show you that in the verification section of Book Three!

Threshold-Equalizing Noise Test

Another test utilizing pure tones (and noise) that can be used in the pre-fitting assessment is the threshold-equalizing noise (TEN) test. This test is designed to detect regions of the cochlea where the inner hair cells are not functional. These areas are commonly referred to as *dead zones* or *dead regions*.

Background

As you probably recall from your ear physiology studies, the basilar membrane is tuned. That is, each place on the membrane is tuned to best respond to sounds of a narrow frequency range—high frequencies toward the base and low frequencies toward the apex. The frequency that induces the maximum vibration for a given region is termed the characteristic frequency. The role of various cells is quite complex with a variety of interactions and sharing of information. A very simplified explanation of the role of various cells is that the outer hair cells sharpen the frequency-specific tuning and amplify the signal, whereas the inner hair cells detect the signal and transmit it to the cranial nerve VIII.

The majority of acquired cochlear hearing losses begin with damage to the outer hair cells. The likelihood that there will also be damage to the inner hair cells typically increases with greater hearing loss. Audiometrically, damage to the inner hair cells is usually present for hearing losses of 55 to 60 dB HL and greater. In some cases, particularly with more severe hearing loss, there may be regions where the inner hair cells become nonfunctional, which we commonly refer to as dead regions. These regions are difficult to detect with traditional pure-tone testing, as a high intensity signal in the area of a dead region will produce enough basilar membrane vibration that there will be a response (the patient hears a tone) at a different region where the inner hair cells are healthy, even though that region is not specifically tuned to the test frequency. This is most notable in steeply sloping hearing losses (either downward or upward). For example, a person with a downward sloping hearing loss with a threshold of 40 dB at 2000 Hz and a dead region at 4000 Hz, may present with a threshold of 80 to 90 dB at 4000 Hz simply because the 4000 Hz tone is being detected by neurons tuned to lower frequencies where hearing is more normal.

Why is this important for the selection and fitting of hearing aids? Research has shown that providing audibility for a frequency range within a dead region is less useful (or maybe not useful at all) than when dead regions are not present. If the clinician if fairly certain that a dead region is present, he or she might:

- Not be as aggressive in trying to provide audibility for this frequency range, which might help eliminate acoustic feedback issues.
- Provide the patient with alternative programs with and without gain for the dead regions for real-world comparison.

KEY CONCEPT: FREQUENCY-LOWERING TECHNOLOGY

- As we discuss extensively in the frequency-lowing chapter of Book Two in this series, most major manufacturers provide the option of frequency-lowering technology in their products. As the name suggests, when a severe-to-profound, high frequency hearing loss exists, this algorithm is designed to transfer important speech sounds from the higher frequencies (e.g., 3000 to 6000 Hz) where they are presumed to be inaudible to lower frequencies where there is less hearing loss, and the probabilities of audibility are greater.
- The signal transfer can be conducted using frequency compression, transposition, or duplication and lowering—different approaches are used by different manufacturers.
- If continued research reveals that this technology provides significant benefit and the magnitude of benefit equals or exceeds that provided by simply providing high-frequency amplification, then TEN test results could help determine when frequency lowering would be applied. The TEN test perhaps could even be delivered by the hearing aid itself.

■ Be more likely to consider hearing aid technology that provides frequency lowering. (This only applies to high-frequency dead regions; see "Key Concept" comments.)

■ Provide the patient specific counseling regarding the realistic benefits of high-frequency amplification.

Historically, the assessment of the tuning capabilities of the damaged cochlea was assessed by measuring tuning curves—a procedure reserved for auditory research laboratories. In 2000, Moore, Huss, Vickers, Glasberg, and Alcántara (2000) introduced the TEN test, a procedure that was relatively easy and quick to administer by clinicians. The first version of the TEN test, however, required the clinician to measure audiometric thresholds twice—once using the tones generated by the audiometer, with level specified in dB HL, and once using the tones from the TEN test CD, with level specified in dB SPL. A few years later, a second version of the TEN test was developed in which the noise was designed to give equal masked thresholds in dB HL for all frequencies from 500 to 4000 Hz for normal hearing people (Moore, Glasberg, & Stone, 2004). This version is called the TEN(HL) test. The basic concept of the TEN test is as follows:

■ The *threshold equalizing noise* is spectrally shaped so that, for normal hearing individuals, it gives equal masked thresholds for pure-tone signals at all frequencies within the test range.

■ When a patient has hearing loss and there are surviving inner hair cells corresponding to the specific test region with elevated audiometric thresholds, the test signal in that frequency region is detected by hair cells with characteristic frequencies close to that region. When this is true, the masked threshold in the equivalent noise will be similar to that for normal hearing listeners (provided that the noise intensity is sufficient to produce significant masking).

■ When the inner hair cells for the test frequency are nonfunctional, however, the signal will be detected by inner hair cells with different characteristic frequencies than the signal frequency. In such a case, it will require a higher equivalent noise level to mask these thresholds, a level significantly higher than normal.

Since the introduction of the TEN test, it has been used in numerous studies to assess the prevalence of dead regions and examine the effects these dead regions might have on speech processing and amplification requirements. Although we often think of dead regions occurring in patients who have severe-to-profound,

---

THINGS TO REMEMBER: ERBS?

If you do some reading on the history of the TEN test, you will see that the expected masked threshold, when a dead region is *not* present, is approximately equal to the nominal level of the noise specified in dB/ERB_N. You might ask, what is an ERB_N? This term is an abbreviation for the equivalent rectangular bandwidth of the auditory filter, measured using normal hearing individuals at moderate sound levels. To understand this better, the loudness perception produced by a sound (or the overall loudness) is computed by adding up the partial loudnesses produced in the ERB frequency groups. The unit of the frequency groups is the equivalent rectangular bandwidth (ERB). In some cases, the older (and now obsolete) bark scale was used instead of the ERB scale. Conversion of the physical unit of frequency F (in kHz) to the frequency group number (in ERB) is based on the following formula:

Frequency group number ERB: ERB = 21.4 log 10 (4.37F + 1)]

steeply downward sloping hearing losses, Hornsby and Dundas (2009) report that it is not quite this straightforward. Using the TEN test, these authors examined the presence or absence of cochlear dead regions for a large group of individuals (59 subjects; 117 ears) who had a wide range of downward sloping hearing losses (varying by both degree of loss and steepness). Some of their findings are summarized in Figure 4–24. Observe in the center panel of Figure 4–24, that when the TEN finding was "no dead region (DR)," there was a clear association with hearing loss. Nearly all ears (>80%) with a hearing loss 40 dB or less had negative findings, whereas very few ears with a hearing loss >80 dB had negative findings. However, if we look at the top panel of Figure 4–24, we see that when a positive finding for dead regions was obtained, there was little difference in dead region prevalence/hearing loss level once the hearing loss reached 50 dB.

Hornsby and Dundas (2009) also examined positive versus negative dead region findings as a function of hearing loss slope (steep, gradually sloping, and flat). The majority of the inconclusive findings (approximately 60%) were for subjects with a steep slope, and only 10% of the negative dead region findings were for this group. However, for conclusive positive dead region findings, the prevalence (approximately 30%) was the same for the flat slope audiograms as for the steep slope.

Clinically, when we consider utilizing frequency lowering algorithms, we usually are interested in the presence of dead regions in the 3000 to 4000 region. Specifically studying the prevalence of dead regions at 4000 Hz using the TEN test (98 ears; hearing loss ranging from 60 to 85 dB HL), Aazh and Moore (2007) report the prevalence of dead regions at 4000 Hz increased with increasing hearing loss and exceeded 50% for hearing losses greater than 70 dB. Using 70 dB HL as the cutoff criteria resulted in a sensitivity of 62% and a specificity of 63%. In agreement with Hornsby and Dundas (2009), they did not find a significant relationship between the presence of the dead region and the slope of the audiogram for the frequency region below 4000 Hz.

Administration and Scoring

Until recently, the TEN(HL) test could only be conducted by use of a CD player connected to an audiometer. In the past few years, the test has been implemented within a few PC-based audiometers including the Affin-

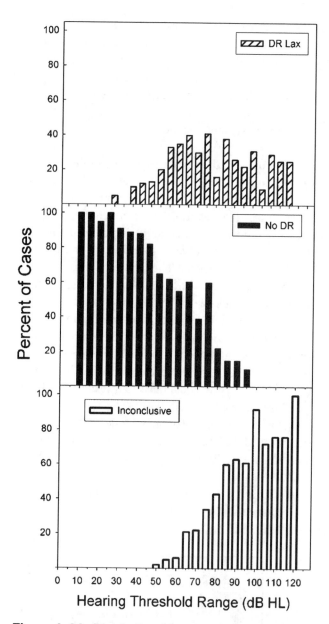

Figure 4–24. Distribution (percent of subjects) of the cochlear dead regions categorized for three classifications. **Top Panel:** Positive for the dead region using lax criteria. **Middle Panel:** Negative for the dead region. **Bottom Panel:** Inconclusive, unable to interpret due to test limitations (adapted from Hornsby and Dundas, 2009).

ity2.0 and Equinox2.0 (version 2.0.4) made by Interacoustics. For the CD version, the tones are recorded on one channel and the equalizing noise on the other. All calibrations are in dB HL, and therefore audiometric thresholds can be measured either using the tones generated by the audiometer or by using the test tones from the CD; the results should be very similar. Moore (2010) states, however, that the first CD version of the TEN(HL) test can only be used with specific (TDH39, TDH49, and TDH50) headphones. More recently, a version has been made available that can be used with the more common ER-3A insert earphones (Moore, Creeke, Glasberg, Stone, & Sek, 2012).

Administration

The test procedure for detecting a test signal in the TEN is determined using the same method as would be used for traditional audiometry, except that a 2 dB step size is used when the tone is in the region of the detection threshold; larger steps can be used initially, to find the approximate threshold. Moore (2010) provides general guidelines for administering the test:

- For frequencies where the hearing loss is less than or equal to 60 dB HL, set the TEN level to 70 dB HL.
- When the hearing loss is 70 dB HL or more at a given frequency, set the TEN level 10 dB above the audiometric threshold at that frequency.
- If the TEN is found to be unpleasantly loud, or if the maximum TEN level of 90 dB HL is reached, then the TEN level can be set equal to the audiometric threshold.
- It may be difficult or impossible to apply the TEN(HL) test when the hearing loss at the test frequency is 90 dB HL or more—although it is quite likely that a dead region would be present with such a severe hearing loss, and this might be apparent from the audiometric configuration.[24]

Scoring the TEN Test

The test is scored as either a positive or negative indicator of a dead region for each ear-specific frequency tested. The following are general guidelines regarding the scoring of the TEN test (from Moore, 2010):

- For a person with normal hearing, the threshold of the test tone in the TEN is typically equal to the TEN level. For example,

if the TEN level is set to 70 dB HL, the threshold for detecting the test tone is about 70 dB HL for any frequency from 500 to 4000 Hz.

- If a patient has a cochlear hearing loss but does not have a dead region at the test frequency, then the threshold of the test tone in the TEN is typically a few dB above the TEN level. For example, if the TEN level is set to 70 dB HL, the threshold for detecting the test tone might be around 73 dB HL. The difference between the reference level and the threshold detection level is referred to as the SNR(T).

- When the test tone frequency falls in a dead region, the threshold for detecting the test tone in the TEN is typically well above the TEN level. The criteria for diagnosing a dead region at a specific frequency are:
  1. The threshold of the test tone in the TEN is 10 dB or more above the TEN level.
  2. The threshold of the test tone in the TEN is 10 dB or more above the audiometric (absolute) threshold.
  3. If the TEN level is selected as we described earlier, then criterion #2 automatically will be satisfied when criterion #1 is satisfied.

- An example of the findings following TEN testing is displayed in Figure 4–25.

TECHNICAL TIP: TEN TEST TIME

The TEN is an ear-specific test, and it usually takes four to six minutes per ear to perform the test for all test frequencies. Typically, however, we only conduct the test for frequencies where dead regions may possibly occur. With the typical downward sloping hearing loss, we would probably only conduct the testing for the frequencies where the hearing loss was greater than 50 dB HL. With upward sloping and *cookie bite* audiograms, however, the pattern of dead regions is less predictable, and it might be wise to also test frequencies with normal or near-normal hearing.

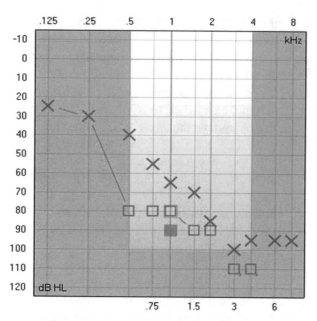

Figure 4–25. Screenshot from the Affinity/Equinox 2.2 PC based audiometer system. The *x*'s show the audiometric (absolute) thresholds. The *box* symbols show the masked thresholds measured for TEN with a level of 80 dB HL. The TEN(HL)-test criteria for a dead region are met at 1.5, 3, and 4 kHz. The result at 2 kHz is inconclusive, as the masked threshold is not 10 dB or more above the audiometric threshold. (Photo courtesy of Interacoustics.)

One consideration is scoring the TEN when the outcome is inconclusive (e.g., only slightly above or below the 10 dB criteria). We know that there are some errors associated with the measurement of the TEN. For example, in the research of Aazh and Moore (2007), of the 36 ears diagnosed as having dead regions, 11 (31%) only just met the criteria, having values of SNR(T) of 10 or 11 dB. Of the 62 subjects diagnosed as not having dead regions, 11 (18%) just failed to meet the criteria, having values of SNR(T) of 8 or 9 dB. In cases like this, it would be worthwhile to repeat the test to determine if a more definitive finding results.

Clinical Application

The clinical applications of TEN test results are based on the assumption that people with cochlear dead regions will not benefit from amplification well inside that fre-

quency region. It is important to explain what we mean by the term *well inside*. Again, we refer to the work of Brian Moore (see summary from Moore, 2010). The recommendations of Moore and his colleagues are that for a high frequency, downward sloping hearing loss, we would only apply amplification up to about 1.7 times the *edge* (beginning) of the dead region (Baer, Moore, & Kluk, 2002). For example, let's take a patient with a very steeply downward sloping hearing loss going from 30 dB at 1000 Hz, 70 dB at 1500 Hz, and 80 dB or worse above 1500 Hz. TEN test results are normal for 1000 Hz but indicate dead regions for 1500 Hz and above—in this example, 1500 Hz would be considered the edge frequency. We would then attempt to restore audibility for frequencies up to about 2500 (1500 × 1.7 = 2550 Hz), but not higher.

The audiogram example that we just used of course is not very common. More common is the audiogram where the severity of the loss does not approach dead region territory until 3000 Hz. If this were the case, according to Moore's recommendations, we then would provide amplification up to 5000 Hz (3000 × 1.7 = 5100 Hz). For the most part, this is no different than what we would do if we did not know the patient had dead regions. If the edge is at 2000 Hz, Moore's guidelines suggest providing amplification up until 3400 Hz, which would be somewhat of an alteration to the typical fitting. For this reason, Vinay and Moore (2007) suggest that for hearing aid fittings for downward sloping losses, we would conduct the TEN for the frequencies of 2000 Hz and below when the hearing loss reaches the level where dead regions may be present (e.g., approximately 60 dB).

These guidelines, however, are loosely interpreted in clinical practice. Many audiologists withhold amplification at the *suspected edge* of the dead region. We say suspected, as this decision usually is made by examining the pure-tone audiogram, not by conducting the TEN test. There are data to suggest that withholding amplification near the edge of the dead region is a mistake, and we address that at the end of this section.

Although we normally encounter high-frequency dead regions, and this is what most research has been concerned with, there also are patients with low-frequency dead regions. Although not as common, the actual impact on the hearing aid fitting might be greater for this population. For low-frequency dead regions, the guidance from research is to only amplify to 0.57 below the edge (Vinay & Moore, 2007; Vinay, Moore, & Baer, 2008).

POINTS TO PONDER: SENSITIVITY AND SPECIFICITY OF THE TEN

Sensitivity and specificity calculations for a given test usually involve a comparative *gold standard*. For the TEN test, the standard commonly used is psychophysical tuning curves (PTC). Summers et al. (2003) compared these two measures and found agreement (presence or absence) for only 10 of 18 cases (56%). The disagreement was because the TEN results suggested the presence of dead regions whereas the PTC results did not, suggesting poor specificity. More recently, Warnaar and Dreschler (2012), using a modified PTC procedure and the TEN(HL) test (*n* = 24), found an agreement between these measures of around 75% when frequency-specific agreement for each test ear was studied. If the comparison was simply the presence or absence of dead regions, then the agreement was quite good—88% (21 of 24 ears).

Consider a patient with Ménières Syndrome, with a severe loss in the lows rising to only a mild loss at 2000 Hz and above. If this patient had dead regions at 250, 500, and 1000 Hz, we then would only amplify down to 570 Hz in the lower frequencies. In this case, amplifying at and *above* the dead region is probably helpful.

Dead regions also are present in other less common audiometric configurations, such as the cookie bite, *V-shaped*, or *inverted V-shaped*. It is difficult to provide amplification rules to these configurations, and it often is helpful to utilize clinical speech testing at different sensation levels to assess the benefits of audibility (see review by Halpin, 2002). This of course is helpful for all configurations.

TEN Test Findings and Hearing Aid Adjustment

Let's talk about how we might use the TEN test results for fitting hearing aids for the typical patient. That is, not the patient with a 50 dB/octave drop in their audiogram with thresholds of >90 dB at 3000 Hz and above, but rather, people with more gently sloping audiograms with losses in the 70 to 90 dB range in the higher frequencies—the kind of hearing loss we more frequently encounter. This has been researched in several studies using real hearing aids in real-world environments (e.g, Cox, Johnson, & Alexander, 2012; Mackersie, Crocker, & Davis, 2004; Preminger, Carpenter, & Ziegler, 2005). In a nicely designed study, Cox and colleagues (2012) used 18 matched pairs to examine the effects of providing prescribed amplification (i.e., NAL-NL1 fitting algo-

rithm) versus rolling off high frequency gain (low-pass) for people with dead regions identified by the TEN test, compared with their matched pair who did not have dead regions (DR). In general, these researchers found:

- For laboratory testing of speech-recognition in quiet, both the DR group and the non-DR group had a significant benefit with the NAL fitting. The benefit was somewhat greater for the non-DR group.
- For laboratory testing of speech-recognition in noise, the DR group did not show a benefit for the NAL fitting (although their performance was not worse either). The non-DR group did show a slight benefit for the NAL fitting.
- For the ratings of speech understanding in real-world environments, both groups showed a benefit for the NAL fitting; the benefit was greater, however, for the DR group. The authors computed standardized effect sizes (Cohen's *d*) to assess the magnitude of the differences between the NAL and low-pass programs for estimated speech understanding. These effect sizes were *d* = 0.65 for listeners with DRs and *d* = 0.19 for listeners without DRs.
- Overall, 66% of the participants favored the NAL program for everyday listening over the low-pass fitting, and this preference increased to 77% for the DR group. The primary reason for favoring the low-pass fitting was the "the other fitting [NAL] was too loud."

ON THE SOAPBOX: POPULARITY OF FREQUENCY LOWERING

Earlier in this section we had a "Key Concept" pull-out about frequency lowering, and we discuss this technology extensively in the features section of Book Two, but that isn't going to stop us from getting "On The Soapbox" now for just a moment regarding this topic. As we mentioned earlier, at this writing, four of the "Big Six" manufactures have some type of frequency lowering as an option, and it may be six of six by the time you read this. Some audiologists fit the majority of their patients with this technology. Why? We know that obtaining good audibility in the high frequencies often is a struggle, fighting feedback is common, and often, even when the goal is met, the patient replies with, "Can't you make it sound less tiny?" But is this reason enough to just give up? We sometimes sense that "there might be a dead region" concept is used as a "free pass" to not try to make these high frequency sounds audible—at the frequencies where they were meant to be audible! As clearly shown in the recent work of Cox and colleagues (2012), even when dead regions are present, audibility usually does some good, and rarely does harm. Let's remember this basic concept.

Cox and colleagues (2012) conclude that "they did not observe any situation in which typical hearing aid patients with DRs were penalized by the provision of high frequency gain similar to the NAL prescription: either they benefited from more high frequency gain or they performed no worse with it."

Because some earlier work has used subjects with dead regions at several consecutive frequencies, it is important to point out that only 17% of the Cox et al. (2012) patients had dead regions below 2000 Hz, 61% only had a dead region at one frequency, and 33% only had dead regions at 4000 Hz. But again, these were typical hearing aid patients, and in their data analysis, the authors did not observe any interactions with these factors.

Our General Recommendations. Our general recommendations, therefore, for using TEN testing to assist in programming hearing aids are as follows:

Probably not too helpful for—

■ Downward-sloping audiometric configuration when the high frequency hearing loss (e.g., 3000 to 4000 Hz) is such that it is not probable that average speech can be made audible (approximately 90 dB or greater). The amplification decision based on the audiogram alone—to give up on these frequencies—will probably be no different than if it was known that dead regions are present.

■ Downward-sloping audiometric configuration when the high frequencies are aidable (e.g., approximately 65 to 85 dB). In this case, it would be reasonable to apply prescriptive gain, whether or not dead regions are present.

■ Determining when to use frequency-lowering algorithms. This would most probably be determined by the degree of high frequency hearing loss, not TEN test results (for the reasons cited in the first two examples).

Maybe helpful for—

■ Upward sloping or flat configurations when the potential exists for low-frequency dead regions or that dead regions exist for several consecutive frequencies.

■ Cookie-bite or V-shaped audiometric configurations when a severe loss exists in the mid-frequencies.

For counseling purposes, we would expect the TEN test findings to be helpful for a greater range of patients, as most research suggests that these patients do not experience the same benefit from audibility as their counterparts without dead regions. Preminger et al. (2005), for example, showed aided APHAB scores

---

TECHNICAL TIPS: SPECIAL CASES

Moore (2010) discusses two special cases regarding interpretation of TEN test findings. He states:

- Patients with auditory neuropathy sometimes have high thresholds for detecting the test tone in the TEN, meeting the TEN(HL) test criteria for diagnosis of a dead region even for frequencies where their audiometric thresholds are near-normal. This does not necessarily indicate that they have extensive dead regions, although they may have only patchy survival of inner hair cells.
- Patients may also have high thresholds for detecting the test tone in the TEN as a result of central problems (e.g., brain injury) in auditory areas resulting from trauma or a stroke. These high thresholds may result from poor *detection efficiency* rather than from dead regions.

Although the TEN test interpretation might be somewhat different in these cases, the positive TEN test finding remains suggestive that these individuals probably will have greater-than-average problems understanding speech in background noise.

---

that were considerably worse than expected (based on degree of hearing loss) for a group of individuals with dead regions. Although this chapter's focus is *pre-testing*, it might be useful to conduct TEN testing *post-fitting* for select patients who do not have the expected benefits for understanding speech when using hearing aids.

Obtaining the TEN Test

For ordering the TEN(HL) CD or the ER-3A CD, contact Brian Moore (hearing.psychol.cam.ac.uk/dead/TENCD.html).

5

Pre-Fitting Testing Using Speech Material

In the previous chapter, we reviewed how pure-tone and narrowband signals can be used to obtain useful information prior to the fitting of hearing aids. And in Chapter 6, we review how pre-fitting self-assessment inventories also assist in treatment planning and counseling. Although both areas certainly are important, it is commonly recognized that the cornerstone of pre-fitting testing lies with speech audiometry. Not only is speech testing part of the routine diagnostic battery, but there are many speech tests available that have direct use for the fitting of hearing aids.

Prior to the fitting, what is it that we would like to know? How the patient understands speech in quiet? Or, how about recognition of speech in background noise? What is his or her annoyance level of background noise when attempting to understand speech? How do patients assess their ability to understand speech in background noise—does this agree with their *true* ability? And what about their central auditory processing capabilities for speech signals? Or cognitive issues related to speech communication?

In this chapter, we review the different areas of pre-fitting speech testing and provide samples of appropriate tests to use, depending on the pre-fitting question that is being asked. Some of the speech tests reviewed also can be used for aided verification (see Book Three of this series on verification), and hence, an application of the pre-fitting test findings will be establishing a

baseline for post-fitting comparisons. But, there also are many other uses. To get us started, we review some general clinical considerations when conducting these tests.

General Considerations

The basic speech test conducted by most audiologists is monosyllable word recognition testing in quiet using phonetically or phonemically balanced (PB) word lists—often simply referred to as *word-rec* testing or *PB-testing*.[25] We discuss this testing in the next section, mostly because the test is so popular for basic diagnostics, not because we believe it is a very useful hearing aid pre-fitting measure. Unfortunately, in some offices and clinics it is the only speech test conducted, so we believe it is important to provide guidelines on the administration and interpretation of this test. The rest of the chapter relates to speech testing in the presence of a competing signal.

Speech-in-Noise Testing

It is common for best practice guidelines related to the fitting of hearing aids to recommend *speech recognition in noise* as a routine measure prior to the hearing aid fitting, and we certainly agree. There are several reasons why these tests are important, besides the fact that the speech recognition score in quiet is a poor predictor of a patient's speech-in-noise performance, including:

- To address the patient's complaints. It is very likely that problems understanding speech in background noise are the primary reason why the patient is seeking assistance. Conducting this testing conveys to the patient that you understand his or her problem.
- To select the best technology. The results of these tests can impact your selection of the fitting arrangement (e.g., unilateral versus bilateral), the hearing aid style, and/or the need for special features such as remote microphones.
- To establish a baseline. The information collected during this testing can be used as a baseline for measuring aided benefit.
- To monitor performance over time. A patient's ability to understand in background noise may become significantly poorer without an associated change in hearing thresholds or speech understanding in quiet.
- To assist with counseling. How does the patient's score compare with individuals with normal hearing, or other individuals with the same degree of hearing loss? As we discuss in detail in Chapter 6, part of the fitting process is to maintain realistic expectations for the patient. The results of speech-in-noise testing will assist in identifying real-world situations where the patient may or may not do well.
- To help a patient make a decision. Many times, a patient may be on the fence regarding the use of hearing aids and maybe has heard that hearing aids do not work. An aided versus unaided speech test during the initial visit provides an example of potential benefit (see example later in this chapter) and often provides that shot in the arm to encourage the patient to move forward.

Words or Sentences?

When conducting speech-in-noise tests, we have the option of using tools that require the recognition of single words, key words embedded in sentences, or entire sentences. There does not seem to be a consensus of what is best, as there are pros and cons of using either words or sentences. As reviewed by Wilson and McArdle (2008), advantages of sentence materials are:

- Better face validity; similar to what the patient experiences in everyday listening.
- Perhaps better approximation of how a person understands conversational speech; monosyllables have a lack of lexical, semantic, and syntactic redundancies and dynamic phonotactic cues.

On the other hand, monosyllables have the following advantages (Wilson & McArdle, 2008):

- With sentence material, context contributes heavily to intelligibility and makes basic auditory function difficult to determine.
- The syntactic and semantic structures of sentence-length stimuli can influence performance.
- Sentences involve more complex cognitive skills; more working memory effort is required. These demands could differentially affect older versus younger patients.

Competing Noises

There are several different types of competing noises used with popular speech tests. The different noises have different characteristics, which can impact the performance for a given test. Most importantly, using the wrong noise can affect list equivalency, resulting in a clinician drawing the wrong conclusion about measured differences between test conditions (e.g., performance for the right versus left ear). It is important, therefore, to use the type of competing noise with each speech test that was used in its development, when normative data were collected. Commonly used competing noises include:

- Speech noise: As the name indicates, this is a broadband, typically non-modulated, noise that usually has been shaped to be consistent with the LTASS. An advantage of this type of competition is that the lack of modulation typically leads to more reliable results for small segments of speech since the SNR is typically more precisely controlled. An example would be the Hearing In Noise Test (HINT), where an effort was made to specifically shape the speech noise so that it was very similar to the LTASS of the HINT sentences.

- Multitalkers: In this instance, the competing signal is competing talkers. We separate this category from our next category, multitalker *babble*, as the conventional definition of speech babble is that none of the background conversations are intelligible. With fewer talkers, however, it is possible to detect meaningful words or strings of words if the patient tunes in to the competing signal. This increases the informational masking (versus energetic masking), which can impact performance. Furthermore, because speech is amplitude modulated, this type of background noise allows listeners who are able, to *listen in the gaps* between competing speech segments improving face validity. Examples of this type of competing signal are the Quick Speech In Noise (QuickSIN) and the Bamford-Kowal-Bench Sentences in Noise (BKB-SIN), which

have a four-talker background competition (one male, three females).

- Multitalker babble: With a mulitalker babble, individual words from the speakers are not recognizable, making it a true babble. This is accomplished by using more talkers, recorded from more loudspeakers, and/or recorded in an uncorrelated manner. For example, the multitalker babble available from Auditec of St. Louis contains 20 talkers. There is some research to suggest that multitalker babble provides more separation between listeners with hearing loss and those with normal hearing than a speech noise competing signal. Examples of tests that use a multitalker babble competing signal are the Words In Noise (WIN) and the Revised Speech-In-Noise (R-SPIN).

- Cocktail party/cafeteria noise: A background that is sometimes used as competition for speech testing is cafeteria or cocktail party noise.[26] These noises are similar to multitalker babble, but usually have greater spectral bandwidth and contain transients, as they typically have the clinking of glasses and dishes as well as multiple talkers. These

---

KEY CONCEPT:
ENERGETIC OR INFORMATIONAL MASKING?

When we conduct speech-in-noise testing, there is a *masking effect* from the background signal. There are different kinds of masking effects, however. As described by Jerger (2006), energetic masking occurs when the neural excitation evoked by the competing signal (speech or noise or both) exceeds the excitation produced by the target speech—for the most part, the masking effect is the energies and the synchrony of the energies of the two signals. There is a second type of masking that can cause an additional interference, or interference independent of energetic masking, which also serves to reduce speech recognition. This is referred to as informational masking (also perceptual or central masking). As the name suggests, this refers to the informational content of the masking signal. To relate these masking effects to clinical testing, the background signal of the HINT and the WIN are strictly energetic, whereas the background signal of the QuickSIN and BKB-SIN also have an informational component. In laboratory studies, Hornsby, Ricketts, and Johnson (2006) found that hearing aid benefit is poorest when the background signal contains both energetic and informational masking. Unfortunately, this is the type of background noise experienced by most listeners in the real world.

background noises are usually recorded at a party or cafeteria, and then overdubbed with time offsets to provide a more unified signal and reduce amplitude fluctuations.

■ Speech: When the goal of the testing is to assess higher level auditory processing, it often is desirable to use single-talker speech as the competition. An early example of this was the Synthetic Sentence Identification Test (SSI), where the competing signal for the synthetic sentences was James Jerger reading a story about Davy Crockett. When dichotic testing is conducted, unless a directed response is used (the patient is instructed to focus on one ear), there is not a defined *competing* signal, as the signal presented to each ear is competing against the other. A couple examples of this are the tests that we discuss later in this chapter, the Dichotic Digit Test (DDT; two digits presented simultaneously to each ear) and the Dichotic Sentence Identification (DSI) test (synthetic sentences presented simultaneously to each ear).

Adaptive Versus Fixed SNR

In the clinic, speech-in-noise testing can be conducted by using an adaptive or a fixed SNR. With adaptive testing, either the speech or the noise level is fixed, and the other signal level is then varied. The variance of the adaptive signal can be at predetermined intervals, with a wide range of SNRs tested (e.g., WIN, BKB-SIN, QuickSIN). Alternatively, the adaptive signal can be varied as a function of the individual's performance on the previous item. An example of this is the HINT, where the target sentence material is raised or lowered in 2-dB steps for each sentence whereas the background noise is fixed. In either case, the purpose of the testing typically is to determine the SNR where the patient is obtaining a score at or near 50% correct. This is referred to as the speech reception threshold (SRT) in noise (often denoted as SNR-50 or SRT_{50}), or in the case of the HINT, it is dubbed the reception threshold for speech (RTS). The QuickSIN and the BKB-SIN compare the patient's 50% correct score with that of individuals with normal hearing, and the score is reported as *SNR loss* (i.e., deviation from normal-hearing norms). Although these SNR loss values are easy to interpret, there are some factors that affect the SNR loss. These factors may include:

■ Age. Patients who are older are more likely to have more SNR loss (Walden & Walden, 2004).

■ Test ear. Even with similar hearing in both ears, on average, patients have less SNR loss in their right ear than left ear (Walden & Walden, 2005).

■ Presence of cochlear dead regions. Patients who have dead regions are more likely to have more SNR loss (Preminger, Carpenter, & Ziegler, 2005).

■ Working memory capacity. Patients who have larger working memory capacity may have less SNR loss (Parbery-Clark, Strait, Anderson, Hittner, & Kraus, 2011).

■ Musical training. Patients who are professional musicians may have less SNR loss (Parbery-Clark et al., 2011).

An alternative method of conducting speech-in-noise testing would be to use a test that has a fixed SNR. That is, the SNR is not adjusted for the individual patient but is presented at the same level for all. Speech tests that use a fixed SNR are the R-SPIN (+8 dB) and the Speech Recognition In Noise Test (SPRINT; +9 dB). The Connected Speech Test (CST) also is a fixed-level test, although the background multitalker babble can be adjusted to different SNRs. For example:

■ We commonly choose speech presentation levels of approximately 53 dB SPL (soft speech vocal effort) when we have the goal of determining the patient's ability to recognize soft speech or when demonstrating to the patient that hearing aids work.

■ We use levels associated with speech produced with average vocal effort (62 dB SPL) or higher when we are demonstrating directional microphone capabilities. In this case, we present the speech from the front and the noise from behind.

■ Based on the guidance provided by Pearson et al. (1977), we typically use fairly positive SNRs (e.g., +10 dB) for lower speech presentation levels and poorer SNRs (e.g., +3 dB) for higher speech presentation levels to reflect what commonly occurs in the real word.

There are clinical advantages to both the adaptive and fixed SNR methods of measuring speech recognition in background noise. First some advantages of the adaptive model:

- Eliminate floor and ceiling effects (i.e., scoring nearly all correct or all incorrect), a common problem when a fixed SNR is used.
- The 50% correct point for most patients can be obtained more reliably and efficiently than a lengthy word list.
- Better able to determine significant differences between patients or between the right and left ears of the same patient.

But, there also are some disadvantages of measuring the reception threshold for speech compared with using a fixed SNR approach:

- Difficult to explain test results to the patient—telling a patient his or her speech reception threshold (SRT) in noise is 10 dB is not very meaningful.
- Difficult for patients to relate their performance to the real world. Because of the way the test is designed, two individuals with very different speech recognition ability would both report that they got about one-half of the words correct.
- Difficult to relate findings to third parties and referral sources. Even audiologists are not always certain if an SNR-50 score of +4 dB is good or bad. And, the SNR-50 score that is good for one speech test might just be okay for another (e.g., see norms for BKB-SIN versus WIN).
- Administration and scoring may be somewhat more cumbersome.

Presentation Level

An important consideration when conducting speech-in-noise testing is to select an appropriate presentation signal. The level selected is directly related to the question being asked and the overall purpose of the testing. Here are some examples:

- Choice #1: Conduct testing at the level at which the norms were collected. This is the most reasonable choice, as it allows for comparison with the norms and should ensure the best interlist reliability.
- Choice #2: Conduct testing at the level at which the best performance is predicted. This should provide the best indication of true recognition ability and best predict potential performance with amplification.
- Choice #3: Conduct testing at the average real-world levels, which should provide the best prediction of how the patient performs in the real world. (Note: We say *best* not *accurate*—clinical testing is not too good at predicting real-world performance.)
- Choice #4: Conduct testing at the specific level that relates to a patient complaint; a patient with a mild hearing loss whose primary complaint is understanding soft speech might be tested at the level of soft speech.

For some individuals and some speech tests, the four considerations above may result in fairly similar presentation levels. In other cases, there may be fairly large differences. Let's take two of the most commonly used speech-in-noise sentence tests, the QuickSIN and the HINT. With the HINT, it is recommended that the background noise be set at 65 dB (A) SPL. For the QuickSIN, it is recommend that the sentences are presented at 70 dB HL if the pure-tone average (PTA) is 45 dB or less and at the patient's *loud but okay* loudness rating, if the PTA is greater than 50 dB—this rating would probably be 85 to 90 dB HL for someone with this degree of hearing loss. Some quick HL to SPL conversions tell us that if standard protocols are followed, the QuickSIN will be presented at a considerably higher levels (e.g., 10 to 20 dB) than the HINT.

What maybe is most important as a clinician is to understand what question really is being answered when the test is conducted, which means we have to know the question being asked. If the question is, "What's the optimum speech recognition performance in background noise?" and the patient has a downward sloping hearing loss, assuring audibility for the high frequencies is a concern, and then a higher presentation level should be selected. On the other hand, if the purpose of the testing is to establish a baseline for aided verification measures a lower presentation level should be used. If a high presentation level is used in this instance, it is very possible that aided measures will be no better than unaided, suggesting to the patient that the hearing aids provide no benefit for understanding speech in background noise.

Earphones or Sound Field?

As with presentation level, the use of earphones versus sound field testing depends somewhat on the purpose of the test and how the test was normed. In general, there are compelling reasons to conduct the testing using earphones:

- Calibration/standardization is much easier.
- Ability to obtain individual ear information.
- Easy to mask non-test ear when necessary.
- Not constrained by upper output limits of sound field speakers.
- Many audiologists fitting hearing aids do not have appropriate sound field systems.

Despite these advantages for earphones, there may be some times when sound field testing is the best choice or required by the test protocol. There are also different ways to do earphone testing. So essentially, we have three options for sound delivery:

- Earphone testing (unilateral): Even people with symmetric hearing loss may have different word recognition (in noise) ability for the right and left ears. Knowledge of this can be helpful during the fitting process (e.g., recommending what ear to use on the telephone) and during post-fitting counseling (e.g., helping explain why the patient notices an ear difference in a bilateral fitting). In most cases, ear-specific testing is recommended.
- Earphone testing (bilateral): This should provide the best indication of optimum recognition ability—although probably not much better than best ear performance from

unilateral testing. The design of some speech tests require bilateral presentation (e.g., dichotic material), and at least one test, the SPRINT, is normed for bilateral earphone presentation. The Acceptable Noise Level Test (ANLT) does not tend to be ear-specific, and although it is normally conducted in the sound field, bilateral earphone testing should work okay.

- Sound field testing: Some speech tests used with fitting hearing aids were normed in the sound field. Also, if the only purpose of the testing is to serve as a baseline for aided verification, if pre-fitting is conducted in the sound field, it is then possible to conduct aided testing using the same test paradigm. We do not recommend attempting ear-specific testing in the sound field, as it is difficult to eliminate the non-test ear, even when using well-fitted earplugs. Unrelated to the fitting of hearing aids, some government agencies, for reasons we do not quite understand, require unaided sound field measures of speech recognition. Obviously, good calibration of the sound field system is critical—something we talk about next.

Sound Field Calibration

As we mentioned, some speech-in-noise tests that we discuss later in this chapter are designed to be conducted in the sound field. It is important to calibrate every signal from every audiometer channel from every loudspeaker position you will use. For example, if you present the competing noise track for a given test from both the front and back loudspeaker, it is important to calibrate the noise track from each one of the two loudspeakers separately. Also, it is important to remember that what is in the test room affects calibration. That is, all equipment and furniture that is typically present should remain in the test room during calibration.

Although not precisely accurate, we find that even cheap sound level meters such as those available from RadioShack for less than $100 are good enough for these purposes and are typically accurate within a decibel or two—and more important, give a repeatable measure. We do not recommend using smartphone applications for this purpose without first verifying their accuracy because the smartphone microphone may not be equally sensitive at all distances and angles, and therefore may be more or less accurate depending on the distance from the loudspeaker.

We have given you several considerations in this section to think about. We encourage you to keep these in mind as you review the many speech tests we have outlined.

Speech Recognition in Quiet

As we mentioned in the introduction, monosyllable word recognition in quiet is probably our least favorite speech test for the fitting of hearing aids, but the fact remains, unfortunately, that it sometimes is the only speech test conducted. There are several monosyllabic word tests available, and we have selected two of them for discussion here. The first is the Northwestern University Test #6 (NU#6; Auditec version)—this choice was easy; it is clearly the most researched and clinically applied speech test of the past several decades. If you are still a fan of the W-22s, consider switching.

The second test we discuss is the Maryland CNCs. Although not as popular as the NU#6, this is the test used by the VA clinics, a group of audiologists who happen to fit 20% of all hearing aids each year in the United States. Moreover, many audiologists not directly affiliated with the VA see veterans on a contract basis, and this test is then also required.

Northwestern University Test #6

The primary monosyllabic word list that we recommend is the NU#6. As the name indicates, this list was developed at Northwestern University in the 1960s.[27] Research at the time was conducted with several lists, all given different numerical designators. Original monosyllabic research was with List #4, which was then expanded to four 50-word lists, categorized as List #6.

Background

Because of the known limitations of the then popular PAL-50 and CID W-22 word lists, Tillman, Carhart, and Wilber (1963) worked to develop a new monosyllabic test. At the time, Lehiste and Peterson (1959) had promoted the notion that monosyllabic word lists should have phonemic rather than phonetic balance. Tillman et al. (1963), therefore, used the word list of Lehiste and Peterson partially for this reason, but also because these were words that had been selected on the basis of a high degree of familiarity,[28] and they were all consonant-nucleus-consonant words.

The early recordings (reel-to-reel tape) of the NU#6 lists that were used clinically had Tom Tillman as the talker, but these were soon replaced by the Auditec recording, released in the early 1970s. One of the first laboratory studies of the Auditec material was by Wilson, Coley, Haenel, and Browning, (1976), who conducted testing for a group of listeners with normal hearing and a second group with sensorineural hearing loss. Their results demonstrated good interlist equivalence for the Auditec version for both groups. They also conducted comparative intelligibility functions for the Auditec and the original Northwestern versions of the NU#6. They did find a slight difference between the two recordings, but they concluded that for clinical purposes the two versions could be considered equivalent. See Appendix L for the NU#6 lists.

There are different versions of the NU#6 recording available. By far, the Auditec recording is the most commonly used among clinicians.[29]

It is important to point out the purpose of conducting traditional monosyllabic testing when used as a hearing aid pre-fitting test. First, we mention three things that this testing is *not* intended to do.

- We are not conducting the testing to determine how this person performs in the real world—monosyllables, under earphones, in quiet, in a test booth are a far cry from the real world (see related "Key Concept").
- Second, this test is also not useful for assessing whether a patient is a good candidate for hearing aids, or for making decisions about what types of signal processing or features the hearing aid should have.
- Finally, we are not conducting the testing to determine how this person performs for *average-level* speech. This approach possibly could be used as a hearing aid verification test, but it is not an important pre-fitting question to answer.

> ### KEY CONCEPT:
> ### POOR PREDICTOR OF BENEFIT AND SATISFACTION
>
> As we have mentioned, we are not encouraging the use of monosyllabic testing in quiet for the purpose of predicting hearing aid benefit or satisfaction. Taylor (2007) conducted an evidence-based review regarding the use of earphone word recognition testing to predict real-world success with hearing aids. He states that out of the 11 studies that met his criteria, only four indicated a weak correlation, and none of the 11 revealed a strong predictive relationship between word recognition scores (in quiet) and success with amplification. Much of the research in this area has been conducted by Larry Humes, PhD, of Indiana University. For review, see his 2003 article on modeling and predicting hearing aid outcomes.

So why are we doing this testing? There are two things that we would like to know: What is the maximum performance possible for this patient? And, is there a significant difference between ears? That is, when we deliver the words at the optimum presentation level—enough, but not too much audibility—what score is obtained? This measure is termed *PB-Max*. We would expect that, if fitted properly, the aided performance will equal or maybe even exceed this value. The task then is to use a test protocol that best assures that the scores we obtain are a close approximation to PB-Max. That is what we discuss in the next section.

Administration and Scoring

Given that clinical monosyllabic word testing has been around for over 70 years and that it is one of the most routine and fundamental tests conducted by audiologists, one might think that a universal test protocol existed. It may exist somewhere in best practice guidelines, but unfortunately audiologists seem to be fond of modifications and shortcuts. This often makes it nearly impossible to compare results conducted at two different clinics, or even compare results for testing conducted at two different times at *the same clinic*.

Although the testing is conducted in many different ways, audiologists do at least agree that the testing is conducted with earphones and that individual ear results are desirable. The scoring is also standard: The patient scores 2% for each word repeated correctly using a 50-word list. An exception to this is when the 10-word or 25-word screening test is used, which we discuss shortly. Most critical for obtaining valid and reliable scores are the presentation level and the presentation format.

Presentation Level. As we mentioned earlier, the goal of this testing is to find PB-Max. In a research lab,

> ### POINTS TO PONDER: THE HISTORY OF PBs
>
> Throughout this section we may sometimes refer to monosyllabic word recognition testing as *PB testing*. We also talk about an important test concept, referred to as *PB-Max*. If you are new to audiology, you might question the history of PB and why it is commonly used (at least by older audiologists). When monosyllabic word lists were first introduced, it was considered to be important that each 50-word list was *phonetically balanced*, abbreviated PB. Since the 1960s, we have used the NU#6 lists, which actually are not phonetically balanced, but phonemically balanced. But, because we maintained the *P*, the terms *PB list*, *PB testing*, and *PB score* have more or less survived.

this would consist of conducting a performance/intensity (PI) function in small steps (2 or 4 dB), with levels ranging from just above the threshold to the patient's loudness discomfort level. In a busy clinic, the audiologist usually will only conduct testing at one level. How do you know what level is best? First, we list three methods that are still sometimes used, which we know are *not* best:

- A fixed SL (30 or 40 dB) added to the patient's SRT.
- A fixed SL (30 or 40 dB) added to the patient's pure-tone average.
- The patient's most comfortable level (MCL) for speech.

There is no single level or procedure that will work the best for finding PB-Max for *all* patients (other than a PI/PB function using small steps). But if we choose to use a single presentation level, we must then pick one that gives us the best chance of being right most of the time. Fortunately, we have some research data to help us make that decision.

In general, the presentation goal relates to audibility of the speech signal, especially the important high frequency signals needed to identify PB words (e.g., 2000 to 3000 Hz region). This is why in many cases, for patients with a downward sloping hearing loss, using a 30 to 40 dB fixed SL approach is not effective. Although maximizing audibility is good, the presentation level also has to be below the patient's LDL (for loudness discomfort level). In 1983, Kamm, Morgan, and Dirks found that, for downward sloping hearing losses, PB-Max most commonly occurred around 95 dB SPL (for average hearing losses of 50 dB or less). This translates to approximately 75 dB HL (earphones), and many clinics that only use one presentation level have selected either 75 dB or 80 dB HL for routine use.

Research by Guthrie and Mackersie (2009) revealed two other approaches, which also seem to work quite well, and in fact in their study these methods were slightly better than the fixed 75 to 80 dB HL method. The first of these two approaches is to measure the patient's LDL for speech and then conduct testing 5 dB below this level. This should accomplish the two goals we stated earlier: maximizing audibility without infringing on the LDL. As we discuss later in this chapter, it has been recommended to conduct some other tests such

as the QuickSIN at the Loud, But Okay loudness level, which for many patients is indeed 5 dB below their LDL. The downside of this approach of Guthrie and Mackersie (2009), however, is that an extra speech test is required—we normally would not conduct an earphone speech LDL (see Chapter 4).

A second approach suggested by Guthrie and Mackersie (2009), the one that we prefer and that was essentially as effective as the LDL minus 5 dB method, is to use a variable sensation level (SL) based on the 2000 Hz threshold. The SL becomes smaller as the threshold becomes worse. The values they recommend are shown in Table 5–1.

It is possible that when using this approach, the speech signal will be "Uncomfortably Loud" for some patients. When this happens, simply reduce the intensity in small steps until the speech signal is judged "Loud, But Okay." We do need to point out that when you first start delivering speech to patients at 75 to 80 dB HL, it is very common for them to act a little startled and say something like, "That's really loud." At this point, it is important to have the patient make the distinction between "Really Loud" and "Uncomfortably Loud." You might say something like, "I realize the speech is loud, but we need to have it loud to obtain the best test results. Is it truly uncomfortable, or just louder than you would like?" In most cases, after some thought, the patient will decide that it's really okay. We suggest using live voice and talking to the patient at the proposed test level intensity to assure that all is well before initiating the actual testing.

List Length. As we mentioned, research has shown that the Auditec recording of the NU#6 lists has a good list equivalency (Wilson et al., 1976). This of course was

Table 5–1. Recommended Presentation Levels for Monosyllabic Word Recognition Testing

The SL values shown below are added to the 2000 Hz threshold to obtain presentation levels:	
2000 Hz Thresholds	<50 dB HL: 25 dB SL
2000 Hz Thresholds	50–55 dB HL: 20 dB SL
2000 Hz Thresholds	60–65 dB HL: 15 dB SL
2000 Hz Thresholds	70–75 dB HL: 10 dB SL

Source: From Guthrie and Mackerzie, 2009.

ON THE SOAPBOX: SRT + 40 dB—JUST SAY *NO*

A little story about a patient evaluated at a large, ear-nose-throat audiology center. The patient, a 55-year-old male, was self-referred, with the complaint of reduced hearing in both ears and some tinnitus. He had a history of noise exposure (hunting without hearing protection since a teenager); his primary reason for the visit was to see if hearing aids would help. His pure-tone thresholds were quite symmetric, with normal hearing in the low frequencies, dropping to a 60 to 75 dB loss in the 3000 Hz to 6000 Hz range. There was a difference between ears, however, at 2000 Hz, where the right ear threshold was 40 dB, and the left ear dropped to 60 dB. The patient had SRTs of 10 dB in both ears, agreeing with his low-frequency thresholds. When the audiologist conducted word recognition testing, she used the *SRT +40* approach (resulting in a 50 dB HL presentation level for both ears) and obtained word recognition scores of 96% for the right ear and 80% for the left—a 16% difference between ears. The patient was then seen for his ear-nose-throat exam, and because of the word recognition asymmetry, an MRI was ordered to rule out a space-occupying lesion.

Does anything about this bother you? We certainly could question why a 16% interaural difference should trigger an MRI, or for that matter, why any monosyllabic finding should trigger an MRI. But, the fact is that these are the guidelines from the American Academy of Otolaryngology (AAO), which are shown in this chart:

Recommendations for Screening MRI for Asymmetric Sensorineural Hearing Loss SNHL

PTA	Speech Discrimination
Mean PTA ≤ 30 dB, then asymmetry of >15 dB at two contiguous frequencies	A difference in speech discrimination scores of greater that 15%
Mean PTA > 30 dB, then asymmetry of >20 dB at two contiguous frequencies	

So, the otolaryngologist was simply following the guidelines from the parent organization. But, does anyone really think those guidelines were intended for word recognition scores obtained from patients who were tested at a presentation level that was 10 dB below their 2000 Hz threshold? On the other hand, shouldn't we be able to assume that values placed in someone's medical records are *correct*?

Testing of this patient a year later at a different facility, using 80 dB HL presentation levels in both ears revealed a 94% score for the right ear and 92% for the left. Our soapbox is directly related to the often cited quote of David Pascoe (1980):

Although it is true that mere detection of a sound does not ensure its recognition . . . it's even more true that without detection, the probabilities of correct identification are greatly diminished.

This unfortunate case begs the question—why would anyone conducting a diagnostic speech test purposely present the speech at a level that would nearly guarantee invalid test results and potentially lead to additional (expensive) testing, not to mention the undue stress to the patient? Selecting the correct presentation level for word recognition testing is not rocket science—let's do it right!

for the full 50-word lists. This does not necessarily hold true for the first or second half of any given list (e.g., the use of a 25-word list)—we have heard that in some clinics, the use of *half lists* is common practice. Consider the following example using the NU#6 List—we limit our discussion to List 1A, as that is the most commonly used. Research by Hurley and Sells (2003) identified the 10 most difficult words for each NU#6 list (actually, all 50 words are rank-ordered for difficulty). For List 1A, it just happens that eight of those words are in the first half and two are in the second half. So let's say a given patient simply misses the 10 hardest words. If a full 50-word list had been used, the score would be 80%. However, if someone were to use a half list and the right ear was tested first, the patient's scores would be 68% for the right ear and 92% for the left. Some otolaryngologists would order an MRI when presented with this degree (24%) of asymmetry for word recognition. If the patient needed hearing aids, and stated that he only wanted to purchase one, some audiologists might fit the left ear because it was the "best," when, in fact, the left ear probably was the same as the right—it just got lucky and got the easy half of the list!

In addition to the validity issue, another reason to use the full 50-word lists is that when the test has more items, critical differences become smaller. We talk about that in detail shortly, but here is a preview. At the .05 level of confidence, for a 50-word list, if a patient has a score of 72% for the right ear, the score for the left ear must be poorer than 54% or better than 86% before the left ear can be considered significantly different from the right. If only 25 words are delivered, then the left ear score must be worse than 48% or better than 92%—the range of *nonsignificance* expands by 12%. This of course is clinically important, as one of the reasons we are doing the test is to determine if there is a significant difference between ears.

We are not certain of all the reasons why some audiologists choose to use a half list, but one thing that is commonly mentioned is time—it does not take as long. We could point out that a *one-word list* is even faster! There is a way to speed up testing and still use 50 words. The NU#6 has a standard interstimulus interval (ISI), however, the list also is available with a shortened ISI. For many, if not most patients, the shortened ISI works fine. If not, it is always possible to pause the test. Specifically, if ordering from Auditec of St. Louis, the CD that you want is: *NU-6 Ordered by Difficulty, Version II, Short Interval*. We explain the "ordered by difficulty" aspect of this title in the next section.

Ten Best (Worse) Words. After just telling you that it is risky practice to only use 25 words, we are now going to say that it is sometimes okay to only use 10—if you use the *right* 10! Some patients with mild losses, but who are still hearing aid candidates, might understand monosyllables in quiet very well and have scores of 96 to 100%. It is possible to identify these patients quickly, and save some valuable clinic time that could be used for counseling, by presenting the 10 most difficult words of a given NU#6 list first.

Research by Hurley and Sells (2003) identified the 10 most difficult words of the four NU#6 lists (Auditec recording). Their research revealed that if patients correctly recognizes 9 or 10 of the first 10 words (which are ordered by difficulty), you can then predict (.05 level of confidence) that their true score using a full 50-word list would be 96 to 100%. Given this high probability, there would be little reason to continue with the other 40 words of the list.

If the patient misses four or more words from the first 10, then conduct the entire 50-word list. If, however, the patient only misses two or three words of the first 10, then compute the score again at the end of 25 words—the next 15 words also are ordered by level of difficulty. If after 25 items, the patient still has only missed two or three words, you can then stop testing, with the prediction (.05 level of confidence) that the true score is 94 to 96%. The NU#6 lists ordered by difficulty can be obtained from Auditec of St. Louis—they even provide an additional 10 second delay after the 10th and 25th words while you are thinking about whether you will go on or stop the test. We advocate always using this version of the NU#6, as the worst case is that you'll present all 50 words, which is what you would have done anyway. This difficulty ordering only applies to the Auditec recording of the words. The NU#6 List ordered by difficulty is displayed in Appendix M.

Presentation Mode. Just as we do not attempt to whistle the pure tones from 250 to 8000 Hz when we conduct air-conduction threshold testing, we also do not use monitored live voice when we conduct word recognition testing. The speaker can have a significant impact on the word recognition score (WRS). Substantial research has been conducted with the Auditec of St. Louis recording of the NU#6, and using this recording has become the standard presentation format. The words are presented from CD or with some computer-based audiometers, from an internal wave file. Using this standard test format allows

---

KEY CONCEPT: THE WORDS ARE *NOT* THE TEST

We've already been "On The Soapbox" once the past few pages, so we'll do this one from ground level. Repeat after us: The words are not the test! The recorded version is the test. This point was made nicely by Fred Bess, in his 1983 book chapter on speech audiometry. He compared four different *recorded versions* of the NU#6, and found that at some sensation levels, average performance varied by as much as 60% for hearing impaired listeners.

---

for the patient's performance to be compared with clinical norms, and for comparisons to be made from clinic to clinic and from visit to visit in the same clinic.

The test is the *recorded* version. Using a haphazard personal modification and then placing these scores into medical records would be considered unethical by many—and certainly could have serious medical-legal consequences.

Clinical Significance: Binomial Model. Once the WRS has been obtained for both ears, we want to decide if the results will impact our decision making regarding amplification. Is the patient's right ear score different from the left? Did the scores change since the patient's last visit? Did the scores change since the patient started using hearing aids? The question then becomes, what percent difference is truly a difference?

In what has become a classic article, Thornton and Raffin (1978) modeled the performance on clinical tests of speech recognition as a binomial variable. This binomial model was tested against data from 4,120 speech recognition scores. They developed tables for determining significant deviations between scores. One of these tables (.05 level of confidence) is shown as Table 5–2 for a 50-word list. As we mentioned earlier, the number of items used is important because variability in scores is inversely related to the number of items in the test. Also inherent in the model is that the variability of the scores is the greatest in the middle of the range (e.g., 50%) and is lowest at the extreme ranges (0% and 100%).

The Thornton and Raffin tables have more or less withstood the test of time, and are commonly used in clinical practice and in the interpretation of research findings. If this sort of thing interests you, however, you might enjoy reading Harvey Dillon's critique of the Thornton and Raffin (1982) model in an *Ear and Hearing* paper and the letters to the editor from both Thornton and Raffin, and Dillon, which followed in a later 1982 issue. Carney and Schlauch (2007) examined a critical difference table for monosyllables using a computer simulation and compared these findings with the Thornton and Raffin table. They did find some small differences, but none greater than the score that would result from missing one word.

If the critical differences shown in Table 5–2 are new to you, we will walk you through an example. Let's say you have a patient with a symmetric hearing loss who has been using a hearing aid in the right ear for several years. The patient is in your office today and tells you that he thinks his left ear (the unaided ear) has been getting worse. The patient particularly notices it on the telephone. You see that when he was tested three years ago, the word recognition score for the left ear was 78%. Today it was 62%. So did his speech understanding get (significantly) worse? To use the chart, first pick one of the two numbers—it does not matter which one—so we will take the higher score of 78%. Locate 78% on the chart and you will see that the critical range (the range where the score is *not* significantly different) is 60 to 92%. Because 62% (the new test score) falls within this range, you would conclude that today's score is not significantly poorer than the score of three years ago. Notice that if you had first picked 62%, the score of the poorer ear, the range would have been 44 to 78% and you would have reached the same conclusion.

We encourage you to use the Thornton and Raffin—or similarly derived—tables whenever comparing word recognition scores. In fact, many audiologists find it is difficult to write a report without it. Some audiologists have expressed concern that the .05 level is too rigid for clinical use—there is a .10 level chart available, if that is more to your liking.

Table 5–2. Thornton and Raffin (1978) Binomial Model Critical Differences at the .05 Confidence Level

Score %	N = 50	N = 25	Score %	N = 50	N = 25
0	0–4	0–8	52	34–70	28–76
2	0–10		54	36–72	
4	0–14	0–20	56	38–74	32–80
6	2–18		58	40–76	
8	2–22	0–28	60	42–78	36–84
10	2–24		62	44–78	
12	4–26	4–32	64	46–80	40–64
14	4–30		66	48–82	
16	6–32	4–40	68	50–84	44–88
18	6–34		70	52–86	
20	8–36	4–44	72	54–86	48–92
22	8–40		74	56–88	
24	10–42	8–48	76	58–90	52–92
26	12–44		78	60–92	
28	14–46	8–52	80	64–92	56–96
30	14–48		82	66–94	
32	16–50	12–56	84	68–94	60–96
34	18–52		86	70–96	
36	20–54	16–60	88	74–96	68–96
38	22–56		90	76–98	
40	22–58	16–64	92	78–98	72–100
42	24–60		94	82–98	
44	26–62	20–68	96	86–100	80–100
46	28–64		98	90–100	
48	30–66	24–72	100	96–100	92–100
50	32–68				

Clinical Significance: Comparison To Pure-Tone Average. Another area where clinical significance is an issue relates to a patient's word recognition score compared to the degree of hearing loss. That is, we often look at a word recognition score, then look at the degree of hearing loss, and form an opinion somewhere between, "Yeah, that's about what I expected" to, "That

just doesn't look right." We do have data, however, to help us make this judgment more precisely. Using the Auditec recordings of the NU#6 word lists and testing over 400 adults with cochlear hearing loss, Dubno, Lee, Klein, Matthius, and Lam (1995) compared PB-Max with the patient's pure-tone average. They then used a best fit regression to provide a 95% confidence limit for these measures. We can then use these data to determine if our patients' word recognition scores are "appropriate" for their hearing loss.

We have audiologist Linda Thibodeau to thank for taking the Dubno et al., 1995 data and putting it into an easy-to-use chart. In fact, you get double-your-pleasure with this chart, as she combined the Dubno data with the Thornton and Raffin chart that we discussed earlier. The chart we are referring to is shown in Figure 5–1; it's dubbed the SPRINT, for speech recognition inter-

SPRINT CHART for 50-WORD LISTS

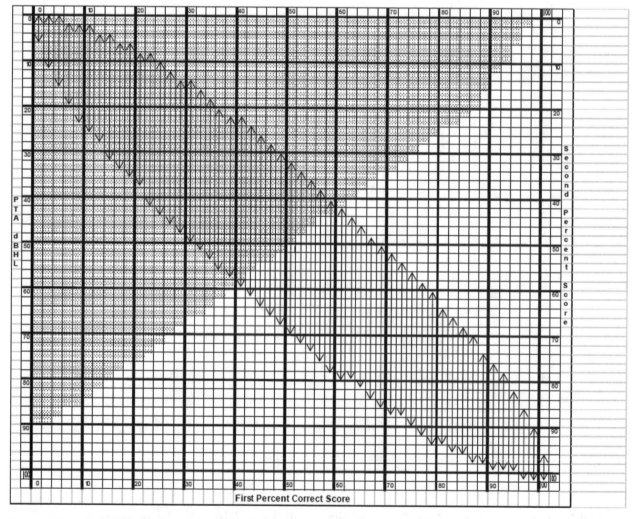

Figure 5–1. SPRINT chart for 50-word lists. To examine the 95% critical difference for two word recognition scores, determine the intersection of the first (bottom x-axis) and the second (right y-axis) score. If the intersection point falls within one of the vertical arrows, the two scores *are not* significantly different from each other (based on work of Thornton and Raffin, 1978). To examine the 95% confidence limit for PB-Max on the Auditec NU#6 list, determine the intersection of the word recognition score on the bottom x-axis, and the patient's PTA on the left y-axis. If the intersection of these two values falls within the shaded area, the word recognition score is considered disproportionately low (based on the work of Dubno et al., 1995). The SPRINT chart is reproduced here with permission from the developer, Linda Thibodeau, PhD (Thibodeau, 2007).

pretation (Thibodeau, 2007). What we are showing in Figure 5–1 is the version for when a 50-word list is used; there also is a version for 25 words (See Appendix N and O for the two different versions). The Dubno data is the same for both charts, whereas the range for the critical differences for the Thornton and Raffin model of course becomes larger for the 25-word chart.

Let's go back to the patient that we discussed earlier. Recall that he originally had a word recognition score of 78%, which had now dropped to 62% We concluded that the difference between these two scores was *not significant* (50-word list). Not surprisingly, we reach this same conclusion when we compare the two scores using the SPRINT (the intersection of 78% found on the bottom abscissa and 62% found on the right ordinate column, which falls within the vertical arrow signifying *non-significance*).

To determine if these word recognition scores agree with the patient's pure-tone hearing loss, we need to use his pure-tone average (500, 1000, and 2000 Hz). The PTA at the time of the first test was 33 dB, and at the time of the second test it had dropped slightly to 36 dB. We now look at the intersection of the first word recognition score (78%) found on the lower "x-axis", and the PTA of 33 dB found on the left "y-axis." Note that the intersection does not fall in the shaded area—the PTA would have to be 24 dB or better for a score of 78% to be disproportionately low. If we now look at this patient's second word recognition score of 62%, and determine the intersection with the second PTA of 36 dB, we see that this indeed does fall into the edge of the shaded area. This could mean that we failed to obtain PB-Max, or perhaps that there is some other factor contributing to his poorer word recognition performance (e.g., auditory processing, reduced cognition, etc.). As you can see the SPRINT chart can be a helpful companion when making day-to-day decisions regarding word recognition performance.

Clinical Applications

As we mentioned earlier, earphone monosyllabic word recognition scores in quiet are poor predictors of who is a candidate for hearing aids and who will benefit from the use of hearing aids. There are some clinical applications, however, where these scores may be helpful in clinical decision making.

Bilateral versus unilateral fitting: In general, we would consider everyone with a bilateral hearing loss a candidate for two hearing aids (see Chapter 7 for review). But what if a person has a relatively symmetrical bilateral hearing loss (e.g., poorer ear falling 10 to 15 dB below the better ear), but the WRSs were approximately 80% in the good ear and approximately 40% in the bad ear? Not a common finding, but it does happen. Is this person still a candidate for bilateral hearing aids? Probably, but if after trying hearing aids, this person reported to us that the bad side just did not seem to be getting much benefit from the hearing aid, our counseling might be different than if both ears had had WRSs around 80%.

Selecting an ear to fit: Although we might encourage most all of our patients with bilateral hearing losses to use two hearing aids, for a variety of reasons, some patients will chose to use only one. When the pure-tone hearing loss is symmetric, what ear do you fit? In some instances, the patient may have specific listening situations that will help you make the decision (e.g., frequently travel as a passenger in the car and need to hear the driver), but in other cases they do not. People typically have similar WRSs in both ears if their hearing loss is symmetrical, but it is possible that you will see an ear

---

KEY CONCEPT: JUST SAY NO TO NOISE

While we are not sure why, given all the well-developed speech recognition in noise tests, some clinicians continue to use standard monosyllable word materials for testing in the presence of background noise. That is, speech noise, white noise, or some other background noise is added to the standard word lists. We urge caution in doing this, as several studies have shown that the standard lists are not equivalent when presented in noise. Moreover, as we mentioned, there are several speech tests that have been designed to be used with background noise—we review most of them later in this chapter.

difference. In this case, you might want to fit the better ear. This of course only applies if the difference between ears is truly a difference (see Table 5–2).

Change over time: An elderly patient of yours, whom you fit bilaterally with hearing aids five years ago, arrives at your office with the complaint that the right hearing aid is not working correctly. You check out the aid and it seems to be fine, so you decide to evaluate the patient's hearing. There has been no significant change in pure-tone thresholds, but the WRS for the right ear has dropped from 84% to 56%—the patient later tells you she had a mild stroke a few months ago. In this case, the results of word recognition testing will make you a better counselor. It is probably obvious, but we say it anyway—comparisons of this type only can be conducted if you follow the test protocol we discussed earlier.

Test Availability

There are several versions of the NU#6, but we recommend using the Auditec of St. Louis recording. As discussed earlier, it makes good sense to routinely use the list ordered by difficulty with the shortened interstimulus interval.

Maryland CNCs

Although this section on speech recognition in quiet focuses on the NU#6, we believe it is also important to briefly discuss a second monosyllabic test—the Maryland CNCs. The primary reason is that this is the standard word recognition measure conducted at all VA hospitals and clinics, where about 20% of hearing aids in the United States are fitted. Also this is the test used for the Compensation and Pension Evaluation Guidelines established by the VA (Speech Recognition and Identification Materials, Disc 2.0, produced in 1998). It is common that clinical audiologists who are not employed by the VA also may be requested to conduct this testing for select patients. The test is very similar to the NU#6, and therefore, all the factors we discussed in the previous section regarding use for the fitting of hearing aids apply to the Maryland CNCs as well.

Background

We assume that the name *Maryland* comes from the location of the Biocommunications Research Laboratory, where Don Causey, PhD, of the VA conducted much of his research. This laboratory was located at the University of Maryland, not far from the VA audiology headquarters in Washington, DC. Causey was the primary researcher in the development of the Maryland word lists. Like the NU#6, the Maryland CNCs rely heavily on the revised CNC lists of Peterson and Lehiste (1962). Causey, Hood, Hermanson, and Bowling (1984) mention some of the goals in the development of the Maryland word lists:

- Uniform distribution of word familiarity.
- Phonetic and/or phonemic balance.
- Maximum interlist equivalence and high test-retest reliability.

THINGS TO REMEMBER:
ALWAYS, ALWAYS, ALWAYS, AND NEVER

If you simply skimmed this section on monosyllabic testing or did not read it at all, at least take a look at our four procedural rules:

1. Always use presentation levels that optimize audibility (see the 2000 Hz threshold + SL approach).
2. Always use 50-word list, unless the patient passes 10-word or 25 word screening.
3. Always use critical differences for decision making when comparing scores between ears or sessions.
4. Never use live-voice presentation.

- Expand the number of equivalent lists available from the four of the NU#6.
- Differentiate satisfactorily among word recognition abilities of individuals with normal hearing versus those with sensorineural hearing loss.
- Account for the effects of consonant-vowel and vowel-consonant transitions. To accomplish this, each key word was embedded in the phrase, "Say the word _____ again." Other monosyllable tests had used either, "You will say _____." or "Say the word _____."

In early research, Causey et al. (1984) studied the performance-intensity function of the Maryland CNCs, and examined the equivalency of the 10 original lists (24-year-old male talker) and test-retest reliability. They found a 2.1% per dB increase in word recognition in the linear portion of the performance-intensity function for normal listeners and a 1.3% per dB increase for hearing impaired listeners. Six of the ten lists were judged to be equivalent (Lists 1, 3, 6, 7, 9, and 10), and good test-retest reliability was reported. Over the years, the original lists have been made available through the work of Richard Wilson, PhD, and colleagues of the VA.

Administration and Scoring

If the Maryland CNCs are simply used as a replacement for the NU#6 list for the pre-fitting of hearing aids, we refer you to the administration and scoring guidelines from the previous section. If the lists are used specifically for a veteran for compensation or pension, however, then the procedures of the VA handbook should be followed. The most current version is: *Handbook of Standard Procedures and Best Practices for Audiology Compensation and Pension Exams* (Version 2-17-2010). We briefly review the test protocol here, although we recommend that you use the most current version of the handbook.

- Both ears must be examined for hearing impairment even if hearing loss in only one ear is at issue.
- The starting presentation level will be the SRT +40 dB. If necessary, the starting level will be adjusted upward to obtain a level at least 5 dB above the threshold at 2000 Hz, if this level does not exceed the patient's LDL.

- When speech recognition is 92% or less, a performance-intensity function must be obtained.

The handbook then provides guidelines for performing the performance-intensity function, which then determines the level that the full 50-word list is delivered:

- Following testing conducted at the starting level described above, present 25 words at 6 dB above and 6 dB below the starting level.
- If recognition performance improves less than 6%, then the maximum word recognition performance has been obtained.
  - Example: Starting level = 50 dB HL. Initial performance = 80%. Decrease level to 44 dB HL. Performance decreases to 76%. Increase level to 56 dB HL. Performance increases to 84%. Test level for full list = 50 dB HL.
- If performance improves by 6% or more at the first 6-dB increment, then word recognition is measured using another 25 words at an additional 6-dB increment.
  - Example: Starting level = 50 dB HL. Initial performance = 80%. Increase level to 56 dB HL. Performance improves to 88% (+8%). Increase level to 62 dB HL. Performance decreases to 84% (–4%). Test level for full list = 56 dB HL.
- A full list (50 words) is then presented at the level of maximum performance. The word recognition performance at this level is reported as the speech recognition score.
- Only the best performance for a full list (50 words) is reported.

Clinical Applications

The Maryland CNCs are commonly used for compensation and pension evaluations for veterans, but the findings certainly would apply to the fitting of hearing aids, in the same manner as we discussed for the NU#6. In fact, if the performance-intensity protocol we described was used, the resulting scores may be more representative of the patient's true performance than if testing was only conducted at a single level, which usually is the case with the NU#6. In general, the clinical applications of these results would be the same as for the NU#6 (see previous section for expanded description):

- When a significant asymmetry exists, use results for selection and counseling guidance related to a bilateral versus unilateral fitting.
- When a significant asymmetry exists, results can be used for a patient who may only want to purchase/use one hearing aid.
- When a hearing aid patient is followed over time, results can be used to determine if significant changes have occurred in speech recognition.

Obtaining the Maryland CNC Test

The Maryland CNC test is available on the Departments of Defense and Veterans Affairs Audiology Materials, Disc 1.0, and also Speech Recognition and Identification Materials, Disc 4.0. See the Eastern Tennessee University website to order (http://www.etsu.edu/crhs/aslp/audiology/resources/VA_CD_Score_Sheets_1.aspx). Frye Electronics also has a CD available containing these lists (http://www.Frye.com). See Appendix P for word lists.

Speech Recognition in Noise

As we described in the introduction of this chapter, when speech testing is conducted for the purposes of fitting hearing aids, we nearly always want to use a speech-in-noise test rather than a speech in quiet test. These tests tend to fall into two general categories: speech recogni-

tion measures with a fixed SNR that result in a percent correct score or the use of a variable speech/noise signal that results in a SNR-50 score. This section reviews three tests that fall in the first of these two categories.

Speech Perception In Noise (SPIN) and R-SPIN

The Speech Perception in Noise Test (SPIN) was developed under contract from the National Institute of Neurological Disorders and Stroke to assess the degree of impairment in auditory reception and/or utilization of context (Kalikow, Stevens, & Elliott, 1977). As we have mentioned before, the problem with traditional tests of speech perception is that they are not good estimates of real-world performance. Considering that the purpose is to assess a person's ability to understand speech in everyday situations, the need for a better test was clear at the time of the development of the SPIN. Instead of examining primarily acoustic-phonetic processing, the authors sought to investigate the *cognitive* aspects such as working memory and receptive language skills (Kalikow et al., 1977).

Background

In the development process, Kalikow et al. began with 285 key words placed each in high-probability (PH) and low-probability (PL) sentences, and then culled the list based on phonetic balance, predictability in the PH condition, and word familiarity. The result was 10 25-sentence list pairs for which only the final word is scored. Initial testing was performed to compare the intelligibility of the low-probability sentences with tradi-

---

TECHNICAL TIP: IS THE SPIN FOR KIDS?

Elliott (1979) conducted a study with children of different ages to identify the age at which children begin to perform at the same level as adults. Results of tests on four different age levels revealed that children younger than 15 to 17 years of age perform significantly poorer than adults on the SPIN. She recommended that the SPIN should not be used in the pediatric population. In related research, Fallon, Trehub, and Schneider (2000) sought to explore the idea that noise affects children's speech understanding more than it does for adults, and they found that children age 11 and younger required more favorable SNRs than adults did, particularly with low-context materials.

KEY CONCEPT: IS THE SPIN A COGNITIVE TEST?

Recall that earlier we mentioned that a design characteristic of the SPIN was to assess cognitive status as well as word recognition. Owen (1981) examined this by using a battery of nonaudiometric cognitive tests to evaluate whether the SPIN test difference score (the difference between low and high predictive sentences) is truly a measure of the listener's use of context. His analysis revealed that the difference score is actually more closely related to audibility, as opposed to contextual cues. Owen (1981), however, suggested that it may be possible to use the low-predictability sentences to evaluate more central auditory processing skills such as auditory closure—the ability to decode a whole word after hearing only part of it.

POINTS TO PONDER: TESTING ABOVE LDL?

Recall that in previous sections of the chapter we have discussed the concept that optimizing audibility is the goal when conducting many of these speech tests. We have also added that one has to be careful not to infringe on the patient's LDL. Dirks, Kamm, Dubno, and Velde (1981) used the SPIN and other speech perception tests to study speech recognition performance at loudness discomfort levels. Their goal was to examine the relationship between LDL and maximum speech recognition performance for people who have sensorineural hearing loss. The rationale was that if maximum speech recognition performance occurred at levels above listeners' LDLs, there may be benefit in allowing hearing aids to amplify beyond that which is comfortable for the listener—an unusual, but interesting concept. The authors found that increasing the signal level beyond the LDL did not increase scores for the SPIN or any of the speech perception tests studied.

---

tional, neutral context words in noise. The results showed comparable intelligibility scores (Kalikow et al., 1977).

The 10 list pairs were further evaluated for equivalency at an SNR of 0 dB to maximize the difference between PH and PL scores. The authors found that two lists were not equivalent, and they therefore were removed from the catalog. The remaining eight lists were evaluated, and although significant differences were identified, the authors stated that considering the conservative statistical model they used, it "should not be regarded as a serious problem" (Kalikow et al., 1977).

A subsequent study from Hutcherson, Dirks, and Morgan (1979) assessed score differences between PH and PL sentences with a range of SNRs. The authors found that for SNRs between –2 and +2, "the difference between the PH and PL score is approximately 40%." They also found that ceiling and floor effects resulted in smaller differences outside of that SNR range. The slopes of the PI functions from this study showed a steeper function for the high-context items, which is evidence for context as a significant contributing factor to speech recognition.

The Revised SPIN. Bilger, Neutzel, Rabinowitz, and Rzeczkowski (1984) set out to standardize the SPIN and posited that normal hearing subjects would not provide a good estimate of the SPIN's reliability. As a consequence, they tested a variety of subjects with hearing loss at a level well above the threshold, with a +8 dB SNR, based on the work of Pearsons, Bennett, and Fidell (1977), who suggested that this was a common SNR encountered in everyday environments. The +8 dB SNR has since become the standard—and basis for normative data—and what typically is used today.

In that study, Bilger et al. (1984) also called attention to the fact that the lists did not meet the qualifications for equivalency. In addition, they stated that "performance reflects two skills that may be largely uncorrelated: ability to listen in noise and to use context." They then revised the test based on the analysis of each test item and removed 31 key words and their corresponding sentences. This resulted in a total of four 50-item list pairs. Today you see this revised version referred to as the R-SPIN or the SPIN-R (Bilger, 1984). Examples of sentences (using the same key words) from the R-SPIN are as follows (see Appendix Q for full list):

High Predictability

- The baby slept in his <u>crib</u>.
- The farmer baled the <u>hay</u>.

Low Predictability

- He can't consider the <u>crib</u>.
- Tom discussed the <u>hay</u>.

We mentioned earlier that the R-SPIN is a fixed SNR test; however, Wilson, McArdle, Watts, and Smith (2012) demonstrated that this test can be configured into a multiple SNR paradigm to estimate SNR-50, but

---

POINTS TO PONDER: NEIGHBORHOOD ACTIVATION MODEL

In this section, we discuss SPIN research that relates to the Neighborhood Activation Model (NAM). This might not be something that you are familiar with, so we provide you with a little background, as this model relates to many of the word recognition tests that we discuss in this chapter.

Luce (1986) and Luce and Pisoni (1998) developed a model of spoken word recognition based on neighborhood probability characteristics of monosyllabic words. This model, known as the NAM, assumes that words are recognized in the context of other similar sounding patterns in the lexicon. NAM predicts that word recognition is dependent on how easy or difficult it is to confuse the stimulus word with phonetically similar words in a lexical neighborhood. The neighborhood is composed of any words in the lexicon that differ from the target by substitution, deletion, or addition of a single phoneme. For example, if the target word was /paid/, neighbors, among others, would be /maid/, /pay/, and /spade/. Consider that word recognition is dependent on the frequency of occurrence of the target word, the number of neighbors, and the frequency of occurrence of the neighbors. The model suggests that the rate at which a word becomes intelligible and recognized in a test condition is inversely related to the confusability of the word with its lexical neighbors in memory.

THINGS TO REMEMBER: THE NAM AND THE R-SPIN

Clarke (2000) designed a study to evaluate the "neighborhood" properties of the final words of both the original and revised SPIN tests. The reasoning behind the need for this effort was Clarke's discussion of Luce's finding in 1986, which detailed that words with higher frequency of use compared with their neighbors tended to have higher intelligibility, and words with lower frequency compared with their neighbors tended to have lower intelligibility. Essentially, when the word was the most frequent option, intelligibility was higher. This characteristic has the greatest effect on the low-probability items. Clarke (2000) ultimately found that both the SPIN and the R-SPIN were statistically equivalent on lexical neighborhood measures and word frequency measures.

that additional research will need to be conducted to develop distinct lists from each of the 200 key words that would be reliable across listeners of representative age and hearing loss.

Administration and Scoring. The SPIN and the R-SPIN take approximately 10 minutes to administer and require a verbal or written response of the last word in each sentence. Both tests are designed for adults but may be used with teenagers as young as 15 years old.

Patient instructions should include the following:

- Listen carefully to each of the following 50 sentences and write down or repeat only the last word. If you are writing your answers down, be sure to put each answer in its corresponding blank space.
- You will have plenty of time, so write legibly and check your spelling.
- The last word will be a common word that you have heard many times before, but some may be easier to understand than others.
- Take a guess if you are unsure. You will not be penalized for wrong answers.

To set up the test, calibrate using the 1000 Hz calibration tone, and then set one channel to the signal, and the other to the babble, and present both to the same ear. Present the sentences with plenty of time in between each item for the patient to respond.

The recommended procedures for selecting the presentation level are as follows:

- Once the babble has been appropriately calibrated, determine the patient's threshold for the babble.
- Set the speech signal to 50 dB above the speech babble threshold.
- Set the babble to 8 dB below the speech signal (SNR = +8 dB).

The R-SPIN score is reported as a percentage. Sum the number of correct high-probability words and the number of correct low-probability words separately. Then, using the scoring nomograph, shown in Figure 5–2 and Appendix Q, find the corresponding number in the high-probability axis and read over to the corresponding number for low probability. That number is called "the percentage hearing for speech" and should fall within the normal region (the outlined area). If the score does not fall within that area, it could be underestimating the patient's hearing for speech. Numbers that are crossed out indicate invalid test results or that the patient may have additional contributing factors that determine the test score. Specifically, as we discussed earlier, non-auditory factors that may contribute to test scores include cognitive declines, difficulty using context, etc.

This scoring and interpretation is quite different from most other speech tests, so to be clear, we include the actual wording of this concept from the R-SPIN manual:

> Scores based on the administration of the R-SPIN test are valid estimates of percent hearing for speech if, and only if, the patient's scores in the high- and low-predictability subtests place her/him in the acceptance region of the scoring nomograph. Scores that fall outside the acceptance region underestimate the patient's ability to hear speech and probably reflect non-auditory factors.

Using the nomograph shown in Figure 5–2, let's take a patient who scored 23/25 for the high-context items (y-axis) and 13/25 for the low-context items (x-axis). The R-SPIN *percent hearing* score would be 76.7 (where the two scores meet on the chart). Note that if the high-context scores were only 15/25, the percent hearing would drop to 56.0%, and observe that this score has been lined out, suggesting that the high-low difference is greater than normal and that there may be contributing factors to the R-SPIN score.

Clinical Applications. There are several potential applications of the R-SPIN related to the selection and fitting of hearing aids:

- To evaluate the degree of handicap for speech recognition in background noise for patients with hearing loss.
- To evaluate whether or not a patient is able to make use of the contextual information to which they have access (difference between low- and high-predictability scores).
- To predict hearing aid benefit. Kalikow et al. (1977) suggest that the comparison of high- and low-predictability scores "has the potential of predicting the ability of a hearing-impaired listener to perform in everyday communicative situations, and thus may help estimate the benefit that the individual is likely to gain from a hearing aid."

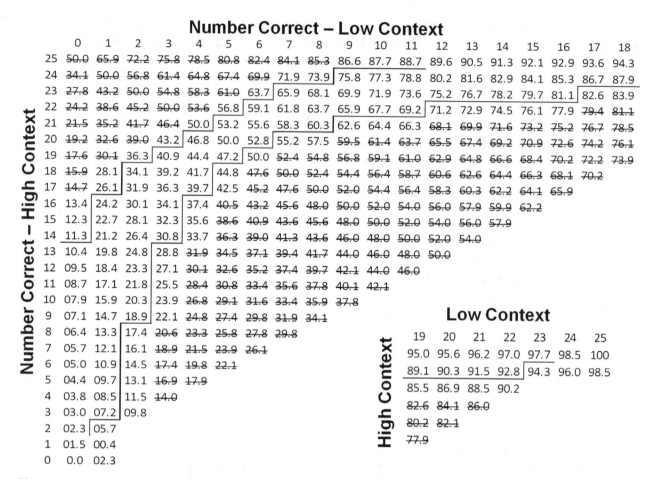

Figure 5–2. Nomograph used for Scoring the R-SPIN. The chart is used to determine the intersection of the number of correct items of the low-probability and high-probability words Adapted from: Bilger RC. (1984) Manual for the Clinical Use of the Revised SPIN Test. Champaign, IL: University of Illinois Press.

TECHNICAL TIP: AGE EFFECTS AND THE R-SPIN

In a large study of speech recognition using different materials, Dubno, Lee, Matthews, and Mills (1997) conducted the R-SPIN for 129 subjects (256 ears) divided into three age groups: 55 to 64 years, 65 to 74 years, and 75 to 84. They found that after the effect of average hearing loss on maximum scores was accounted for, 11.6% of the remaining variance in scores for males can be explained by age, whereas the corresponding value for females was 0.3%. For the R-SPIN, statistically significant decreases in scores for males were observed for words in high-context sentences; a declining trend with age was also observed for words in low-context, but this was not significant. These results suggest that, for male patients, you may expect to see an effect of aging, in addition to auditory effects of hearing loss.

To evaluate ear-to-ear differences or differences over time, if using a complementary list pair.

Unfortunately, the R-SPIN only contains 25 items of each type per list, and therefore, is not sensitive to small changes and is vulnerable to variability. In addition, it tests only monosyllabic nouns, and the test is relatively time-consuming compared with other available tests of speech perception. The R-SPIN has been used in considerable research related to hearing aid verification, often using different SNRs than the standard +8 dB, and because of ceiling effects, only the low-predictability sentences—see Book Three for a review of these test procedures.

Obtaining the R-SPIN. The R-SPIN can be obtained for a nominal charge through the Department of Speech and Hearing Science, University of Illinois, Champaign, IL 61820.

Connected Speech Test (CST)

Developed in the Hearing Aid Research Laboratory at the University of Memphis, the CST is a sentence recognition test designed to approximate everyday conversations in which contextual cues are usually available and includes both audio-only and audiovisual versions (Cox, Alexander, & Gilmore, 1987; Cox, Alexander, Gilmore, & Pusakulich, 1988). That is, the CST can be administered with or without the talker's face visible.

Background

The CST test consists of 24 equivalent pairs of passages of speech. Each passage has 9 or 10 sentences about a familiar topic, such as windows, an umbrella, grass, etc. These sentences, spoken by a female talker, were constructed to be syntactically and semantically simple. The topics and vocabulary were based on children's reading materials. The CST also includes 8 practice passages and 16 learning passages. An example of a CST passage about a woodpecker is shown in Figure 5–3.

The CST was designed to be used primarily as a criterion measure for research studies of hearing aid benefit. Because the test has a high number of equivalent lists, good test-retest variability, and high content validity, it has been used extensively in hearing aid research (e.g., Arehart, Kates, & Anderson, 2010; Boike & Souza, 2000; Picou & Ricketts, 2011; Wu & Bentler, 2010) and has been recommended to be an integral part of a standardized research test battery (Walden, 1997).

Administration and Scoring

The CST is a sentence recognition test, during which a patient hears a sentence and repeats that sentence as precisely as possible. The clinician scores the patient's response based on standardized key words in each

The woodpecker is a bird with a **STRONG BEAK**.
It bores **HOLES** in **TREES** looking for **INSECTS**.
Woodpeckers **LIVE** in all parts of the world.
The **TOES** of woodpeckers **ARE VERY UNUSUAL**.
Two **POINT FORWARD** and two face **BACKWARD**.
This allows the **BIRD** to cling to **TREES**.
The **TAIL FEATHERS** of a woodpecker are **STIFF**.
THEY can **USE** their tails as a **SUPPORT**.
They also use their tails to grasp **TREES**.
Woodpeckers **HAVE** long **TONGUES** with pointed **TIPS**.

Figure 5–3. This is a sample CST passage. The general topic of the passage is woodpeckers (the patient is informed of this), with the key words in bold. Note that the passage contains 25 key words (Adapted from the Hearing Aid Research Lab, University of Memphis, Memphis, TN).

sentence. There are 25 key words in each passage; standard administration is to use two passages at a time, yielding 50 key words. Whether presenting the materials as audio-only or audiovisual, it is important that the patient be told the passage topic before presentation of every list. Note that in Figure 5–3, the key words are bolded in caps for ease of scoring.

The speech sentences and background noise are on separate tracks on the disc, which allows for presentation in quiet or in any SNR the clinician chooses. The selection of the speech level and SNR for this test should be based on your clinical goal, as we discussed earlier in this chapter.

The two-channel calibration noise contains steady state noise in both channels for use in calibration. Most important, these are not the same noises in each channel, as one matches the spectrum of the CST babble and the other matches the spectrum of the speech. Furthermore, Sherbecoe and Studebaker (2002) showed that the key words are about 1 dB higher in level than all the words taken together. As a consequence, the authors indicate that the test should be calibrated by adjusting the VU meter to –5 dB when playing the noise channel and –4 dB when playing the speech channel.

Manual scoring is accomplished by counting the number of key words the listener misses out of 50 for each passage pair. We simply make tick marks for every word missed on a piece of scrap paper. Alternatively, one could print out copies of the passage pair text and mark out the actual words missed. The recordings contain pauses after each sentence presentation, so that the patient has time to repeat the sentence and to facilitate scoring. As a consequence, test administration and scoring after calibration simply consists of telling the patient the passage topic, pressing play, and keeping track of the number of key words that are not correctly repeated.

The speech track of the CST can be routed to one earphone or to a loudspeaker, and the noise track can be routed to the same earphone or loudspeaker to evaluate speech recognition in noise without spatial separation, or to another loudspeaker (e.g., behind the patient) to evaluate speech recognition in noise with spatial separation—for example, to evaluate directional benefit for counseling purposes. The video track of the DVD can then be routed from the DVD player to either a television or other video monitor using the appropriate video cord (e.g., S-video, DVI, HDMI, etc.). A sound level meter will be required to calibrate the level at the position of the listener's head for loudspeaker presentation.

Obtaining Speech Intelligibility Ratings

As an alternative to use as an objective speech recognition measure, the CST materials can also be used to estimate subjective perception of performance. Although the same corpus of sentences is used, a male talker is used instead, the instructions are different, and the test is referred to SIR (for Speech Intelligibility Ratings; Cox & McDaniel, 1989). In this test, listeners rate the intelligibility of test passages on an equal-appearing interval scale from 0 to 100. A rating of 0 should reflect a situation in which none of the words is understood and a score of 100 would represent a situation in which all of the words are understood.

**THINGS TO REMEMBER:
THE HARL AT THE UNIVERSITY OF MEMPHIS**

As we mention here, both the CST and the Speech Intelligibility Ratings (SIR) are available from the Hearing Aid Research Laboratory (HARL) at the University of Memphis, headed by Robyn Cox, PhD. Both tests can be ordered from their website, which is a treasure trove for audiologists needing tests related to hearing aid selection and fitting. Besides the tests we just mentioned, this is also where you find other fitting applications such as VIOLA and the Contour Test (Chapter 4), as well as pre-fitting measures that we discuss in Chapter 6 such as the APHAB and ECHO, and also popular outcome measures like the SADL, IOI-HA, and DOSO, which we discuss in the validation section of Book Three of this series—all in all, it is a useful website to visit.

Asking participants to estimate the percentage of words they understood yields very similar results as objective speech recognition scores. Although listeners with hearing loss generally underestimate their performance, they do so consistently. Therefore, to estimate objective hearing aid benefit, one could gather subjective data on the perception of intelligibility in both aided and unaided conditions. Listeners who underestimate their performance unaided will also underestimate their performance aided, giving similar estimates of hearing aid benefit (Cox, Alexander, & Rivera, 1991). Similar results have been reported with the SIR (Cox & McDaniel, 1989) test and the Revised SIR (Cienkowski & Speaks, 2000). In total, these results suggest that subjective impression of perceived intelligibility may be a useful measure for evaluating the effects of hearing aids on speech recognition. Therefore, one may choose to use the SIR instead of the CST if interested in the performance with a male, instead of a female talker.

Clinical Applications

The CST was designed for, and is used most often in, hearing aid research studies. Although we find it is a bit long for routine clinical use, there are some specific clinical situations where the CST is useful. Many speech recognition in noise measures are limited in the context they provide, which in turn limits their face validity relative to the continuous discourse that is often present during typical conversations. Even more striking, the vast majority of speech recognition measures are presented without the visual cues that are commonly available during typical communication. One reason for this limitation is there are more logistical challenges and greater costs associated with presenting audiovisual materials than just the audio.

Despite these challenges, it is sometimes of interest to determine either the benefit to speech recognition from visual cues or, more likely, the performance advantage provided by a hearing aid with visual cues present. This latter question may be of interest especially in listeners with very poor speech recognition (typically severe-to-profound loss) who are unable to understand speech without visual cues. For example, for counseling purposes, during the pre-fitting visit, you may be interested in showing a patient with profound hearing loss that a directional hearing aid might be able to provide benefit. Unfortunately, this patient is unable to accurately repeat any words in noise without having visual cues. With the audiovisual presentation of the CST and presentation of the noise from behind, you can demonstrate how the directional microphone can make things

---

TECHNICAL TIP: CRITICAL DIFFERENCES FOR THE CST

If you are conducting the CST using earphones for ear-specific findings, you might want to know if there is a significant difference between ears. If you conducted this pre-fitting testing as a baseline for later amplification, you might want to know if aided findings are better than unaided. When is a difference really a difference? Cox et al. (1988) reported that the 95% critical difference for scores based on mean performance across two pairs of passages (100 key words) is 14 rau (rationalized arcsine units, a measure similar to percent correct). For adults with hearing impairment, the critical difference is 15.5 rau. This means that, for a hearing aid to have a significant effect for a listener, the difference between aided and unaided speech recognition should be approximately 15% or more. This difference of course will need to be larger if only two passages are used.

You might have noticed we use the term rau. What is a "rau" you might ask? For starters, it is the abbreviation for rationalized arcsine unit. Arcsine transformations are used to transform proportions to make them more suitable for statistical analysis. These arcsines, however, sometimes do not have an obvious relationship to the original proportions. The *rationalized* arcsine provides values that are numerically close to the original percentage values over most of the percentage range. They still, however, retain the desirable statistical properties of the arcsine transform. See Studebaker, 1985, for review.

THINGS TO REMEMBER: HOW CHANGING SNR AFFECTS PERFORMANCE

Cox et al. (1988) reported that, for normal hearing listeners, the slope of the performance-intensity function of the CST is 12 rau per dB. For listeners with hearing loss, the slope of the function was 8.5 rau per dB. This means that, for every change in dB, we might expect approximately a 10 % change in speech recognition. This information can be used to adjust the SNR and avoid floor and ceiling effects.

---

easier to understand even when the talker's face is visible. Repeating this testing at a very challenging SNR can help you demonstrate how an FM system or remote microphone may be needed instead in difficult listening situations. Such demonstrations can provide a useful starting point when counseling patients on the use of different microphone technologies.

Obtaining the CST

The audio-only version of the CST and the SIR Test are included on the HARL Speech Intelligibility Tests audio CD. The audiovisual version of the CST is available on DVD and organized into six-passage, audiovisual-equivalent sets as discussed in Cox & McDaniel (1989). Both versions can be obtained from the HARL website at the University of Memphis (http://www.memphis.edu/csd/harl/cstest.htm). Also available is an automated scoring system for the audio-only CST. See Appendix R for passage lists.

Speech Recognition In Noise Test (SPRINT)

For many years, the SPRINT was considered a test that only was of interest to military audiologists, as it was developed by U.S. Army audiologist researchers to assist in determining fitness for duty. In recent years, however, this test has found its way into civilian audiology clinics, and therefore, we believe it is important to include a summary of the test in this chapter. The reason that some civilian audiology clinics have started using the test is that they find themselves testing military personnel, particularly reservists and National Guard members, through contractual arrangements. It can also be used

for any patient to simply examine more thoroughly the effects of high frequency hearing loss on speech recognition. However, the test is lengthy (200 words), so the time commitment could be a deal breaker for some clinics.

Background

As mentioned, the SPRINT was developed at Walter Reed Army Medical Center for use in the U.S. Army. To understand the reason for its development, it is first necessary to briefly review the fitness for duty requirements. Soldiers in the army are profiled in six different categories, referred to as PULHES:

- P = Physical capacity
- U = Upper extremities
- L = Lower extremities
- H = Hearing-ears
- E = Vision-eyes
- S = Psychiatric

In each of these categories, a numerical rating of 1, 2, 3, or 4 is assigned. An H-1 profile indicates normal function, while an H-4 profile indicates *"unfit for duty."* Clearly, these profiles have a huge impact on a soldier's career.

The four profile categories for hearing are summarized below:

- H-1: PTA ≤ 25 dB @ 500, 1000, and 2000 Hz with no single threshold > 30 dB; ≤ 35 dB @ 3000 Hz, ≤ 45 dB @ 4000 Hz
- H-2 (bilateral criteria): PTA ≤ 30 dB @ 500, 1000, and 2000 Hz with no single threshold > 35 dB; ≤ 45 dB @ 3000 Hz, ≤ 55 dB @ 4000 Hz

■ H-2 (unilateral criteria): Hearing loss in better ear cannot be > 30 dB @ 500 Hz, > 25 dB @ 1000 and 2000 Hz, and > 35 dB @ 4000 Hz. Hearing loss in poorer ear is not considered—soldier can have no measureable hearing in poorer ear.

■ H-3: SRT in better ear ≤ 30 dB with or without hearing aid.

■ H-4: Hearing loss worse than H-3.

Individuals need to meet the H-2 profile guidelines to be inducted. Retention standards are not as rigid. Primarily because of the occurrence of noise-induced hearing loss in the military, it is common for soldiers who enter active duty having an H-1 or H-2 profile, to suffer high frequency hearing loss and, as a consequence, have thresholds exceeding H-2 levels at 3000 and/or 4000 Hz. This bumps them into the H-3 category. In most cases, their SRT will be ≤ 30 dB without hearing aids and nearly always with hearing aids, so it is unlikely that soldiers with noise-induced high-frequency hearing loss will be classified as H-4.

As reviewed by Cord, Walden, and Atack (1992), soldiers with H-3 profiles may be required to go before a Military Medical Retention Board (MMRB) that makes a determination to retain, reclassify, or separate the soldier from active duty. This is based on the soldier's ability to perform his or her duties. As a result, the H-3 profile generates the most discussion and was the motivation for developing the SPRINT.

If you consider the profiling system, which is based on pure-tone thresholds, two different soldiers, both with H-3 profiles, could have very different speech understanding abilities. We know that speech understanding cannot be predicted reliably from the pure-tone audiogram. Moreover, soldiers have very different duties, which also need to be considered. As a result, there has long been concern among army personnel that some soldiers have been unnecessarily reclassified or separated from the army, whereas others have been retained in assignments that may further jeopardize the soldier's fitness for duty (Cord et al., 1992). It was determined, therefore, that a clinical test of speech recognition in noise should be developed that could be easily implemented by audiologists to provide MMRB's with information regarding a hearing impaired soldier's potential communication handicap on the job.

The SPRINT consists of the 200 monosyllabic words from Form C of the NU#6 lists. The words are prerecorded in a background of multitalker babble noise, with a +9 dB speech-to-babble ratio. Cord et al. (1992) explains that this level was chosen so that normal hearing soldiers score 95 to 100% on the test. The goal of this word recognition in noise test is to provide information to the MMRBs for fitness of duty and also to allow for the comparative evaluation of different people holding the H-3 profile.

Normative Data. In early research with the SPRINT, 319 soldiers with H-3 profiles were evaluated. The mean score for the group was 163 items correct (81.5%) with a range of 65 (32.5%) to 196 (98%). A frequency distribution of the scores (i.e., number of words correct) for the 319 H-3 profile soldiers is shown in Figure 5–4. This illustrates the wide range of performance that we mentioned earlier.

Outside of the military, there has not been much research with the SPRINT. One exception is the work of Wilson and Cates (2008), which compared the SPRINT with the WIN test (a test that determines SNR-50, reviewed later in this chapter) for normal hearing and hearing impaired subjects. They report that listeners with normal hearing obtained 92.5% correct on the SPRINT with a WIN-50 score of 2.7 dB SNR. The listeners with hearing loss obtained 65.3% correct on the SPRINT and a WIN-50 at 12.0 dB SNR. The SPRINT and WIN were significantly correlated ($r = -0.81$), indicating that the SPRINT had good concurrent validity. As expected, these authors also report that the high frequency, pure-tone average (1000, 2000, 4000 Hz) had higher correlations with the SPRINT and WIN than did the traditional three-frequency, pure-tone average (500, 1000, 2000 Hz).

Administration and Scoring

Some general guidelines for administering the SPRINT are as follows:

■ The test is delivered using standard audiometic equipment via earphones, using standard calibration procedures. (Note: Given the purpose of this test and the relatively low presentation level, correct calibration of the signal is essential.)

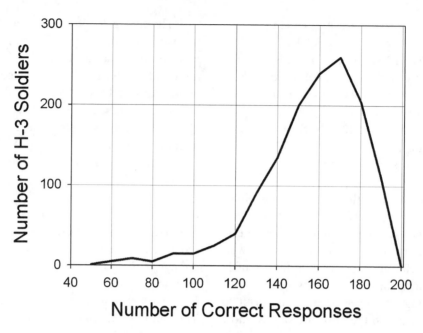

Figure 5–4. Distribution of scores (number of items correct per 200) for the SPRINT for 319 soldiers with high frequency hearing loss (Adapted from Cord et al., 1992).

- The monosyllabic words and the multitalker babble are prerecorded at the +9 dB speech-to-babble ratio on the same track of the CD; therefore, only one channel is needed.
- The test is conducted using a *bilateral presentation* (i.e., separate ear scores are *not* obtained).
- The presentation level is 50 dB HL.
- The complete 200-word test must be administered for this test to be valid.

The recommended instructions for the test are as follows:

You will be hearing a recording of a man's voice saying some words. In the background, there will be the sound of several people talking at once. I want you to repeat back the words that the man is saying. Some of the words may be difficult for you to hear. If you're not sure what the word is, take a guess. There are 4 lists containing 50 words each for a total

---

TECHNICAL TIP: PRACTICE EFFECT FOR THE SPRINT?

Although performance for all 200 words of the NU#6 list is used for scoring the SPRINT, Wilson and Cates (2008) examined scores for each 50 word list independently. They found that for the normal hearing group, the scores for Lists 1 to 4 were: 89.0, 93.7, 92.8, and 94.4%. The respective scores for the hearing loss group were: 62.1, 66.8, 67.3, and 65.2%. In both cases, there appears to be about 4% poorer performance for List 1, reflecting a possible learning effect for the speech-in-noise task. An alternative explanation would be poor interlist equivalency; however, Wilson et al. (1976) showed good interlist equivalency for these Auditec NU#6 recordings.

of 200 words. This will take about 20 minutes. You will be hearing the words and the background talkers in both ears.

The patient's SPRINT score is simply the number of monosyllabic words that were correctly identified (i.e., 0 to 200). To compare the score with the standardization sample, it is necessary to convert the score to a percentile ranking within the frequency distribution depicted in Table 5–3. For example, if the patient only correctly identifies 133 of the 200 monosyllabic words, the patient would then fall in the 10th percentile, and therefore, we would predict that 90% of all patients with similar hearing losses will score higher than he or she on the SPRINT. When used in the military, other charts and considerations are used to determine fitness for duty (see SPRINT manual).

Clinical Applications

As we mentioned in the introduction, the SPRINT was designed to provide additional information regarding fitness for duty for army personnel. In the military, it is usually administered to all active duty soldiers who are identified as having a permanent H-3 profile and retested when soldiers with an H-3 profile demonstrate a significant, permanent threshold shift.

When making fitting decisions based on the results of speech tests, we normally are looking at results from testing conducted at a relatively high presentation level—we discussed why this is important earlier in this chapter. The SPRINT is delivered at 50 dB HL (around the level of average conversation speech), considerably softer than we would normally use for other pre-fitting speech tests. There would be one benefit, however, of using this lower level. Although we are not aware of real-world validation, we would expect that patients with a significantly poorer SPRINT score are having more difficulty in their everyday communication than the patients with the higher SPRINT scores. This difference, in fact, likely would be greater for the SPRINT, than other tests administered at higher presentation levels. Recall, however, that the SNR for the SPRINT is +9 dB. Individuals with a high SPRINT score, therefore, could be having significant problems in more adverse listening situations—a high SPRINT score does not necessarily mean the patient is not a candidate for hearing aids.

Table 5–3. Conversion Table for the SPRINT*

Score	Percentile	Score	Percentile
0–75	1	162	37
76–100	2	163	40
101–107	3	164	42
108–116	4	165	45
117–122	5	166	48
123–124	6	167	49
125–126	7	168	51
127–128	8	169	53
129–130	9	170	55
131–135	10	171	57
136–138	11	172	59
139–140	12	173	62
141	13	174	64
142	14	175	67
143–144	16	176	70
145	17	177	72
146	18	178	74
147	19	179	76
148	21	180	78
149–150	22	181	80
151–152	23	182	83
153	24	183	86
154	26	184	89
155–156	28	185	92
157	29	186–187	95
158	30	188	96
159	32	189	97
160	34	190	98
161	35	191	99

*Using this table, the item correct score is converted to a percentile.
Source: Adapted from Cord, Walden, & Atack, 1992.

The 200 items of the SPRINT makes it one of the longer speech tests, so it is unlikely an audiologist would adopt this for routine testing when fitting hearing aids.

TECHNICAL TIP: TEST-RETEST RELIABILITY

Cord et al. (1992) report test-retest data for 30 individuals. The mean score for the initial administration of the SPRINT was 164.6 words correct ($SD = 15.46$), and the mean score for the retest was 166.8 words correct ($SD = 14.21$). The authors found a correlation coefficient of .93 ($p < .01$), suggesting good test-retest agreement. The slightly better (approximately 2%) mean performance for the second administration could be related to the apparent learning effect reported by Wilson and Cates (2008), which was observed following the first 50 words.

But, if the testing is already being conducted for military reasons, then it seems worthwhile to consider the patient's performance on the SPRINT along with other pre-fitting measures.

Obtaining the SPRINT

The SPRINT can be obtained from Auditec of St. Louis. If using the test for military purposes, we suggest obtaining the test guidelines: militaryaudiology.org/site/2009/01/sprint-test/.

Reception Thresholds for Speech-in-Noise

In the preceding section, we discussed speech-in-noise tests that were designed to use a fixed SNR. These tests answer the clinical question regarding how a patient performs for a given listening situation. These tests, however, often are not good at differentiating patients, primarily because of floor and ceiling effects. Consider two different patients, both with similar high frequency hearing losses. One of these patients does very well in background noise and does not start to have problems until the SNR reaches 1 to 2 dB. The other patient starts to have problems when the SNR is around 6 to 7 dB. These two patients, with the same hearing losses and fitted with the same hearing aids, might have different real-world outcomes impacting hearing aid satisfaction. But, if the speech-in-noise test selected had a fixed SNR, and that SNR was relatively good (such as the R-SPIN at +8 dB), these two patients might appear more similar than they really are due to ceiling effects.

Adaptive speech tests, as the name indicates, vary either the speech or the background noise level for each patient. Rather than a percent correct, the test is scored as the SNR where the patient obtained 50% correct. As mentioned previously, this is referred to as the speech reception threshold (SRT) in noise (often denoted as SNR-50 or SRT_{50}), or in the case of the HINT, it is dubbed the reception threshold for speech (RTS). We describe four of these tests in this section.

Finally, it is important to point out that it is risky to generalize the 50% correct for speech-in-noise performance for a given patient without referring back to the test itself and performance for that test for individuals with normal hearing and hearing loss. Fortunately for our discussion in this chapter, Wilson, McArdle, and Smith (2007) just happened to compare the four SNR-50 speech tests that we describe. They found that for a group of individuals with hearing loss, the mean SNR-50 results for the four different tests were as follows:

BKB-SIN	SNR-50 = 5.0 dB
HINT	RTS = 8.9 dB
QuickSIN	SNR-50 = 12.3 dB
WIN	SNR-50 = 14.0 dB

The above mean values are from the same patients, so that if we only knew that a given patient from this group had an SNR-50 of 8 dB, it would not tell us much. That performance would be considerably better than average for the WIN but worse than average for the BKB-SIN. As you might expect, these scores from hearing impaired individuals differed significantly from people with normal hearing, but the degree of difference also varied for the different tests. The difference was as

> ### TECHNICAL TIP: VARY THE SPEECH LEVEL OR THE NOISE LEVEL?
>
> In this section, we discuss adaptive procedures for determining the speech reception threshold in noise (i.e., SNR for 50% correct). For some tests, the noise is fixed and speech varies (e.g., the HINT), and in others, the speech is fixed and the noise varies (e.g., BKB-SIN). In most real-world listening situations, it is the noise that is fixed, so that approach would seem to have to the most face validity. But, there also are certain advantages of having a fixed-speech signal. One might ask if the test outcome differs depending on which of the two is the variable signal? Wilson and McArdle (2012) did ask this question using modified versions of the R-SPIN, and they found, at least for this test, that it *does not* matter. The mean 50% points were slightly lower (better) on the speech-variable, babble-fixed condition, but the small differences (0.1 to 0.4 dB) are not clinically significant. Larger differences might be expected however, if lower presentation levels are used and there is an interaction with the audibility of the speech signal.

low as 4.2 and 5.6 dB for the BKB-SIN and the HINT (which have more context in the material) compared with 7.9 and 10.1 dB for the QuickSIN and the WIN.

Hearing In Noise Test (HINT)

For audiologists working with hearing aids, the HINT is one of the most well-known speech-in-noise tests, because for the past 15 to 20 years, it has been the favorite test of researchers when comparative hearing aid performance is conducted. Hence, audiologists are accustomed to thinking about things like the benefit from directional technology in terms of HINT scores—manufacturers often use these scores in promotional literature.[30] The test is favored by researchers of course, because of the adaptive nature of the HINT, floor and ceiling effects are avoided. Moreover, using the SNR-50 approach, which zeros in on the steepest portion of the performance-intensity function, it is more probable that small differences in true performance will be observed.

Although most audiologists know about the HINT, it is not commonly used in the routine hearing aid fitting protocols for adults. This is probably because of several reasons including, administration and scoring is more cumbersome than most other tests, the results are in SNR rather than percent correct, and availability of the test has been spotty. Nevertheless, it is one of the most researched speech tests and certainly could be

adopted for routine clinical use. Conversely, the version for children (HINT-C) is used more commonly, likely because it is more readily available.

Background

The HINT was originally developed for testing related to the evaluation of bilateral versus unilateral hearing aid fittings. Prior to the HINT, one of the only adaptive speech reception threshold tests reported was the Dutch test developed by Plomp and Mimpen (1979)—which influenced the development of the HINT. The now-classic article describing the development of the HINT at the House Ear Institute of Los Angeles was published by Nilsson, Soli, and Sullivan (1994). The following are some details regarding the development of this test (Nilsson et al., 1994; Vermiglio, 2008):

- The HINT material was derived from the BKB (for Bamford-Kowal-Bench) sentences, which were from British children. The language level is approximately a first-grade reading level.
- The 336 BKB sentences were revised, roughly equated for sentence length, rated for naturalness by native speakers of American English, and were rescaled to obtain equal intelligibility. Following these measures, 252 of the 336 sentences remained Figure 5–5 shows the sample sentences.

1. (A/the) **boy fell from** (A/the) **window**

2. (A/the) **wife helped her husband**

3. **Big dogs can be dangerous**

4. **Her shoes** (are/were) **very dirty**

5. (A/the) **player lost** (a/the) **shoe**

6. **Somebody stole** the **money**

7. (A/the) **fire** (**is/was**) **very hot**

8. **She's drinking from her own cup**

9. (A/the) **picture came from** (a/the) **book**

10. (A/the) car (**is/was**) **going too fast**

Figure 5–5. Sample of a 10-item list from the HINT (Adapted from HINT Manual Two, House Ear Institute).

- The CD version of the HINT has 25 lists of 10 sentences. It is common (and recommended) to use two lists/test (20 sentences). Each list is phonemically balanced and the 12 20-sentence lists are equivalent.
- The HINT masking noise is a speech spectrum noise that was spectrally matched to the long-term average spectrum of the stimulus sentences.

As we have discussed, there are several adaptive speech tests available for the audiologist to choose from. Are these tests all pretty much the same? Mueller, Johnson, and Weber (2010) tested a group of adults with mild-moderate downward sloping hearing loss using both the HINT and the QuickSIN. They found a relatively strong 0.75 correlation between these two measures. Wilson et al. (2007) sought to determine which adaptive speech test would be the best for separating hearing impaired listeners from individuals with normal hearing using four different adaptive speech tests: HINT, QuickSIN, BKB-SIN, and the WIN—the later three tests are discussed in detail later in the section. They concluded that separation between groups was greater for the QuickSIN and the WIN (8 to 10 dB), compared with the HINT and the BKB-SIN (4 to 6 dB). These results suggest that, although there is a strong correlation between these adaptive tests, the QuickSIN and the WIN may be most sensitive to the effects of hearing loss.

Administration and Scoring

The recommended instructions from the HINT manual are as follows:

> This is test of your ability to hear soft speech in a noisy situation. First you will hear background noise. Then you will hear a man reading a sentence. The loudness of the man's voice will change during the test. Sometimes it will be very faint. Please repeat anything you hear, even if it is only part of the sentence. I will stop after each sentence to allow you to repeat what you heard. It is all right to guess.

The HINT is recorded on two separate tracks of the CD. For test administration:

- Deliver the right channel output to channel 1 input of the audiometer and the left channel output to the channel 2 input of the audiometer.

THINGS TO REMEMBER: THE HINT GOES INTERNATIONAL

There is little question that the HINT is the most internationally used speech test. In a special issue of the *International Journal of Audiology* (2008), there were summaries of research and norms published for the HINT for the following different languages: Latin American Spanish, Brazilian Portuguese, Turkish, Castilian Spanish, Bulgarian, French, Korean, Norwegian, Malay, Japanese, Canadian French, Cantonese, Taiwanese Mandarin, and Mainland Mandarin.

- Use calibration tone to set the VU (for Volume Unit) meters for both channels.
- Play the noise signal and adjust the HL until the calibration microphone measures 65 dB SPL. Make note of this dial setting. Conduct this measure for both channels.

Once the patient is ready to take the test:

- Set the noise channel to the HL dial reading that was determined to deliver 65 dB SPL.
- Begin with a sentence presentation level 5 dB below the noise.
- Play and repeat the first sentence, increasing the level in 4-dB increments until the patient responds correctly. Record this level on the score sheet.
- Begin testing at this level with Sentence #1 using the adaptive approach for the intensity of the sentences—increase the intensity when the patient does not provide a correct response and decrease the intensity when

the response is correct. Use 4-dB steps for Sentences #1 to 4.
- Use 2-dB adaptive steps for Sentences #5 to 20.

Scoring the HINT. If you are using the standard CD/paper and pencil version of administering and scoring the HINT, the process requires a bit more attention than for most recognition measures. First, you will need to listen carefully to the patient's response and determine if the patient got all the words of the sentence correct. All words must be correct for the sentence to be scored correct. If correct, a "+" is placed on the score sheet; if not correct, "−" is recorded. Then quickly, the intensity level must be lowered or raised, so that the next sentence is presented at the correct level. To help illustrate this method, we have a completed score sheet shown in Figure 5–6 (see Appendix S for blank score sheet). This paper-to-dial visual task, and remembering that for "plus" turn dial down, "minus" turn dial up activity, is not the kind of speech recognition scoring that allows you to simultaneously sip coffee or read text messages, or even daydream. (Note: There are automated

---

POINTS TO PONDER: WHEN IS THE HINT NO LONGER THE HINT?

In various published research studies related to the evaluation of hearing aids and hearing aid candidates, we have observed numerous modifications of the HINT. Often, in these studies it is reported that the HINT was used as the speech material, although we question if it is really the HINT if the test is not administered and scored as originally intended? Some modifications we have observed include:

- Presentation levels of the fixed noise signal are lower or higher than the recommended 65 dB SPL.
- Multitalker babble, cocktail party noise, ISTS (for International Speech Test Signal), and other noise signals are used as competition instead of the standard HINT noise.
- The silent gap between the sentences is filled in with noise.
- An introductory phrase is used for each sentence.
- Rather than an adaptive presentation, the background noise is presented at a fixed SNR or in quiet. This is a common procedure for patients with cochlear implants.
- Rather than scoring each sentence as all or nothing, each word of each sentence is scored.

What really gets confusing is that we have even heard mention of using the HINT *with no background noise*, which would then seem to make it the HIQT rather than the HINT.

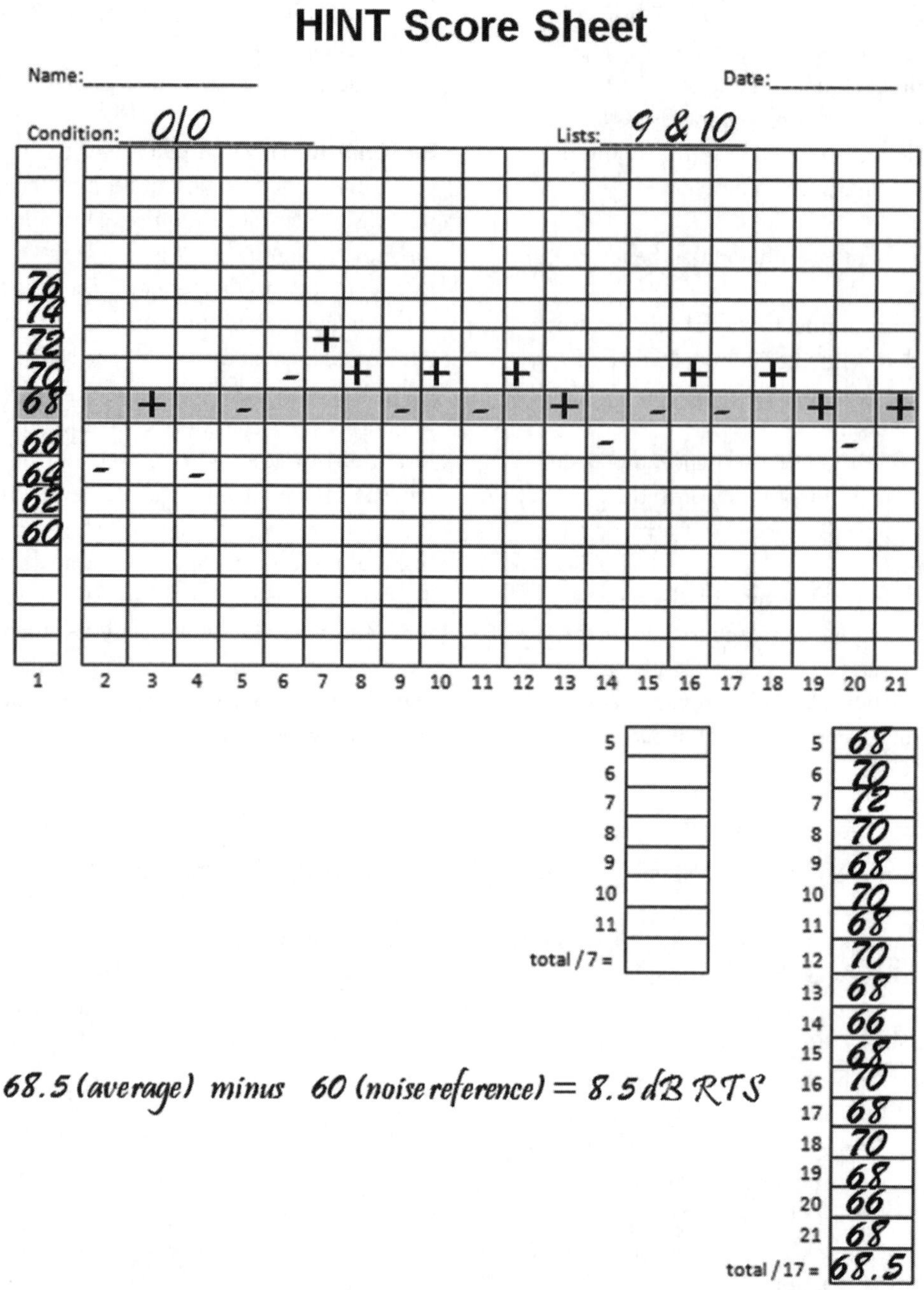
HINT Score Sheet
Name:
Date:
Condition: 0/0
Lists: 9 & 10
76
74
72
70
68
66
64
62
60
1 2 3 4 5 6 7 8 9 10 11 12 13 14 15 16 17 18 19 20 21
total / 7 =
5 68
6 70
7 72
8 70
9 68
10 70
11 68
12 70
13 68
14 66
15 68
16 70
17 68
18 70
19 68
20 66
21 68
total / 17 = 68.5
68.5 (average) minus 60 (noise reference) = 8.5 dB RTS

Figure 5–6. Sample of completed score sheet from the HINT. The "+" and "–" markings indicate when the patient had a correct or incorrect response for a sentence for a given presentation level. The RTS value shown was calculated by subtracting the level of the backgound noise (60 dB HL) from the average of the last 17 presentations levels (68.5)

programs that simplify this process, but these are not always available to the clinician.)

Details regarding the scoring (20-sentence list):

- The score placed for the column 21 is based on the patient's performance for Sentence #20. If the patient got Sentence #20 correct, the score for column 21 is 2 dB lower than what was recorded in column 20. If the patient missed Sentence #20, then the score placed in column 21 is 2 dB higher.

- The presentation levels for columns 5–21 are then summed and divided by 17 to obtain an average. For example, we see in Figure 5–6 that the total of the 17 presentations was 1,164.5; divided by 17 we have an average value of 68.5 dB.

- To obtain the RTS, we need to subtract the HL reference level that was used for the 65 dB SPL calibration. In this case, that value was 60 dB HL, and therefore our RTS is 68.5 dB minus 60 dB or 8.5 dB.

Clinical Applications

TECHNICAL TIP: PERFORMANCE-INTENSITY FUNCTION OF THE HINT

When using the HINT, it is sometimes desirable to think of different HINT RTS scores in terms of predicted intelligibility change. This is, if a person experienced a 3 dB reduction in his HINT RTS, how could we express that as a percent of reduced speech recognition? To obtain an estimate, we can look at performance as a function of the SNR. Nilsson and Soli (1994) reported a slope of 9.5%/dB between 10% and 90% of the range. Eisenberg, Dirks, Takayanagi, and Martinez (1998) reported the slope of the PI function as 11.8% between 20% and 80%. Roughly then, 10 to 12%/dB SNR for the midrange of the function would be a reasonable estimate to remember.

One of the clinical applications of the HINT is to determine how a given patient's score differs from people with normal hearing. Shown in Table 5–4 are norms from the HINT manual for sound field testing with both the signal and noise presented from a 0 degree azimuth. Shown in Table 5–5 are HINT norms for bilateral earphone testing (Vermiglio, 2008). Also included in

Table 5–4. HINT Norms for Sound-Field Testing with Both Sentences and HINT Noise Delivered from a Loudspeaker at 0° Azimuth

Percentile	Hint RTS
90th	−4.2
70th	−3.4
50th	−2.8
30th	−2.3
10th	−1.5

Source: Adapted from Koch, Nilsson, & Soli, 2004.

Table 5–5. HINT Earphone Norms For Bilateral Presentation, Noise Front Condition. Also shown is the expected intelligibility change from the mean (50th percentile).

Percentile	Hint RTS	Intelligibility Change
90th	−3.9	14%
70th	−3.3	7%
50th	−2.6	0%
30th	−1.9	7%
10th	−1.3	14%

Source: Adapted from Vermiglio, 2008.

Table 5–5 is the expected intelligibility change from the mean (50th percentile). Note that these two different sets of norms are very similar, within 0.2 to 0.3 for the 90th, 50th, and 10th percentiles.

If we look at the norms for normal hearing individuals, we then have an estimate of where our patient falls. For example, if the HINT RTS is 7 dB, we would then assume that the patient would need the speech turned up or the noise turned down about 9 to 10 dB compared with normal hearing individuals (see 50th percentile for Tables 5–4 and 5–5). This is similar to the SNR loss designator that is used for the QuickSIN, which we explain in the next section. The degree of this SNR loss can be used in pre-fitting counseling. We also know that a patient with an RTS of 2 dB may require different counseling than one with a 10 dB RTS. The same would apply to large ear differences for the HINT.

There are not norms per se for people with sensorineural hearing loss, primarily because there is such variance in the hearing losses studied. Also, many of the studies have modified the HINT, using different background noises, loudspeaker arrangements, and presentation levels. It is common, however, with typical downward sloping hearing losses, to see scores in the +3 to +9 dB RTS range—in the research we mentioned earlier from Mueller et al. (2010), who used the standard HINT format, they reported the mean RTS was 6.4 dB with a range of 0.4 to 16.3 dB.

In addition to providing useful information for counseling, pre-fitting HINT measures can serve as a baseline for later hearing aid verification. Because of the adaptive nature and the 2-dB steps, the sensitivity of the HINT is better than many speech tests for detecting differences in hearing aid performance, for example, the benefits of directional technology. We should mention that if the patient only has a mild-to-moderate hearing loss and the HINT was conducted at a fairly high presentation level, it is very possible that the aided HINT RTS will be no better than the unaided—more on this in the verification section of Book Three of this series.

Obtaining the HINT

Many clinics already have the HINT CD, either obtained when the test was licensed by Starkey Laboratories or from Cochlear Corporation, as the HINT has been a common speech test used in the evaluation of the cochlear implant candidate.[31] Ten years ago or so, the HINT for Windows was developed, which for some time was distributed by Bio-Logic, a division of Natus

---

KEY CONCEPT: APPLICATIONS OF THE HINT

In this chapter, we address the use of the HINT for the pre-fitting of hearing aids. We have also mentioned that the HINT is a commonly used test in research for assessing and differentiating hearing aid performance, and evaluating new hearing aid algorithms. However, perhaps the major application of the HINT is outside the world of hearing aids. It is used for screening functional hearing ability in occupational health settings. This application is primarily with government agencies that have public safety and law enforcement jobs. Federal, state (provincial), and local agencies in the United States and Canada are using the HINT for this purpose.

THINGS TO REMEMBER: THE HINT TEST FOR KIDS?

The focus of this chapter is testing for adults, but it is worth mentioning that there is also a HINT-C version of the HINT for children (see Gelnett, Sumida, Nilsson and Soli, 1995). This research found that the HINT-C test can be used for children as young as five years old.

Medical Incorporated, with the market name of "HINT Pro." It is important to note that the Windows version is a complete system that includes both hardware and software. This significantly streamlines administration and scoring. A more basic version of this system currently is available from the Californian company, Hearing Test Systems, in 13 languages (three more in development), with long-time HINT purveyor Sig Soli, PhD, chief scientific officer. At the time of this writing, the HINT CD version was not distributed commercially, although the HINT-C was available on CD in American English, Canadian French, Norwegian, Mandarin, and Cantonese. Unrelated to hearing aid fitting, a Web-based version of the HINT for use in occupational hearing screening is also available.

Quick Speech In Noise (QuickSIN) Test

As we have discussed, understanding speech in background noise is not predictable from a patient's pure-tone thresholds (Dirks et al., 1982; Killion & Niquette, 2000; Lyregaard, 1982; Walden & Walden, 2004). Some early attempts to create clinical tests such as the Speech in Noise test (SIN; Killion & Villchur, 1993) and the R-SPIN (Bilger et al., 1984) turned out to be less than ideal because they were lengthy, and in some cases, the lists were not equivalent or they were too difficult for some patients (Bentler, 2000). The QuickSIN was developed to overcome some of these limitations (Killion, Niquette, Gudmundsen, Revit, & Banerjee, 2004).

Background

The QuickSIN was designed to be short enough for routine clinical use, but yet provide a quick and reliable way to measure a listener's speech understanding ability in noise (Duncan & Aarts, 2006). The test certainly is quick, as a single list only requires about a minute to administer after instructions. It should be noted, however, that not all lists are equivalent as described in our "Things to Remember" passage in this section, so only eight of the lists should be used for routine clinical testing. When introduced, the QuickSIN joined the HINT as a measure that tests multiple SNRs by design. As a result, a threshold SNR for which approximately 50% of the material is correctly repeated is determined (commonly referred to as an SNR-50), and the difficulty of

choosing a single, correct SNR that avoided floor and ceiling effects is eliminated.

The QuickSIN consists of 12 standard lists and 3 practice lists. Each list contains six sentences with five key words per sentence. Sentences are spoken by a female talker who is reading sentences from the speech corpus of the IEEE (1969). The IEEE sentences were designed to be syntactically appropriate and meaningful, but to provide limited contextual information. For example, a practice sentence is:

"One step more and the board will collapse."

The QuickSIN sentences are presented in a multitalker background at six predetermined SNRs, which become progressively more difficult with each sentence in 5-dB steps. That is, the first sentence is presented at a +25 dB SNR, and the second sentence is presented at a +20 dB SNR. The final sentence is the most difficult and is presented at a 0 dB SNR. The presentation level of the speech is fixed, and the level of the multitalker background varies when SNR is adjusted. The competing signal is somewhat unique, as it is not a true babble as used with some of the other tests we describe. It is only four talkers, and one of the talkers, a female, is the same talker who is reading the target sentences. At the adverse SNRs (when the multitalkers become louder) many patients report that they have a tendency to try to follow the woman in the competing noise. We discussed information masking earlier in this chapter, and of course, this type of background noise is not unlike what many of our hearing aid patients frequently experience.

The standard QuickSIN lists are available in both a mixed version (target sentences and competing talkers on same track) for standard testing through a headphone or single loudspeaker and a "separated" version where the noise and speech are on separate tracks so they can be routed to separate loudspeakers. The mixed version is helpful, as you do not have to be concerned with the calibration of two different channels to maintain the correct SNR.

The standard QuickSIN lists were also modified to generate High Frequency Emphasis (HFE) and High Frequency Emphasis-Low Pass (HFE-LP) lists. These lists are designed to be used in combination to assess the importance of maximizing high frequency gain for patients with steeply sloping high frequency hearing loss (see "Clinical Applications"). Both HFE lists are the standard lists with approximately 30 dB of high frequency gain applied to simulate the hearing aid gain that might be applied for a listener with 60 to 70 dB of hearing loss. To generate the HFE-LP lists, a low-pass filter was applied with a cut-off frequency of 3,000 Hz to simulate a hearing aid that provides high frequency gain, but only through approximately 3000 Hz.

Administration and Scoring

The easiest method of administering the QuickSIN is using the commercially available CD in a CD player routed to a clinical audiometer. The QuickSIN manual describes specific calibration and scoring methods.

- For standard measurement of the SNR-50, the presentation level should be 70 dB HL (83 dB SPL) for patients with pure-tone averages 45 dB or less and should be set to "loud but okay" (just below the patient's LDL) for patients with more hearing loss.
- The test can be administered under headphones (bilaterally or unilaterally) or in the sound field, depending on the desired use (see "Clinical Applications").
- The patient's task is to repeat the sentence spoken by the female talker. Each sentence consists of five key words, and patients receive credit for each key word correctly

repeated—unlike the HINT, which we discussed earlier, they do not need to get the entire sentence correct.
- The test is easily scored (with minor math applications) using the standard score sheet, copies of which are available online. The clinician simply marks the number of key words correctly repeated for each sentence and then sums these numbers to calculate a total score, shown in Figure 5–7.

To determine the SNR-50 or what the authors refer to as the SNR loss (because the score is adjusted based on average performance for normal hearing individuals), the number of correctly repeated key words is subtracted from 25.5 (SNR loss = 25.5 – Correct Key Words). This number reflects the SNR at which a patient correctly repeats approximately 50% of the key words, with the normal hearing correction (Killion et al., 2004). For example, let's say a patient repeated all the words correctly for the first four sentences (a total of 20 words; 5 key words/sentence), and was not able to get any of the words correct for the last two more difficult sentence presentations (SNR of +5 dB and 0 dB). We would then subtract 20 (words correct) from 25.5, and this patient would have an SNR loss of 5.5 dB.

Critical difference values for the QuickSIN are shown in Figure 5–8. You can see that these values drop pretty rapidly as the number of lists per condition

---

TRACK 21

Practice List A   Score

1. The <u>lake</u> <u>sparkled</u> in the <u>red</u> <u>hot</u> <u>sun</u>.   S/N 25   _____

2. <u>Tend</u> the <u>sheep</u> <u>while</u> the <u>dog</u> <u>wanders</u>.   S/N 20   _____

3. <u>Take</u> <u>two</u> <u>shares</u> as a <u>fair</u> <u>profit</u>.   S/N 15   _____

4. <u>North</u> <u>winds</u> <u>bring</u> <u>colds</u> and <u>fevers</u>.   S/N 10   _____

5. A <u>sash</u> of <u>gold</u> <u>silk</u> will <u>trim</u> her <u>dress</u>.   S/N 5   _____

6. <u>Fake</u> <u>stones</u> <u>shine</u> but <u>cost</u> <u>little</u>.   S/N 0   _____

                                                                    TOTAL   _____

Figure 5–7. Sample list from the QuickSIN (Adapted from the QuickSIN manual, Etymotic, Inc.).

Lists per Condition	1	2	3	4	5	6	7	8	9
95% C.D. +/-, in dB	3.9	2.7	2.2	1.9	1.7	1.6	1.5	1.4	1.3
90% C.D. +/-, in dB	3.2	2.2	1.8	1.6	1.4	1.3	1.2	1.1	1.1
80% C.D. +/-, in dB	2.5	1.8	1.5	1.3	1.1	1.0	1.0	0.9	0.8

Figure 5–8. Critical differences for the QuickSIN for different number of lists used (Adapted from the QuickSIN manual, Etymotic, Inc.).

increases from one to three. Given the very fast test time of giving one list, we believe it is worthwhile to present at least two lists per condition when comparing conditions (e.g., HFE versus HFE-LP or right ear versus left ear). In this case, the time investment is still less than five minutes and critical differences approach 2 dB with 90% confidence. For a single condition (e.g., measuring the patient's SNR loss), it is probably worth your time to present three lists to gain a more accurate and reliable measure.

KEY CONCEPT: BACKGROUND FOR SCORING THE QUICKSIN

Audiologists often ask why is it that for scoring the QuickSIN, we use the number 25.5? Why not subtract the missed words from 30, as this is the number of items. Let us explain. This calculation was modeled after the Tillman and Olsen (1973) spondee threshold method. The math is kept simple by using five words per step and a 5-dB step size—in other words, one word per dB. In this case, one-half of the step size (2.5 dB) is added to the starting SNR (+25 dB) and then 2 dB is subtracted from this value because normal hearing listeners score +2 dB SNR on the average. As the authors explain, "if someone repeats all the words correctly down to 15 dB SNR and then misses everything beyond that point, they gave 15 correct responses (five each at 25, 20, and 15 dB SNR). Because they scored 100% correct at 15 dB SNR and 0% correct at 10 dB SNR, their SNR-50 would be about 12.5 dB, halfway between 15 and 10."

THINGS TO REMEMBER:
DO NOT USE THESE QUICKSIN LISTS

For a standard administration, the QuickSIN is a quick and reliable method of estimating a patient's ability to understand speech in noise. As we have mentioned, you will want to use two or three lists per ear when conducting your testing. It is important, therefore, that all lists are equivalent. Research by McArdle and Wilson (2006) suggests that they may not be. In studying individuals with hearing loss, they found that the range among lists was 10.0 to 14.3 dB SNR. The data from their study indicated that for purposes of homogeneity of test results, only the following eight lists should be used: 1, 2, 3, 5, 6, 8, 9, 10, 11, and 12.

Clinical Applications

There are several ways that the QuickSIN findings can be used to assist in hearing aid selection and patient counseling. We review a few of them here.

Hearing Aid Selection. One of the most obvious clinical uses for the QuickSIN may be as a pre-fitting measure to aid in hearing aid selection and counseling decisions. Once a clinician has determined the SNR loss, this information can be combined with knowledge of the patient's communication needs to provide evidenced-based recommendations to the patient regarding hearing aid features, in particular microphone technology. For example, let's assume a patient has the communication goal of better speech understanding in a noisy mall, which you estimate the SNR to be +4 dB. If the patient has a QuickSIN score indicating the SNR at which they can repeat 50% of words in sentences (SNR-50) of +6, they might expect to obtain large and important benefits from directional technology. Conversely, if the patient has a goal of communicating in a noisy club in which you estimate the SNR to be +1 dB and their QuickSIN SNR-50 is +15 dB, an FM system or remote microphone may need to be considered, and you may have some counseling about realistic expectations to do as well!

We find that information regarding SNR loss as it relates to goals and realistic expectations for counseling purposes is one of the best uses for the QuickSIN—this counseling then ties into the pre-fitting completion of the Client Oriented Scale of Improvement (COSI), which we discuss in the next chapter. There is some evidence that unaided SNR loss may be a significant predictor of amplification success in everyday living. That is, people who have more SNR loss may report less success with hearing aids (Walden & Walden, 2004).

High Frequency Gain. An additional clinical use of the QuickSIN capitalizes on the HFE (for high frequency emphasis) lists (Tracks 36 to 47) and HFE-LP (for high frequency emphasis-low predictability) lists (Tracks 52 to 63). As we discussed in Chapter 4, there is some question as to whether or not people with steeply sloping high frequency hearing loss, particularly those with cochlear dead regions, can benefit from high frequency amplification. Although data suggests that, on average, benefit is expected, it does not occur for all listeners; it appears that the degree to which a patient can make use of high frequency cues depends on the individual. For some patients, providing high frequency amplification may actually impair speech recognition, and for others, high frequency amplification provides additional speech cues, improving speech recognition (Hornsby, Johnson, & Picou, 2011; Rankovic, 1991; Turner & Cummings, 1999). Therefore, a clinician could use the HFE and HFE-LP QuickSIN lists to determine if an individual patient would benefit from high frequency gain, or if that patient would be better served to not have the prescription gain and instead have less high frequency gain. The advantages to not providing high frequency gain for a patient, who would not benefit from it, are that providing high-frequency gain may actually impair speech recognition for some patients, especially with steeply sloping high frequency hearing loss. Feedback is generally easier to manage if maximizing high frequency gain is not essential. Therefore, using a couple of QuickSIN lists to determine the usefulness of maximizing high frequency gain could potentially save a clinician (and the patient) lots of time and energy, if high frequency gain proves to be not helpful.

Unilateral Versus Bilateral. The QuickSIN may also be helpful in determining whether to fit unilateral or bilateral amplification. For some patients, especially those that are older, it is possible that using only one hearing aid allows them to understand speech better than with two hearing aids (Walden & Walden, 2005). Whether or not a patient will benefit from two hearing aids is not necessarily predictable from their audiogram. That is, even patients with symmetric hearing loss may perform better with only one hearing aid. Therefore, using the QuickSIN under headphones to evaluate SNR loss in each ear and also a bilateral SNR loss could help guide clinical recommendations for hearing aid selection. For example, if a patient has an SNR loss of 4 dB in the right ear, 9 dB in the left ear, and 12 dB bilaterally, the best clinical recommendation may be to fit only the right ear with a hearing aid. Because the SNR loss in the left ear is worse than the right ear and because the bilateral SNR loss is worse than either ear alone, the right ear is a prime candidate for amplification. Dichotic speech testing also will be helpful in making this decision—see our discussion later in the chapter.

> ### THINGS TO REMEMBER: RELIABILITY OF THE QUICKSIN
>
> For HFE and HFE-LP administration, it may be necessary to test a patient with eight lists—four HFE lists and four HFE-LP lists. By using eight lists, the 95% confidence interval is 1.9 dB. In other words, if the average difference between the HFE and HFE-LP scores is 2 dB or greater, you can assume that the difference is real. So, if a patient achieves a score that is more than 2 dB better with the HFE lists than with the HFE-LP lists, you can conclude that this patient is likely helped by high frequency gain and you should strive to provide the recommended high frequency gain for this patient. The research of Johnson and Cox (2009) revealed lists 1, 4, 5 and 10 of the HFE and HFE-LP lists were the most sensitive to reduction of high-frequencies and should give the most valid information regarding about benefit from high-frequency cues. Therefore an alternative procedure would be to only use these four lists (two per condition).

Obtaining the QuickSIN

The QuickSIN CD is available from Etymotic Research at http://www.etymotic.com/pro/.

Bamford-Kowal-Bench Sentences in Noise (BKB-SIN)

The BKB-SIN (Etymotic Research, 2005) is another speech-in-noise test that uses the SNR-50 approach. Like its cousin the QuickSIN, it was developed to quickly and accurately assess speech recognition performance in background noise during a routine clinic visit. See Appendix T for sentence lists.

Background

The BKB-SIN consists of sentences from the Bamford-Kowal-Bench corpus spoken by a male talker with a multialker babble background noise (the same four-talker background that is used for the QuickSIN). The sentences should be appropriate for use with pediatric populations because the sentences were derived from language samples taken from young children (Bench, Kowal, & Bamford, 1979) and are at approximately a first-grade reading level (Nilsson & Soli, 1994). Recognition of the words in the sentences in each list progressively becomes more difficult by increasing the noise +3 dB for each sentence. That is, the SNR progressively changes in 3 dB steps from +9 to –6 dB (List Pairs 1

to 8) and from +21 to 0 dB (List Pairs 9 to 18). Each list pair consists of two lists, each with 8 to 10 sentences. A sample list is displayed in Figure 5–9.

Although not quite as quick as the QuickSIN, it is still quite fast. In addition, the BKB-SIN holds several other advantages including: better reliability, better list equivalency, and more normative data including norms for cochlear implant users. For these reasons, we favor the BKB-SIN over the QuickSIN for most of the clinical applications we described earlier for the QuickSIN. There are two caveats to this recommendation. First, there are currently no HFE or HFE-LP lists available for the BKB-SIN, so the QuickSIN still must be used for assessing benefits for high frequency amplification. Second, and perhaps more importantly, the Quick-SIN results in larger differences between normal and hearing impaired listeners, likely due to differences in talker gender and sentence complexity, and is therefore more sensitive to difficulties understanding speech in noise.

Administration and Scoring

Administration and scoring is nearly identical to the QuickSIN, which we detailed in the previous section. In brief, the easiest method of administering the BKB-SIN is using the commercially available CD in a CD player routed to a clinical audiometer. The BKB-SIN manual describes specific calibration and scoring methods. For determining an SNR loss and comparison with normative data, the presentation level should be 70 dB HL for patients with three-frequency pure-tone averages 45 dB

List 9A	Key Words	# Correct	SNR
1. The <u>football</u> <u>player</u> <u>lost</u> a <u>shoe</u>.	4	_____	+ 21 dB
2. The <u>painter</u> <u>used</u> a <u>brush</u>.	3	_____	+18 dB
3. The <u>lady</u> <u>sat</u> on her <u>chair</u>.	3	_____	+15 dB
4.The <u>milkman</u> <u>brought</u> the <u>cream</u>.	3		+12 dB
5. The <u>dog</u> <u>chased</u> the <u>cat</u>.	3	_____	+9 dB
6. <u>Mother</u> <u>shut</u> the <u>window</u>.	3	_____	+6 dB
7. The <u>apple</u> <u>pie</u> was <u>good</u>.	3	_____	+3 dB
8. <u>Rain</u> <u>falls</u> from the <u>clouds</u>.	3	_____	0 dB
	Total Key Words Correct	_____	
	SNR – 50 = (23.5) – (# correct)	_____	

Figure 5–9. Sample list from the BKB-SIN (Adapted from the BKB-SIN manual, Etymotic, Inc.).

or less and should be set to "loud but okay" for patients with more hearing loss. The test can be administered under headphones (bilaterally or unilaterally) or in the sound field, depending on the desired use (see "Clinical Applications"). The patient's task is to repeat the sentence spoken by a male talker. The instructions are as follows:

Imagine you are at a party. There will be a man talking and several other talkers in the background. The man will say, "Ready" and then will say a sentence. Repeat the sentence the man says. The man's voice is easy to hear at first because his voice is louder than the others. The background talkers will gradually become louder, making it difficult to understand the man's voice, but please guess and repeat as much of each sentence as possible.

The BKB-SIN contains 18 equivalent list pairs, but both lists in the pairs must be administered and included in the score to retain maximum reliability and equivalency. Each sentence consists of three or four key words—the first sentence has four, the rest have three—and patients receive credit for each key word correctly repeated. The number of key words correct is

subtracted from 23.5 to determine the SNR-50, or the SNR at which a patient understands 50% of the words (SNR loss = 23.5 – Correct Key Words). Calculate an SNR-50 for each list and then average the values for both lists in a list pair to calculate an overall SNR-50. This number reflects the SNR at which a patient correctly identifies approximately 50% of the key words.

Once the SNR-50 is obtained, the BKB-SIN manual contains normative values that can be used to calculate an SNR loss, which is analogous to the SNR loss derived using the QuickSIN. SNR loss is calculated by subtracting the average SNR-50 for a population from the patient's SNR-50 (SNR loss = Patient's SNR-50 – Normative Data SNR-50). These normative values are found in the BKB-SIN manual and are displayed in Table 5–6. For example, if you tested an adult hearing aid candidate and calculated the SNR-50 to be 10 dB, you could then calculate the SNR loss (SNR loss = 10 dB – (–2.5 dB) = 12.5 dB). The same data interpretation can be used for the BKB-SIN as the QuickSIN (see Table 5–6). That is, for this patient, you have discovered a moderate SNR loss, relative to adult listeners with normal hearing.

There are some important points to note relative to these data interpretations. First, these normative values are only applicable when using the CD, a calibrated

Table 5–6. BKB-SIN Test Norms (List Pairs 1–8)

	Adults		Children		
	Normal Hearing	**CI Users**	**Ages 5–6**	**Ages 7–10**	**Ages 11–14**
Mean SNR-50	–2.5	*	3.5	0.8	–0.9
St. Dev.	0.8	1.6	2.0	1.2	1.1

Source: Adapted from Etymotic Research, 2005.

audiometer, List Pairs 1 to 8, and moderate-to-loud presentation levels. These data are not to be used if testing was completed with a system that has not been calibrated, soft presentation levels (35 to 40 dB HL), or the Split Track tests. The Split Track CD contains recordings with the speech and noise on separate channels and is useful for sound field testing.

Clinical Applications

Like the QuickSIN, the BKB-SIN can be used to estimate SNR loss to assist in hearing aid selection, to guide realistic expectations counseling, to demonstrate the benefits of amplification, and to evaluate directional microphones. There are some notable differences between the BKB-SIN and the QuickSIN. First, the BKB-SIN takes approximately three minutes to complete, whereas the QuickSIN is only one minute per list. In addition, recent evidence suggests that the BKB-SIN is easier than the QuickSIN (Wilson, McArdle, et al., 2007). Because it is easier, the BKB-SIN may be more appropriate than the QuickSIN for use with patient populations who would otherwise struggle with speech-in-noise testing, like children, patients with severe hearing losses, or patients with cochlear implants. Although the BKB-SIN contains normative data for a variety of ages, the interpretation of the results is more difficult for children. Because speech, language, and academic skills and experience can play a role in susceptibility to background noise and learning, the same general categories of SNR loss for adults probably does not apply to children.

Similar to the QuickSIN, the BKB-SIN may be related to other self-reported outcomes. More specifically, some investigators have reported that higher SNR losses, as measured with the BKB-SIN, are significantly related to self-perceived communication difficulties for adults who use cochlear implants. That is, people who have more significant SNR loss, are more likely to report

---

THINGS TO REMEMBER: RELIABILITY OF THE BKB-SIN

Because one use for the BKB-SIN is to compare hearing aid features (e.g., omni-directional, directional modes), it is important to consider how different scores need to be to be considered reliably different. This minimum difference score varies based on patient population. Figure 5–10 displays the critical differences for the BKB-SIN for each patient population and for each confidence interval. The confidence interval indicates how certain you can be that the difference you have found is real. If the difference between two lists is larger than the 95% confidence interval, you can assume that there is only a 5% chance that the difference between the lists is not real. For example, let's say you test a hearing aid candidate and find a score of 10 dB SNR-50 for the right ear and a score of 7 dB for the left ear. Using the table shown in Figure 5–10, you can see that there is better than a 95% chance that the difference between the two ears is real. To obtain meaningful differences that are smaller than the values listed, a clinician would need to use more than one list pair per condition.

Number of Lists =	1	2	3	4	5	6	7	8	9	
Adults										
95% C.D. Test +/-	2.2	1.6	1.3	1.1	1.0	0.9	0.8	0.8	0.7	dB
80% C.D. Test +/-	1.8	1.3	1.0	0.9	0.8	0.7	0.7	0.6	0.6	dB
Adult CI Users										
95% C.D. Test +/-	4.4	3.1	2.6	2.2	2.0	1.8	1.7	1.6	1.5	dB
80% C.D. Test +/-	3.6	2.6	2.1	1.8	1.6	1.5	1.4	1.3	1.2	dB
Children by Age										
5–6										
95% C.D. Test +/-	5.4	3.9	3.1	2.7	2.4	2.2	2.1	1.9	1.8	dB
80% C.D. Test +/-	4.4	3.1	2.6	2.2	2.0	1.8	1.7	1.6	1.5	dB
7–10										
95% C.D. Test +/-	3.5	2.5	2.0	1.8	1.6	1.4	1.3	1.2	1.2	dB
80% C.D. Test +/-	2.9	2.0	1.7	1.4	1.3	1.2	1.1	1.0	1.0	dB
11–14										
95% C.D. Test +/-	3.2	2.3	1.9	1.6	1.5	1.3	1.2	1.1	1.1	dB
80% C.D. Test +/-	2.6	1.9	1.5	1.3	1.2	1.1	1.0	0.9	0.9	dB

Figure 5–10. Critical differences for the BKB-SIN for the different number of lists used (Adapted from the BKB-SIN manual, Etymotic, Inc.).

difficulties communicating in daily life, even with a cochlear implant (Donaldson et al., 2009). This information can be used to help guide expectations counseling for both hearing aid and cochlear implant users.

Obtaining the BKB-SIN

The BKB-SIN is available from Etymotic Research and can be obtained from http://www.etymotic.com/pro/. See Appendix U for sentence lists.

THINGS TO REMEMBER: THE BKB-SIN FOR KIDS?

The focus of this chapter is testing for adults, but it is worth mentioning that there is also BKB-SIN normative data for children provided in the user manual. This research found that the BKB-SIN test can be used for children as young as five years old. However, reliability is considerably lower for children under 7 years old.

Words In Noise (WIN) Test

So far in this section, we have discussed three different SNR-50 tests which easily could be used for hearing aid pre-fitting testing. The HINT is a sentence test (all words in the sentence must be correct for the sentence to be correct); the QuickSIN and the BKB-SIN also use sentences, although the scoring is for individual key words within each sentence. The final test in this category is the WIN (for Words in Noise Test), which uses the NU#6 monosyllables. Recall that in the beginning of this chapter, we reviewed some benefits of using sentences material for speech-in-noise testing, but there also are associated limitations:

- With sentence material, context contributes heavily to intelligibility and makes basic auditory function difficult to determine.
- Sentences involve more complex cognitive skills; more working memory effort is required. These demands could differentially affect older versus younger patients.

These factors could lead us to select a monosyllable test for speech-in-noise testing, and if so, the WIN seems to be the most carefully researched tool available.[32]

Background

Wilson (2003) describes that several factors entered into the development of the WIN test, including: a test that would use traditional word stimuli, that would fit a clinical protocol, that would evaluate recognition performance at multiple SNRs, and that would generate a performance metric that was easy to compute and easy to interpret. The WIN then evolved with the following characteristics (Wilson, 2003):

- The NU#6 monosyllabic materials recorded by a female speaker were selected. This test was already in widespread use in VA clinics and, therefore, familiar to clinicians. This word list also was selected because of its sensitivity to the variety of word-recognition performances in quiet exhibited by individuals with hearing loss. This enables word-recognition data to be obtained in quiet and in the background noise using the same speaker, speaking the same words.
- The justification for selecting multitalker babble as the competing background noise was based on evidence that multitalker babble is the most common environmental noise encountered by listeners in everyday life (Plomp, 1978). The multitalker babble used with the WIN test was recorded by audiologist Donald Causey and consists of three female and three male speakers talking about various topics (Sperry, Wiley, & Chial, 1997).
- The level of the multitalker babble is fixed relative to the varied level of the speech signal. This is designed to mimic the real world, in which background noises are maintained at fairly constant levels for given listening situations.. To reduce test variability, the words were time-locked to a unique segment of babble for reduced variability.
- To achieve the goal of *clinical time efficiently*, the test was designed to use multiple speech presentation levels in which 10 words were presented at each of seven levels (a total of 70 words).
- Finally, the WIN test design was amenable to quantification in terms of percent correct at each signal-to-babble ratio, of the overall percent correct, and of the 50% correct point of the signal-to-babble function.

The above provides some of the original goals, and the clinical WIN test of today is mostly the same. It has been shortened to 35 monosyllables (see Wilson & Burks, 2005), which are presented in seven groups of five with a fixed babble level; the level of the words change in 4-dB steps equating to SNRs ranging from 24 to 0 dB, see score sheet shown in Figure 5–11.

POINTS TO PONDER: WHAT TYPE OF NOISE WITH THE WIN?

We have mentioned that the WIN test uses a multitalker babble. An alternative would be speech spectrum noise, such as that used with the HINT. Wilson, Carnell, and Cleghorn (2007) constructed such a noise to use with the WIN test and compared it with the standard multitalker babble for both normal hearing and hearing impaired individuals. They found no significant differences for either group as a function of the background noise. They concluded, therefore, that the use of multitalker babble is warranted, as it has more face validity —patients with hearing loss frequency complain of difficulty understanding speech in noisy backgrounds, especially when the noise is composed of multiple people talking such as a restaurant or party environment. It is important to remember, however, that the competing noise of the WIN was adjusted for each word to control SNR precisely. Therefore one cannot simply use whatever noise they wish when administering the WIN.

Words-in-Noise (WIN)

Name_____SS#_____Age_____

Date_____By_____Ear_____Level_____

# Correct	Threshold
1	25.2
2	24.4
3	23.6
4	22.8
5	22.0
6	21.2
7	20.4
8	19.6
9	18.8
10	18.0
11	17.2
12	16.4
13	15.6
14	14.8
15	14.0
16	13.2
17	12.4
18	11.6
19	10.8
20	10.0
21	9.2
22	8.4
23	7.6
24	6.8
25	6.0
26	5.2
27	4.4
28	3.6
29	2.8
30	2.0
31	1.2
32	0.4
33	-0.4
34	-1.2
35	-2.0

Categories (alongside threshold scale): PROFOUND, SEVERE, MODERATE, MILD, NORMAL

Track 25, List 1, Random 1

24-dB S/B		12-dB S/B		0-dB S/B	
1	pain	16	hate	31	gaze
2	youth	17	shack	32	life
3	wheat	18	tool	33	get
4	dodge	19	voice	34	read
5	cool	20	rush	35	bath

20-dB S/B		8-dB S/B	
6	ditch	21	turn
7	ring	22	young
8	kick	23	bite
9	chair	24	pick
10	luck	25	half

Correct
Threshold (50%)
dB S/B

16-dB S/B		4-dB S/B	
11	base	26	far
12	wire	27	learn
13	red	28	mood
14	time	29	talk
15	judge	30	note

Ear_____Level_____

Track 25, List 2, Random 1

24-dB S/B		12-dB S/B		0-dB S/B	
1	food	16	good	31	back
2	road	17	search	32	dab
3	juice	18	pass	33	kill
4	late	19	witch	34	nice
5	hire	20	chief	35	calm

20-dB S/B		8-dB S/B	
6	tire	21	sour
7	such	22	doll
8	shawl	23	deep
9	haze	24	soap
10	gun	25	make

Correct
Threshold (50%)
dB S/B

16-dB S/B		4-dB S/B	
11	live	26	beg
12	date	27	mess
13	gas	28	long
14	have	29	mouse
15	dog	30	sheep

Figure 5–11. Example of score sheet used for the WIN test (Adapted from the Clinical Protocol for Speech Testing, Eastern Tennessee State University, Johnson City, TN).

KEY CONCEPT: PRESENTATION LEVEL EFFECTS

Wilson (2003) examined the effects of presentation level of the WIN for two different levels (70 versus 90 dB SPL) for groups of normal hearing and hearing impaired individuals. He found that for the listeners with normal hearing, 20% of the performances were better for 70 dB SPL than for 90 dB SPL; 32% were better for 90 dB SPL than for 70 dB SPL; and 48% of the performances were equal at the two presentation levels. The same analysis for the listeners with hearing loss revealed 33% of the performances were better for 70 dB SPL than for 90 dB SPL; 30% were better for 90 dB SPL than for 70 dB SPL; and 36% of the performances were equal at the two presentation levels. As shown, there was a fairly even distribution for both presentation levels, with no clear winner.

In 2011, Wilson published a summary of WIN test results for a rather impressive number of test subjects—3,430! In this study, he compares the WIN findings with age, degree of hearing loss, and performance on the NU#6 test in quiet. One of the major findings supports our statements at the beginning of this chapter —it is very difficult to predict a patient's speech understanding in noise from their speech recognition in quiet. Wilson reports that 70% of the participants had recognition performances in quiet (NU#6) that were good or excellent, but only 6.9% of these same patients had normal performance for the WIN. For the 222 participants who had normal performance for the WIN, 218 (98.2%) also had excellent word recognition in quiet (92% correct or better). And perhaps most important, 1,383 (46.1%) of the 3,000 participants with abnormal performances on the WIN had excellent performances on the NU#6 in quiet (92% or better). In other words, normal performance on the WIN pretty much assures normal performance for speech in quiet, but the opposite is not true. The general relationship between word recognition in quiet and the WIN is shown in Figure 5–12. As expected, WIN performance also became poorer when the hearing loss became greater. This relationship is shown in Figure 5–13 for both the 500, 1000, and 2000 Hz pure-tone average and the high frequency average (1000, 2000, and 4000 Hz).

Administration and Scoring

The WIN test protocol that we describe here is that developed by Richard Wilson, PhD, and is available from the Eastern Tennessee State University (ETSU) website. The protocol is for the use of the VA CD, Speech Recognition and Identification Materials, Disc 4.0.

This protocol suggests testing the patient in quiet first, so that a comparison between performance in quiet and in noise can be made. If your only interest is performance in background noise or if you have already conducted speech testing in quiet, this step can be skipped. It is recommended to test the better ear

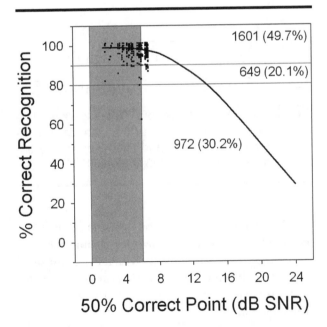

Figure 5–12. Bivariate plot of WIN test performance as it relates to word recognition scores in quiet (Adapted from Wilson, 2011).

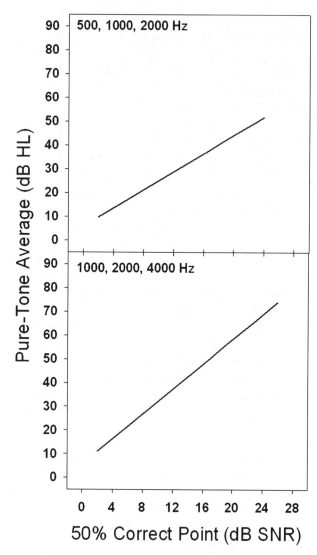

Figure 5–13. Bivariate plot of WIN test performance as it relates to hearing loss for both standard pure-tone average (500, 1000, and 2000 Hz) and for the high frequency average (1000, 2000, and 4000 Hz).

first. The mixed speech in noise is in one channel and only the test stimuli are on the other channel which is not used for testing. This second channel can instead be used by the clinician to clearly hear the words for monitoring and scoring purposes. Test administration is about 6 minutes.

Testing in quiet:

- For the NU#6 in quiet, half-lists are presented at the two levels that approximate the highest

and the lowest presentation levels of the words-in-babble.

- For a pure-tone average ≤40 dB HL, lists in quiet are presented at 60 and 84 dB HL.
- For pure-tone averages >40 dB HL, lists in quiet are presented at 70 and 94 dB HL. (Ensure that the 94 dB HL presentation is below the LDL.)

For the WIN:

- With the pure tone calibrated to 0 VU (0 dB), the babble is 20 dB below the level of the calibration tone indicated on the monitoring meter.
- The words-in-noise testing is completed under headphones. The words-in-noise are on the left channel, and the words-in-quiet at a constant level are on the right channel (for monitoring purposes only). Therefore, the left channel should be routed to whichever ear is being tested.
- The score sheet selected determines the tracks that are presented (i.e., if the next score sheet is for Tracks 3 and 4, then those tracks are presented to the patient).
- The presentation level for the WIN is determined from the following:
  - Pure-tone average ≤40 dB HL: the HL is set to 80 dB. This puts the babble at 80 dB SPL (60 dB HL) with the words ranging from 104 dB SPL (84 dB HL) to 80 dB SPL (60 dB HL).
  - Pure-tone average >40 dB HL to 59 dB HL: the HL is set to 90 dB. This puts the babble at 90 dB SPL (70 dB HL) with the words ranging from 114 dB SPL (94 dB HL) to 90 dB SPL (70 dB HL).
  - Pure-tone average ≥60 dB HL: The ETSU protocol recommends not conducting the WIN when hearing loss reaches this level, as background data are not available.

To score the WIN, the number of words repeated correctly is counted for each signal-to-babble ratio (five possible for each of seven levels). Some audiologists also plot the number of correct responses on the WIN normative chart; the shaded region represents the 90th percentile for people with normal hearing, shown in Figure 5–14. This graphic representation can be helpful

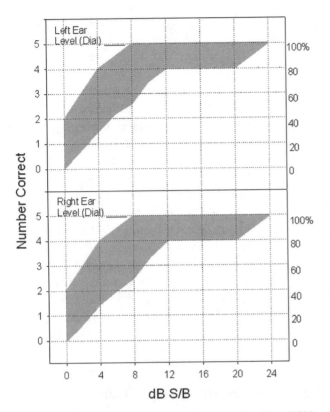

Figure 5–14. Chart for plotting the results of the WIN. The shaded area represents the 90th percentile cutoff (Adapted from the Clinical Protocol for Speech Testing, Eastern Tennessee State University, Johnson City, TN).

THINGS TO REMEMBER: LIST 3 FOR PRACTICE ONLY

Presently there are two 35-word WIN lists, for a total of 70 words. When the WIN test was developed, researchers originally had identified 150 words from the NU#6 list that potentially would be appropriate. Wilson and Watts (2012) examined the possibility of constructing a third list of 35 words for the WIN test from the 80 that were left over. There are times, both in the clinic and in research, when a third list would be useful. In their research, the authors found that the 90th percentiles for Lists 1 and 2 for the listeners with normal hearing were both 6.0 dB SNR, which is exactly the 90th percentile established with the original WIN (Wilson, Abrams, & Pillion, 2003). In contrast, the 90th percentile for List 3 was 10.6 dB SNR. A large difference also was present for List 3 for individuals with hearing loss. The authors recommend, therefore, that the List 3 could be used as a practice list but should not be used for clinical testing.

---

for patient counseling. The scores for each level are then added to determine the total correct and the SNR-50 (SNR for 50% correct) is then obtained from the chart on the right hand side of the score sheet (see Figure 5–11). These thresholds correspond to the descriptors used in the threshold chart on the score sheet (e.g., normal, mild, moderate, severe, or profound), and these terms can be used to describe the patient's performance.

If the look-up SNR-50 chart is not available or if you just enjoy doing a little math, the following equation can be used to calculate the WIN SNR-50 based on the raw score:

WIN Score = 26 − (80% of total correct words)

Thus, the best WIN score that can be attained (35 correct) is −2.0 dB SNR-50 (80% of 35 = 28; subtracted from 26 = −2 dB SNR), and the worst WIN score possible (0 correct) is an SNR-50 of 26.0 dB (80% of 0 = 0;

subtracted from 26 = 26 dB SNR). Lower WIN scores, therefore, are indicative of better performance on this test, as is also the case for other measures of SNR-50, such as the BKB-SIN, QuickSIN and HINT.

Clinical Applications

As we mentioned in the introduction of this chapter, SNR-50 scores for a given patient must be interpreted relative to the test that was used. The following are general interpretation guidelines provided by Wilson and Burks (2005):

- Normal: ≤6.0 dB.
- Mild: 6.8 to 10.0 dB.
- Moderate: 10.8 to 14.8 dB.
- Severe: 15.6 to 19.6 dB.
- Profound: >20 dB.

Armed with the chart above and with the average data from the large sample of patients displayed in Figures 5–12 and 5–13, the patient's WIN findings can be used to assist in making fitting decisions and providing appropriate counseling. For clinical purposes, we usually consider a difference of 3 dB significant for the WIN test. Here are some examples of how WIN test results might be used:

■ The patient's WIN scores are 6 to 8 dB in both ears. The speech-in-noise recognition is at or near that of people with normal hearing. We would expect the patient do quite well in background noise with the hearing aids if we provide appropriate audibility.

■ The patient's WIN scores are 16 to 18 dB in both ears. We would expect this patient to have significant problems in background noise even with properly fitted hearing aids. They should be counseled accordingly and strongly encouraged to use FM or other assistive listening technology.

■ The patient's high frequency pure-tone average is 30 dB and the bilateral WIN score is 17 dB. A patient with a high frequency average of only 30 dB typically has a WIN score around 10 dB. The 17 dB score, therefore, suggests that the patient may have cognitive and/or auditory processing difficulties that impact the ability to understand in background noise.

■ The patient has relatively symmetrical hearing and word recognition in quiet, but the WIN score is 8 dB for the right ear and 14 dB for the left. If this patient has a strong preference to only purchase one hearing aid, consider aiding the right ear. If this patient is fitted with bilateral amplification, consider that the hearing aid for the left ear may not be helpful for listening in background noise.

KEY CONCEPT: WIN AND QUICKSIN—SAME OR DIFFERENT?

Earlier in this chapter, we talked about another SNR-50 test, the QuickSIN, which is a sentence recognition task. McArdle, Wilson, and Burks (2005) compared the recognition performances of 36 listeners with normal hearing and 72 listeners with sensorineural hearing loss on the WIN test and the QuickSIN. Two different lists were used for each test. The listeners with hearing loss had mean SNR-50s for both tests that were 7 to 8 dB higher than those of the listeners with normal hearing. The mean SNR-50 performance for the WIN for the two lists was 12.3 and 12.4 dB; for the QuickSIN 10.1 and 13.3 dB. The difference between the WIN and QuickSIN performances was not significant, suggesting that at least for these two tests, words and sentences in multitalker babble provide the same differentiation between performances by listeners with normal hearing and listeners with hearing loss. Therefore, both the WIN and QuickSIN would seem to be equally sensitive to the effects of hearing loss.

THINGS TO REMEMBER: THE WIN TEST FOR KIDS?

The focus of this chapter is testing for adults, but it is worth mentioning that the WIN test also has been normed for children (see Wilson, Farmer, Gandhi, Shelburne, & Weaver, 2010). This research found that the WIN test can be used for children as young as six years old. Suggested upper cutoffs for each of the seven age groups ranged from 13.2 dB SNR-50 (6-year-olds) to 8.4 dB SNR-50 (9- to 12-year-olds).

Obtaining The WIN

The VA Auditory and Vestibular Research Laboratory have three audio compact discs available. The WIN is included on Disc 4.0, Speech Recognition and Identification Materials, available through the East Tennessee State University Foundation, Johnson City, TN.

Speech-Based Subjective Ratings

To this point, we have discussed several tests that are objective measures of speech recognition in noise—some use sentence material and others use monosyllables. Some have a fixed SNR, whereas others use an SNR-50 approach. What these tests all have in common, however, is that they require a response from the patient that is then objectively scored by the audiologist. In this upcoming section, we discuss two speech-in-noise tests that are somewhat different. Both of these tests utilize a subjective response from the patient. In one case, the patients relate at what point they are bothered by background noise; in the other instance, the patients report how well they believe they are understanding speech.

Acceptable Noise Level (ANL)

It is possible to combine speech and noise and have the patient make judgments regarding the signal. One such measure is the *acceptability* of the level of the background noise while listening to speech. This is the design of the acceptable noise level (ANL) test. Although the ANL is a relatively new *clinical* procedure, it has been used in research for over 20 years. The development of the ANL is credited to the research of Anna Nabelek at the University of Tennessee.[33]

Background

The first publication describing the ANL procedure was by Nabelek, Tucker, and Letowski in 1991. At that time, the test was called the *tolerated SNR*. And, speaking of names, it is important to point out that the term ANL is somewhat of a misnomer, as the test score is a *difference value*, not a *level* per se. More precise, it is an SNR, as

indicated by its original name. The test consists of two measures and a calculation:

- Measurement #1: Most Comfort Level (MCL). The patient first adjusts running speech in quiet, using a bracketing procedure, until the MCL has been determined.
- Measurement #2: Background Noise Level (BNL). Leaving the running speech set at the patient's MCL, multitalker babble is introduced. Again, a bracketing procedure is used, and the listener adjusts the babble to the maximum level that is deemed acceptable and that still enables the listener to follow the speech passage *without becoming tense or tired*. This determines the BNL.
- Calculation: Acceptable Noise Level (ANL). The BNL is subtracted from the MCL, which provides the ANL. For example, if the patient's MCL is 72 dB HL and the BNL is 64 dB HL, then the ANL would be 8 dB.

As apparent from the procedure just described, small ANLs (e.g., 5 dB or less) are normally considered good, as this means that the patient is willing to put up with a considerable amount of noise while listening to speech. On the other hand, big ANLs (e.g., >15 dB) are not so good, as it means that the patient is easily bothered by background noise. As reported by Plyler (2009), data from years of ANL research at the University of Tennessee laboratory show ANL values ranging from −2 to 38 dB for listeners with normal hearing and from −2 to 29 dB for listeners with hearing impairment. Plyler (2009) reports that their most common ANL value is around 10 dB for both groups of listeners, and both groups have similar ANL distributions.

An interesting factor associated with the ANL test is that the patient's ANL seems to be unaffected by many test variables that sometime do affect objective speech recognition measures. For example, research has shown that there are several things that *do not* appear to affect ANL scores—see Freyaldenhoven (2007) and Plyler (2009) for a complete review. What has been shown *NOT* to affect the ANL:

Age, gender, primary language, degree of hearing loss, acoustic reflex thresholds, otoacoustic emissions contralateral suppression, type of speech material, type of background noise, patient's speech recognition in quiet or in background noise, whether the testing is aided or unaided, and experience using hearing aids.

We talk about some of these factors in more detail shortly. Given the list above, at this point you might be asking, what *does* affect the ANL or what is related to the ANL? Limited research suggests association could exist with the following (Freyaldenhoven, 2007; Plyler, 2009):

- Presentation Level: ANLs tend to be larger (worse) as the presentation level of the speech signal becomes higher (although ANL growth patterns are the same for normal hearing and hearing impaired individuals). One study revealed a 4-dB increase in speech presentation level yielded a 1-dB increase in ANL. Given that the MCLs for individuals being fitted for hearing aids usually fall in relative small range (e.g., 20 dB or so), this factor should not have a large impact on ANL clinical interpretation.
- One study revealed that normal hearing listeners classified as Type B personality had significantly smaller ANL values than listeners classified as Type A personality. That is, people who are more "high strung," prefer a higher level of control, and are more detail

oriented (Type A personality) tend to have larger ANL values—more easily bothered by background noise.
- Research with patients diagnosed with ADHD/ADD found that ANLs improved while the patients were on stimulant medication.

A point we make in in this chapter and others regarding pre-fitting testing is that it is not feasible to do all the tests, so when you select your test battery you will want to use tests that provide *different* information. Because of this, it has been common to compare ANL findings with more commonly administered objective speech recognition measures. The results of these studies have been in agreement, showing that the patients' ANL was not significantly related to their performance on the SPIN (Nabelek, Tampas, & Burchfield, 2004), the HINT (Mueller et al., 2006), or the QuickSIN (Mueller et al., 2010). Although it may seem that a patient with hearing loss, who has an excellent aided score on the QuickSIN (e.g., SNR loss around 2 dB) would also have a small aided ANL, this relationship does not exist consistently. This suggests that, at least for some individuals in a controlled clinical setting, the desire to perform well on a speech recognition test trumps the annoyance of the noise. In real-world listening, however, the patient may avoid those situations, develop stress or fatigue in those situations, or not use the hearing aids. Therefore, the inclusion of the ANL into a clinical test battery may give a clinician additional valuable information.

THINGS TO REMEMBER: HEARING AID TECHNOLOGY AND THE ANL

Given that we usually think of small ANLs as good, it is reasonable to question if hearing aid technology can improve the ANL. Freyaldenhoven et al. (2005) showed that directional microphone technology resulted in an average 3 dB improvement (lowering) of the measured ANL. Note, the patient's ANL is not really changing; the SNR in the ear canal is. Regardless, we would expect that the patient would now accept 3 dB more of background noise. Mueller, Weber, and Hornsby (2006) reported similar findings for digital noise reduction (DNR); an approximate 4 dB improvement. These DNR findings should be interpreted with caution, however, as the noise was the competing speech-shaped broadband signal of the HINT. The magnitude of the benefit would likely be smaller if a more speech-like noise was present.

Administration and Scoring

Research suggests that the speech signal and the type of background noise that is used for the ANL measurement does not matter too much; however, given the large body of research conducted with the *standard material*, we recommend that you obtain this CD if you are going to use this test. The primary speech signal is a male talker reading a travelogue about Arizona and the background noise is a multitalker speech babble; specifically, the babble from the revised SPIN test we discussed earlier in this chapter.

Given that the calculation of the ANL only requires two measurements and some first-grade math skills, a standard *test form* or score sheet is not really necessary. Most clinics do develop their own worksheet, however. This is helpful for repeat testing, as then you also will know the measured MCL and BNL. The test commonly is presented sound field, although using earphones (bilateral presentation) is okay too. Because the ANL is not affected by the degree of hearing loss or speech recognition ability, there usually are not ear differences, and you can save a little time by conducting the test bilaterally. In the case of a unilateral fitting, you might want to test each ear just to confirm that there are not significant ANL differences. For example, if all other audiometric results are symmetrical and if there were an interaural ANL difference, you might consider fitting the ear with the lower ANL score. When conducted in the typical sound field manner, the test will take no longer than two or three minutes to conduct. The instructions for the MCL portion of the test are as follows:

You will listen to a man reading a story through the loudspeaker. After a few moments, select the loudness of the story that is most comfortable for you, as if you were listening to a radio. I will adjust the loudness for you—just signal to me if you want it turned up or down. But first, I'd like you to have me turn the loudness up until it is too loud and then down until it is too soft. Then, have me turn the loudness up and down until we find the loudness level that is the most comfortable for you.

We suggest starting the test at around 30 to 40 dB HL and initially using 5-dB steps to establish the general upper and lower limits. Then switch to 2-dB (or 2.5-dB) steps for more precise final bracketing. Once this value is obtained, provide the instructions for the BNL procedure, which are as follows:

Now you will listen to the same story as before, except there now will be background noise of several people talking at the same time. After you have listened to this for a few moments, select the level of background noise that is the MOST you would be willing to accept or "put-up-with" without becoming tense and tired while following the story. First, have me turn the noise up until it is too loud and then down until the noise is soft and the story becomes very clear. Finally, adjust the noise (up and down) to the MAXIMUM noise level that you would be willing to 'put-up-with' for a long time while still following the story.

TECHNICAL TIP: HOW GOOD IS TOO GOOD?

As we have described, the task for the patient when setting the noise level is to adjust it to "the most you would be willing to accept or 'put-up-with' without becoming tense and tired while following the story." The key point here is that the patient must still be able to follow the story. We have found that some patients are focusing so intently regarding what they can put up with that they forget this other important part of the instructions. The result will be unusually low ANL scores, maybe even a negative ANL score. Consider that few people will be able to follow the story when the noise is equal to the signal. If you see scores that seem unusually low, we suggest reinstruction and repeating the test. If you continually see small ANLs—check out your calibration, especially if you do not commonly conduct two-channel speech testing.

THINGS TO REMEMBER: RELIABILITY OF THE ANL MEASURE

Given that the BNL portion of the ANL procedure is a somewhat unique measure (e.g., most patients are not accustomed to assessing what they can put up with), Mueller et al. (2006) examined the test-retest of this component of the ANL calculation (during a single test session). In all, the BNL was repeated three times for each of three different test conditions for 22 subjects, a total of 66 ANLs. They found that in 15% of the cases, the BNL did not change at all; in 61%, the largest difference among the three measures per person was 2 dB (2-dB steps were used in the research); and in 13%, the BNLs differed by 4 dB. The largest test-retest difference observed was 6 dB, present for 11% of the 66 ANLs calculated.

The findings of Mueller et al. (2006) suggest that the BNL is a relatively reliable measure, although these researchers did not address the variability of the MCL, which has the potential to be unreliable in that for most patients, it is a *range*, not single dB value. Considering the minimal time it takes to conduct the MCL and BNL (and calculate an ANL), we would suggest repeating both measures and taking an average of the two ANLs.

Clinical Applications

For starters, the thing to remember is that small ANLs are good; large ANLs, are not so good! Good for what, you might ask? And what constitutes a good ANL? The cutoffs that generally are used, based on studies from the University of Tennessee that we discussed previously are:

- Low: 7 dB or less
- Midrange: 8 to 12 dB
- High: 13 dB or higher

Intuitively, it would seem that someone who is not bothered much by background noise would be a more successful hearing aid user. That may be true. A large-scale study (*n* = 191) on this topic was reported by Nabelek, Freyaldenhoven, Tampas, Burchfield, and Muenchen (2006). Unaided ANLs were compared for individuals who had been fitted with hearing aids. Based on a questionnaire regarding hearing aid use, the subjects were divided into three groups: full-time users (*N* = 69), part-time users (*N* = 69), or nonusers (*N* = 59). The authors found that full-time users had significantly smaller ANLs than the other two groups (mean ANL of 7.7 dB); however, there was little difference in mean ANLs between the part-time users and nonusers (13.5 and 14.4, respectively). When the part-time and nonuser groups were combined (considered unsuccessful) and compared with the full-time users, the authors

report that the unaided ANL predicted success with hearing aids with 85% accuracy.

Figure 5–15 was generated from the logistic regression analysis of the Nabelek et al. (2006) data. It shows a predicted probability of success (full-time hearing aid use) as a function of the patient's ANL. For example, if a patient's ANL was 8 dB (a fairly common clinical finding), we would predict they had about an 80% change of being a successful full-time user. Although the Nabelek et al. (2006) predictive data are impressive, hearing aid use does not necessary equate to benefit or satisfaction. These two outcomes also have been compared with the ANL. Freyaldenhoven, Nabelek, and Tampas (2008) examined the relationship between ANLs and the APHAB. They found that there was *not* a significant relationship between either the unaided or aided ANLs and aided benefit scores for any subscale on the APHAB. Taylor (2008) used the International Outcome Inventory for Hearing Aids (IOI-HA) questionnaire and found a weak but significant correlation with the ANL. More specific, the high ANL group (ANLs >12; *n* = 4) had poorer overall IOI-HA scores, primarily due to lower scores for the Factor 1 questions (which does include a question regarding hearing aid use).

The work of Schwartz and Cox (2011, 2012) has been less encouraging regarding the clinical utility of the ANL. Although they do report that is was significantly correlated to the aversiveness scale of the

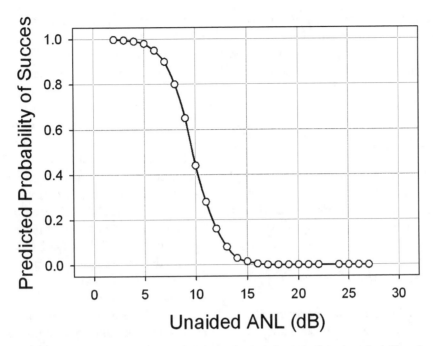

Figure 5–15. A regression curve displaying the predicted probability of success with hearing aids as a function of unaided ANL score. (Adapted from Nabalek et al., 2006)

APHAB—people with large ANLs are more bothered by loud noises—it was not significantly correlated to the other outcomes of the APHAB or findings from the HHIE or the SADL. Looking at several domains, such as benefit, satisfaction, quality of life, and so forth, they found the prediction accuracy to range from 52% to 64%, with the highest accuracy for hearing aid use (64%).

So what is the practical take-home message from these ANL studies? First, given that there is not a consensus, it appears that more research is needed before we make a strong recommendation. But for the moment, let us assume that there is at least a weak relationship between the ANL and hearing aid use. So going back to the Nabelek et al. (2006) data shown in Figure 5–15, if someone has an ANL of 20 dB do you simply tell them that they'll probably never use their hearing aids, so they might as well save their money? Of course not, but you might put a "red X" by their name and target them for more intense counseling and post-fitting audiologic rehabilitation. It would be reasonable to consider them at risk for not being successful with amplification. If they tell you that loud noises are bothering them, that would be a predictable outcome. If you normally only

have your new hearing aid patients come back for follow-up visits once or twice during the first month after the fitting, you might consider seeing the high ANL patients more frequently.

Finally, you might ask if a patient's ANL score would alter the hearing aid technology that you will select or the way special features will be adjusted? The answer is—usually not. Although we would agree that someone with a large ANL probably needs directional technology and DNR, we are going to fit this technology to someone with a small ANL too. Adjust the DNR to maximum strength rather than medium? Maybe, but there is no evidence to suggest that this will make a difference. Remote microphone technology, of course would be beneficial, especially if they are avoiding noisy listening situations.

Given the significant relationship between large ANLs and real-world annoyance from loud sounds (Schwartz & Cox, 2011), if your patient's ANL is significantly larger than average, you might spend more time than usual during the fitting process assuring that environmental sounds are not "Uncomfortably Loud" (see Cox loudness anchors in Chapter 4). As we discuss in detail in the verification section of Book Three of this series, we recommend presenting loud environmental sounds (e.g., 85 SPL dBA) with the patient aided bilaterally and making frequency-specific output limiting adjustments to assure that loudness ratings fall no higher than "Loud, But Okay."

Obtaining the ANL Test

The standard CD with the travelogue and the R-SPIN competing noise is available from Frye Electronics (http://www.frye.com). The instructions, especially for the BNL measure are important—see Appendix X.

Performance-Perceptual Test (PPT)

As the name suggests, the Performance-Perceptual Test (PPT), also requires the patient to make a subjective judgment. In this case, however, the *perceptual* part is a judgment regarding speech recognition. That is, the patients *self-score* their performance. The measure of most interest is not the perceptual score itself, but how the perceptual score differs from the true performance score, and this difference is referred to as the performance-perceptual discrepancy, or PPDIS.

Background

Saunders (2009) explains that the PPT originally was developed to study individuals with obscure auditory dysfunction (OAD). Persons with OAD report difficulties hearing speech in noise, yet have clinically normal hearing. In her early research, Saunders found that people with OAD tended to underestimate their hearing ability. This led to the notion that the misjudgment of speech understanding ability also could be related to hearing aid satisfaction.

The speech test that is the basis for measuring the patient's perceptions of word recognition and calculating the PPDIS, is the HINT, which we discussed earlier in this chapter. The performance score of the PPT, therefore, is obtained using the standard HINT protocol—that is, the background noise is constant, and the intensity level of the sentences are adaptively raised or lowered depending on the patient's response for the preceding sentence. The patients repeat back what they hear, and the audiologist determines if all words of the sentence are correct. For the perceptual portion of the

PPT, the intensity of the sentences is altered based on whether patients *think* that they correctly recognized all the words of the sentence. Rather than repeat back the sentence, the patient simply responds with a *Yes* or *No*.

We discuss the norms later but in general, the average patient tends to have similar scores for the performance and perceptual administration of the HINT. What we are interested in are those who do not, and for that reason, we calculate the PPDIS. This defines the extent to which the patient misjudges his or her hearing ability. If the perceptual HINT RTS is more adverse (a more difficult SNR) than the performance RTS, it suggests that patients overestimate their speech recognition ability. If, on the other hand, the perceptual RTS is less adverse (an easier SNR) than the performance RTS, this indicates someone who underestimates their speech recognition ability. Ideally, we want patients who have a PPDIS around 0 dB, as there could be problems associated with both significantly positive and negative PPDIS scores.

You might wonder how this unique speech test correlates with patient characteristics or other hearing aid pre-fitting measures that might be conducted. Here is a brief summary of some related findings:

- PPDIS is not related to age or degree of hearing loss (Saunders & Forsline, 2006).
- PPDIS is not significantly related to other pretests, such as the ANL or QuickSIN (Mueller et al 2010).
- PPDIS is related to self-perceived hearing handicap. Saunders, Forsline, and Fausti (2004) examined the relationship between unaided HHIE/A scores (see Chapter 6 for description) and the PPT. They found a significant relationship, in that people whose HHIE/A scores were worse than what would be expected from their hearing loss tended to have PPT scores that underestimated their speech recognition ability.
- PPDIS may be related to hearing aid dissatisfaction. Saunders (2009) reports that negative PPDIS scores (underestimators) tend to associated with more hearing aid dissatisfaction.

Although at this point we are talking about using the PPT for pre-fitting testing, it of course also can be a valuable outcome measure. Of interest, Saunders and Forsline (2006) reported that when the unaided PPDIS was compared with the aided PPDIS, the aided score had less variance. The mean unaided and aided PPDIS did not differ significantly. That is, although the patient's absolute scores may have changed, the use of hearing aids did not influence the relationship between their measured and perceptual judgments.

Administration and Scoring

As we mentioned, the PPDIS consists of using the standard HINT material. Refer back to the HINT section of this chapter for the recommended test procedure. The PPT is administered in the sound field, although bilateral earphone administration would probably yield similar results. The scoring of the PPT, using 20-sentence HINT lists, is as described earlier in this chapter for the HINT and illustrated in Figure 5–6. The perceptual portion is always administered first. The reason for this, as described by Saunders, is that if you do the performance portion first, the patient will know that you already have scored them on the same test and are probably trying to catch them out (which is somewhat true), which could influence their perceptual judgments (see Mueller, 2010, for review).

To calculate the PPDIS, we want to know the difference between the two HINT scores. The basic rules for calculation and interpretation are as follows:

PPDIS = HINT *Performance* RTS minus HINT *Perceptual* RTS

Positive PPDIS = Patient *overestimates* speech recognition ability

Negative PPDIS = Patient *underestimates* speech recognition ability.

Clinical Applications

It is first important to consider how the average patient performs regarding their PPDIS. Data from Saunders and Forsline (2006; $n = 94$) are shown in Figure 5–16. It appears that on average, the perceptual and performance scores are fairly similar, with a mean unaided PPDIS of –1.4 dB, indicating a slight trend for individuals to underestimate their speech recognition ability. These data are similar to those reported by Saunders et al. (2004), and these authors offer the following interpretation guidelines:

- Underestimation: PPDIS < 33rd percentile of normative data (value ≤ –3)
- Accurate: PPDIS between 33rd and 66th percentile of normative data (value> –3 and < +0.2)
- Overestimation: PPDIS> 66th percentile of normative data (value of ≥ +0.2)

Mueller et al. (2010), however, reported mean values that were 2 to 3 dB higher than shown above—their subjects had a slight tendency to overestimate their speech recognition ability. The authors speculate that this may be because their subject sample only included hearing aid users who were satisfied with their hearing aids—recall that dissatisfaction with amplification is associated with negative PPDIS scores. In general, your primary counseling efforts will be directed toward patients who fall significantly outside of these normative values (e.g., PPDIS more negative than –3 dB or more positive than +3 dB).

It is unlikely that a patient's PPDIS score will be helpful for selecting fitting arrangements or different technology; however, there are certainly counseling

---

TECHNICAL TIP: TEST-RETEST RELIABILITY OF PPT

Saunders et al. (2004) report good test-retest reliability for the PPT. The authors reported reliability data for the perceptual ($r = 0.95$), the performance ($r = 0.97$), and the PPDIS ($r = 0.88$), all in unaided listening conditions. As mentioned by the authors, it is somewhat surprising that patients are as reliable with the perceptual task as they are with performance, as we usually do not think of subjective measures as being as reliable as objective ones. The reliability of the PPDIS is of course somewhat lower, as it is derived from the two other measures, each with their own variability, but it still is considered excellent for a test like this.

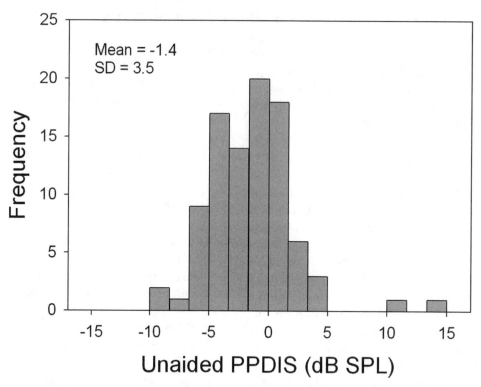

Figure 5–16. Distribution of PPDIS scores. PPDIS = HINT *Performance* RTS minus HINT *Perceptual* RTS. Positive PPDIS = Patient *overestimates* speech recognition ability. Negative PPDIS = Patient *underestimates* speech recognition ability (Adapted from Saunders and Forsline, 2006).

insights that can be gained. Particularly for the new hearing aid users who either overestimate or underestimate their speech recognition ability, the PPDIS score can provide general areas for discussion regarding the patient's adjustment to amplification. For example, if you know that someone is an underestimator, before they leave your office with their hearing aids you might encourage them to try guessing when they do not understand or assume they understand when they are uncertain. Sanders (2009) provides a summary of how PPDIS scores can be used in patient counseling, shown in Figure 5–17. Because we know that negative PPDIS scores are associated with hearing aid dissatisfaction, special attention should be paid to this group.

A somewhat different pre-fitting use of the PPDIS would be for those individuals with significant communication problems who believe that they do not really need hearing aids. In many cases, these people are over-estimators. By conducting the PPT, it is possible to show

the patient the difference between the true score and perceptual score, which might be helpful in initiating the trial of hearing aids.

In a 2009 article, Dr. Saunders was asked why it was that some people judge their speech understanding different from what it really is. Her response is as follows:

I don't have a definitive answer for that, and most likely the reasons vary from person to person. The explanation might be related to personality (being perfectionist, anxious, or lacking self-confidence) or to past experiences. Or it might be associated with expectations about hearing. It might be specific to hearing, or it might not be.

From a practical perspective, I suggest that being aware that not everyone has an accurate perception of their own ability to understand speech is more important than figuring out why—unless, of course, the reason why can be used to fix the prob-

UNDERESTIMATORS	ACCURATE ESTIMATORS	OVERESTIMATORS
Provision of information		
This test shows you hear better than you think you do	You accurately assess your hearing ability	This test shows you overestimate how well you can hear
Suggested explanation		
High expectations, cautious, reluctant to take risks, lack of confidence, not want to fail		Denial of self and others, slow onset of HL, overconfident
Subject exposition		
Response to above, other explanations?	Response to above, comments?	Response to above, other explanations?
Discussion/ramifications		
Fearful of social interaction, withdrawal dependency	Accepting of hearing loss and the limitations it imposes	Frustrate others, appear, unintelligent or arrogant, misunderstandings or wrong information
Solutions		
Try guessing, take risks, assume you heard correctly, rephrase to clarify and boost confidence, use communication strategies	NA. Discuss use of communication strategies	Ask for clarification, admit to difficulties to self, use communication strategies

Figure 5–17. Illustration of how the PPDIS can be used for patient counseling (Adapted from Saunders, 2009).

lem. If misjudgment is personality-based, changing that trait is going to be difficult. Therefore, I propose that we address the implications of misjudgment of hearing, not its causes. That's why PPT-based counseling focuses on behavioral changes—not explanations.

Obtaining the PPT

All the normative data to date for the PPT have been with the HINT; see our comments regarding obtaining this test in that earlier section of this chapter. It is possible that a different speech test could be used, although norms would need to be established.

Dichotic Speech Tests

The 1960s were an exciting time for diagnostic audiology. We were moving beyond simple air and bone conduction threshold testing, and beginning to construct diagnostic tests that would allow us to identify pathologies of nerve VIII, the brain stem, and yes . . . even the brain. In James Jerger's now classic 1969 book, *Modern Developments in Audiology*, there was an intriguing review chapter on central auditory processing by Italians Bocca and Calearo. It was there that many audiologists first read about the *redundancy principle*—extrinsic, the linguistic redundancy of the test stimuli, versus intrinsic, the multiplicity of auditory processing pathways. Simply stated, when conducting clinical speech testing, the principle reminds us that the more subtle the auditory disorder, the more the redundancy of the test stimuli needs to be reduced for the speech test to be sensitive.

Certainly, one way to reduce redundancy is to present different speech stimuli to the two ears simultaneously, which we refer to as dichotic testing. It was more than 50 years ago—in 1961—when Doreen Kimura published two articles describing how dichotic digit testing could be used to help describe central auditory processing. Her explanation of the crossed auditory pathways, ipsilateral suppression, and the *right ear effect* has withstood the test of time, and laid the groundwork for the design and interpretation of many audiologic speech tests that followed.[34] We review a revised version of her dichotic digit test later in this section.

So what does all this have to do with hearing aid selection and fitting? Although dichotic speech tests can be used to help identify a specific auditory pathology or disorder, the results of this testing also can be used in a more general framework to gauge a patients overall processing ability. In many cases, especially with older adults, cognitive factors contribute to the poor performance on dichotic tests. When used in conjunction with fitting hearing aids, there are two primary results that might impact the fitting and/or patient counseling:

■ Performance for both ears is significantly reduced, more so than expected based on pure-tone thresholds and other monaural speech-in-noise tests. When this finding occurs, the patient would be counseled

---

TECHNICAL TIP: TERMINOLOGY

When describing the presentation mode for auditory processing tests, specific terminology usually is used, which is somewhat different from what is used for other speech testing.

■ Monotic: The signal, or signals (e.g., speech and competition), is presented to only one ear. This essentially is the same as a unilateral or monaural presentation. Tests such as the QuickSIN or WIN are presented unilaterally for hearing aid pre-fitting testing.

■ Diotic: The same signal is presented to both ears. The SPRINT, which we discussed earlier, is presented diotically. The QuickSIN and BKBSIN can also be presented diotically via headphones.

■ Dichotic: Two different competing speech signals are presented to each ear simultaneously (often carefully timed to have the same onset). The task is to identify both signals, or in some cases, the signal for a pre-cued ear. The two tests that we discuss in this chapter, the DSI and the DDT, are examples of clinical dichotic tests.

regarding realistic expectations for hearing aid benefit in background noise or when multiple talkers are present, and FM technology or other wireless assistive listening devices would be strongly encouraged.

■ Performance for one ear is significantly worse than the other, more so than predicted by pure-tone thresholds or other monaural speech tests. This patient would be considered at risk for optimum benefit with bilateral amplification. This finding would probably not negate a bilateral fitting, because of the potential advantages unrelated to dichotic speech understanding, but these results do alert the audiologist to pay close attention to patient comments in this regard on post-fitting visits and to perhaps have some specific suggestions for hearing aid use (e.g., only use one hearing aid for parties). Moreover, if the patient only desires to purchase one hearing aid, it would be reasonable to fit the ear with the best dichotic speech score (assuming the between ear difference was significant).

Free-Recall Versus Direct-Recall

There have been two different types of recall patterns used when dichotic speech testing has been conducted:

■ Free recall: In the free-recall condition, the patient has to attend to and report the speech signal(s) heard in both ears. The ear-order of report is not cued (for difficult dichotic tasks, most patients do tend to report the right ear signal first).

■ Directed recall: For this response mode, the patient is instructed to only report the signal for one ear. They hear the speech signals presented to each ear but can focus on the signal heard in the cued ear while disregarding the signal presented to the non-cued ear. This results in a reduced demand on cognitive processing.

Clearly, the free-recall condition places greater stress on attentional resources than the directed-recall condition. When recognition performance is below nor-

mal in the free-recall condition but improves substantially in the directed-recall condition, then we assume the problem is primarily in the cognitive domain because memory and attention abilities are insufficient for successful performance when both ears must be monitored simultaneously.

When performance is below normal in both the free- and directed-recall conditions, then the problem is interpreted to be primarily in the auditory domain because performance does not improve by reducing cognitive demands (Jerger, Stach, Johnson, Loiselle, & Jerger, 1990).

Effects of Peripheral Hearing Loss

One concern in the clinical interpretation of all auditory processing tests is the influence of a concurrent peripheral hearing loss. That is, how is one certain that results showing an ear difference or reduced overall performance are not because of cochlear damage, rather than related to higher processing function? In the general population, this is not so much an issue, as often the patient suspected of having an auditory processing disorder has normal hearing. When these tests are used as part of the hearing aid pre-fitting battery, however, it is always something that must be considered in test interpretation. Although it is very difficult to eliminate the influence of a peripheral hearing loss when using these speech tests, we have selected two tests to discuss in this section that appear to be the most resilient to hearing loss and, therefore, the best choice for use in the hearing aid selection process.

The Dichotic Sentence Identification Test

As we have mentioned throughout this chapter, the purpose of adding speech tests to the pre-fitting battery is to obtain unique information about the patient. In the case of the DSI (for Dichotic Sentence Identification Test), the new information that might be gathered, particularly for older adults, is the presence of a more central processing deficit than what might be detected using tests such as the QuickSIN or the WIN. Research has shown that the DSI may be successful in making this identification.

TECHNICAL TIP: THE PROBLEM WITH DICHOTIC CVs

A popular dichotic speech test over the years among cognitive psychologists and neuroscientists, as well as research audiologists, has been dichotic CVs. In this case, the vowel /a/ is paired with six different stop consonants, resulting in the following stimuli: pa, ta, ka, ba, da, ga. These stimuli are then paired with each other and presented dichotically—one syllable to each ear for each single presentation. Because of the similarly of the syllables and their short duration, it is possible to have very close alignment for dichotic presentation, making this a difficult test for even young individuals with normal hearing; mean performance of approximately 75% correct for the right ear and approximately 55 to 60% for the left (Mueller, 1985). Because of this difficulty, it also is the clinical test that is the most likely to reveal an ear advantage and is the most sensitive to processing difficulty. However, as apparent from the construct, correct identification of these stimuli easily can be compromised by even a mild high frequency hearing loss. Hence, this is a poor dichotic test to use for hearing aid pre-fitting measures.

Background

The DSI was introduced by Fifer, Jerger, Berlin, Tobey, and Campbell (1983). The test used the 10 sentences of the well-established Synthetic Sentence Identification (SSI) test.[35] These 10 sentences were paired with each other and presented dichotically (one sentence to each ear). To make the sentences more appropriate for dichotic pairing, the items were edited and equalized for overall intensity. Also, to enhance timing alignment, the duration of each sentence was adjusted to equal two seconds, by editing out or expanding the vowel segments of the sentences. The authors stated that one of the goals was to design a dichotic test that was relatively resistant to the effects of peripheral hearing loss. In this early work, the authors report that the DSI indeed was resistant to the influence of hearing loss until the pure-tone average (average of 500, 1000, and 2000 Hz) exceeded approximately 50 dB HL. In a later study (Jerger, Chmiel, Allen, & Wilson, 1994), DSI testing was conducted on individuals with ear PTA asymmetry as great as 30 dB. Even with this lax criterion of symmetry, analysis showed that only 5% of variance in the DSI ear differences could be accounted for by the PTA average.

Shortly after the introductory report by Fifer et al. (1983), a shortened clinical version of the DSI was developed, which only included 6 of the original 10 sentences of the SSI. These sentences are shown in Figure 5–18.

Each sentence is delivered five times to each ear and paired accordingly with each of the other five sentences, resulting in a total of 30 test items.

Because of its relative resistance to hearing loss, the DSI has been used to study processing in older individuals. Chmiel and Jerger (1996), for example evaluated 115 elderly subjects over the age of 60 years with high frequency sensorineural hearing loss. Using the free- and directed-recall conditions for the DSI test, they found that 29% of the subjects were categorized as having an auditory-specific processing deficit. In an earlier study using a similar DSI procedure, Jerger et al. (1990) administered this dichotic test to 172 elderly hearing

---

1. Agree with him only to find out.
2. Down by the time is real enough.
3. Go change your car color is red.
4. Women view men with green paper should.
5. Built the government with the force almost.
6. Small boat with a picture has become.

Figure 5–18. The six sentences used for DSI testing. Sentences were taken from the original sentences of the SSI test.

impaired subjects (60 to 90 years). In this study, 58% showed below-normal performance in one ear in the free-recall condition, with a significant improvement in the directed-recall condition, suggesting a cognitive-based disorder. Another 23% showed a deficit in both response modes. Only 19% of this sample showed no deficit in either ear for either DSI condition.

The 60 to 90 year age group studied in the Jerger et al. (1990) study is pretty representative of the individuals we fit with hearing aids. If it is true that 80% of these individuals have a cognitive or auditory specific deficit that is preventing them from processing speech

effectively, how do we account for that during the hearing aid fitting process?

Administration and Scoring

In general, the DSI can be given to individuals with a pure-tone average (500, 1000, and 2000 Hz) of 50 dB HL or less. General test procedures are as follows:

- The test is conducted under earphones.
- The patient is given the card with the six sentences printed on them (large bold print should be used).

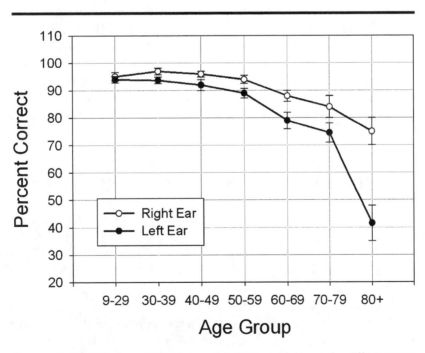

Figure 5–19. Display of DSI scores for right and left ears for different age groups (Adapted from Jerger et al., 1994).

- The patient is then instructed to listen for two different sentences presented to both ears simultaneously, to find the two sentences from among the six on the printed list and to call out the corresponding numbers of the sentences heard.
- The test items are delivered at 50 dB SL relative to the pure-tone average (500, 1000, and 2000 Hz) for the respective ears. If this level exceeds the patient's LDL, lower the intensity to the "loud but okay" loudness rating of the patient.
- With the intensity set at desired levels for both channels/ears, talk to the patient (bilateral presentation) to assure a relative loudness match between ears is present. Your voice should be localized to the center of the head. Adjust intensity if necessary.

We typically deliver the test using free-recall. If the findings are abnormal, the test certainly could be repeated using directed-recall to gather additional information—although it probably will not alter your counseling to a great degree. As we mentioned, the DSI consists of 30 sentence pairs and scoring for each ear is reported in the percent correct (each correct item is multiplied by 3.3%). A sample score sheet in shown in Figure 5–20. Given that there are only six sentences, one might think that the patients would guess a lot, given the probability of a correct guess. It is surprising that this does not happen very often. When they do not get it, they simply do not respond. It is true of course that they really only need to identify one key word of the sentence, and this is okay

The chart shown in Figure 5–21 can be used to assist in test interpretation. Because we know that the results will be impacted by hearing loss, this is accounted for in this chart. For example, note that for PTA up to 25 dB, DSI scores of 75% or better are considered normal—we would expect younger patients to fall closer to the top of this range. As the PTA increases, the cutoff for normal decreases. Notice that a 50% score would be in the normal range for someone with a PTA of 40 dB. If the hearing loss is relatively symmetric, we would expect DSI scores to be within 16 to 20% between ears. An exception might be patients older than 80 years, where we would expect a left ear deficit.

Clinical Applications

As we discussed in the introduction portion of this section, there is a general belief that dichotic speech tests such as the DSI can be used to help predict who might show the greatest benefit from amplification. Chmiel and Jerger (1996), for example, used the HHIE outcome measure (see Chapter 6) to examine the reduction of handicap for new hearing aid users after six weeks of first-time hearing aid use. They compared the improvement for the HHIE to the patients pre-fitting DSI performance and found that there was a significant improvement in average HHIE scores but only for the DSI-normal category. In the subgroup with dichotic deficits (DSI-abnormal group), average HHIE scores did not change significantly after hearing aid use.

TECHNICAL TIP: SCORING OF DOUBLE CORRECTS

We often see that patients who are having trouble with the DSI will attempt different listening strategies. One of these is to self-impose a directed-ear response. That is, they will focus on the right ear for a period of time, and you will notice that they are getting all the right ear sentences correct. Then, they will switch their focus to the left ear, and they will get all the left ear sentences correct. But, they never (or seldom) get both correct. For this reason, we find it useful to also score *double corrects*. That is, the percent of time that the patient gave the correct response for both ears. We suspect that a patient who scores 50% in both ears with 50% double correct responses is different from the patient who scores 50% in both ears with no double correct responses.

DICHOTIC SENTENCE IDENTIFICATION TEST

Name_____Age_____Sex_____Date_____

Presentation: Ch. 1 _____Ear @ _____dB HTL; Ch. 2 ____Ear @ _____dB HTL

Score percent correct: _____% Right Ear; _____% Left Ear

_____

1.   AGREE WITH HIM ONLY TO FIND OUT
2.   DOWN BYTHE TIME IS REAL ENOUGH
3.   GO CHANGE YOUR CAR COLOR IS RED
4.   WOMEN VIEW MEN WITH GREEN PAPER SHOULD
5.   BUILT THE GOVERNEMTN WITH THE FORCE ALMOST
6.   SMALL BOAT WITH A PICTURE HAS BECOME

_____

	CH. 1	CH. 2			CH. 1	CH. 2
1.	1	4		16.	3	5
2.	3	1		17.	4	3
3.	4	2		18.	1	2
4.	6	5		19.	2	5
5.	6	2		20.	2	1
6.	5	3		21.	5	4
7.	3	4		22.	5	1
8.	3	6		23.	2	6
9.	1	6		24.	4	5
10.	1	3		25.	2	4
11.	1	5		26.	3	2
12.	5	6		27.	6	1
13.	5	2		28.	6	4
14.	4	1		29.	2	3
15.	4	6		30.	6	3

Figure 5–20. Example of score sheet used for DSI testing (Adapted from Auditec of St. Louis).

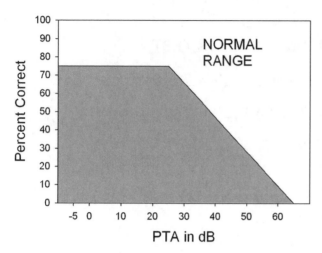

Figure 5–21. Normative data as a function of hearing loss for interpreting DSI findings (Adapted from Auditec of St. Louis).

In their 1994 article, Jerger et al. suggest that a patient's score for a particular ear for the DSI is the linear contribution of four different factors:

- Speech Recognition: The patient's ability to recognize a target sentence in the presence of contralateral competition by a difference sentence. This factor is assumed to be equivalent for right and left ears.
- Left Ear Deficit: This is a performance difference favoring input to the right ear due to left hemisphere dominance for speech signals. This factor favors the right ear score over the left ear score and operates in both the free-recall and directed-recall modes.
- Task Deficit: A deficit in performance resulting from the cognitive demands of the instructional set. This is associated with the demands on memory and speed of mental processing inherent in the behavioral response in the dichotic paradigm. It is assumed to be equivalent for right and left ear scores, but operates primarily in the free-recall mode.
- Interaction Effect: An additional task deficit resulting from the interaction between the patient's report bias and the task deficit. If, for example, the patient is biased toward responding first to the right ear input, then

the left ear score might be more affected by the task deficit factor than the right ear score. This is primarily a factor in the free-recall mode.

Although understanding *why* reduced DSI scores are present is important, the clinician will want to know how a given score impacts the fitting process. It is certainly possible that a patient could score well on tests such as the QuickSIN or the WIN, yet have an abnormal DSI score. At the beginning of this section, we outlined some of the uses of dichotic speech results—to briefly review:

Low scores in both ears:

- This patient will probably be less successful using hearing aids than the average patient —especially for any situation when there are competing signals. Informing the patient of this could be part of the pre-fitting process.
- Also, encourage the use of FM, remote microphone, and other assistive listening devices.

Low performance in one ear:

- This patient also may be less successful than average when using hearing aids, but in this case, we need to decide if it is worthwhile to aid the ear with the low DSI score. Poor performance on dichotic speech tasks has been related to poorer performance with bilateral amplification.
- We would probably still fit the patient with two hearing aids but monitor success closely, and perhaps have the patient try only using the hearing aid in the good ear when involved in listening in competing noise.

Obtaining the DSI

The DSI can be obtained from Auditec of St. Louis. It also can be found on Audiology VA CD, Disc 2 (http://www.etsu.edu/crhs/aslp/audiology/resources/Aud_VA_CD_Disc_2.aspx).

The Dichotic Digit Test (DDT)

As we discussed with the DSI test, there may be instances during the pre-fitting process when a dichotic test is needed to assess the cognitive and/or central

> ### KEY CONCEPT: TIMING IS EVERYTHING!
>
> In construction of a dichotic listening task, the timing of the two different signals to the two ears can have a significant impact on the test outcome. Musiek (1983) reports that his version of the DDT was recorded so that two digits on one channel of the tape recorder were aligned with two digits on the other channel by using a timing cue for the onset of the talker. The onsets of the digits were within 70 milliseconds, which is within the range of onset times critical for maintaining dichotic perception. Intensity levels (by VU meter readings) of individual items were within ± 4 dB for intra- and interchannel comparisons [the difference in mean intensity (by VU meter) of the digits for channels 1 and 2 was less than 1 dB]. The inter-digit interval was approximately 0.5 seconds.

auditory processing integrity of the patient. The DDT (for Dichotic Digit Test) is an easy to administer auditory processing test that can be used for this purpose. In general, the test is similar to the DSI, and similar results would be expected. It is unlikely that you would administer both to a given patient.

Background

As we mentioned in the introduction of this section, much of the early work with dichotic listening, dating back to the early 1960s, utilized dichotic digits. The test was seldom used in clinical audiology, however, until the 1980s. The rediscovery of this processing test among clinicians was due in large part to an article by Frank Musiek (1983). In this article, he presented his version of a DDT, norms for both normal hearing and individuals with mild to moderate cochlear hearing loss, and also 21 subjects with intracranial lesions. Unlike some of the earlier dichotic digit tests, which used three digits per ear, Musiek's version only used two digits per ear. The digits from 1 to 10, excluding the number 7 (the only two-syllable digit in this range) were paired to form 20 test items, 40 for each ear.

To establish cutoff values for clinical differential testing, Musiek (1983) used the means and two standard deviations (with some rounding, to obtain easy-to-use numbers) for the normal hearing and cochlear hearing loss group. Although it is known that a right ear advantage is sometimes observed for dichotic speech testing, this effect was very small for the normative data, and therefore, no ear-specific norms are necessary. The following normative values were reported:

- Normal hearing: 90% or better
- Hearing loss: 80% or better.

For clinical use today, there are three different dichotic digits tests to choose from: the Musiek version we just discussed, an Auditec of St. Louis version, and a version developed by Richard Wilson and colleagues of the VA system. The VA version has one, two, and three digit pairs available. Table 5–7 shows the mean values reported by Strouse and Wilson (1999) for the two-pair dichotic digit presentations (similar to Musiek DDT) for different age groups for the free-recall paradigm.

Notice that for these mean values, there is an age-related decrease in performance, especially for the left ear, similar to what was displayed in Figure 5–19 for the DSI. Strouse and Wilson (1999) also tested these same subjects using a directed-recall mode. As expected, the

Table 5–7. Mean Values for the Two-Pair Dichotic Digit Presentations for Different Age Groups for the Free-Recall Paradigm

Age Group	Right Ear	Left Ear
20–29	97.6	96.9
30–39	95.1	86.5
40–49	94.3	88.3
50–59	90.7	78.4
60–69	91.9	83.8
70–79	90.6	74.3

Source: Adapted from Strouse & Wilson, 1999.

results were considerably better. The poorest performance was again for the oldest group, but the mean values were 95.7% for the right ear and 90.7% for the left. One might question if the reduced performance shown in Table 5–7 for the older groups was simply because these subjects had greater hearing loss? They did indeed have greater hearing loss, but Strouse and Wilson (1999) addressed this issue and provided three convincing reasons why this probably was not related to the poorer performance for the dichotic digits: (1) reduced performance was not observed for the one-digit dichotic presentation, (2) reduced performance was not observed for the directed response, and (3) scores for monosyllabic word testing, delivered at the same HL (70 dB), were not reduced.

As we discussed earlier, from a clinical standpoint, it is meaningful to have a general idea of what percent of our older patients have some sort of processing deficit. Recall that one study (Jerger et al., 1990) suggested it may be as high as 80%. To examine this for their sample, Strouse and Wilson (1999) looked at a subsample of their population, the subjects in the 60 to 79 age range ($n = 60$). They report that within this group, 48% had a deficit in at least one ear for free-recall condition, and 7% of these subjects also showed the deficit for the directed recall. Although the free-recall versus direct-recall differences are academically interesting, when we relate the test results to hearing aid fittings, they become less important, as our fitting and counseling strategies will be very similar for both a cognitive-based and an auditory-based cause.

Administration and Scoring

The administration of the DDT is similar to our previous discussion for the DSI. As mentioned, there are different dichotic digit tests available—we base our review here to the Musiek Auditec version, which seems to be the most commonly used (for further information regarding administration of this test, see Guenette, 2006):

- A two-channel audiometer is required, and the test is presented from a CD. It is important that the audiologist is certain of what channel is going to each ear (confer with the patient if necessary) and that each channel is calibrated.
- In most cases, a presentation level of 50 dB above the SRT is appropriate. If the SRT was

not conducted, use 50 dB above the pure-tone average (500, 1000, and 2000 Hz). Exceptions to this include the following:

- If the patient has normal hearing in the low frequencies (resulting in an SRT of approximately 10 dB) and a sharply falling hearing loss (e.g., resulting in >50 dB for 2000 Hz and above), 50 dB SL may not result in a high enough setting.
- In a relatively moderate flat hearing loss (SRT approximately 40 to 45 dB), using a 50 dB SL may place to test signals at the patient's LDL.
- For both of the above situations, we recommend using a presentation level of 75 to 80 dB HL, or the patient's "Loud, But Okay" loudness rating for speech, which should be about 5 dB below their speech LDL.

- With the intensity set at desired levels for both channels/ears, talk to the patient (bilateral presentation) to assure a relative loudness match between ears is present. Your voice should be localized to the center of the patient's head. If the patient reports that one ear is louder than the other, raise the intensity of the softer ear to match the loudness of the louder ear.
- Deliver the three pairs of practice items. Repeat if the patient seems to have trouble understanding the task.
- Deliver the 20 test items.
- Give the patient ample time to respond, even though this probably will require pausing the CD occasionally (the norms were established allowing patients as much time as they wished to respond).
- If a patient cannot respond orally, they can write the digits or point to them on a large response board.

The following are sample instructions:

You will be hearing two numbers in each of your ears. Listen carefully in both ears and repeat all the numbers you hear. The order that you repeat them doesn't matter. If you are unsure of the numbers, please guess. The first few items will be for practice. At this point the audiologist might also want to give the following example: "You might hear the numbers 3 and 9 in your right ear, and the numbers 4 and 8 in your left ear. What you then would repeat back to me is all four numbers: 3, 9, 4, and 8. Any questions?"

The DDT is scored by percent correct. The Musiek version has 20 pairs or 40 items, so the patient is given 2.5% for each correct digit per ear. An example of the score sheet is shown in Figure 5–22.

	Version 1 **Practice Items**				Version 2			
	Channel 1 to R L Ear (Circle)		Channel 2 to R L Ear (Circel)		Channel 1 to R L Ear (Circle)		Channel 2 to R L Ear (Circle)	
TRIAL #	Stim.	Resp.	Stim.	Resp.	Stim.	Resp.	Stim.	Resp.
A	5		2		5-4		2-1	
B	1		8		8-3		6-4	
C	3		10		2-8		3-5	

	Version 1 **Test Items**				Version 2			
	Channel 1 to R L Ear (Circle)		Channel 2 to R L Ear (Circle)		Channel 1 to R L Ear (Circle)		Channel 2 to R L Ear (Circle)	
TRIAL #	Stim.	Resp.	Stim.	Resp.	Stim.	Resp.	Stim.	Resp.
1	1		7		6-1		8-2	
2	8		3		2-5		10-4	
3	2		6		4-3		9-5	
4	3		4		8-6		3-1	
5	1		3		9-2		4-6	
6	7		5		3-10		2-4	
7	5		3		5-8		1-10	
8	1		2		2-9		5-3	
9	3		10		10-5		4-9	
10	10		7		1-9		6-4	
11	6		2		3-1		8-6	
12	4		9		5-3		2-9	
13	8		1		2-4		3-10	
14	3		5		8-2		6-1	
15	8		10		10-4		2-5	
16	6		2		9-5		4-3	
17	9		4		4-9		10-5	
18	1		9		6-4		1-9	
19	2		8		1-10		5-8	
20	10		3		4-6		9-2	
# Correct	___ x 2.5 = %		___ x 2.5 = %		___ x 2.5 = %		___ x 2.5 = %	

Figure 5–22. Example of score sheet used for the Musiek DDT (Adapted from Auditec of St. Louis).

Clinical Applications

The DDT is similar to the DSI, and we would expect similar results. Hence, the clinical applications are essentially the same as we discussed in the DSI section. As with the DSI, the DDT can be conducted in both a free-recall or a directed-ear mode. In some cases, we see large improvement for one ear in the directed-ear condition, but not for the other. This finding may give some indication of what ear to fit for patients who only are purchasing one hearing aid.

In general, bilaterally reduced DDT scores are a red flag that additional counseling may be needed. Included would be guidelines for effective listening and encouragement to use assistive listening devices. As with the DSI, a significantly low DDT score in one ear only may influence decisions and counseling regarding bilateral amplification.

Obtaining the DDT

There are two different versions of the DDT available from Auditec of St. Louis. A third version of the DDT is available from Audiology VA CD Disc 2 (http://www.etsu.edu/crhs/aslp/audiology/resources/Aud_VA_CD_Disc_2.asp).

In Closing

In this chapter we have attempted to give you a review of the most commonly used speech-in-noise tests and a few pointers on testing speech in quiet as a bonus. It should now be obvious why all hearing aid best practice guidelines include the use of speech-in-noise measures.

Two More Just for Fun

And just when you thought we had covered all the speech tests that could be used with hearing aid fitting, we have a few more to mention. These are not tests that are commonly used today in the fitting of hearing aids, but you will probably want to at least know that they exist and they may be useful for some special purpose fittings.

AzBio Sentences

The AzBio sentences are perhaps the newest member of our ever growing list of speech-in-noise tests. These sentences are commonly used with cochlear implant patients. The AzBio sentences were first described by Spahr and Dorman (2004) and were developed in the Department of Speech and Hearing Science at Arizona State University. The development of these sentence materials was enabled by a grant from the Arizona Biomedical Institute at ASU (currently known as the Biodesign Institute), and in appreciation, the resulting speech materials were dubbed the AzBio sentences (see Spahr et al., 2012 for review).

The AzBio sentence materials are available on an audio CD designed specifically for use with a clinical audiometer and consist of 15 lists of 20 sentences each. There is a 10-talker babble on the second track of the CD. Unlike some other sentence tests we have discussed, the AzBio sentences differ considerably in length. For example, for List 1, three sentences only have 5 words and three contain 10 words. Some lists have sentences of 4 or 11 words, but most are 7 to 9 words. The total words possible for each 20-sentence list then also varies and ranges from 133 to 154 (for sample score sheet, see Appendix V).

Schafer, Pogue, and Milrany (2012) examined the equivalency of the 15 AzBio Sentence Test lists on the commercially available CD at two SNRs. They tested participants with normal hearing and a second group with cochlear implants. These authors concluded that when the AzBio Sentence Test is used with the background noise for clinical or research purposes, only Lists 2, 3, 4, 5, 8, 9, 10, 11, 13, and 15 are recommended.

As far as we know, the AzBio test is not used much with the typical hearing aid patient, but if your goal is to select a sentence test with a fixed SNR, we do not see why it could not be. The AzBio is available from www.auditorypotential.com.

Beautifully Efficient Speech Test

We had to include this test if for no other reason than because of the clever name. Really, who would not want to use something that is *beautifully efficient*? This test was developed at the National Acoustic Laboratories and has been used in several research studies conducted at this facility (Schmitt, 2004). The Beautifully Efficient Speech Test (BEST) is designed to efficiently estimate a listener's speech recognition performance in noise using an adaptive SNR procedure. An important design feature is that the intelligibility of individual words in the sentence is equalized by varying the SNR from one word to the next. It has been shown that the slope of the performance-intensity function of the BEST is as steep as 34% per dB, which would enable the SNR-50 to be found with high accuracy in a very short time. Background information on the BEST is a bit scarce, and we are not sure if it is available for commercial distribution. But we like the name. See Appendix W for example score sheets.

Cognitive Measures

We certainly all would agree that the patient's cognitive function will impact the hearing aid fitting process and will influence our counseling during the pre-fitting testing. Some might even suggest that cognitive function can be used to help determine the best signal processing (see Book Two of this series on technology for a discussion of this topic). It seems reasonable, therefore, to perhaps include a cognitive test in our pre-fitting battery. We did not specifically include any cognitive speech tests here. However, recall that comparing free recall versus directed recall for dichotic speech tests such as the DSI may provide insight into cognitive function.

There are other speech tests available that are designed to assess cognitive function. One recommended by Pam Souza (2012) for clinical use is the Reading Span Test (although it sometimes is given as a reading test first so that the results are not contaminated by reduced speech recognition). This test was designed to measure simultaneous storage and processing capacity. The patient is asked to determine if a particular sentence makes sense, and then after several sentences have been presented, the patient is asked to recall the first or last words of those sentences. The number of sentences presented prior to recall increase during the test, and the final score is the percentage of correctly recalled words (Souza, 2012). This is just one example of cognitive testing that one day may be fairly routine in hearing aid pre-fitting testing.

So there you have it. Quite a buffet of speech tests to choose from. We reviewed two speech tests that are given in quiet, four that use a fixed SNR, four more that use an adaptive SNR-50 approach, a couple tests that require a subjective response, two dichotic speech tests, and a few bonus tests at the end. You certainly have several to choose from—we have our favorites and hope you will find yours.

6

Self-Assessment Scales for Pre-Fitting Testing

To this point, we have discussed objective pure-tone, narrowband, and speech recognition tests that can be used during the assessment prior to the fitting of hearing aids. We recommend also using self-assessment inventories to complement the objective findings. That is, some type of formal questionnaire completed by the patient that relates to their hearing difficulty, communication needs, the use of hearing aids, and their candidacy in general should be included in this pre-fitting battery.

In some ways, these scales are not much more than an extended case history, but they allow the clinician to collect information in an organized manner, and in most cases, the patient's responses can be compared with average data from large samples. The information collected using these inventories can significantly influence pre-fitting counseling and in some instances alter fitting decisions. In some cases, the scores collected before the fitting serve as a baseline, as they may be compared with results measured after a patient wears hearing aids for a period of time to directly quantify subjective hearing aid benefit, reduction in hearing handicap, or other outcomes of interest—we talk about this extensively in Book Three in the validation section.

As we reviewed in the previous chapter, there are many speech tests to choose from, and the notion is that we select a specific test to answer a specific question we might have about the patient (e.g., How much are they bothered by background noise? How well do

they understand speech in background noise?). The same is true regarding self-assessment inventories. There are pre-fitting inventories that are geared toward determining communication difficulty, whereas others are geared toward examining the patient's expectations. Others may be focused toward perceived handicap, how the patient judges loudness, or their motivation to use hearing aids. Once the audiologist determines the types of questions that need to be answered, an inventory that addresses these specific issues can be selected.

Reasons to Use Pre-Fitting Self-Assessment Scales

To get us started, we first list a few areas where self-assessment pre-fitting tests might be helpful for the overall hearing aid fitting process. Our examples include names of specific tests. You might not be familiar with these tests just yet, but all are explained in detail later in the chapter. Here are seven general uses for standardized scales as part of the pre-fitting process:

- Assist in determining if a patient is a candidate for hearing aids.
  Example: A patient has a very mild hearing loss; normal hearing through 2000 Hz,

dropping down to a 40 dB loss in the 3000 to 6000 Hz range. The HHIE or APHAB scores, however, show significant handicap and considerable communication problems. This might lead us to make a different decision regarding amplification than if the HHIE or APHAB scores were consistent with someone with normal hearing.

■ Determine the need for pre-fitting counseling. Example: On the STHP, the patient does not pass 7 of the 11 items on the adjustment subscale. Before being fitted with hearing aids, it might be wise to spend some time talking with the patient about how he or she has adjusted to having a hearing loss, or what other issues are driving this failing score.

■ Assist in determining if a patient is ready to be helped.

Example 1: A patient has a bilateral downward sloping hearing loss ranging from 30 dB in the lows to 70 dB in the highs. The AI (for Audibility Index) is 38% for the right ear and 32% for the left. The scores for the HHIE and the APHAB, however, are consistent with someone with normal hearing. If this person denies these communication problems, will he or she accept the use of hearing aids? Is counseling needed before even attempting to move forward?

Example 2: A patient with a mild hearing loss scores in the 10th percentile for the motivation subscale of the HASP. Is this patient ready to accept and use hearing aids, or is the patient a *return for credit* waiting to happen? Why did the patient make the appointment for the hearing aid evaluation? Or did someone else make the appointment?

■ Assist in establishing realistic expectations. Example: A patient with a moderately severe bilateral hearing loss is being fit with hearing aids for the first time. The results of the ECHO show that the patient believes that the use of hearing aids will resolve 100% of the communication problems, including understanding speech in

adverse background noise situations. It is probably best to readjust the patient's expectations before he or she begins to use hearing aids.

■ Assist in establishing a baseline. Example: The patient's results for the PAL and for the aversiveness scale of the APHAB reveal a low tolerance for loud sounds (e.g., the patient judges sounds to be Uncomfortably Loud when most individuals consider these sounds to be Loud, But Okay). This information might be helpful in setting the AGCo kneepoints at the time of the fitting and will be useful in interpreting the post-fitting ratings on these scales (e.g., the patient may complain that sounds are too loud despite seemingly appropriate hearing aid output settings).

■ Assist in establishing goals to select and prioritize technology as well as providing topics that may require further counseling. Example: A patient lists specific goals related to telephone use and listening in noisy restaurants on a COSI. This information is combined with the patient's speech recognition in noise performance and threshold information to make decisions related to prioritizing hearing aid features, appropriate expectations counseling, and appropriate telephone listening technologies. Establishment of specific hearing aid goals is critical for developing an intervention plan that targets each individual patient's listening needs and leads to increased patient satisfaction and use.

■ Quality Assurance Management Example: An audiology private practice has three different clinics in a large metropolitan area. The HASP is administered to all potential hearing aid candidates over a six-month period. The results from each clinic are analyzed to determine if the patient population is different. Motivation? Physical limitations? Cost? These findings could be used to change staff, test protocols or

---

TECHNICAL TIP: A GOOD "QUICK SIX"

Although we recommend the use of validated self-assessment scales, there will be times, for one reason or another, when administration will not be possible. Here are six open-ended questions that can be used to quickly obtain information similar to that obtained with related scales (adapted from Taylor & Mueller, 2011). It is actually reasonable to use these questions with all patients, as it will help establish your concern for the patient's problems and supplement the pre-fitting information gathered from other more formal measures. Remember, as we discussed in Chapter 2, once you have asked the question, you will need to sit back, quietly listen to the response, and make sure that you really hear the individual patient's answers without leading them to the most common answer.

1. Tell me what brought you into the office.
2. How long have you been noticing difficulty with communication?
3. Do other people notice you are having difficulty with communication?
4. Tell me about the areas you are having difficulty with communication.
5. Would you be willing to accept help or assistance with the difficulties you are having?
6. On a scale of 1 to 10, 1 being I don't need help and 10 being I need help right away, how would you rate your ability to communicate?

---

office procedures, or could be helpful in explaining different dispensing patterns among offices.

In this chapter, we review several different self-assessment scales that can be used in the pre-fitting process. Clinically, it is common to only use one or two of these with any given patient, although that is often related more to time constraints than the clinical value of the scales themselves. Most clinicians are likely to mainly use a favorite one or two with most patients and save the others for special cases. However, it is important to be familiar with as many as possible because all the measures we describe can provide unique and important information for at least a small number of patients.

Some clinicians comment that it would be nice to use pre-fitting scales more routinely, but they just don't have the time. Given how much information these scales can provide, however, we find that spending the time on appropriate pre-fitting measures up front can in fact save time by helping in the selection process and providing a focus on the most important counseling issues. In addition, there are some ways to facilitate administration to make the process as streamlined as possible. Ways to streamline the process include mailing the scale

to the patient so they can complete it at home before arriving at the clinic or having them complete the scale in the waiting room, with assistance from support personnel if needed. Although having the patient complete the scale on their own is certainly preferable to skipping the scale altogether, we have to be aware that data clearly show this leads to significantly less reliable answers than when questions are given to patients in interview form. Another way to increase efficiency is to administer a scale orally as part of the case history.

Regardless of the administration method, we highly recommend the use of modern computer technology to automate scoring. Without this, there may simply not be enough time to score the scale in an efficient enough manner to easily use the data during the selection appointment to facilitate selection and counseling. As the average patient becomes more computer savvy, this technology can also be used to facilitate administration—that is, the patient can simply complete a couple scales using a tablet (e.g., iPad), which is then handed to you when you begin your initial pre-fitting counseling. In some cases, a tablet can be used to complete the scale through an interactive interface that would be expected to improve reliability when compared with old-fashioned pen and paper administration.

> ### SOAPBOX:
> ### SOME THINGS YOU JUST HAVE TO MAKE TIME FOR!
>
> We have all heard the old saying, "You can't judge a book by its cover." A saying that is maybe not as well-known, but is even more true is, "You can't judge a hearing aid candidate by his audiogram." Patients differ in so many ways that are not displayed in Xs and Os or word recognitions scores. There is an excellent battery of validated preselection self-assessment inventories available. They are easy to administer and score. The results of these scales will shape the fitting process, assist in technology decisions, and are invaluable for developing counseling strategies along the way. The routine use of these scales is not only a good thing to do, it is the right thing to do.

A One Question Assessment?

It is even possible to obtain useful information from a pre-fitting questionnaire containing only one question. An example of this was reported by Palmer, Solodar, Hurley, Byrne, and Williams (2009). In a retrospective study of over 800 adults aged 18 to 95 years, these authors examined the relationship between the patient's rating of his or her hearing ability, and their subsequent decision to purchase hearing aids. The patients were asked the following question:

"On a scale from 1 to 10, 1 being the worst and 10 being the best, how would you rate your overall hearing ability?"

The answer to the above question was then compared with whether the patient purchased hearing aids. Table 6–1 is a probability chart that resulted from the data analysis. Note that the results showed that there appear to be two distinct groups: those who are very likely to purchase hearing aids (ratings #1 to #5) and those who are likely not to purchase hearing aids (rat-

> ### KEY CONCEPT:
> ### SPOUSES, RELATIVES, AND FRIENDS WANTED!
>
> In most cases, the pre-fitting self-assessment scales are completed during the pre-fitting appointment. Most professionals who have fitted hearing aids for a while say that it is important to have the patient who is seeing you for the first time to bring a companion with them. The companion, is someone who can make the consultative appointment more comfortable for the patient. In fact, subjective pre-fitting measures have been developed that are specifically targeted to significant others such as the HHIE-SP, described later in this chapter. Some reasons why we recommend having a significant other present during the pre-fitting appointment:
>
> 1. Provide details about the general health of the patient.
> 2. Give a second opinion about how the patient is communicating in daily living.
> 3. Facilitate discussion during the needs assessment and testing phase of the appointment.
> 4. Help the patient remember what was said during the evaluation.
> 5. Assist in making treatment and purchasing decisions.

Table 6–1. The Relationship Between the Patient's Self-Rating of Hearing Ability and Probability of Purchasing Hearing Aids

Patient Rating of Hearing Ability (#1 = Worst, #10 = Best)	Predicted Probability of Hearing Aid Purchase
1	98%
2	96%
3	92%
4	83%
5	73%
6	58%
7	7%
8	20%
9	10%
10	6%

Source: From Palmer et al., 2009.

ings #8 to #10). Palmer and colleagues suggest that these initial ratings can be used to determine the best counseling approach for a potential hearing aid user.

A Preview of the Assessment Scales

There have been a large number of inventories that have been introduced over the years. Rather than reviewing every measure, we have selected a subset that we believe are useful, and each of which provides unique information. More specific, we have selected seven different self-assessment inventories that can be used in the pre-fitting process. Here is a brief summary:

- Hearing Handicap Inventory for the Elderly/ Adult (HHIE/A). Measures the degree of handicap for emotional and social issues related to hearing loss.
- Abbreviated Profile of Hearing Aid Benefit (APHAB). Provides the percent of problems the patient has for three different listening conditions involving speech understanding (in quiet, in background noise, and in

reverberation) and problems related to annoyance of environmental sounds (aversiveness scale).

- Expected Consequences of Hearing Aid Ownership (ECHO). Measures the patient's expectations for four different areas: positive effect, service and cost, negative features, and personal image.
- Client Oriented Scale of Improvement (COSI). Requires patients to identify three to five very specific listening goals/communication needs for amplification. Can then be used to measure patients' expectations related to these specific goals.

THINGS TO REMEMBER: THE HANA HISTORY

If you review the literature related to the testing prior to hearing aid fittings, you may see mention of the HANA (Hearing Aid Needs Assessment). As far as we know, it is not a pre-fitting measure that has ever been used clinically, but here is a little history nonetheless. In 1999, Don Schum published a paper regarding the development of the HANA, in which it was used in conjunction with the Hearing Aid Performance Inventory (HAPI) outcome measure to determine if there was a relationship between patients' perceived communication needs and expected benefit from hearing aids, and the benefit that actually was obtained two to three months following the fitting. Eleven items from the HAPI were used as the assessment questions. The test was designed so that subjects answered three questions for each test item, with a three-point rating scale for each (e.g., very little, some, very much). The three questions were: (1) How often are you in this type of situation?, (2) How much trouble do you have in this listening situation?, and (3) How much help do you expect the hearing aids to provide? Not too surprising, the overall findings revealed that expectations exceeded benefit, but it is interesting to note that those subjects with higher expectations for listening in noise had significantly higher benefit.

- Hearing Aid Selection Profile (HASP). Assesses eight patient factors related to the use of hearing aids: motivation, expectations, appearance, cost, technology, physical needs, communication needs, and lifestyle.
- Characteristics of Amplification Tool (COAT). Nine questions designed to determine the patient's communication needs, motivation, expectations, cosmetics, and cost concerns.
- Profile of Aided Loudness (PAL). Assesses the patient's loudness perceptions and satisfaction with these perceptions for 12 different everyday environmental sounds.

Hearing Handicap for the Elderly/Adult (HHIE/A)

Perhaps the oldest and most well-known self-assessment scale related to the pre-fitting of hearing aids is the HHIE. As the name suggests, this scale assesses handicap—specifically related to the emotional and social aspects of having a hearing loss.

Background

There have been some modifications to the HHIE scale over the years, so to get started, here is a brief summary:

- HHIE: The original 25-item questionnaire (Ventry & Weinstein, 1982), designed for the elderly—people 65 and older.
- HHIE-S: S=Screening. A modification of the HHIE containing only 10 items (Weinstein, 1986).
- HHIA: A=Adult. A 25-item of the HHIE for individuals younger than 65 years (Newman, Weinstein, Jacobson, & Hug, 1990).
- HHIA-S: S=Screening. A modification of the HHIA containing only 10 items (Newman, Weinstein, Jacobson, & Hug, 1991).

Research has shown the shortened versions have comparable reliability and validity with the longer 25-item version, with an adequate internal consistency, and have high test-retest reliability (Newman et al.,

1991; Ventry & Weinstein, 1983). For clinical use, therefore, we recommend the 10-item versions of both the HHIE and the HHIA. If we look at the 10-item versions, there are only two items that are different between the elderly and adult scales:

Question #3

- HHIE: Do you have difficulty understanding when someone speaks in a whisper?
- HHIA: Does a hearing problem cause you difficulty hearing/understanding coworkers, clients, or customers?

Question #6

- HHIE: Does a hearing problem cause you to attend religious services less often than you would like?
- HHIA: Does a hearing problem cause you problems in the movies or theater?

As you can see from the comparative questions, the adult version is geared more to someone who is still employed. If your 70-year-old patient is indeed still actively employed, there are no rules (that we know of) that say you cannot give him the HHIA-S rather than the HHIE-S. One might even question if the age cutoff is the same today as it was when the scales were developed—is age 65 "elderly?"

The HHIE was designed to have questions that fall into two general areas: emotional and social/situational. These questions are sometimes designated by an "E" or an "S" on the form; there are five of each category on the HHIE-S and HHIA-S. The emotional scale examines the patient's attitudes and emotional feelings related to their hearing loss:

"Does a hearing problem cause you to feel embarrassed when you meet new people?"

The social/situation scale measures the perceived effects of hearing loss for a variety of communication situations:

"Does a hearing problem cause you difficulty when in a restaurant with relatives or friends?"

Many of the self-assessment scales that we describe in this chapter are designed to provide additional infor-

---

TECHNICAL TIP: AN HHIE SCALE FOR THE SPOUSE TOO!

In addition to the HHIE and the HHIA and their screening companions, there is also the HHIE-SP, described by Newman and Weinstein (1986). The HHIE-SP is identical to the HHIE except that the substitution of your spouse for you in each question. This then provides an indication of how the spouse views the hearing problem. Newman and Weinstein (1986) report the husband's score (they used all male subjects in the study) were significantly higher (worse) than the wives for both the social and emotional scale (31 versus 24 points for the 25-item, 100-point version). Correlations between the HHIE and the HHIE-SP revealed a stronger relationship for the social/situational scale than for the emotional scale—probably because the hearing impaired person's handicap in social situations is often observable, whereas his or her thoughts about the situation might not be as obvious. It is important to remember that differences in the perceptions of hearing handicap between the patient and his or her spouse do not indicate that either party is right or wrong. It can be useful, however, to examine areas of discrepancy or agreement and use these emotional or social situations to shape counseling objectives.

---

mation to assist in hearing aid selection and counseling for the candidate. The HHIE, on the other hand, often has been used to determine *if* the patient is a candidate. For example, the HHIE-S is recommended by the ASHA (1997) as a screening tool for hearing disability in older adults. In some instances, the HHIE even is used in marketing in an attempt to convince a potential hearing aid user that they have communication problems. For example, you might see the HHIE as part of a full-page hearing aid promotional ad in the Sunday newspaper. The readers are encouraged to answer the questions, score themselves, and rate their handicap.

Considerable research has been conducted comparing HHIE scores with the patient's audiogram. For example, Lichtenstein, Bess, and Logan (1988) validated the HHIE-S against pure-tone audiometry for 178 patients over age 65. They report that an HHIE-S score from 0 to 8 resulted in a likelihood ratio of 0.36, 13% probability of hearing loss (95% confidence interval, 0.19 to 0.68;), and a score of 26 or more yielded a likelihood ratio of 12.00, 84% probability of hearing loss (95% confidence interval, 2.62 to 55.00).

In one of the largest studies of this type, Wiley, Cruickshanks, Nondahl, and Tweed (2000) used the HHIE-S in the study of 3,471 adults (1,963 women, 1,508 men), as part of a large epidemiologic study of hearing disorders in older adults. Participants were divided into four groups based on age, which ranged from 48 to 92 years. Figure 6–1 illustrates the percent of significant hearing handicap (HHIE-S >8) as a function of the degree of hearing loss. While you might assume that as people age, their hearing handicap will become worse, the authors report that after accounting for the degree of hearing loss in men and women, self-reported hearing handicap was *lower* for older age groups. After adjusting for the degree of hearing loss, handicap declined 24% for every five-year advancement in age. There are several possible reasons for this:

- Elderly individuals may minimize or ignore health problems.
- The older population is simply less bothered by problems such as hearing loss, and may cope more successfully. Some may simply accept hearing loss as a natural part of aging.
- The generation of older individuals studied may have experienced greater hardships during their life, which led to lower expectations and stronger tolerance.
- The younger individuals are more active and place greater demands on their communication skills.
- The younger individuals are not as accepting of having a hearing loss.

Another large-scale study that utilized the HHIE was the Blue Mountains Hearing Study, conducted in a representative older, Australian community during the

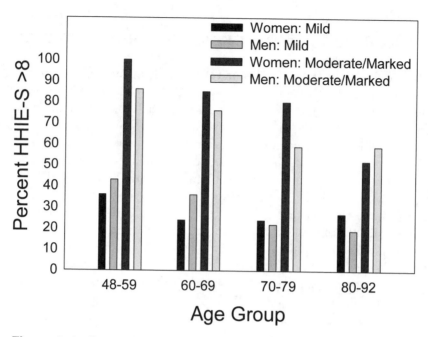

Figure 6–1. Illustration of the percent of significant hearing handicap (HHIE-S>8) as a function of the degree of hearing loss, separated for men and women. (Adapted from Wiley et al., 2000.)

years 1997 to 1999 (Sindhusake et al., 2001). The study included 1,817 individuals who had both audiometric threshold testing and completed all questions on the HHIE-S (scores >8 were considered indicative of hearing handicap). Using the audiogram as the gold standard, a receiver operating characteristic (ROC) curve

for HHIE-S score, for mild, moderate, and marked hearing impairment was computed, shown in Figure 6–2.

The authors consider that the ROC curves shown in Figure 6–2 confirmed the usefulness of an HHIE-S score >8 in identifying moderate hearing loss, but suggest that a lower HHIE-S cut point score (e.g., >6) might

---

TECHNICAL TIP: ROC CURVES

We mention the study using the HHIE-S findings and the audiogram to construct ROC curves. Here is a little information to help interpret Figure 6–2.

- Sensitivity: The percent of time that a positive test finding will result for people who have the disease/pathology in question.
- Specificity: The percent of time that a negative test finding will result for people who *do not* have the disease/pathology in question.

In signal detection theory, a receiver operating characteristic (ROC), or simply ROC curve, is a graphical plot of the sensitivity, or true positive rate, versus the false positive rate (1-specificity). These curves then allow for comparison of the trade-off between sensitivity (hit rate) and 1-specificity (false positive rate) as the pass or fail criteria of the test is manipulated. In this case, we are looking at the sensitivity of the HHIE to detect hearing loss.

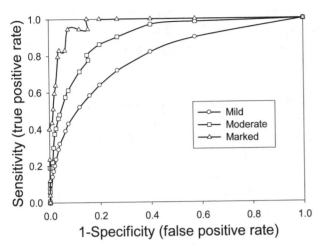

Figure 6–2. Illustration of the receiver operating characteristic curve (ROC) for HHIE-S scores (scores >8 were considered indicative of hearing handicap) for mild, moderate, and marked hearing impairment. Based on data from 1,817 individuals who had both audiometric threshold testing and who completed all questions on the HHIE-S. (Adapted from Sindhusake et al., 2001.)

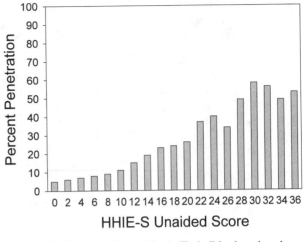

Figure 6–3. Data from MarkeTrak IV, showing how unaided average HHIE scores relate to hearing aid ownership for individuals who state they have hearing loss. (Adapted from Kochkin, 1997.) Although, as expected, hearing aid ownership increases as HHIE scores become worse, even when HHIE scores are 30 or more, ownership is only around 50%.

be more useful in screening for mild hearing loss and a higher cut point score (e.g., >14) for marked hearing loss. It is interesting to note that the HHIE-S performed best in younger male subjects. Overall prevalence of hearing loss in the study was 39.4%. The prevalence was lower, however, for the moderate and marked hearing loss groups, and therefore, the HHIE-S had higher negative predictive rates and lower positive predictive rates for these subject samples.

The HHIE-S also was used in the ongoing hearing study of the Framingham Heart Study cohort. The gold standard used in this study was an audiogram showing a pure-tone threshold of 40 dB HL or poorer at 1 and 2 kHz in one ear or at 1 or 2 kHz in both ears. Gates, Murphy, Rees, and Fraher (2003) reported that the HHIE-S (cutoff score >8) had a sensitivity of 35% and a specificity of 94% for detecting the criterion hearing loss.

Given the significant correlations that have been shown between HHIE score and degree of hearing loss, it is reasonable to assume that the HHIE score also is correlated with the decision to use hearing aids. As part of MarkeTrak IV, Kochkin (1997) included the HHIE-S in a survey of 3,000 hearing aid owners and 3,500 hearing impaired nonowners (response rate approximately 80%

for each group). The relationship between hearing aid ownership (percent penetration) and the HHIE-S score is shown in Figure 6–3. As illustrated, there is a systematic (and significant) relationship between the HHIE-S score and the decision to own hearing aids. However, note that even when HHIE scores are 30 or greater, approximately 50% of this group did not own hearing aids.

Administration and Scoring

One feature of the HHIE that has contributed to its popularity is that it is very easy to administer and score. It is recommended that the HHIE be delivered face-to-face to help prevent patients from skipping questions because of the belief it is not applicable to them. In this regard, the instructions also state, "Do not skip a question if you avoid a situation because of your hearing loss." For each of the 10 questions of the HHIE/A-S, the patient has the choice of three answers:

- Yes (scored 4 points)
- Sometimes (scored 2 points)
- No (scored 0 points)

KEY CONCEPT:
THE IMPORTANCE OF CONSISTENT INSTRUCTIONS

Clinicians should keep in mind that different instruction sets should not be used interchangeably. There are a large number of studies that clearly have shown that the specific instructions and response scale used can greatly affect the measured results of subjective questionnaires. Therefore, if the goal is to compare your patient to normative data, the specific instructions and response scale used when collecting the normative data must be used. It's very likely that using "Frequently" versus "Always" versus "Yes" for the 4-point HHIE response might all result in different scores for the same patient.

We have seen forms where these answers have been changed to Always, Sometimes, and Never. In the MarkeTrak IV survey we discussed earlier, Kochkin (1997) used Frequently, Sometimes, and Never.

Once completed, the scores for the 10 items simply are added, with 40 representing the highest (worst) score, a significant handicap. A separate score can be calculated for each of the two different subscales (emotional and social), although typically just the overall score is used (especially for the screening version).

The general guidelines for interpreting the results are:

- 0 to 8: No significant perception of a hearing handicap
- 10 to 22: Mild to moderate perception of a hearing handicap
- >22: Perception of a severe handicap

Clinical Application

Like some of the other scales we will discuss, the unaided HHIE often is used as a baseline for the measure of hearing aid benefit following the fitting of hearing aids. Hopefully, with the use of hearing aids, we will observe the scores improve from the unaided findings. The HHIE also is a very useful tool for pre-fitting counseling. Assume our patient is a 74-year-old male who is semi-retired. He has a history of noise exposure and a bilaterally symmetrical downward sloping hearing loss, with near-normal hearing in the lows, dropping to 50 dB at 2000 Hz and 70 dB in the 3000 to 4000 Hz range. His HHIE-S scores are 16 for social/situational and 4 for emotional, giving him a total score of 20. The total score of 20 places him in the moderate perception of handicap category. The 16 score for the social subscale indicates that he is having problems in several

---

POINTS TO PONDER: AN HHIE-HHIA MERGING?

If you have used the HHIE/A in a busy clinic, you know that it is somewhat of a pain to use the two different forms and make sure the patient receives the correct form based on their age or employment status (or whether they attend religious services). Help is on the way. Barbara Weinstein tells us that a single, merged screening form for the HHIE/A is now available and is being used in at least one research project. Forms and normative data will be available soon, although the data undoubtedly will be very similar to what we have been using, given that most questions are the same, and the scoring has not changed. Be on the lookout for this new form!

different communication settings. It would be worthwhile to discuss these problems more, as they might make good items for the COSI. It is a little unusual that his emotional score is as low as it is, given the 16 score for social. It could indeed be that although he is having considerable difficulty, it really does not bother him or his family. On the other hand, he simply may be denying that he is frustrated and embarrassed, or he maybe has not really accepted his hearing loss. This too would warrant discussion prior to the fitting.

What if a patient with this same hearing loss had an overall HHIE-S score of 36? It seems unlikely that this degree of hearing loss would cause that much handicap. Could it be that this patient is purposely exaggerating his handicap for some other reason? Why did he make the appointment? Other health problems? This takes us back to many of the issues we discussed in Chapter 2—except you are now armed with HHIE findings to assist in the counseling process.

Obtaining the HHIE/A

The HHI-E and HHI-A are reprinted in Appendix X through AA. The HHIE/A is not copyrighted.[36] Because most clinicians use the screening versions and because it is only 10 questions, clinics or individuals often design their own template of the questionnaire.

Abbreviated Profile of Hearing Aid Benefit (APHAB)

In the previous pages, we discussed the HHIE, perhaps the most utilized hearing aid fitting pretest over the past few decades. We would guess that the second most popular, and gaining ground, is the APHAB, a scale developed by Robyn Cox and colleagues at the University of Memphis.

Background

Although normally thought of as an outcome measure, the APHAB also is a popular pre-fitting tool for one main reason: To calculate benefit with hearing aids, we need an unaided baseline. As we discuss shortly, there

---

THINGS TO REMEMBER: THE APHAB AND THE IHAFF

In the early 1990s, a group of 12 audiologists banded together to form what was dubbed the IHAFF (for Independent Hearing Aid Fitting Forum).[37] The goal was to develop a better way to fit hearing aids and provide a step-by-step protocol that could be adopted by audiologists across the United States (and maybe the world). Critics (or perhaps they were realists) suggested that the complete name should have been: "IHAFF-A-DREAM." Regardless, in 1994, after a couple of years of meetings, the IHAFF group indeed did emerge with a complete fitting protocol (Mueller, 1994b). Robyn Cox was a member of the IHAFF, and her APHAB, launched as part of this protocol, was a key component to the overall IHAFF fitting philosophy. Today, the IHAFF is mostly forgotten, but the APHAB is still going strong.

---

are several good reasons why the APHAB should be used as a measure prior to the hearing aid fitting other than simply obtaining baseline unaided information.

As you might predict from the word *abbreviated*, the origins of the APHAB are from other more extensive self-assessment scales, also developed at the University of Memphis. The first of these was a scale designed to assess hearing aid users' opinions about the helpfulness of their hearing aids. This scale was the Profile of Hearing aid Performance (PHAP; Cox & Gilmore, 1990). This questionnaire consisted of 66 items distributed among seven subscales. Five subscales addressed the problems people have communicating in daily life, and two subscales related to the unpleasantness of everyday sounds. The PHAP was then modified so that the questions could also be answered by the unaided listener, which could then assess opinions regarding the benefit of using hearing aids. This revision of the PHAP was dubbed the Profile of Hearing Aid Benefit (PHAB; Cox, Gilmore, & Alexander, 1991). It was comprised of the same items and the same subscales as the PHAP. The PHAP and the PHAB were developed as research tools; the 66 questions and scoring for seven subscales were not generally considered *clinically friendly*. This led to the development of the shortened (or abbreviated) version of the PHAB, the 24-item, four subscale APHAB (Cox & Alexander, 1995).

The APHAB is composed of 24 items that are scored in four subscales (six questions each). The subscales are:

- Ease of Communication (EC): The strain of communicating under relatively favorable conditions. (e.g., "I have difficulty hearing a conversation when I'm with one of my family at home.")
- Reverberation (RV): Communication in reverberant rooms such as classrooms. (e.g., "When I am talking with someone across a large empty room, I understand the words.")
- Background Noise (BN): Communication in settings with high background noise levels. (e.g., "When I am listening to the news on the car radio and family members are talking, I have trouble hearing the news.")
- Aversiveness (AV): The unpleasantness of environmental sounds. (e.g., "The sounds of running water, such as a toilet flushing or a shower, are uncomfortably loud.")

Cox, Alexander, and Gray (2003) compared unaided APHAB scores with four different audiometric variables: pure-tone hearing loss and three speech recognition tests—speech reception thresholds, monosyllables in quiet, and the revised Speech-In-Noise (R-SPIN) test. They report that for EC and RV subscales, 4 to 5% of additional variance was accounted for by combining a second variable with the one most strongly related to the subscale. For these subscales, the combined audiologic variables accounted for 45% (EC) and 51% (RV) of the variance in APHAB scores. For the BN subscale scores, however, combining audiometric variables did not improve their ability to predict APHAB scores. And it is interesting to note that it was not the R-SPIN, but rather monosyllabic word recognition in quiet that was the most closely related to the BN score. Differences in word recognition accounted for 26% of the differences in BN scores. As we might expect, scores for the AV subscale were not significantly associated with any audiometric variable.

The authors remind us, however, that although there was a modest correlation between audiometric findings and the EC and RV subscales, it is still risky to attempt to predict communication problems from audiometric data on an individual basis. This is clearly shown in Figure 6–4. If there were a close relationship, all data points would be clustered along the diagonal regression line. Instead, as shown, it was common for the true APHAB score to differ by 30% or more from the predicted. For example, if we observe the results for an unaided predicted score in the 50% to 60% range (a common clinical finding), note that true APHAB scores range from 20% to over 80%. Differences such as this one are precisely why we believe that in addition to objective tests, subjective tests such as this are an essential component of selecting hearing aids.

As part of MarkeTrak IV, Kochkin (1997) questioned if the unaided APHAB was related to hearing aid ownership. For this analysis, he averaged the three subscales, EC, RV, and BN, and referred to this as *percent disability*. The APHAB was completed by 5,954 individuals with self-admitted hearing loss. The results showed a strong relationship between ownership and the unaided score, as illustrated in Figure 6–5. These data suggest that average unaided APHAB scores would need to exceed 65% before hearing aid ownership reaches 50% of individuals admitting to having a hear-

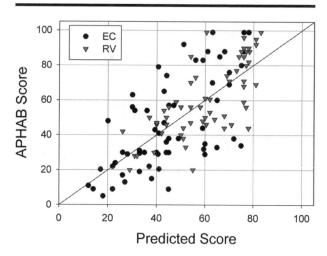

Figure 6–4. The APHAB score for the EC and BN subscales, predicted from audiometric measures, compared with the patients' true APHAB score for the same two subscales. (Adapted from Cox et al., 2003.)

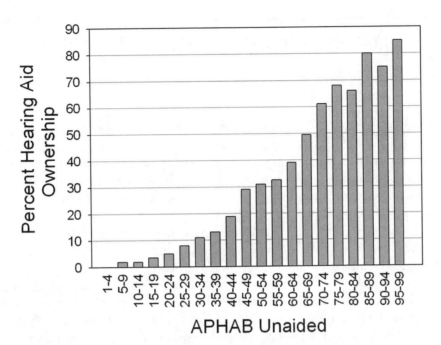

Figure 6–5. The relationship between the unaided APHAB score (percent of problems) compared with hearing aid ownership. (Adapted from Kochkin, 1997.)

ing loss. We can compare this with the norms for satisfied users of hearing aids (Johnson, Cox, & Alexander, 2010). These data show the 50th percentile average for the combined EC-AV-BN scales is 69%.

Administration and Scoring

The APHAB can be administered as a paper and pencil test, or using a computer software version (e.g., the APHAB is included in the Questionnaire Module of the NOAH software). The 24 items of the APHAB are scored on a seven-point scale. A percent value, shown on the form, is designated for each letter answer:

- ■ A: Always (99%)
- ■ B: Almost Always (87%)
- ■ C: Generally (75%)
- ■ D: Half-the-time (50%)
- ■ E: Occasionally (25%)
- ■ F: Seldom (12%)
- ■ G: Never (1%)

If a computer version of the APHAB is used, scoring is automatic and the results are displayed with comparative normative data. It is a little tedious and you might need a calculator, but it is relatively easy to score the APHAB by hand. Guidance for this can be found at the HARL website and is included in Appendix AC. However, if you plan to administer this test during the hearing aid selection visit, computer scoring is highly recommended so that the information can quickly and efficiently be used to aid in selection.

The instructions for completing the APHAB are as follows:

"Please circle the answers that come closest to your everyday experience. Notice that each choice includes a percentage. You can use this to help you decide on your answer. For example, if a statement is true about 75% of the time, circle 'C' for that item. If you have not experienced the situation we describe, try to think of a similar situation that you have been in and respond for that situation. If you have no idea, leave that item blank."

TECHNICAL TIP: ADMINISTERING THE APHAB

In her 1997 article describing the administration of the APHAB, Cox provides tips regarding two potential problems that could arise.

- Patients sometimes have difficulty responding to a particular item because they do not experience the specific situation described in their daily life. She states that in this case, we should attempt to help them identify a similar situation in preference to leaving the item blank. If we must leave items blank, Cox states that we probably should not give much weight to subscale scores derived from fewer than four responses.
- A second important point is to tell the patient that each item must be read carefully because sometimes a response of *always* means a lot of problems, and sometimes it means few or no problems. Cox reports that the items were written this way to make sure that patients pay close attention to their content, and not simply read the first one or two and then give the same answer to all the rest. She states that if we tell the patients about this feature of the questionnaire and perhaps even show them some items that demonstrate the point, the great majority of people will complete the questionnaire successfully.

Clearly these issues suggest that reliability and validity of the APHAB can be enhanced by face-to-face administration, or at the least, reviewing the answers with the patient.

KEY CONCEPT: LOOKING AT PREVIOUS ANSWERS IS OKAY!

Like some of the other pre-fitting scales we discuss, one of the primary uses of the pre-fitting APHAB is to serve as a baseline for the *aided* APHAB that will be conducted following the fitting. Be sure to use the same form for both, as Cox (1997) states that to maximize the validity and reliability, the patient should be allowed to see his or her responses to the Without Hearing Aid portion while he or she is completing the With Hearing Aid part. Cox further states that the patient should be *encouraged* to review the earlier responses, and they are allowed to change responses to the Without Hearing Aid part retrospectively. Seeing the unaided answers tends to recalibrate the patient and improves the quality of the With Hearing Aid answers.

Clinical Application

Cox (1997) states that there are four potential clinical uses of the APHAB:

1. Predict success from unaided scores.
2. Compare results with different hearing aids.
3. Evaluate fittings in an absolute sense.
4. Measure benefit from the fitting.

Both the first and fourth of these clinical uses apply to this chapter. We discuss the fourth one first. The most common use of the APHAB is to calculate the benefit with amplification. To do this, one must first have the unaided baseline for comparison. This is best obtained before the patient begins to use the instruments. We question if the patient really remembers accurately how they were doing *without* hearing aids after a month of hearing aids use. Before actually using the unaided APHAB for pre-fitting patient counseling, it is helpful to compare these scores with other tests of the pre-fitting test battery that you might have conducted. Here are a few examples:

- Do the EC subscale problems agree with the pure-tone audiogram or the AI scores from the count-the-dots calculations (see Chapter 4)?
- Does the BN subscale score agree with the WIN or the BKB-SIN SNR Loss (see Chapter 5 for review of these tests)?
- Does the AV subscale score agree with the patient's LDLs or unaided PAL findings?
- Do the patient's problem areas identified on the APHAB (e.g., lectures, grocery store, in car, etc.) agree with the items nominated on the COSI?

When using the APHAB for pre-fitting counseling, it is helpful to examine the scores for each one of the four subscales. Below are the results for a 74-year-old man with a mild-to-moderate downward sloping hearing loss (the same patient who we discussed in the previous HHIE section). He still works part-time in his office-supply business, which involves frequent meeting with clients. His average APHAB percent of problems for each subscale are:

- EC: 27%
- BN: 58%
- RV: 62%
- AV: 19%

Once these scores have been obtained, you will then want to compare them with normative data (norms). One counseling approach is to compare the patient with individuals with normal hearing. We prefer to plot the findings on a chart, provided by Cox when the APHAB was first introduced (Cox, 1997)—they are also part of the APHAB module included with the NOAH software.

We have included these charts in Appendix AD and they are shown here in Figure 6–6, with our patient's scores included. Our patient is 74 years old, which some consider elderly, so we are using these norms, as well as those for young people with normal hearing for this patient. As shown in Figure 6–6, this patient's problems for both the BN and RV subscale exceed the 95th percentile of people with normal hearing—that is, more than 95% of people with normal hearing do not have this large of an amount of problems.

Another way to view this patient's unaided APHAB scores is to compare them with norms of successful

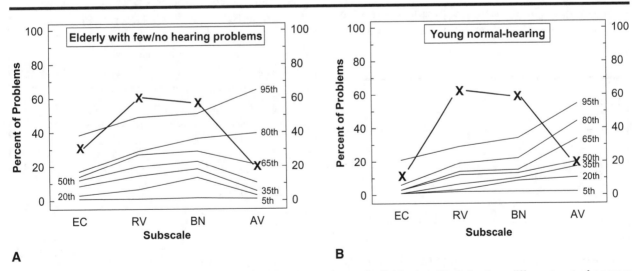

Figure 6–6. The plotting of the unaided APHAB scores for an individual patient, for two different set of norms: elderly with few or no hearing problems (*Panel A*) and young normal hearing individuals (*Panel B*).

THINGS TO REMEMBER:
USING PERCENTILES FOR POST-FITTING COUNSELING

Although we are focusing on the use of the APHAB for pre-fiting testing, it is important to point out that the charts shown in Figure 6–6 can be very helpful for post-fitting counseling. The patient's *aided* APHAB can be plotted just as we plotted the unaided scores. It often is pleasing to see how closely our patients are performing compared with people with normal hearing, which we eagerly share with the patient. The graph also is a helpful reminder that a patient who still has 20% problems in background noise following hearing aid use is actually only slightly higher than the 50th percentile of young normal listeners.

---

hearing aid users. This can be done by using a table available from Robyn Cox's HARL (for Hearing Aid Research Laboratory) website (see Appendix AE) and displayed in Figure 6–7 (adapted from Johnson et al., 2010). Using this table, we see that our patient falls around the 5th percentile for the EC subscale, 30th percentile for RV, 20th for BN, and 60th for AV. In general, the patient's problems are not as severe as the average hearing aid user.

Obtaining the APHAB

See Appendix AB through AE, for information related to the APHAB. Complete APHAB information can be obtained from Robyn Cox's website (http://www.memphis.edu/ausp/harl/). APHAB scoring software also is available. Some hearing aid manufacturers have included the APHAB as part of their software, and the

Percentile	EC	RV	BN	AV
95	99	99	99	70
80	83	87	89	35
65	75	81	81	21
50	63	71	75	14
35	56	65	67	9
20	46	58	58	3
5	26	47	41	1

Figure 6–7. Percentiles of unaided APHAB scores for successful hearing aid users. (Adapted from Johnson et al., 2010.)

TECHNICAL TIP: PERMISSIONS FOR USING THE APHAB

Many audiologists like to post the APHAB (and other self-assessment scales) on their website. Here is the word regarding APHAB permissions, straight from the developer, Robyn Cox, PhD:

You do not need permission to post the APHAB on your website for use by your patients as long as you follow certain procedures. The APHAB is under copyright which means that no one but the authors can legally copy, distribute or adapt the questionnaire without permission. We make the questionnaire freely available on HARL's website (http://www.memphis.edu/ausp/harl/). This means that we have given you permission to download it and use it. However, you cannot change it, sell it, or claim to have created it. I suggest that you download the "Form A-New Format" version to post to your website because it has a few additional instructions that would help patients complete the questionnaire correctly before their appointment.

Thank you Robyn!

APHAB is part of the Questionnaire Module of NOAH, a free add-on for registered NOAH users, available for download from http://www.himsa.com.

Expected Consequences of Hearing Aid Ownership (ECHO)

As the name indicates, the Expected Consequences of Hearing Aid Ownership (ECHO) is all about *expectations*. It is generally believed that expectations can impact satisfaction. Overly high expectations can lead to disappointment. And on the other hand, it seems reasonable that a person with low expectations may be more apt to be satisfied. We are reminded of Benjamin Franklin's often repeated statement: "Blessed is he who expects nothing, for he shall never be disappointed." Anecdotal reports suggest that most audiologists would prefer to have a patient with relatively low or, at the least, moderate expectations, and some audiologists might even attempt to lower the patient's expectations if they appear to be too high. The ideal would seem to be *realistic* expectations as we discuss below. But unless we measure expectations and compare our findings to realistic norms, it may be difficult to know what counseling on this topic is needed.

Background

The ECHO was introduced by Cox and Alexander in 2000. It was designed to be a companion scale for the Satisfaction of Amplification in Daily Life (SADL; Cox et al., 1999). The SADL is an outcome measure of satisfaction, designed to be used following the hearing aid fitting (see the validation section of Book Three for a detailed description). The questions used on the ECHO are essentially the same as those of the SADL, only slightly reworded. The items on the SADL are questions, whereas for the ECHO, the sentence is transformed into a statement of expectation. Here is an example:

- SADL: How natural is the sound from your hearing aid?

POINTS TO PONDER: ARE HIGH OR LOW EXPECTATIONS GOOD?

We probably all have had the experience of going into an unknown seedy restaurant, only to walk out incredibly satisfied with our dinner. But if we had had the same meal at Ruth's Chris or the Palm, our satisfaction might have been considerably lower. When it comes to dining at restaurants, it is reasonable to conclude that it is more likely to be satisfying if our expectations are low. But does this also apply to obtaining hearing aids? Many clinicians are concerned that if their patients' expectations are too high (e.g., my new hearing aids will help me do better in *all* listening situations), amplification may not meet the expectations, and the patient will not be satisfied. This seems reasonable. On the other hand, some people are simply optimistic. They may have high expectations, but their attitude toward the use of hearing aids (and life in general) is such that they will make good things happen. If they believe that a positive outcome will result, it probably will. Limited research shows that the latter example might be the most true for hearing aid fittings. For example, Schum (1999), in his work developing the HANA, found that patients who expected more help in noisy situations reported that they received more help in this listening condition. And relative to our discussion here of the ECHO, Cox and Alexander (2000) report that for the *Positive Effect* subscale, there was a significant positive correlation between higher expectations and greater satisfaction. (The other subscales were not significantly correlated in either direction.) This is not necessarily a cause and effect finding, however, and could likely be related to a third variable such as optimism. In related research, Cox, Alexander, and Gray (1999) found that extroverted individuals tended to report more hearing aid benefits in all types of listening settings. The bottom line: If your patient believes that the new hearing aids are going to work well, that is probably okay (as long as expectations are within reason)![38]

■ ECHO: My hearing aid will have a natural sound.

The ECHO consists of 15 items, which are divided among four subscales. A description of the subscales is as follows (Cox & Alexander, 2000):

Positive Effect: This subscale comprises six items addressing the domain of improved performance and function. Two items concern acoustic benefit, one is about sound quality, and three address psychological dividends accompanying hearing aid use (e.g., getting hearing aids is in my best interest). Cox and Alexander (2000) report that this domain appears to be the largest single contributor to the variance in overall post-fitting satisfaction with amplification.

Service and Cost: This subscale includes two items about service and one item on cost. If the individual is not paying for the hearing aids, the cost item is omitted.

Negative Features: Each of the three items in this subscale addresses a different potentially negative aspect of hearing aid use. All three were often identified by hearing aid users as relatively unsatisfactory. This subscale provides an estimate of the status of matters that can often detract from an otherwise highly satisfactory fitting.

Personal Image: The fourth subscale, also three items, addresses the domain of self-image and hearing aid stigma. The image or stigma content area has been implicated repeatedly over time as highly influential in the decision to try amplification and in ultimate hearing aid satisfaction.

The background research in the development of the ECHO consisted of four separate experiments. The following are some general observations and conclusions taken from the Cox and Alexander (2000) paper:

■ The data gathered regarding expectations only represent a small portion of *potential* hearing aids candidates. The ECHO data are from individuals who decided to seek help, who probably have different attitudes toward their hearing loss and toward the psychosocial impact of using hearing aids than those who do not.

■ The typical novice hearing aid user does not have a realistic view of the hearing aid's strengths and weaknesses.
■ Expectations differ significantly among patients.
■ Informational counseling is warranted for individuals who do not understand the potential negative features of hearing aids or have unrealistic expectations related to personal image.
■ A high score for the Positive Effect subscale was significantly correlated with increased satisfaction. Cox and Alexander caution, however, that this does not mean you should try to raise expectations, as we do not really know that it was these higher expectations that *caused* the better outcome. They support the common thought that unusually favorable opinions about the anticipated benefit from hearing aids might predispose the patient to disappointment.

Administration and Scoring

There are 15 questions, and each question is scored on a seven-point scale indicating the extent that the patient agrees with the statement. The subject simply circles the best answer for each question. The seven answers for each item are as follows (points assigned are 1 through 7 for answers A through G, respectively):

A: Not At All

B: A Little

C: Somewhat

D: Medium

E: Considerably

F: Greatly

G: Tremendously

The appropriate subscale for each question and scoring guidelines are displayed in Appendix AG and available at Robyn Cox's HARL website. For each subscale, the values of the three or six answers (for the Positive Effect subscale) are then averaged. For example, if for the three items of the Service and Cost subscale, the patient answered Considerably (5 points), Greatly

(6 points), and Considerably (5 points), the score for this subscale would be 5.3 (5 + 6 + 5 = 16; 16/3 = 5.3). Four of the 15 items of the ECHO are *reversed scored*, meaning that an answer of Not At All would receive 7 points rather than 1 point. This is clearly explained in Appendix AG. An overall *Global Score* (average of the four subscales) also is calculated, although for clinical use, you will probably want to focus more on each individual subscale to know where to focus your counseling. The ECHO easily can be scored by hand, and scoring software also is available. Again, the use of scoring software is highly recommended if the ECHO is to be administered during the selection appointment.

Once the answers have been scored, the average values are plotted on the ECHO Reality Norms form shown in Figure 6–8. *Reality Norms* meaning that this is what you might expect from the average patient seeking amplification. The black circles on the form for each category represent the mean, and the gray bars illustrate the 20th to 80th percentile score.

TECHNICAL TIP: WHAT DO HIGH ECHO SCORES MEAN?

We have found that when clinicians first start using the ECHO and see the patient's scores plotted on the Reality Norms form, it is not always intuitive to interpret what a deviation from the norm is telling us. It is easy to interpret the Positive Effects scale: a high score means that the person has high expectations regarding the performance of hearing aids and the benefits of amplification. This makes sense. But what about the Personal Image scale? Do high scores mean that the person has high expectations regarding the appearance of hearing aids (e.g., that he or she thinks the hearing aids will be invisible?) That might be a difficult individual to work with. But look at a question from that subscale: "I will be content with the appearance of my hearing aids." If the person answers Greatly or Tremendously, a high ECHO score will result and that is the answer most clinicians would like to hear. So, a high score is *good*. Likewise, with the Negative Features scale, a high score does *not* mean that the patient highly expects negative things to occur, but rather, they do not believe that there are negative features (which is not always good either if their beliefs are unreasonable).

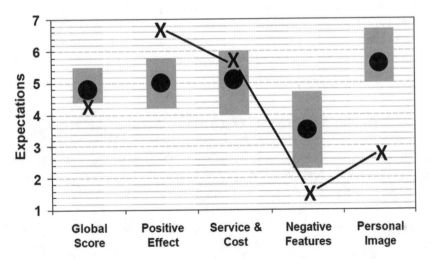

Figure 6–8. Score sheet for the ECHO. Black dots represent mean performance for average individuals with hearing loss (Reality Norms). The gray bars represent the 20th to 80th percentile score. The "Xs" on the chart are the scores for a given patient.

Clinical Application

It is reasonable to believe that that when pre-fitting counseling is targeted toward specific attitudes of the patient, post-fitting use and satisfaction will follow. The ECHO questionnaire is an excellent tool to target specific issues that need to be addressed. The Reality Norms provide a convenient way to compare your patient's expectations with average. In general, low scores are more problematic than high scores, but if unusually high ratings are based on erroneous information or beliefs, this may require additional counseling as well.

A sample case is plotted on Figure 6–8. First, observe that the patient has an average Global Score, although ratings are *not average* for three of the four subscales. Recall that the gray bars represent the 20th to 80th percentiles. The patient has a very optimistic approach toward the potential benefits of amplification (Positive Effects), which is probably okay, and the score for Service and Cost is average. The very low score for negative features indicates that the patient has either experienced or heard several negative things regarding hearing aids. This is a topic that should be explored further before fitting. For example, many of the past negative concerns regarding acoustic feedback no longer apply given the sophisticated feedback reduction circuitry now routinely available. The extremely low score for personal image is also a concern, as it indicates the patient rated all three questions low. This means that the patient believes that people will notice the hearing loss more when wearing the hearing aids, that the patient will not be happy with the appearance of the hearing aids, and that using hearing aids will make the patient appear less capable. These attitudes easily could sabotage the fitting, as they might outweigh the patient's positive attitude regarding hearing aid benefit. This is clearly something that needs to be discussed with the patient.

Obtaining the ECHO

See Appendix AF through AH. The forms for the ECHO can be obtained at HARL's website (www.memphis.edu/ausp/harl/). Software scoring also is available.

Client Oriented Scale of Improvement (COSI)

The COSI is probably the most commonly used *outcome* measure among clinicians. However, it is also very useful for formalizing the specific listening goals a patient has for hearing aids, which is why we've included it here as a pre-fitting assessment tool. As we discuss in this section, the specificity of these goals can be particularly important as we prioritize hearing aid features and consider hearing assistive technology (HAT). In addition, we have found that this scale also is useful for assessing expectations. Because it already is being used for outcome assessment, expectations easily can be assessed without introducing a new scale to the patient.

Background

One issue related to most all standardized self-assessment scales is that the item must be relevant for the

---

TECHNICAL TIP: CATEGORIZING COSI SITUATIONS

If the COSI will be used as an outcome measure, and the information is going to be quantified and analyzed according to each listening situation, then the listening category for each also should be recorded. On the bottom of the COSI form, there are 16 different general listening situations that can be used for this purpose. The item number is then placed in the category column on the form for each situation. This information is most useful when conducting research (or for some group analysis). If you're simply going to use the nominated items clinically, to assess expectations, benefit, and a guide for counseling, then this categorization isn't needed.

hearing aid user. Asking about understanding speech at church or at a noisy restaurant is not useful if the patient does not go to either. To some extent, scales have tried to account for this by adding shortened versions—the APHAB is a shortened version of the PHAB; the HHIE-S is a shortened version of the HHIE—or by having somewhat different scales for different groups (e.g., the HHIE and the HHIA). This somewhat reduces irrelevance, but not completely, as patients still often omit items. Stuart Gatehouse (1994) weighed in on this issue, and he suggested that when assessing unaided disability, we should consider such factors as how often the patient is in a given situation and how much trouble they have communicating in this situation. The COSI was designed to accomplish these goals, as well as eliminate irrelevancy. Furthermore, it allows patients to identify and rank order listening goals that are most important to them as an individual. For example, two patients may both have the goals of understanding speech in a noisy restaurant and understanding small children speaking. However, the importance of these two goals, and which one is most important, may be very different for the two patients.

The COSI was introduced in an article by Dillon, James, and Ginis in 1997. In short, the COSI allows patients to design their own questionnaires. The patients provide specific listening situations that are important for them. Making situations very specific is useful because it allows patients to easily remember and

pay attention to situations when asked about hearing outcomes. From a hearing aid selection and counseling standpoint, however, it can also be quite useful as demonstrated in the clinical example we present later. After providing three to five specific situations, they are then rank ordered for importance. Recall that the COSI was designed for measuring outcomes, but the rationale for relevancy and situation importance also applies to selection and expectation ratings. Dillon et al. (1997) cite four goals related to the development of the COSI: (1) acceptable reliability (test-retest stability), (2) acceptable validity (correlations to other scales believed to be valid), (3) convenient to use, and (4) capable of improving, as well as measuring, rehabilitation outcomes.

If you have worked with the COSI but never used it for measuring expectations, you might be curious regarding how benefit after hearing aid use compares with the patient's initial expectations. Palmer and Mueller (2000) provide some insight in this area in their study of 50 individuals (25 experienced users and 25 new users), who were fitted bilaterally with hearing aids as part of a larger study. Each subject completed a Patient Expectations Worksheet (PEW; a scale developed at the University of Pittsburgh that is very similar to the COSI) and listed five different communication situations where they would like to obtain improvement (a total of 250 items). Their expectations were obtained using the five-point scale of the COSI, in which they

---

THINGS TO REMEMBER: FROM GAS TO COSI

The COSI is based on experience that Dillon and colleagues had with an earlier self-assessment scale, the Goal Attainment Scaling (GAS; Dillon et al., 1991). At one time, the GAS was used throughout the many National Acoustic Laboratories (NAL) hearing centers. Like the COSI, the GAS had patients nominate situations in which they were experiencing difficulty in hearing and in which they would like to improve their ability to hear. Following this, the patients, working with the audiologist, established performance goals for each item with which they would be satisfied. The goals were negotiated with the audiologist to assure that they were realistic. Dillon et al. (1997) state that the GAS was replaced by the COSI in part because clinical audiologists did not like negotiating and quantifying goal levels, or quantifying the degree of difficulty experienced by the client when they first met the patient. The importance of establishing goals to aid in selection and counseling remains, however. Further, when using the COSI for expectation ratings, the audiologist may want to do a little *negotiating* with the patient, to assure that the patient does not leave the office with totally unrealistic expectations for a given listening situation.

identified the percent of time that they believed they would be successful in a given situation following the use of hearing aids: Hardly Ever, Occasionally, Half the Time, Most of the Time, or Almost Always. Following a month of hearing aid use, the subjects rated their benefit for each situation using the same rating scale.

The results from Palmer and Mueller (2000) are shown in Figure 6–9. Note that expectations were met for a large percentage of the items (slightly greater for the previous user group, who may have had more realistic expectations), and moreover, expectations were exceeded for approximately 20% of the items. If we combine the Met and Exceeded categories, we have about a 70% success rate for all the items. That research was conducted almost 15 years ago, so we might expect even better results with today's technology.

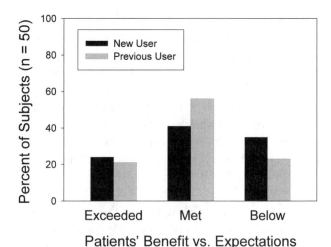

Figure 6–9. The degree that new and previous users exceeded, met, or fell below expectations when the COSI was used as a pre-fitting expectations tool.

Administration and Scoring

Unlike any other scale, the COSI starts off as a blank sheet. It is certainly possible that after seeing hundreds of patients, no two COSIs will look the same. The process begins by having the patient identify up to five specific listening situations in which he or she would like to hear better. It is important to stress these are *listening situations* and not necessarily just communication. For some patients, the listening goals may all focus on communication, but for other listeners (e.g., a patient with a severe hearing loss), the goal may be to better hear when someone knocks at the door. Some patients will happily list six or seven, but for other patients, it is a struggle to come up with three. We suggest having at least three whenever possible. We find some patients are simply not talkative and are somewhat unresponsive in the interview process. For these individuals, it may be more productive to administer a more closed set questionnaire such as the APHAB, HHIE, or another in lieu of the COSI.

It is important to make each item as specific as possible. "Hearing in background noise" would not be specific enough. After some questioning, this could be narrowed to, "Hearing my friends while playing cribbage at the bar at the Elk's club." Once one situation is identified, you then move on and establish other situations. After all situations have been identified, it is then helpful to go back, review all situations, and rank order them. Simply place a 1 for most important, 2 for the second most important, and so on in the box to the left of the item. Often, the item that the patient mentions first is something that just happened recently and is not the most important.

Shown in Figure 6–10 is the completed COSI form for a 68-year-old male patient with a moderate downward sloping bilateral hearing who was being fitted with his first set of hearing aids. With some prodding, he

THINGS TO REMEMBER: NUMBER OF COSI ITEMS

As discussed, we usually have the patient nominate as many as five COSI items. It is important to have the patient then rank order the items and, in particular, identify the two most important. Why is this? Research by Elaine Mormer and Catherine Palmer (2001) revealed that when people were asked again to nominate items two to three weeks later, 96% identified two of the same, but only 64% named three of the same. None of the individuals who initially listed four items named the same four items on retest. It appears that there probably is a recency bias for items of lesser importance, but at least two items remain constant.

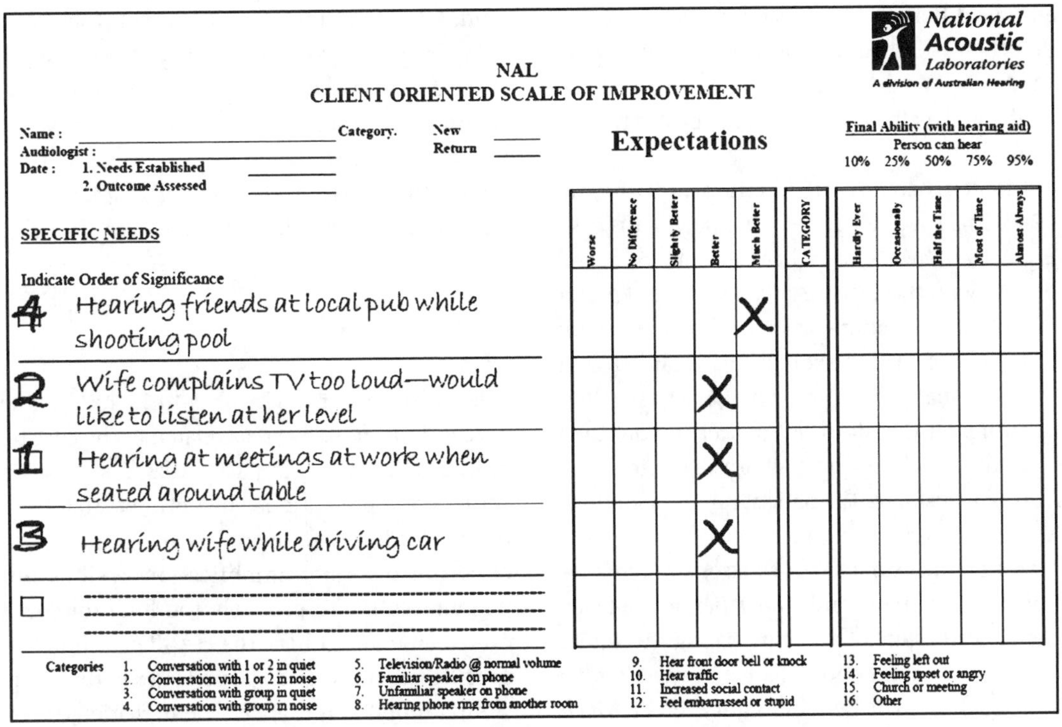

National Acoustic Laboratories
A division of Australian Hearing

NAL
CLIENT ORIENTED SCALE OF IMPROVEMENT

Name : ____ Category. New ____ Return ____
Audiologist : ____
Date : 1. Needs Established ____
2. Outcome Assessed ____

Expectations

Final Ability (with hearing aid)
Person can hear
10% 25% 50% 75% 95%

SPECIFIC NEEDS

Indicate Order of Significance

Specific needs	Worse	No Difference	Slightly Better	Better	Much Better	CATEGORY	Hardly Ever	Occasionally	Half the Time	Most of Time	Almost Always
4 Hearing friends at local pub while shooting pool					X						
2 Wife complains TV too loud—would like to listen at her level				X							
1 Hearing at meetings at work when seated around table				X							
3 Hearing wife while driving car				X							
☐											

Categories
1. Conversation with 1 or 2 in quiet
2. Conversation with 1 or 2 in noise
3. Conversation with group in quiet
4. Conversation with group in noise
5. Television/Radio @ normal volume
6. Familiar speaker on phone
7. Unfamiliar speaker on phone
8. Hearing phone ring from another room
9. Hear front door bell or knock
10. Hear traffic
11. Increased social contact
12. Feel embarrassed or stupid
13. Feeling left out
14. Feeling upset or angry
15. Church or meeting
16. Other

Figure 6–10. Completed pre-fitting COSI form showing the four nominated items by the patient, the patient's 1 to 4 ratings of the importance of these items, and the patient's expectations of how much benefit will be obtained when the patient starts using hearing aids ("X" markings in rating boxes). The "Expectations" heading is our modification of the standard COSI form.

TECHNICAL TIP: NOMINATING COSI ITEMS

As discussed, the items for the COSI are obtained by having a discussion with the patient, and having them nominate situations where they have problems and would like improvement. On occasion, a patient will seem to only focus on the most difficult situations, often situations where normal hearing individuals have difficulty. This can be a problem for three reasons: (1) These situations possibly are not really the most important, (2) These situations probably occur infrequently, and (3) It will be difficult to meet expectations as these are the very situations where we expect the least benefit from amplification. Often, a quick glance at the audiogram tells us that the patient must be having trouble in other listening situations—like hearing conversations involving soft speech—even though the patient is not mentioning this. One way to *calibrate* the nomination process is to have the patient account for time. You might say: "Bob, you have named four different situations involving listening in background noise. In any given week (month), about how much time do you spend in these situations?" It is not unusual for Bob to answer, after some thought, that it is only four hours per week. Your next question then is: "So Bob, what do you do the other 96% of your waking hours?" This may uncover some other real, and perhaps even more important, listening situations where Bob has difficulty.

nominated four different items, listed in the order that he provided them (he had just been out playing pool the night before). We then went back and prioritized the items, reflected by the numbers in the box to the left of each item.

Once the items are identified and prioritized, we normally then make a photocopy of the page. This is so we will have a clean sheet to use when he comes back and rates his benefit with the hearing aids—we would prefer that he not see his expectations when he does the benefit rating—this is different from comparing unaided with aided, where we usually *do* want the patients to see their pre-fitting ratings. If that does not matter to you, then you have saved some time and you are ready to move ahead. We usually just have the patient rate expectations for the Degree of Change section.

Observe that this patient's expectations were *Better* for three of the four items and *Much Better* for hearing his friends at the pub. The *Better* ratings are quite reasonable, and we have a good chance of meeting his expectations for these. The benefit might even be *Much Better* for the TV listening situation. His expectations for the pub, however, are a little concerning. We have been to the Blarney Stone; it has a cement floor and exposed brick walls, and the evening noise levels are nearly always 80 dBA or greater. If you look back at our discussion of communication in background noise in Chapter 3, you see that with this noise level it is unlikely to experience a positive SNR for an average conversation. This patient's QuickSIN score was 6 dB SNR loss. This expectation, therefore, is something we will want to talk to him about before he leaves the office with his new hearing aids. It may also lead us to discuss additional assistive technology that may allow him to communicate in this situation.

Obtaining the COSI

See Appendix AI. The form for the COSI can be downloaded (http://www.nal.gov.au/pdf/COSI-Question naire.pdf).

Hearing Aid Selection Profile (HASP)

The Three-Clinic HASP was developed by researchers (clinicians) at the Henry Ford Hospital in Detroit, Michigan; the Cleveland Clinic Foundation in Cleve-

land, Ohio; and the Mayo Clinic in Rochester, Minnesota (Jacobson, Newman, Fabry, & Sandridge, 2001).[39] Although many pre-fitting scales focus directly on communication problems and the effects of having a hearing loss, we know that there also are many *non-auditory* factors that can impact the benefit from and satisfaction with hearing aids. That's what the HASP is all about.

Background

The purpose of the HASP, is to include patients' self-perceptions in many areas related to the core beliefs and attitudes that might impact the successful selection and fitting of amplification. The notion is that the results of the HASP improve overall hearing aid satisfaction by choosing the right amplification options for a given patient. Although probably too long for routine clinical use in many clinics, the HASP has clinical utility for specific situations as discussed later in this chapter. For a similar tool that is more efficient, readers are referred to the COAT, which is described in the next section.

The HASP is a 40-item self-report measure containing eight subscales, each consisting of five items. The response format is a five-point Likert scale with anchors of *Strongly Agree* and *Strongly Disagree* yielding a maximum score of 20 points per subscale. The following is adapted from the Sandridge and Newman (2006) review regarding the construction of the HASP:

Three of the eight subscales address issues directly related to hearing aids:

- Motivation to wear hearing aids (e.g., "I want to wear a hearing aid even if I have difficulty in some situations.")
- Expectations regarding hearing aid performance (e.g., "A hearing aid will restore my hearing to normal just as eyeglasses restore vision to normal.")
- General communication needs (e.g., "It is very important for me to hear conversations when I am in a larger group, for example at a party.")

The remaining five subscales contain items that assess a patient's perceptions and attitudes about issues not directly related to the use of hearing aids:

- Importance of physical appearance to others (e.g., "There is nothing wrong with using

plastic surgery to improve one's appearance.";
this subscale is reversed scored.)

■ Attitude toward cost of commercial goods and
services (e.g., "I don't think that I need the
best money can buy."; this subscale is reversed
scored.)

■ Attitude toward technology (e.g., "I feel that
new technology has improved our lives.")

■ Physical functioning and manual dexterity
(e.g., "It is easy for me to use small objects
such as paper clips, coins, small buttons, and/
or zippers.")

■ Lifestyle (e.g., "I consider myself to be an
active, busy, on-the-go kind of person.")

In the original research with the HASP, there were
some preliminary observations about the effect that
subject characteristics had on subscale scores. These
factors are reviewed by Jacobson et al. (2001) and Jacobson, Newman, Sandridge, and McCaslin (2002):

■ Elderly patients tended to be less comfortable
with high technology (Technology), had more
physical constraints (Physical Function), and
fewer communicative needs (Communicative
Needs) than younger patients.

■ Men tended to be less motivated (Motivation),
less comfortable with high technology
(Technology), had reduced expectations
(Expectations), had fewer communicative
needs (Communicative Needs), and were
more appearance-conscious (Appearance)
than women.

■ Patients who were previous hearing aid
users tended to be more highly motivated
(Motivation) than patients who had not worn
hearing aids previously.

■ Individuals with less formal education
tended to have more physical constraints
(Physical Function) and a less active lifestyle
(Lifestyle).

■ Self-perceived hearing handicap affected
scores on the Motivation and Communicative
Needs subscales. Patients who had greater
self-perceived hearing handicap were more
highly motivated to obtain hearing aids
and had greater communicative needs than
patients with lesser amounts of self-perceived
hearing handicap.

Jacobson et al. (2002) used the HASP to retrospectively study the characteristics of individuals who
rejected hearing aid use and returned their hearing aids
for credit. There were three significant findings:

■ The return-for-credit group fell at the 20th
percentile for the Motivation subscale.

■ The return-for-credit group demonstrated
greater problems with manual dexterity,
scoring between the 20th and 50th percentile
for the Physical Functioning subscale.

■ The return-for-credit group also had reduced
listening needs, where scores also fell
between the 20th and 50th percentile for the
Communicative Needs subscale.

Administration and Scoring

Like many other pre-fitting tests, the HASP usually is
administered (paper and pencil test) before discussing
the use of hearing aids with the patient (see Appendix
AJ and AK). As mentioned, there are 40 total items on
the HASP, and each item is answered on a five-point
scale ranging from Strongly Agree (4 points) to Strongly
Disagree (0 points). There are eight subscales with five
questions per scale; therefore, the total potential score
for each scale is 20 points. The questions for each subscale are randomized within the questionnaire, with an
identifying letter by the number of the question to sig-
nify the subscale. Table 6–2 is an example of how the
scoring would work for the five questions of the Motivation subscale. If you total the points for the five questions (far right column), we see that this patient has a
score of 15 for this subscale. A simple pencil and paper
score sheet like that in Table 6–2 easily could be used for
each subscale. We recommend, however, using the Excel
spreadsheet that is available through www.audiologyon-
line.com (see specifics at the end of this section).

Once the score for a given subscale has been determined, you would then compare this score with the
HASP norms. These are shown in Figure 6–11, along
with all the subscale scores for our patient (see open
circles). Notice that the subscale score we calculated
in Table 6–2 (15 points), places this patient exactly at
the 50th percentile for Motivation. For clinical use, you
could have a copy of these norms printed, and then each
subscale score could be marked by hand on this chart.
However, as mentioned earlier, we would recommend

Table 6–2. Sample of Questions and Scoring for the Motivation Subscale of the HASP

Q#	Question	Answer	Points
16	I want to wear a hearing aid even if I still have difficulty hearing is some situations.	Neutral	2
20	I know that a hearing aid will help me.	Agree	3
29	I am prepared to do what it takes to improve my hearing.	Strongly Agree	4
34	I am certain that I want a hearing aid	Agree	3
35	I am having a significant problem understanding speech.	Agree	3

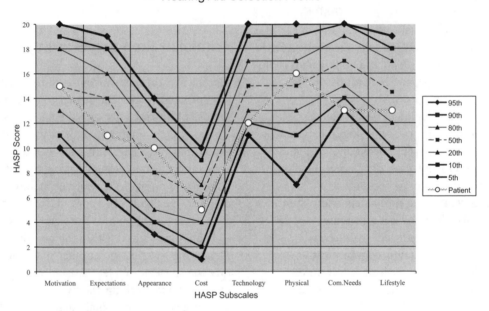

Figure 6–11. HASP norms (5th to 95th percentile) for the eight subscales. The white circles represent performance for a given individual.

the use of a spreadsheet and electronic graphing and printing for efficient clinical use.

It is important to point out that the Appearance and Cost subscales are *reversed scored*. That is, the total points from the five subscale questions are *subtracted* from 20—the questions are worded so that Strongly Disagree is the answer most consistent with good hearing aid candidacy. This way, greater diversions from the 0 baseline will always have positive connotations regarding hearing aid candidacy for all eight subscales.

Clinical Application

In general, the HASP was designed to provide the audiologist with a wide range of information that could be useful in the hearing aid selection process. As obvious from the names of the subscales, this could involve such things as listening needs, dexterity problems, concern with cost of the instruments, or cosmetics issues. Certainly, some of these factors could impact on the selection of hearing aid style or special hearing aid features.

The results of the HASP also could be used as a predictor of who is at risk for unsuccessful use of hearing aids. For example, we know from the research of Jacobson et al. (2002) that people who returned their hearing aids for credit tend to have below average HASP subscale scores for Motivation, Physical (hand and finger dexterity), and Communication Needs. If this is known before the patient leaves with the hearing aids, counseling can be focused on these areas, and the patient can be targeted for more attention during the first few weeks of hearing aid use. In general, most all subscale scores that fall significantly below the 50th percentile need to be addressed.

In addition to targeting patient counseling, Jacobson et al. (2001) also suggest some other applications of the HASP:

- Audiologist accountability: At present, hearing aids are available with a wide range of features and at various price points. Often, the audiologist's recommendation for a specific set of features or model is haphazard and based on little data. There usually is no objective information to support the fitting decision. The HASP would help identify patients who were interested in the latest technology or price conscious, or concerned about cosmetics—all of which could assist in the selection of the hearing aid model and features.
- Hearing aid selection guide: Jacobson et al. (2001) suggest that the findings of their factor

analysis could possibly be used to develop an *expert clinician* algorithm that could generate, based upon results of audiometry and the HASP, a pool of best hearing aid fittings. This could be especially useful for individuals just beginning to dispense hearing aids.

- Quality improvement projects: If your practice involves more than one practice or more than one site, the HASP could be used to determine if there are differences in the perceptions of patients seen at the different locations. For example, if the HASP scores from one site showed that the patients had significantly reduced score for Physical, this might explain why this clinic had a higher return-for-credit rate. Taking this one step further, average HASP scores could be compiled for the patients of each staff audiologist. This would help answer the often-asked question "Why do I always have to see the tough patients?"

Let us return to Figure 6–11 and discuss how we might use this person's HASP scores in counseling or hearing aid selection. One way to approach it is to ask, how is this patient different from average (deviation from the 50th percentile)? That is, how will you differ from your average counseling and average selection procedure? Note that for Motivation, Expectations, Cost, and Physical, the patient is fairly close to the 50th percentile. The patient is somewhat less than average regarding concerns about appearance—this is good, as

---

POINTS TO PONDER: THE HASP AND EXPECTATIONS

The authors of the HASP state that scoring is designed so that "greater diversions from baseline have positive connotations." This is why the Appearance and Cost subscales are reversed scored (e.g., we usually would prefer that a patient was *not* concerned about either, and on the HASP, this person will have a *high* score). But what about expectations? Do you want your patient's expectations to be high or low? One HASP question is: "A hearing aid will make it possible for me to understand speech in all situations." How would you like your next hearing aid patient to answer that? If he or she answers Strongly Agree to this and other similar HASP questions, they will have a high Expectations score. So, big HASP subscale scores may not always be good. The point is that it is important to look at the individual's HASP score for each subscale, compare it with the average patient's score, and conduct counseling accordingly.

it allows you to offer a wide range of styles. The patient is at the 10th percentile for technology, significantly below average. This suggests that simple might be better. This probably is not someone who will be comfortable with five memories, a remote control for training the hearing aid, and extensive wireless connections. The Communication Needs are minimal (5th percentile), which agrees with the patient's lower Lifestyle scores. As these pieces fall together, it is much easier to determine the best fitting options.

Obtaining the HASP

The HASP questionnaire along with the normative template is in Appendix AJ and AK. The form and the Excel spreadsheet for scoring and graphing are available at http://www.audiologyonline.com (askexpert/display_question.asp?question_id=815).

Characteristics of Amplification Tool (COAT)

The COAT is a pre-fitting test that was developed by two of the four developers of the HASP, Sharon Sandridge and Craig Newman of the Cleveland Clinic. These authors recognized the documented psychometric adequacy and clinical usefulness of the HASP; however, they mention that it is not the most time-efficient tool, limiting its application in a busy clinical practice. For this reason, they developed a new tool, the COAT.

Background

For time efficiency, the COAT can be more or less used as a replacement for the HASP. It is based on the following criteria (Sandridge & Newman, 2006):

- Similar constructs to the HASP
- Short in length so that it could be completed in 10 minutes or less
- Easy to administer and interpret
- Ability to obtain the critical nonaudiologic information useful in determining the style and level of technology required by the patient
- Function as a basis for counseling during the hearing aid selection process
- Serve as a measure for clinician accountability in this era of evidence-based practice
- Useful as a teaching tool for student externs

The COAT consists of nine items. Sandridge and Newman describe the rationale for including each item (Sandridge & Newman, 2006):

Item 1: Please list the top three situations where you would most like to hear better. This item is similar to the COSI. When patients are allowed to indicate specific areas of desired improvement, they play a more active role in the fitting process and in selecting the hearing aids that will meet their individual needs.

Item 2: How important is it for you to hear better? This item assesses the patient's global priority of hearing. For example, the retired individual whose primary activity is reading may not place as much importance on hearing as the individual involved in a variety of social activities.

Item 3: How motivated are you to wear and use hearing aids? A patient without motivation to use hearing aids sets the stage for failure; therefore, it is critical to assess motivation levels.

Item 4: How well do you think hearing aids will improve your hearing? Unrealistically high or low expectations regarding the use of hearing aids may lead to poor outcomes. Unrealistic expectations can result in decreased satisfaction with or complete rejection of the devices.

Item 5: What is your most important consideration regarding hearing aids? Four important considerations when selecting hearing aids are ranked, ordered by the patient. These include:

- Cosmetics (hearing aid size and the ability of others not to see the hearing aids)
- Audibility of speech (improved ability to hear and understand speech)

- Listening in background noise (improved ability to understand speech in noisy situations such as restaurants/parties)
- Finance (cost of the hearing aids)

Item 6: Do you prefer hearing aids that: are totally automatic, allow you to adjust the volume and change listening programs, or no preference? This question provides insight into the patient's locus of control regarding hearing aid functionality.

Item 7: Indicate which hearing aid style(s) you would not *be willing to use.* Pictures illustrating six styles of hearing aids are displayed. The six styles include: traditional BTE, mini BTE with open ear tubing, full-shell ITE, half-shell ITE, ITC, and CIC. The patient is asked to indicate which style(s) of hearing aids is *not* acceptable.

Item 8: How confident are you that you will be a successful hearing aid user? The degree of self-efficacy (i.e., domain-specific belief that one can successfully complete a task) can be a predictor of successful hearing aid use. If a patient indicates low self-efficacy (i.e., lack of confidence), the audiologist can explore what concerns the patient has regarding hearing aid use.

Item 9: Select the cost category that represents the maximum amount you are willing to spend. This last item focuses on the patient's willingness to pay, guiding the clinician to select a level of technology consistent with the patient's desired financial investment.

Clinical Application

The items on the COAT cover a large range of pre-fitting areas including patient-specific listening needs, motivation, expectations, financial concerns, and cosmetics. The audiologist can easily use this form to focus on areas that need to be discussed or use the response to narrow the pool of products that are appropriate.

In the 2006 original article describing the COAT, authors Sandridge and Newman present a case study, which nicely describes how the COAT can be used clinically to assist in the hearing aid selection:

Case study is a 59-year-old male who is being seen for a Hearing Needs Assessment appointment. His audiometric results indicate a mild-to-moderate sensorineural hearing loss, bilaterally. Upon review of his responses on the COAT, the following is noted:

- Wants to hear his customers in restaurants, his grandchildren at family gatherings, and coworkers at company social functions (Item 1).
- Hearing better is very important to him (Item 2); he is very motivated to use hearing aids (Item 3); and he expects that they will greatly improve his hearing (Item 4).
- Rates hearing aid size as the most important consideration followed by cost, understanding in background noise, and improved ability to hear speech (Item 5).
- Prefers hearing aids that are automatic (Item 6).
- Unwilling to use any style of hearing aids except CICs (Item 7).
- Indicates high level of confidence for successful hearing aid use (Item 8).
- Did not complete the cost item (Item 9).

Combining all factors (age, hearing loss, responses on the COAT), a mini-BTE would be recommended with open ear fitting. He is initially uncomfortable with this recommendation because of the cosmetics. The advantages and disadvantages of an open-ear fitting over the CIC are discussed, and he agrees to try the recommended style of device. The level of technology is discussed. He needs devices that have multiple microphone (directional) technology and noise-reduction processing to provide him better hearing in restaurants and social events. This increases the level of technology needed and hence the device cost. He is not willing to commit to the recommended level of technology. Lower-end devices are chosen with the understanding that his hearing in background noise may be compromised to a certain degree. He understands that and wishes to proceed with the devices that fall within his budget.

Obtaining the COAT

See Appendix AL. The COAT is available for general use and the form can be downloaded from a link contained in the original 2006 COAT publication at http://www.audiologyonline.com/articles/article_detail .asp?article_id=1541.

Profile of Aided Loudness (PAL)

The PAL was introduced by Mueller and Palmer (1998), with administration and scoring details provided the following year (Palmer, Mueller, & Moriarty, 1999). Additional data for test interpretation (loudness rating distributions for test items for normal hearing individuals) were provided in 2000 by Palmer and Mueller.

Background

As discussed, there are many goals involved in the overall fitting. A primary one of course is improvement of speech understanding, which relates to the questions asked on inventories such as the APHAB. Another goal of the fitting, at least for mild-to-moderate hearing losses, is appropriate loudness perceptions for everyday sounds. That is, after the fitting of hearing aids, we would expect that the patient would now judge the loudness of speech, noise, and environmental sounds similarly to listeners with normal hearing. This is one of the underlying concepts behind the use of wide dynamic range compression (e.g., to make soft sounds audible, average sounds comfortable, and loud sounds loud but not too loud). The PAL was designed as an outcome measure to determine if this fitting goal had been accomplished. There are several reasons, however, to also use this scale during the pre-fitting process.

The selection of the 12 items on the final version of the PAL began with a list of 95 sounds that new hearing aid users had reported hearing during their first few weeks of hearing aid use. Normal hearing subjects between the ages of 20 and 65 rated the loudness of each sound based on the seven-point loudness scale of the Cox Contour Test (see Chapter 4). It is important to note that this was not a laboratory measure, but rather each subject rated the loudness as they remembered hearing it. The 95 items were reduced to the current 12 items using the following criteria:[40]

■ Items were consistently rated the same: Items that did not have a test-retest 0.7 or greater

Pearson correlation coefficient and had a two-tailed *p* value of >0.05 were not included.
■ Items were rated the same across age groups: Items that did not have the same ratings across age groups were eliminated.
■ Items had clustered loudness ratings: Items that did not have ratings clustered around three loudness categories were eliminated.
■ Items met desired ratings: The loudness ratings for the final items needed to cluster around targets of either #2 (soft), #4 (average), or #6 (loud), with an equal number of items for each category.
■ Items experienced by the majority of hearing aid users: A small subset was administered to hearing aid users, and the final 12 items were based on: (1) an acceptable test-retest, and (2) that the item was experienced by most hearing aid users.

The 12 items of the PAL include four items relating to soft sounds (target is a #2 rating), four items for average (target is a #4 rating), and four items for loud (target is a #6 rating). Because of the rigid criteria used for item selection, it is possible that your patient may have a poor memory of the loudness of some of the items (e.g., it is not common to routinely encounter a marching band, which is one of the items).

In addition to the loudness categories, there also are satisfaction ratings for each item ranging from #5 (best) to #1 (worse). There are not norms *per se* for satisfaction, although when it is used as an outcome measure, any satisfaction rating below a #3 (okay) needs to be discussed. The highest satisfaction rating of #5 is not necessarily good (for the patient). For example, a patient could rate Your Own Breathing as a #0 (cannot hear; desired rating is #2) on the loudness scale, yet rate this as #5 (just right) for satisfaction.

Administration and Scoring

The PAL is a scale administered by paper and pencil and can be conducted in the waiting room prior to the clinic visit, or it could be mailed to the patient. Some audiologists administer it *knee-to-knee* by reading the questions to the patient. The 12 items from the three different loudness categories are randomized on the form (i.e., the four items with a normative rating of #2 do not follow each other). The instructions are as follows:

Please rate the following items by both the level of loudness of the sound and by the appropriateness of that loudness level. For example, you might rate a particular sound a #1 (Very Soft). If Very Soft is your preferred level for this sound, then you would rate your loudness satisfaction as Just Right. If on the other hand, you think the sound should be louder than Very Soft, then your loudness satisfaction rating might be #2 (Not Too Good) or even #1 (Not Good At All). The loudness satisfaction rating is not related to how pleasing the sound is to you, but rather, the appropriateness of the loudness. Here is an example:

Sample Item: The hum of a refrigerator motor:

Loudness Rating	Satisfaction Rating
0. Do Not Hear	5. Just Right
1. Very Soft	4. Pretty Good
2. Soft	3. Okay
3. Comfortable, But Slightly Soft	2. Not Too Good
4. Comfortable	1. Not Good At All
5. Comfortable, But Slightly Loud	
6. Loud, But Okay	
7. Uncomfortably Loud	

In this example, the patient rated the loudness level of a refrigerator motor running as Comfortable, But Slightly Soft and rated his loudness satisfaction for this sound as Just Right. This satisfaction rating indicates that the patient believes that it is appropriate for a refrigerator motor to sound Comfortable, But Slightly Soft.

It is also important to inform the patient that it is okay to skip an item if it is simply not something the patient recalls hearing and, consequently, does not have a loudness perception.

Once the patient has completed the inventory, scoring is quite straight forward. Using the form shown in Figure 6–12, enter the patient's loudness and satisfaction ratings for each of the 12 items and then calculate an

PATIENT SUMMARY
Profile of Aided Loudness (PAL)
Unaided Performance

Soft sounds	Q3	Q4	Q5	Q8	Category average
Loudness	1	1	1	1	1.0 (target = 2)
Satisfaction	5	5	3	3	4.0

Average sounds	Q1	Q6	Q7	Q12	Category average
Loudness	3	2	2	3	2.5 (target = 4)
Satisfaction	4	1	3	3	2.7

Loud sounds	Q2	Q9	Q10	Q11	Category average
Loudness	5	6	5	6	5.5 (target = 6)
Satisfaction	4	5	3	3	3.7

Figure 6–12. Example of patient scoring for the PAL. Ratings are obtained for loudness perceptions (1–7) and satisfaction with the perceptions (1–5) for 12 environmental sounds.

average of the four. The example shown in Figure 6–12 is for a patient with a mild-to-moderate downward sloping hearing loss. Observe that this patient is rating soft sounds somewhat below norms (1.0), but the satisfaction rating is quite good (4.0). The loudness ratings for average are considerably below those of normal hearing individuals (2.5; 4.0 is target rating), and satisfaction also is poor. Ratings for loud sounds and satisfaction are okay.

In some cases, it might be useful to go into more detail regarding the patient's judgments. The distribution table shown in Figure 6–13 can be helpful. These are the data from the original normal hearing subjects used in the development of the PAL. The vertical bars displayed for each item represent the percent of subjects that gave that specific loudness rating (e.g., about 75% of individuals consider a marching band to be Loud, But Okay). This table is especially useful for counseling the patient when the PAL is used as an outcome measure but also is helpful during pre-fitting. For scoring, we usually just put an "X" for the patient's rating for a given item. It easily can then be visualized what type of amplification needs are present. For example, note that this patient rated the loudness of a religious leader during the sermon as #2 (Soft). The majority of people with

Normative data for PAL

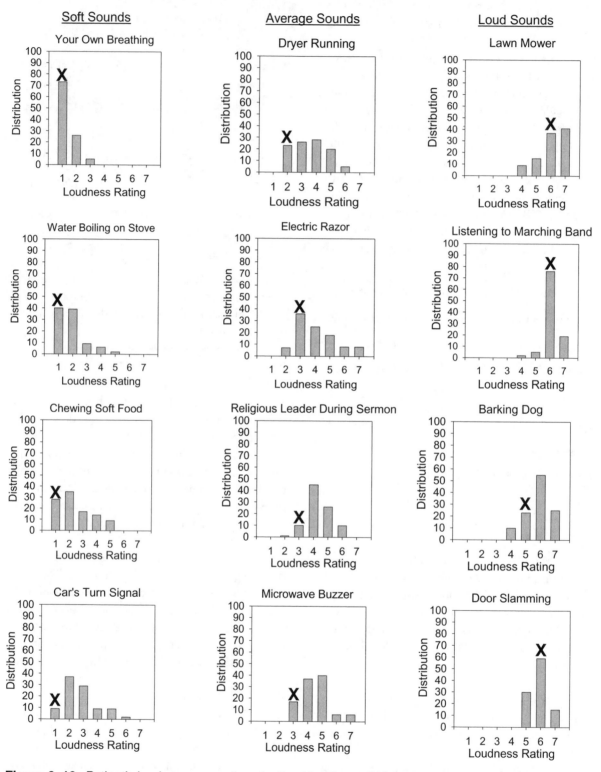

Figure 6–13. Patient's loudness perceptions for the 12 different PAL items are plotted ("X" markings) on the normative distribution scale for each item.

THINGS TO REMEMBER: THE ENVIRONMENTAL SOUNDS QUESTIONNAIRE, A COUSIN OF THE PAL

In several studies of a hearing aid signal processing scheme termed ADRO (for adaptive dynamic range optimization), Peter Blamey and colleagues used a modification of the PAL inventory to obtain loudness ratings and satisfaction (see Blamey and Martin [2009], for review). Their self-assessment scale is the Environmental Sounds Questionnaire (ESQ). The ESQ utilizes the same loudness and satisfaction scaling as the PAL and includes 9 of the 12 PAL items. Nine additional items were added for an ESQ total of 18. It is interesting to note that several of the nine new items of the ESQ were included in the original PAL research but were not included in the final version as they did not meet the selection criteria.

The items from the PAL that were deleted for the ESQ were:

- The dryer running
- The religious leader during a sermon
- Listening to a marching band

The nine items added to the ESQ were:

- Traveling in a car with the windows closed
- Traffic noise when standing on the curb of a busy road
- Washing machine
- Running water, such as a toilet or a shower
- A motorbike passing by
- Vacuum cleaner
- Telephone ringing close by
- Refrigerator motor
- Birds twittering

---

normal hearing, however, rate this item a #4 or #5, and only 2 to 3% rate it the same as this patient. This chart is included in Appendix AN.

Clinical Applications

When the PAL is used as a pre-fitting measure, the primary utility is to quickly observe where loudness perceptions need to be changed and to determine the patient's satisfaction for their current loudness perceptions. Although the case could be made that the PAL is a useful scale for *all* patients, we have found it is most useful for new hearing aid users—especially those who believe that with hearing aids, they will be hearing things that no one else hears, or that that all environmental noises will be way too loud. This of course is not always easy to predict prior to the actual fitting. However, when these comments are immediately made on the day of the fitting, it is not too late to administer the PAL before the patient leaves the office.

Using the charts shown in Figure 6–13, the patient can be counseled regarding how they differ from people with normal hearing. The PAL findings might also serve as a warning of potential problems down the road. If all the items that typically are rated #5 or #6, are rated #7, it may be important to assure that little or no hearing aid gain is provided for inputs of this intensity range.

One of the most important reasons for using the PAL as a pre-fitting measure is to establish a baseline

---

TECHNICAL TIP: HOW GOOD IS TOO GOOD?

When using the PAL for pre-fitting testing, one possible outcome is that a potential hearing aid candidate (based on pure-tone threshold results) will have the same loudness ratings as someone with normal hearing and will have high satisfaction scores. This begs the question: Does this person then need hearing aids? If loudness perceptions are normal, why are they in the office? These finding do occur occasionally, and usually it is because of one of two reasons. First, the patient may have normal hearing in the low frequencies. These patients often have relatively normal loudness perceptions yet have significant problems with speech understanding, which is why you would not interpret the PAL results in isolation—what are the patient's QuickSIN or unaided APHAB scores?

Another reason why some patients present with a significant hearing loss but normal unaided PAL scores is that the PAL questions do not specifically address what they perceive as their problem, and maybe they do not think about the questions carefully enough. We are reminded of a recent patient whose primary reason for obtaining hearing aids was so she could hear her young grandchildren, who she reported spoke softly. Yet, her ratings for the four Soft questions on the PAL revealed a rating similar to that of someone with normal hearing (mean of 1.7). The COSI will help you identify these patients.

In general, the PAL is not a good measure to determine who should be fitted with hearing aids. There probably is not any single measure that is. The downside of course, for someone who provides normal ratings for the pre-fitting PAL, is that there is no room for improvement *after* the fitting of hearing aids. The PAL still can be used as an outcome measure, however, to assure that the fitting did not make things worse.

KEY CONCEPT: THE PAL AND THE APHAB

The reason to conduct a battery of pre-fitting tests is to collect new information with each measure. There is some overlap, however. If you conduct both the PAL and the APHAB, for example, we would expect to see agreement between the PAL ratings for the four Loud, But Okay questions and the APHAB subscale score for aversiveness. This is something that you will also want to compare when you use these scales as outcome measures. If the results from these scales indicated the patient had a low tolerance for louder sounds, you might take a look at your pre-fitting LDL and ANL findings (see Chapters 4 and 5). Same patient, same ears, and same brains used for all testing—things should (and usually do) fit into a predictable pattern.

---

for which *aided* PAL responses can be compared. Once your patients start using hearing aids, it is a bit risky to then have them go back and rate how they heard when they were unaided. They may find that what they once thought was comfortable was really soft.

Obtaining the PAL

The PAL is not copyrighted. We suggest you simply use the forms in Appendix AM and AO. There is not a computerized version or scoring system for this scale.

In Closing

We have reviewed several different self-assessment scales, all of which measure somewhat different aspects regarding the potential use of hearing aids. We recognize that it is not feasible, or probably even necessary, to conduct all of them for a single patient; you will need to develop a battery that works the best for your situation, or different batteries for different patients.

And how many scales really are enough? In part, that depends on what we want to measure, how well we want to do it, and how much time we are willing to invest? New pre-fitting scales continue to be introduced; the most recent is the Screening Test for Hearing Problems (STHP; Demorest, Wark, & Erdman, 2011). The STHP is 20-item scale modeled after the Communication Profile for the Hearing Impaired (CPHI), which is a lengthy 163-item instrument yielding 25 scale scores. The authors caution, however, that the STHP should not be thought of as simply a shortened version of the CPHI. A major difference is while the patient answers each item on a five-point scale like the CPHI, each item is scored pass or fail. The STHP has two subscales, Communication and Adjustment Problems, and each subscale also is scored pass or fail. Because the Communication and Adjustment Problems are relatively independent, Demorest et al. (2011) emphasize the need to screen for both, and the patient must pass both to pass the STHP. For example, in their sample, 87 participants fell in the bottom quartile on Communication only, 79 fell in the bottom quartile on Adjustment only, and only 29 fell in the bottom quartile on both factors. Although the STHP is somewhat similar to other pre-fitting self-assessment inventories we have discussed (e.g., APHAB, HHIE), does it provide *new* information? Maybe. More valid and reliable information? Maybe. We have included this new scale in Appendix AP. Try it out!

The most important take-home point from this chapter is that there are many aspects of a patient's communication needs that cannot be predicted by routine audiometric measures. It is important to allow the patient to tell his or her story, and one effective way to do this is through the use of pre-fitting self-assessment scales.

7

Hearing Aid Styles and Fitting Applications

To this point, we have discussed the general attributes of the hearing aid candidate, the importance of speech information and how it interacts with the environment, several objective tests that we can use to assess the candidates ability to process speech, and additional tests to refine our fitting. We have also reviewed the self-assessment scales that further define the patient's problems and listening needs, and also provide insight regarding the patient's handicap, motivation, and expectations. We are now ready to sit down with the patient and start making collaborative decisions. The first of these is selecting the best hearing aid style. Although the signal processing of the hearing aid is often of utmost concern, packaging this processing in an unacceptable style can lead to rejection of amplification.

Although the most obvious differences in hearing aid styles are cosmetic (size and shape), it is important to understand that style choices also impact hearing aid acoustics, comfort, and ease of use. There are several benefits and limitations that are tied to hearing aid style that are unrelated to cosmetics. It often is the audiologist's job to strike a reasonable balance between *form* and *function*. We start by considering the look and physical characteristics of different hearing aids styles. Then, we continue by discussing bilateral versus unilateral fittings, and reviewing fittings aimed at specific special populations and applications.

Despite differences in style, hearing aids share several commonalities. At their most basic levels, all hearing aids include three stages that can be generally described as shown in Figure 7–1.

- The sound pick-up stage usually consists of a microphone or telecoil.
- The sound processing and amplification stage is where the bulk of the signal processing

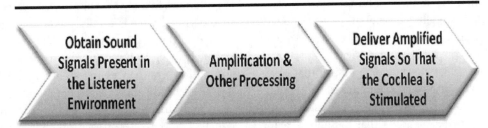

Figure 7–1. Three general stages of a hearing aid.

work is done to change the signal into the desired level and form.

■ The sound delivery stage is primarily made up of a tiny loudspeaker (along with supporting processing) referred to as a receiver. Instead of a receiver, the output stage may include a vibrating oscillator that stimulates the cochlea through bone conduction or a variety of other specialized transducers including those associated with middle ear implants.

Although there may be multiple goals, the primary function of the electronic components and sound processing is to work together to increase the level of sounds in a frequency specific manner. The frequency specific increase in sound level for a signal at the output of a hearing aid in comparison with the sound level at the input is referred to as gain. Gain is really just the opposite of attenuation (a frequency specific level decrease, commonly expressed in dB). In fact, gain can be thought of as negative attenuation, whereas attenuation can be thought of as negative gain. This is an important concept to understand because some styles of hearing aids seal into the ear canal very well, and although they provide positive gain for a wide range of frequencies, negative gain (attenuation) may also occur in some frequency regions—more on that later in this chapter.

Unilateral Versus Bilateral Amplification

At some point in the hearing aid selection process, a joint decision must be made between the clinician and the patient regarding whether one or two hearing aids will be fitted. This sometimes is dictated by the audiogram (hearing in one ear is either too good or too bad for hearing aid use), but the majority of patients (e.g., 85 to 90%) are potential candidates for bilateral amplification. Although the intuitive notion that two ears are better than one is usually true, not all patients benefit from bilateral amplification, and not all patients who do benefit want to wear two hearing aids.

It might be surprising to some of you that bilateral fittings have not always been embraced by audiologists. As recent as the early 1970s, it was common for audiologists to tell patients that a single hearing aid was adequate, and in some cases, when the patient returned from a dispenser (hearing instrument specialist) wearing two hearing aids, the audiologist accused the dispenser of simply trying to double the profit. Contributing to the *unilateral-is-okay* belief was a 1975 ruling by the Federal Trade Commission regarding the hearing aid industry, which stated:

No seller shall prepare, approve, fund, disseminate, or cause the dissemination of any advertisement which makes any representation that the use of two hearing aids, one in each ear, will be beneficial to persons with a hearing loss in both ears, unless it is clearly and conspicuously disclosed that many persons with a hearing loss in both ears will not receive greater benefits from the use of two aids, one in each ear, than the use of one hearing aid.

The importance for children to be fitted bilaterally, however, was beginning to be widely accepted about this time, and the general understanding of bilateral fittings then gradually transferred to adults. This move to consider bilateral the *routine* fitting probably was also fueled by the large number of audiologists who began direct dispensing in the late 1970s (see Chapter 1 for details). It was not until the 1990s, however, that the majority of people in the United States were fitted bilaterally. Currently based on MarkeTrak data, about 75% of the U.S. fittings are bilateral (slightly less for first-time users), and about 90% of those with bilateral hearing loss are fitted bilaterally. This of course does not mean that they are using two hearing aids, or even using *one* hearing aid.

Potential Advantages of Bilateral Amplification

There are several benefits of *binaural hearing*, and many of these benefits will be experienced with *bilateral fittings*. These benefits are assuming that you have selected an individual who is a reasonable bilateral candidate from an audiometric standpoint. That is, there must be aidable hearing in both ears, adequate speech recognition and central processing ability, and not too much asymmetry. How much is too much asymmetry? A rule of thumb is that we would like to have the *aided* speech signals within 15 dB of each other (see our Technical Tip on this topic). We would expect the greatest bilateral

---

KEY CONCEPT: BILATERAL VERSUS BINAURAL

You may have noticed that in our discussion here and in other chapters that both the words bilateral and binaural have been used in reference to hearing with two ears. There is an important difference, however, between these two terms. When we refer to the auditory system, we use terms binaural hearing and monaural hearing. The concepts of binaural hearing, and the related advantages, are mostly based on research with normal hearing individuals. When we are talking about hearing aids, we use the terms bilateral fittings and unilateral fittings. For example, if you presented the same speech signal to both ears (referred to as a diotic presentation), your patient would have *bilateral* processing, but not the same phase and amplitude differences observed in *binaural* processing. In general, you can presume a *bilateral fitting* improves *binaural hearing*, but this is not always the case, which is why we have this differentiation.

KEY CONCEPT: HEARING AID VERSUS HEARING AIDS (WITH AN "S")

As we discuss in this section, there indeed are some patients with a bilateral hearing loss where a single hearing aid is the best solution. The majority of patients, however, are best served with a bilateral fitting. Many of these patients will come to you, with the belief that they need only one hearing aid. Following a diagnostic procedure, it is not uncommon for a patient to say, "So do you think I need a hearing aid?" but rarely do they say, "Do you think I need a pair of hearing aids?" Why is this? Perhaps they have a friend who only uses one? Perhaps they have a mild loss and think two hearing aids are only for people with severe loss? Maybe it is simply wishful thinking (one hearing aid is less hassle, less money). We have found, however, that a common reason is that the patient has been told at one time or another that they only need *one* hearing aid. Maybe not directly, but they have heard the word *aid* used in the singular, rather than the plural form. For example, the family physician said, "Your hearing is getting worse; I think you probably need a hearing *aid*." Or, the clinic receptionist said, "We have you scheduled for a hearing *aid* evaluation." For some individuals, when they arrive at their appointment and hear that two hearing aids are recommended when they were expecting to be fitted with only one, this new concept requires some time to digest (see review of effective pre-fitting counseling in Chapter 2). So what is our point? Like most things that come in pairs (e.g., eyeglasses, shoes, chopsticks, and turtle doves), using the plural term *hearing aids* or *pair of hearing aids* early on in your discussions with patients might reduce the need for extended counseling down the road.

---

benefit when the amplified signals are relatively equal. With that in mind, we review the primary bilateral benefits here. It is important to have a basic understanding of each advantage, as in many cases you will want to explain these to your patients and provide real-world examples. Some audiologists even use take-home handouts.

Elimination of the Head-Shadow Effect

Sounds arriving from one side of the head, particularly high-frequency sounds, are reduced or attenuated by 10 to 15 dB for reception in the opposite ear. In the case of a unilateral fitting, patients may then still lack important audibility if they are not able to turn their head to face the talker when the origin is from their unaided ear. This is illustrated nicely in Figure 7–2, which shows the attenuation effects for different key frequencies as a function of the presentation angle. Assuming a relatively symmetrical hearing loss, a bilateral fitting will eliminate the head shadow effect. This will have an impact on speech understanding, as the patient no longer has a bad side.

Loudness Summation

This refers to the auditory system's ability to integrate and fuse sounds from each ear. That is, the sound level has to be reduced to produce the same loudness when listening with two ears in comparison to listening with one. Much of the research on this topic has been conducted with people with normal hearing, but the results for individuals with cochlear hearing loss appear to be similar. In general, summation effects become greater as a function of the degree that the signal occurs above the person's threshold. At threshold, summation effects are 2 to 3 dB, but summation may be 6 to 8 dB, or even higher at suprathreshold levels (depending on symmetry, individual variances, listening paradigm, and input level). The expected practical advantage for the hearing aid user is that less amplifier gain is needed to reach the preferred loudness level, and the hearing aids are therefore less prone to feedback. If lower gain levels are used, there also would be less likelihood of loud sounds

exceeding the patient's LDL. And, for some patients with severe hearing loss, the extra loudness might be the only way to achieve the desired overall loudness level.

Improved Auditory Localization

We discuss auditory localization later in this chapter. In brief, localization requires the comparison of phase and amplitude differences between the two ears to determine the location of a sound. Research has clearly shown that this is accomplished more effectively in a bilateral fitting than in a unilateral one (see Simon [2005] for review). In fact, a person with a mild-moderate symmetrical hearing loss could have worse localization after being *aided unilaterally*, then when they were unaided, especially when they are first fitted. There is evidence to show that it is possible that patients fitted bilaterally may have localization ability rivaling that of those with normal hearing (Drennan et al., 2005).

Improved Speech Understanding in Noise

Bilateral amplification and binaural processing allows for an improvement in speech understanding in background noise. We expect this advantage to be a 2 to 3 dB improvement in the SNR. There are two factors that account for this:

- Binaural redundancy: There is an advantage of hearing the same signal in both ears. The brain essentially has two chances of extracting the correct information—see *diotic* condition in Figure 7–3. For high input levels, this bilateral advantage may not be present, as the signal might be heard in the unaided ear for a unilateral fitting.
- Binaural squelch: Through central auditory processing, the brain can compare two individual speech-in-noise signals, and the result will be a fused signal with a better SNR than either of the two. As pointed out by Dillon (2001), the squelch effect will already be present if the low frequency components of both the speech and noise are above thresholds in both ears for a unilateral fitting.

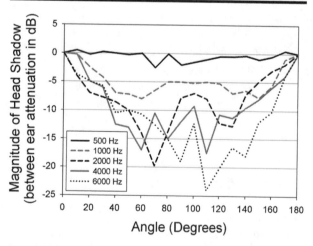

Figure 7–2. Effects of head shadow as a function of frequency. Attenuation shown for signals presented from 0 to 180 degrees.

Although there has been a general belief that bilateral amplification is superior to unilateral for understanding speech in background noise for the past 25 to

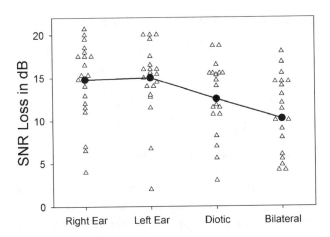

Figure 7–3. Average performance (SNR loss) for four different conditions: right ear, left ear, diotic (same signal to both ears), and bilateral (separately recorded signal to each ear). (Adapted from McArdle et al., 2012.)

30 years, there has not been much study of this topic recently. An exception is the publication of McArdle, Killion, Mennite, and Chilsolm (2012). These finding are summarized in Figure 7–3. This figure shows speech recognition in background noise (uncorrelated) for a group of hearing impaired listeners. The signal was recorded from the Knowles Electronics Manikin for Acoustic Research (KEMAR) and played to the subjects via earphones. Both the redundancy and squelch effects are apparent. Note that for the diotic presentation (signal recorded from a single ear, but presented to both ears), there is an approximate 2 dB advantage, compared with either the right or left ear. We expect this advantage due to redundancy. When the subjects listened to the speech and noise signals that were recorded bilaterally (reflecting phase and amplitude differences), and these two different recordings were played to the two different

SOAPBOX: CLINICAL SPEECH MEASURES FOR BILATERAL FITTINGS

Some audiologists conduct bilateral speech testing following the standard unilateral testing to determine if the patient will benefit from two hearing aids. Clinicians also are sometimes tempted to conduct aided speech testing in the clinic to demonstrate to the patient why two hearing aids are better than one. There are several reasons why we do not recommend these practices:

- We would only expect to see the bilateral advantage when noise is present and the listening task is difficult. For a test such as monosyllables in quiet, we would expect the outcome to be no better than that of the best ear (unless PB-Max was not correctly obtained during the initial unilateral testing).
- We would only expect the bilateral benefit to be obtained if the person was in a distributed noise field and the noise was uncorrelated (e.g., a typical real-world environment). Most clinics do not have the sound field loudspeaker arrangement or recorded speech and noise material to conduct this type of testing.
- The bilateral benefit we are observing is small, and may be smaller than the test-retest and critical differences of the speech material used (see the critical differences discussed in Chapter 5).
- The speech-in-noise advantage only will be noticeable with clinical speech testing when an SNR improvement of 3 dB has an impact on a given patient's speech recognition—that is, when testing is conducted around their 50% intelligibility point. If the clinical test condition is too difficult or too easy (and this will vary from patient-to-patient), the benefit will not be observed. A variable or adaptive SNR test as described in Chapter 5 is required.
- Even though a substantial portion of patients may choose unilateral amplification after a bilateral trial, it does not appear that clinical tools are sensitive enough to predict which individuals these will be. Moreover, the decision to use only one hearing aid often is related to factors other than speech recognition.

ears, another 2 dB improvement was observed, for a combined 4 dB advantage when compared with the right or left ears. (Note that the measure is SNR loss, so lower numbers indicate an SNR improvement.)

Improved Sound Quality and Better Spatial Balance

If you have ever compared one versus two earphones while listening to your iPod, we do not have to tell you that bilateral listening provides better sound quality than unilateral. There is sense of fullness, and the sound seems in your head rather than at the ear. This also applies to the hearing impaired and hearing aids, and has been substantiated by research (e.g., Balfour & Hawkins, 1992).

It is difficult to measure *spatial balance* in the clinic, but what we mean by this is the general sense of being in sync with your surroundings. We frequently hear from bilateral hearing aid users who had to be without one hearing aid because of a repair issue, that they felt *unbalanced* by only wearing one hearing aid. Cox, Schwartz, Noe, and Alexander (2011) reports that when individuals compared two versus one hearing aid in the real world, *balance* was the leading reason for preferring the bilateral fitting.

Avoidance of the Unaided Ear Effect

We recall hearing stories from the 1970s of unscrupulous hearing aid dealers telling potential customers that they needed to buy two hearing aids, because if they only used one, the other ear would become lazy, and their hearing in that ear would get worse. Once viewed as merely a sales tactic, science now tells us that there was some truth to what these salesmen were saying. An article published by Silman, Gelfand, and Silverman (1984) garnered attention when these authors reported that a sizeable percent of people who once had a symmetrical hearing loss and word recognition scores, suffered a reduction in word recognition in the unaided ear after being aided unilaterally for several years (with no significant change in pure-tone thresholds). In a retrospective study, Hurley (1999) reported that this effect was present for about 25% of unilateral hearing aid users.

This often has been referred to as auditory deprivation, or late onset auditory deprivation, although we prefer the term *unaided ear effect*. The reason for this is that it does not seem to happen unless the opposite ear is aided. We say this because people with a bilateral hearing loss who are not fitted with a hearing aid do not experience *deprivation*, even though their hearing loss is the same as the unaided ear of the people who were

---

TECHNICAL TIP:
THE UNAIDED EAR EFFECT (AUDITORY DEPRIVATION)

The unaided ear effect is an intriguing topic, which is still in need of considerable research. Much of what we know is from retrospective reports or illustrative cases, not controlled studies. Here is a brief summary, however, of what we believe to be true:

- The unaided ear effect will occur in about one-quarter to one-third of the people with symmetrical hearing loss fitted unilaterally.
- A significant effect (decrease in word recognition) may be noticed as soon as within one year, or may occur more gradually over three to five years (possibly related to daily hearing aid use? Degree of hearing loss in unaided ear?).
- At some point, the effect seems to plateau, and no further reduction in speech recognition occurs.
- When the unaided ear is fitted with amplification after the effect has occurred, recovery in word recognition occurs for some individuals but not others—possibly related to age and/or duration of the effect.

fitted unilaterally. Why is this? Part of it indeed may be due to deprivation. When people start wearing a hearing aid on one ear, their world generally becomes softer (people do not have to talk to them as loud, the TV is softer, etc.). Hence, there probably is less audibility for the unaided ear than if they were not wearing a hearing aid. But also, the use of amplification in one ear leads to a mismatch in central timing, with the aided ear having the stronger signal. Over time, the brain may become more dominant for the stronger signal and pays less attention to the signal from the weaker ear. Regardless of the cause, the effect rarely occurs in bilateral fittings (Hurley, 1999), which is why this is often considered a compelling reason to use two hearing aids.

Potential Contraindications for Bilateral Amplification

Although there certainly are many reasons to think of the routine fitting as bilateral, there also are some reasons why a unilateral fitting might be the best choice. We have listed the most common:

Degree of Hearing Loss

Simply put, to be a candidate for bilateral hearing aid amplification, the hearing for each ear cannot be too good, or too bad. Regarding minimal hearing loss, there are no rules regarding how much hearing loss is

---

TECHNICAL TIP: COMMON FITTING DILEMMA

Regarding bilateral fittings, a common dilemma is when a patient has one ear with a 30 to 40 dB loss (PB-Max around 85 to 90%), and the other ear has a loss of 60 to 70 dB (PB-Max around 50 to 60%). You could decide to give up on the poorer ear and give the patient one close-to-normal ear by fitting only the best ear. Or, you could decide to give the patient pretty good symmetry and fit only the bad ear. Or, you could fit the patient bilaterally. Our choice would be a bilateral fitting, for a couple of reasons. First, the patient probably thinks that the good ear is normal. If you only aid the better ear, the patient will always wonder why you did not aid the ear with the hearing loss. Given that the good ear has a 30 to 40 dB hearing loss, if only the bad ear is aided, the patient would still be lacking audibility for soft speech; it would be tough to achieve enough gain to make soft speech audible in the bad ear—which then leaves us with a bilateral fitting.

Although this patient probably will not experience all of the desired binaural benefits, we would expect improved localization, simply because you are now making many sounds audible in the poorer ear. It is true, the decision would be easier if word recognition was better for the poorer ear. But, we do know that in general, patients will achieve an aided bilateral word recognition score equal to the best ear. In other words, you do not have to be concerned that amplification of the poorer ear will *pull down* overall speech understanding (unless this patient falls into the 5 to 10% of people with binaural interference). In fact, the brain might be able to use loudness from the poorer ear, combined with speech clarity from the better ear to provide the patient with overall benefit, especially when people are talking from the bad side and the patient cannot turn their head (such as while driving or riding in a car). And also, you might find that when aided, the word recognition score for the poorer ear is better than what you obtained with earphones.

Another alternative we have not mentioned is a BiCROS, which we discuss in a later section. But for a patient like this, we would always try a bilateral fitting first. We would put our chances of success at fifty-fifty or better, which makes it worth the effort. The success will depend somewhat on the resulting aided symmetry for speech. If the aided asymmetry is too great, the patient will simply perceive all sounds in the good ear and consider the hearing aid in the poorer ear a useless nuisance.

necessary to justify hearing aid use—we would expect, however, some hearing loss (>20 dB) in the speech range. It is relatively common today to fit hearing aids to someone with normal hearing through 2000 Hz if they are experiencing communication difficulty. Individuals with open fittings and normal low frequency hearing may be able to use audible low frequencies to provide adequate localization, binaural squelch and binaural redundancy even when fitted unilaterally. Consequently, their remaining bilateral benefit will be more limited and mostly be related to head shadow and a sense of balance for high frequency sounds. Conversely, one of the causes for rejection of bilateral amplification, increased occlusion effect will not be present in the open fittings so many of these patients will still be excellent candidates for bilateral amplification (see the section on open fittings later in this chapter for more details).

Regarding severe hearing losses in cases with a large asymmetry between the ears, sophisticated feedback reduction systems allow us to provide more feedback-free gain than ever before, and with smaller instruments. This allows us to fit the poorer ear in the vast majority of cases. The rules, however, for this population keep changing as advancements occur with cochlear implants.

Cost

Hearing aids are expensive. The patient's income level impacts hearing aid adoption in general and also influences the purchase of one versus two hearing aids. In many clinics, the cost of two entry level products is about the same as one premier product. Given that the standard features on most entry-level products are quite satisfactory, if the patient only has a fixed amount of funds, we would recommend two lower priced instruments rather than one super instrument. But, even two entry-level hearing aids might be more than some people can afford.

Convenience

Some patients have considerable trouble putting the hearing aids in and taking them out, changing batteries, and making adjustments. Some consider the wearing of a hearing aid uncomfortable or annoying. A bilateral fitting doubles the problems. Wireless connectivity helps somewhat with this—a single button adjusts the volume or changes programs on both instruments. Remote controls also can be helpful. But the patient will still have the other issues of dealing with two instruments.

Binaural Interference

There is a small portion of the population (approximately 5 to 10%) who has a *reduction* in speech recognition when they experience bilateral amplification. Believed to be due to an auditory processing deficit, this is referred to as binaural interference. This would not necessarily be a contradiction for a bilateral fitting, however; the patient simply would only use one hearing aid when listening in background noise or competing signals. We would expect this person to obtain all the other benefits of bilateral amplification for other listening environments; the average user spends the majority of their time in situations without significant background noise.

Perceived Benefit

Earlier, we described several real and potential benefits of bilateral amplification. One might think, therefore, that if we selected people with symmetric hearing losses, who audiometrically were candidates, who were able to easily handle two hearing aids, and allowed them to experience using one versus two hearing aids in the real world, there would be a large preference for bilateral amplification. This does not appear to be true. Cox et al. (2011) reports that after three months of real-world use of bilateral versus unilateral amplification, only 54% ($n = 94$) of the participants selected bilateral amplification. The research included assessing potential predictors of bilateral versus unilateral preference such as demographic, audiometric, auditory lifestyle, personality, and binaural processing variables. The authors concluded, however, that at this time, there is no accurate method that will predict which patients will prefer one hearing aid rather than two. Because this cannot be predicted, hearing aid returns are possible, and many listeners will prefer two hearing aids. Many clinicians will select bilateral amplification as the default and then return one of the instruments if the patient indicates unilateral amplification is preferred. This emphasizes the need for appropriate counseling at the time of the fitting and during the first few weeks of hearing aid use.[41]

> ## TECHNICAL TIP: SCREENING FOR BINAURAL INTERFERENCE
>
> As we mentioned, research suggests that as many as 10% or so of patients may have binaural interference when using two hearing aids. This is not something that likely would be detected prior to the fitting, as it often is not reflected in the pure-tone audiogram or routine speech recognition testing. As we discussed in Chapter 5, possible screening tests for binaural interference are the DSI and the dichotic digits. It seems reasonable to expect that significant ear asymmetry observed with these earphone dichotic tests also could impact a bilateral hearing aid fitting. Unfortunately, these are not tests conducted routinely in the hearing aid fitting process. This would be something, however, that could be implemented in post-fitting visits when a patient has an otherwise unexplained negative experience understanding speech in background noise using two hearing aids.

Two Overriding Factors Influencing Hearing Aid Style Selection

Several style related factors affect hearing aid acoustics including position of the microphone, position of the receiver, separation of the receiver and microphone, type of coupling to the ear, etc. Two considerations, however, that cut across all hearing styles are acoustic feedback and the occlusion effect. Before reviewing specific styles, we review some of the problems associated with feedback and the occlusion effect, and offer a few solutions.

Acoustic Feedback

Acoustic feedback occurs when amplified sound from the receiver finds a pathway back to the microphone and is reamplified by the hearing aid repetitively in a feedback loop. In this case, the transfer function measured when comparing the sound input with the sound output is referred to as the *closed loop* response. It is differentiated from an *open loop* response that is measured when the receiver and microphone are acoustically isolated from each other. With typical hearing aid fittings, acoustic feedback is almost always present; however, the level is usually not high enough to result in oscillation that produces *audible* feedback. That is, acoustic feedback is not a problem if the amount the signal level is reduced (attenuated) when it travels the feedback pathway (from the receiver to the microphone) is greater than the amount of amplification provided by the hearing aid. In other words, feedback will become a problem when the output of the receiver that reaches the microphone exceeds the original input level (unity gain exceeds 0 dB). It is important to note that a feedback loop can occur regardless of the level of the original sound in the environment (even ambient noise). For most hearing aid styles, the microphone is somewhat isolated from the receiver, providing attenuation to this looped signal that helps to reduce the likelihood of feedback.

On occasion, the feedback path does not provide enough attenuation to offset the hearing aid gain, and there is the potential for the signal to become larger (amplified) on every loop. This amplification will only occur, however, if the reamplified sound adds in phase with the original sound. That is, for the signals to add in phase the duration of the entire loop must be equal to, or an integer multiple of, the period of the signal. If this *in-phase* addition occurs, it can generate an audible oscillation commonly described by the patient as squealing, howling, or whistling. A hearing aid will generate audible feedback at any frequency that has a period that is an integer multiple of the travel time required for sound to travel the entire feedback and gain loop (the duration of the closed loop response) if hearing aid gain amplification is greater than the feedback loop attenuation (unity gain exceeds 0 dB). In Figures 7–4 and 7–5, we walk you through two examples of how acoustic feedback might occur. Although in both cases, the input signal is the same, note that in Figure 7–4, we have more amplifier gain and less attenuation, and as a result, we have feedback.

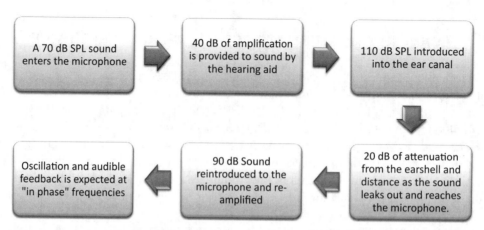

Figure 7–4. Simplified schematic of a possible feedback path with arbitrary numbers. The exact amount of gain in each case will depend on the hearing aid, and the exact amount of attenuation of the feedback loop will depend on the specific earshell and venting used.

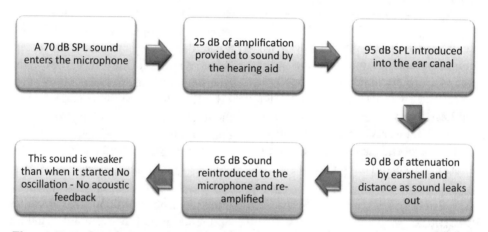

Figure 7–5. Schematic example of a hearing aid for which attenuation of sound traveling the feedback loop is attenuated through distance and limited venting, so that audible feedback does not occur.

Critical Gain Measures

In the past few years, it has become common practice for audiologists to conduct *open loop gain* or *critical gain* measures with the hearing aid fitted to their patient. It is called *open loop* because in this case the hearing aid signal processing path is split between microphone and receiver; the microphone signal is not forwarded to the receiver. This measure provides a good estimate if feedback is probable, and changes to hearing aid gain

can be made if the audiologist believes that the risk of feedback is too great (or, the fitting software will make these changes automatically if that choice is selected). Basically, this measurement is the attenuation between the ear canal SPL and the microphone, and is an estimate of maximum stable gain. For example, if a tone was generated by the hearing aid with a known output of 80 dB SPL, and the microphone picks up the tone via the feedback path and it is measured to be 20 dB SPL, then we would predict that the stable gain would be 60 dB at this frequency. This value, however, should not be interpreted as the maximum gain provided by the hearing aid that was used to conduct the measurement—that is a different measure.

Examples of real-ear open loop gain measurements are shown in Figure 7–6, Panel A and Panel B. These measures are from the same hearing aid, with the same hearing aid settings, but using two different types of coupling systems for a patient's real ear. Note in Panel A, when an open custom tip was used, the output of the hearing aid exceeds the stable gain reference by 10 dB in the 3500 Hz region. As expected, stable gain was the lowest for the frequency region where the output of the hearing aid was the highest. This is a clear indication that feedback will be present. Hearing aid fitting software can be set so that it will automatically reduce the output for this region and minimize the potential for feedback. This might not be a wise choice, however, if the patient needs gain in this region for audibility of speech. An alternative choice would be to use an earmold with a tighter fit, which will serve to increase the stable gain values. This is shown in Panel B. All parameters of the hearing aid were set the same, except in this case, a tighter fitting custom dome was used. Note that we now have the same output peak for the 3500 Hz region, but we are 5 dB below the stable gain values—a good probability we will *not* have feedback.

Feedback Problems and Solutions

Acoustic feedback is undesirable for a number of reasons as it has the potential to lead to: loudness discomfort, annoyance, embarrassment, reduced sound quality, and in many cases, it will limit gain. Individuals who wear hearing aids that are prone to feedback often will use feedback as the determining factor in adjusting the volume—they will increase the gain until they hear feedback, then turn it down a little from this point. Unfortunately, in a poorly fitted hearing aid, this setting may be less than what is needed for appropriate audibility for the patient.

In addition to the annoyance caused by audible feedback, acoustic feedback that is present at gain levels just below those resulting in oscillation (approximately 1 to 3 dB) can result in a *peaky* response (e.g., Cox, 1982). This is sometimes referred to as suboscillatory feedback. The peaky response occurs because suboscillatory feedback can cause both increases and decreases in the hearing aid output, depending on frequency. Specifically, addition will occur for in-phase frequencies (period = integer multiple of the travel time), and reduction will occur for frequencies that are exactly out of phase (period = one-half integer multiple of the travel time).

In addition to an acoustic feedback pathway, a mechanical feedback pathway is also present. That is,

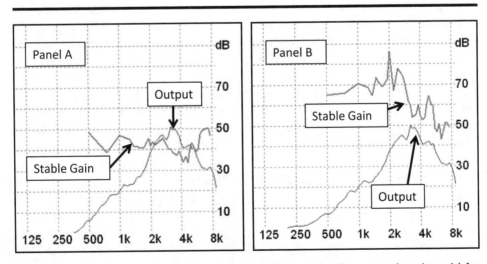

Figure 7–6. Example of open loop gain measured for the same hearing aid for an open fitting (*Panel A*) and a more closed fitting (*Panel B*). Note that the output remains similar whereas the stable gain values change considerably.

POINTS TO REMEMBER: FEEDBACK AND STIGMA

We would like to expand a little on the embarrassment issue we mentioned related to feedback. Most hearing aid users do not want to draw attention to the fact that they wear hearing aids. A whistling hearing aid, especially in a quiet room, clearly works against this concept. Some patients simply then do not wear their hearing aids in these situations. This relates to the stigma issue that we discussed in Chapter 2. A driving factor related to the stigma is the common belief among average consumers that hearing aids do not work very well. A whistling hearing aid disturbing a church service confirms this belief, which then only adds to the stigma. Who among us would want to be that person known for spending thousands of dollars for something that does not work? As we explain in detail in Book Two in this series on technology, the advancement of sophisticated feedback reduction algorithms in recent years has helped us make significant strides in showing people that hearing aids really do work and can provide the desired amount of amplification without feedback!

---

sound vibration from a receiver can travel through any number of mechanically linked pathways (through an earshell, up a wire and through plastic case, up tubing and through a plastic case, etc.) back to the hearing aid microphone. Although the mechanisms responsible for mechanical feedback are similar to those of acoustic feedback, other than the travel path, the solutions are different. Mechanical feedback must be accounted for in the manufacturing process by mechanically isolating the microphone from the receiver, using rubber and other vibration dampening materials to limit mechanical linkage.

To differentiate between acoustic and mechanical feedback, simply plug the microphone and/or receiver ports. If the feedback is still present, it is likely to be mechanical in nature. If not mechanical, this feedback is likely an *internal acoustic feedback* due to acoustic leakage within the case. In either situation, the solution requires a mechanical repair. Mechanical feedback is not commonly observed in routine hearing aid fittings. When observed, it often is with very high gain instruments or with a hearing aid that has been damaged (e.g., dropped on a hard surface).

In contrast with solutions for mechanical and internal feedback, acoustic feedback can often be reduced using simple clinical manipulations such as reducing leakage of the signal from the ear canal (caused by venting). All hearing aids or earmolds allow for at least a small amount of sound to leak out of the residual ear canal space (the sound that escapes around the borders

of the hearing aid/earmold in the concha is referred to as *slit leak*). Venting simply refers to the *intentional* process of increasing the amount of this leakage, usually by creating an additional sound channel—see Chapter 8 for details.

Given the cause of feedback, it should not be surprising that the simplest ways to eliminate oscillation caused by acoustic feedback include reducing the hearing aid gain at the feedback frequencies or by further isolating the sound output from the receiver from sound input to the microphone (e.g., reduce venting or increasing the distance between the microphone and receiver). Both of these techniques are used in Figure 7–5. More attenuation by using a tighter earshell and greater microphone to receiver distance (30 dB instead of 20 dB) is a big reason. However, gain was also reduced from 40 dB to 25 dB. Reducing gain, however, could present a major problem if this patient actually requires more gain than 25 dB for this input level at this frequency and is being under fit.

The bottom line is that acoustic feedback can impact style selection, and this most frequently happens when high levels of gain are needed. As discussed, one technique for reducing feedback is to increase the distance between the microphone and the receiver. A person who desires a small hearing aid that fits totally in the ear canal (very short distance between microphone and receiver) might be best served using a hearing aid where the microphone is above the ear, so that the necessary feedback-free gain can be obtained. Selecting a hearing aid with a good feedback reduction system, of course, is

---

TECHNICAL TIP: CHECKING FOR FEEDBACK PROBLEMS

In our examples in Figures 7–4 and 7–5, for simplicity we used a hearing aid with linear gain. In clinical practice, however, we will nearly always be fitting hearing aids with wide dynamic range compression (WDRC). Consider that with a common WDRC fitting (e.g., 40 dB SPL kneepoint; 2:1 compression ratio), gain is reduced as input increases, to the point that at high inputs (e.g., 80 dB SPL or so) gain may only be 5 or 10 dB, and the output will be relatively equal to the input. The point where gain is the highest and feedback is the most probable, is at the compression kneepoint (commonly an input of approximately 40 dB SPL). Why is this important for identifying potential feedback problems? Quite often, the hearing aid fitting is conducted in a room with a relatively high ambient noise level (caused by several computers running, heating and air conditioning, reverberant conditions, etc.). When the patient then goes home and uses the hearing aids in a quiet setting (e.g., their living room), feedback occurs. We suggest, therefore, that before you send the patient home with the hearing aids, you take them to a quiet place in your clinic or office (a test booth if necessary) to ensure that feedback does not occur for this type of listening situation.

---

also a big factor—yes, they do vary considerably among manufacturers.

The Occlusion Effect

Although we have described how decreasing venting can be a solution for reducing feedback, it can create a problem of its own related to the occlusion effect. Notice that we are using the term *occlusion effect*, not simply occlusion.[42] You can have occlusion without the occlusion effect—more on that later. The occlusion effect may increase the level of sounds in the lower frequencies (e.g., 200 to 500 Hz) by up to 20 to 30 dB in the occluded ear canal when compared with the level in the open ear canal. The occlusion effect causes the hearing aid user to report, "My head sounds like it is in a barrel when I talk" or that their own voice sounds hollow or booming (see Mueller [2003] for review). In addition, this problem can make chewing food sound noisy or unpleasant. To experience this sensation yourself, simply tightly plug your ears and then speak, or better yet, chew a raw carrot or eat a few kettle cooked potato chips.[43]

Why the Occlusion Effect Happens

So what causes the occlusion effect? The process goes like this:

- When we talk, certain sounds, especially vowels, reach 120 to 130 dB SPL or more in the back of the throat.
- The high intensity sounds travel via the mandible (bone conduction) to the condyle, which is positioned adjacent to the ear canal.
- This bone-conducted signal then becomes an air-conducted signal by setting up vibrations (primarily low frequency) of the cartilaginous portion of the ear canal.
- In normal situations, this low-frequency energy escapes out the open ear canal and does not contribute significantly to our perception of our own voice.
- If the lateral portion of the ear canal is plugged with a hearing aid or earmold, this signal cannot escape, and the resulting trapped energy in the residual ear canal volume is reflected back to the eardrum and transmitted to the cochlea in the typical air-conducted manner.
- These sounds will then change the perception of our own voice and can also enhance sounds of chewing, and even breathing.

Note that the occlusion effect process is not related to the signal going through the hearing aid. In fact, the occlusion effect will be the same whether the hearing aid is turned on or off. This is important to remember if you are ever tempted to treat the occlusion effect by turning down low frequency gain. If turning down low frequency gain solves the problem of the patient's voice sounding funny, then the problem was not the occlusion effect. The problem was too much low frequency gain.

Magnitude of the Occlusion Effect

Prior to the common use of probe-microphone measures, it was necessary to rely on the patient to describe the magnitude of the occlusion effect and inform us if our treatment strategies were working. Since the 1980s, however, we have used probe-microphone measures to provide an objective measure (see Mueller and Hawkins [1992] and Book Three of this series for complete review). Because the effect is directly related to the energy contained in the residual ear canal cavity, it can be measured precisely by placing a probe-microphone at this location.

There seems to be a general belief among clinicians that males have more occlusion effect problems than females; perhaps this simply is because their voices tend to be more booming to begin with. To examine this and to obtain general objective data regarding the average occlusion effect, Mueller, Bright, and Northern (1996) compared the occlusion effect for males and females. The subjects were fitted with custom, full-concha ITE instruments that were not vented but were somewhat loose fitting. The mean occlusion effect measured for this group is shown in Figure 7–7 (the bars represent the *range*). As shown, the greatest average effect was at 500 Hz (approximately 17 dB), although a substantial amount of occlusion also was present at the other key frequencies. Observe that except for 125 Hz, the average occlusion effects were essentially the same for males and females. Most notable is the large range for all frequencies for both genders (see bars in Figure 7–7). The authors comment that although some individuals had 0 dB of occlusion effect at some frequencies, all subjects had at least 8 dB of occlusion effect for one key frequency. It could be that the perception that men have more problems with the occlusion effect is related to the fact that male hearing aid users are more apt to have normal hearing in the lows (e.g., a high-frequency, noise-induced loss). Although the true magnitude of the male occlusion effect may be the same as for females, it is therefore more bothersome for this population.

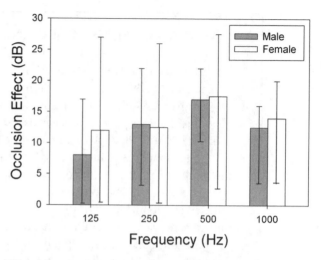

Figure 7–7. Average occlusion effect for four key frequencies comparing gender differences. Individuals fitted with closed custom instruments. Vertical lines within each bar represent the range for that frequency. (Adapted from Mueller et al., 1996)

In the Mueller et al. (1996) research, the occlusion effect was measured by having the patient vocalize the /ee/ sound. This is a common approach in both research and clinical practice. This is because the effect is greatest for the vowel sounds /ee/ and /eye/, and not very significant at all for /ah/. This contributes to why the effect can be annoying, as not only is there the increased emphasis of the low frequencies, but it only occurs for certain vowels.

An example of the outcome of using probe-microphone measures to measure the occlusion effect shown in Figure 7–8. This patient was wearing a CIC with a pressure vent, with the tip of the shell about 12 to 15 mm deep in the ear canal. The initial measure was for the open ear /ee/ vocalization (75 dB SPL measured at 12 inches); the tip of the probe tube was located near the eardrum. What you see in Figure 7–8 is the primary energy of this vocalization around 250 to 300 Hz and then a secondary peak around 3000 Hz, which is reflective of the ear canal resonance. We then insert the CIC instrument, but *do not* turn it on. The upper curve that you see in Figure 7–8 is the ear canal output from the vocalization with the hearing aid in place. Observe that in the lower frequencies, we have a 15 to 20 dB increase, and the output is as high as 100 dB (ear canal SPL). Because the hearing aid was turned off, we can be assured that this increased

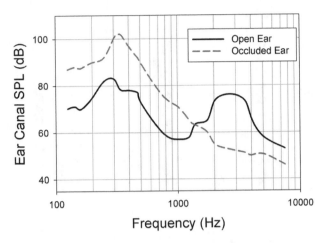

Figure 7–8. Example of the occlusion effect measured using probe-microphone equipment. Output from patient vocalization of the /ee/ sound at 75 dB for open ear and ear occluded with CIC hearing aid (turned off).

output is caused by signal traveling via bone conduction to the ear canal, and then the resulting air-conducted vibrations not being able to escape. Note that the peak in the higher frequencies is gone, as the ear canal no longer has its natural resonance. This degree of occlusion effect is somewhat greater than average but certainly not uncommon when a closed fitting is employed.

Given that this was a CIC, there is not too much we can do to fix this problem. Maybe the vent could be slightly bigger, or the fitting could be looser (slit leak venting). Maybe the shell could have gone somewhat deeper, but then we might have had a comfort issue. It is unlikely, however, that any of these methods would reduce a 20 dB occlusion effect to the point that it would not be annoying. If we do make modifications, however, probe-microphone measures are an excellent way to monitor progress (if any). Look for our complete description of using probe-microphone measures for assessing the occlusion effect in the troubleshooting sectin of Book Three of this series.

Identifying and Treating the Occlusion Effect

As we mentioned, it is important to differentiate between the true occlusion effect and too much low frequency gain from the hearing aid. The easiest way to make this differentiation is to conduct probe-microphone measures of the patient's vocalizations with the hearing aid turned off. Most probe-microphone systems allow you to listen in, and you also will be able to hear the patient's occlusion effect yourself. If you do not have probe-microphone capabilities, or are pressed for time, a quick check to allow you to differentiate is to have the patient read a passage with the hearing aid turned on

---

POINTS TO PONDER: AMPCLUSION—WHAT IS IT?

You might have seen the term *ampclusion* used in articles about the hearing aid occlusion effect. And unfortunately, the term has led to some misunderstanding regarding the treatment of the occlusion effect. The term was coined by Steve Painton in a 1993 article. According to Painton (1993, p. 152), ampclusion is "the combination of occlusion and low-frequency amplification that results in the 'hollowness' or 'head in the barrel' complaints." So, if we are understanding this correctly, if you know that the patient's problem is caused by the occlusion effect, then the patient *would not* have ampclusion, as there is no combined effect.

We do not use the term ampclusion because usually the combined effects are not the major clinical issue. First, consider that if the occlusion effect and the hearing aid output were at the same frequency range and the same intensity, the combined effect would be no more than 3 dB (and that is only if the two signals were equal). True, it is possible that there could be an occlusion effect problem at 200 Hz, and too much gain at 500 Hz, but usually the problem is one or the other. For effective treatment and management, you really need to determine which of the two factors is the prime contributor to the problem.

versus off. If the problem is amplifier gain, the "hollow voice" perception will go away when you turn the hearing aid off. If it is the occlusion effect, the voice will still sound hollow. You can use most any passage, but it helps if there are a lot of /ee/ sounds. If you want to make it a bit fun, have your patient read this passage:

"Through three cheese trees three free fleas flew."

The easiest way to alleviate the occlusion effect is to vent the space between the hearing aid/earmold/tubing tip and the eardrum. Of course, larger vents increase susceptibility to feedback. It is often a compromise. In addition, venting has a little or no effect on occlusion occurring in the 500 to 750 Hz frequency region and above, unless very large vents (3 to 4 mm or greater) are used—see the effects of venting described in Chapter 8. Fortunately, a large occlusion effect in this higher frequency range is somewhat rare. The frequency-specific probe-microphone evaluation of the occlusion effect will give you a quick indication of how easy it will be to reduce the output by venting—a 250 Hz or below effect can be treated fairly easily.

Open canal (OC) fittings have become popular in recent years, and although this is not venting as we traditionally know it, it is equivalent acoustically to a very large vent. And indeed, this fitting approach is very successful in reducing and, in many cases, eliminating the occlusion effect. The occlusion data from MacKenzie (2006) are shown in Figure 7–9. He compared an occluding earmold with four different sizes of vents and a totally open fitting (the open fitting data is from the mean of the open domes of three different manufacturers). Note that the occlusion effect for the closed earmolds was similar to the data shown in Figure 7–7 from Mueller et al. (1996). Also, observe that as the vent was made bigger, the degree of occlusion decreased, especially for 250 Hz (low frequencies are most affected by venting—see Chapter 8). The effects for the open fittings, however, are quite dramatic. There was essentially *no* occlusion effect present.

A second method for alleviating the occlusion effect is to fit the hearing aid or earmold tightly and deeply in the ear (down to the bony portion), very close to the eardrum (Killion, Wilber, & Gudmundsen, 1988; Mueller & Ebinger, 1996). This method decreases the magnitude of the occlusion effect by increasing impedance at the tympanic membrane, increasing the resonant frequency of the residual ear canal space and reducing

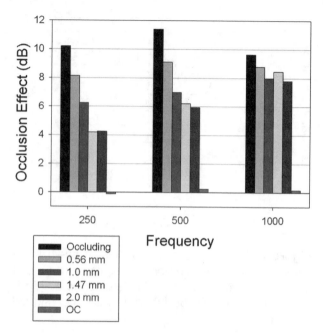

Figure 7–9. Average occlusion effect at key frequencies as a function of the tightness of the earmold plumbing. Most notable is the absence of the occlusion effect when open-fit stock eartips are used. (Adapted from MacKenzie, 2006.)

how well the ear canal wall can vibrate. Although laboratory studies have shown that this method is effective, unfortunately it is uncomfortable for a large percentage of patients. Moreover, with some products, it requires a deep earmold impression, which some audiologists shy away from. There continues to be new solutions for deep fittings proposed using different types of shell material, earmolds, or extended tips. None of the methods proposed prior to the time of this writing really have a proven track record of success.

We have already told you that reducing low frequency gain is *not* a solution for the occlusion effect, but we mention it again, as it seems to be the most common treatment used. Part of the problem is that this notion is promulgated by the fitting software of several manufacturers. As we said before, if turning down gain solves the problem, the problem probably was not the occlusion effect.

An interesting twist, however, in the treatment of the occlusion effect is to *add* low frequency gain, rather than reduce it. This does not reduce the occlusion effect per se (it will still be the same if you measured it with your probe-microphone system), but with

---

KEY CONCEPT:
THE REAL EAR OCCLUDED RESPONSE MEASURE

There is sometimes confusion regarding the occlusion effect, and the real ear occluded response (REOR) measure, which is conducted with your probe-microphone equipment. The two terms do sound similar. There is a big difference, however. The REOR is conducted by delivering an air-conducted signal to the ear, with the hearing aid turned off. It typically is used to observe how this response differs from the open-ear real ear unaided response (REUR). It is common to see the reduction or elimination of the normal ear canal resonance, and if it is a relatively tight fitting, attenuation caused by the earmold or hearing aid also will be observed. This is only indirectly related to the occlusion effect. If for example, the REOR looks very similar to the REUR (as it does in an open fitting), then you can be fairly certain that there will not be a significant occlusion effect. But, on the other hand, you could have an REOR that fell significantly below the REUR, by 20 or 30 dB, but this also could be for a hearing aid that caused little occlusion effect if it were a deep fitting instrument. In general, the REOR cannot be reliably used to predict the occlusion effect, except when it approximates the REUR. Much more on the REOR in the probe-microphone section of Book Three of this series.

---

some patients, it reduces the complaint of the occlusion effect. Why is this? It seems that the added gain tends to mask out the annoyance—the person's voice arriving via amplification sounds more natural, perhaps because the consonant/vowel intensity ratios are better maintained with the amplified signal. The down side of course is that this extra low frequency gain may have a negative effect on sound quality and speech understanding in background noise.

It is important to note that the occlusion effect can be a problem for any hearing aid style for which a tight fit (minimal venting) is required, and a very deep fitting is not desirable or possible. Therefore, the occlusion effect can be highly problematic when high amounts of gain are needed for audibility, especially when the patient desires the smallest hearing aid style possible. Sometimes patients will have complaints that are similar to those from occlusion when there is a significant amount of low frequency amplification. This is particularly common when the patient has low frequency hearing thresholds in the mild-to-moderate range; the close proximity of the hearing aid user's mouth to the microphone allows for their voice (particularly the low-frequency components) to be picked up and amplified more than is desirable. In this case, reducing low frequency gain may indeed be the solution.

Hearing Aid Styles

Hearing aid styles have been grouped in various ways throughout history. The most common grouping scheme is based on where the amplifier is worn (e.g., Dillon, 2001). Specifically, instruments are categorized as behind-the-ear (BTE) or over-the-ear (OTE), eyeglass BTE, in-the-ear (ITE), in-the-canal (ITC), completely-in-the-canal (CIC), and all other styles including Body Worn (Body). Using this scheme the majority of mini-BTE instruments including those referred to as receiver-in-the-canal (RIC) or receiver-in-the-ear (RITE), and receiver in the aid (RITA) instruments (described in detail later in this chapter) also fall into the BTE category.

This classification scheme is commonly used by organizations such as the Hearing Industries Association (HIA) when they report the percentage of hearing aids sold for each style as shown in Figure 7–10. More recently, the HIA has begun to differentiate RIC instruments from other BTEs; however, this still lumps mini-BTE RITA instruments with more traditional full-sized BTEs. The reason for tracking the RIC separately appears to be related to popularity, as this style accounts for more than 45% of the total hearing aids sold at the time this was written.

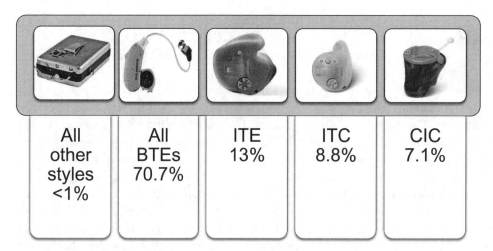

Figure 7–10. Hearing aid market share by style in the United States at the end of 2012.

A less common, but perhaps more useful naming scheme differentiates hearing aids by aspects of their *design* and/or *function*. It is most important to note that this scheme differentiates hearing aid styles by how they affect hearing aid *acoustics* caused by interactions between the hearing aid and user. In the following, we use this second scheme in combination with the more traditional amplifier position–based naming scheme (i.e., BTE, ITE, ITC, CIC) to provide guidance in hearing aid style selection.

If we consider the functional differences of today's hearing aids, then they tend to break down into larger classifications such as body hearing aids, traditional BTE, mini-BTE, traditional custom, and smaller custom products such as CIC instruments, but there also are several subcategories, which we discuss.

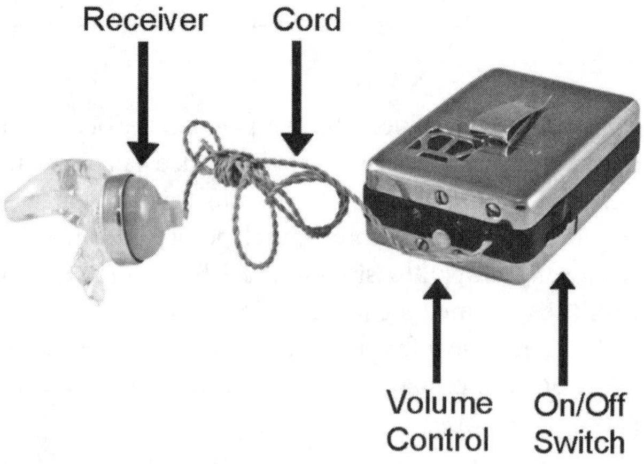

Body Hearing Aids

This style is partially included for historical reasons, although there are still one or two manufacturers that produce it. Body aids, as you might guess from the name, are worn on the body. They are relatively large and include a box-like case (approximately 2 inches high by 2 inches wide by 0.5 inches thick), which contains the microphone and amplification stages, and a receiver that is worn in the ear and is attached to the case by a cord, shown in Figure 7–11. Access to the hearing aid

Figure 7–11. Example of a body style hearing aid with an attached external receiver.

battery and user controls including the volume control wheel and the on and off switch are provided on the case surface (see Figure 7–11), usually on the top and/or bottom. The case can be worn in a variety of positions including on a cord around the neck, in a shirt pocket, or attached to another part of the user's clothing.

At one time, as recent as the 1950s, essentially all electric hearing aids were body aids. These were even larger than today's body aids, and considerable effort was expended to make them invisible or, at the least, more comfortable to wear. Early body aids also required a rather large battery pack, which further complicated the issue. A manufacturer's example of how to accessorize discretely with your hearing aid and battery pack is shown in Figure 7–12.

Functionally, body aids are different than all others in that the microphone is worn on the body. The fact that the microphone is not near the position of the ear is not optimal because picking up sound at, or very near, the normal position of the two tympanic membranes is necessary for the brain to process signals binaurally. Binaural processing of sound is necessary for opti-mal sound localization and also can assist with speech understanding in background noise as described earlier in this chapter. Early body aids utilized what was called a *Y-Cord* that allowed the signal to be transmitted to two receivers—a bilateral (diotic) presentation, not true binaural hearing. In later years, body aids were designed with two different microphones; however, the separation was minimal, and the effect was not what we would achieve with microphones at the two ears.

The position of the microphone on the body also leads to a so-called body-baffle effect that increases gain

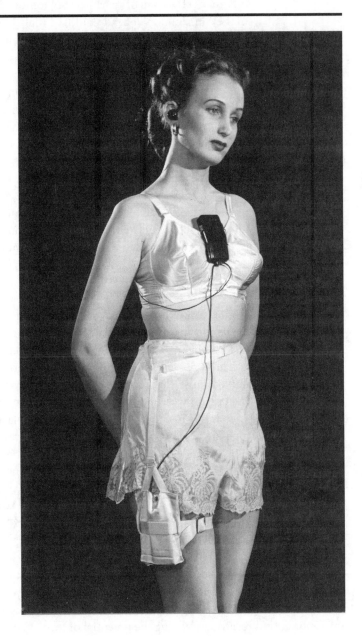

Figure 7–12. Magazine ad from the 1950s illustrating discrete arrangement of body hearing aid and battery pack (Photo courtesy of Washington University School of Medicine).

THINGS TO REMEMBER: AUDITORY LOCALIZATION

In our discussion of body hearing aids, and earlier on the topic of bilateral hearing aid benefit, we mention localization. Later in this chapter, we talk about localization again, as it relates to CIC fittings. Here is a brief review of some localization basics:[44]

■ We are able to localize sound well primarily because we have two ears that sample sound in two different places and a sophisticated binaural processing system. The level and timing differences of a sound as it arrives at the two ears are used as the primary cues for sound location in the horizontal plane.

■ Intreraural Level Difference (ILD) cues, also known as the interaural intensity difference (IID), are primarily useful for localization of high frequencies, because of the contribution of head shadow—high-frequency sounds act more like a beam and do not bend around corners as well as low-frequency sounds. This is illustrated in Figure 7–2. Note that for 90 degrees, low frequencies are only attenuated a few dB, whereas high frequencies are reduced by 10 to 15 dB.

■ Interaurual Time Difference (ITD), sometimes referred to as Interaural Phase Difference cues, are primarily useful for localization of low frequencies. The shorter wavelength of high-frequency sounds can lead to an ambiguous phase cue.

■ Our ability to localize in the vertical plane is primarily due to monaural filtering effects. That is, the head, shoulders, torso, and most important, the outer ear/pinna act to filter and scatter sound in different ways depending on its angle and elevation of arrival.

■ In addition to leading to accurate localization, the binaural cues of ILD, ITD, and monaural filtering effects are also used by our brains to aid in speech recognition in the common cases in which speech and noise arrive from different angles.

---

in the frequency region below 800 Hz and decreases amplification for the frequencies from 1000 to 2500 Hz. The body style is also problematic because of obvious cosmetic concerns. The cords are subject to breakage; there may be unwanted noise due to clothes rustling against the case; and certain wearing positions such as around the neck may result in food and other debris clogging the microphone port—this can be especially problematic in children and those elderly adults with limited remaining self-care abilities. Partially because of these concerns, the body aid style is rarely recommended by current practitioners.

Although the body style hearing aid represents less than 1% of total hearing aid sales, there are some aspects of this style that make it of some interest to some hearing aid users. One historical advantage of the body aid style relates to acoustic feedback. Specifically, the design of the body aid results in a large separation between the microphone and receiver providing the potential of the highest amplified levels without feedback of any of the available styles. The introduction of modern feedback reduction systems, however, have virtually eliminated effective advantages in usable gain and output in comparison with other large hearing aid styles. In addition to the advantage of less susceptibility to feedback, the placement and size of the user controls on the top of the case makes them the easiest to see and manipulate of all the hearing aid styles.

Traditional Behind-the-Ear (BTE) Hearing Aids

By the mid-1970s, most people were wearing the BTE style because it offers several advantages over its body-worn counterpart. In BTE hearing aids, all the electronics are inside a plastic case that is fitted behind the ear, shown in Figure 7–13. Access to the hearing aid battery and user controls are provided on the case surface, usually on the back and/or bottom. Sound is routed from the receiver through an earhook that also is used to help retention. The sound is then directed to the ear through tubing and a custom-made earmold, shown in Figure 7–14.

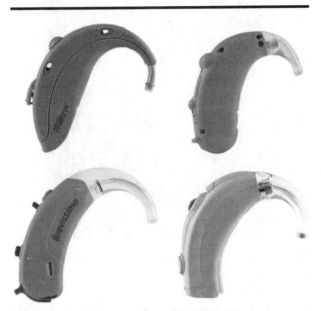

Figure 7–13. Four examples of traditional BTE hearing aids.

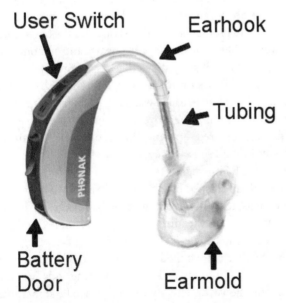

Figure 7–14. External features of a BTE hearing aid with tubing and earmold attached (Photos courtesy of Phonak and Westone).

As discussed in detail in Chapter 8, an added advantage to the BTE design is that the earmold, tubing, and earhook can all be used to modify the frequency response of the amplified signal. Unlike the body aid, the microphone port in the BTE is nearer to the position of the tympanic membrane, as it is usually positioned between the case and the earhook placing it on top of the pinna when worn. This provides the potential for some binaural cues. This design also provides the greatest separation between the sound output (at the end of the tube in the ear) and the microphone of any of the designs other than the body aid. Therefore, when used with an appropriate earmold and modern feedback suppression, this style is able to provide adequate amplification without the presence of feedback for any magnitude of hearing loss for which a listener is expected to benefit from amplification. The larger size of the traditional BTE case also makes it possible to apply various other technologies that we discuss in detail in Book Two of this series. These include directional microphones, wireless signal routing, strong telecoils, and direct auditory input (DAI). Improved miniaturization has also allowed for frequency modulated (FM) receivers to be attached directly to a BTE via a boot, shown in Figure 7–15, or be directly integrated into the BTE case. Most of these features also are available in the larger custom instruments but are often implemented more effectively in the BTE style. Because traditional BTEs can provide considerable amplification, are relatively large and easy to manipulate, and have a high degree of flexibility, they

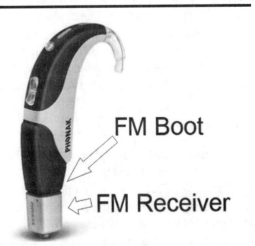

Figure 7–15. Example of an FM receiver and boot that is designed to snap onto the bottom of a BTE hearing aid (Photo courtesy of Phonak).

are appropriate for a wide range of hearing losses and populations. Clinically however, their most common use is for adults with severe or greater hearing loss and in children.

The fact that only the earmold is custom fitted to the ear and it contains no electronics also provides other advantages for the BTE style. Specifically, for children who are still experiencing growth of their ear canals, the earmold can be remade relatively inexpensively without requiring any change to the hearing aid itself. In addition, the separation of the electronic components from the warm, moist, cerumen-producing environment of the ear canal can lead to improved durability.[45] This is important because cerumen clogging the receiver continues to be the number one cause of hearing aid repairs for ITE, ITC, RIC, and CIC styles. The BTE tubing can still become clogged with moisture and debris, but it can be cleaned out or changed without approaching any of the electronic components. Finally, an advantage of the BTE style over custom instruments is that they can be stocked in the clinic. This means that if necessary (or desired), a stock ear piece can be used, and the patient can be fitted with a pair of hearing aids on the same day he or she walked in the door for a diagnostic exam.

Although traditional BTEs are among the largest of the hearing aid styles, it should be pointed out that they are not necessarily the least cosmetically appealing. The right hair style, especially those styles that cover the top of the pinna, in conjunction with the use of a clear earmold and tubing can result in an instrument that is actually much less visible—shown in Figure 7–16—than some of the custom styles such as the ITE, which completely fill the concha with colored plastic. Moreover, as we discuss later, it is now common to use barely noticeable thin tubing with mini-BTEs, and there are adaptors that allow the use of this thin tubing with the larger BTEs, making the overall fitting even less noticeable.

Eyeglass BTEs

Functionally, most *eyeglass* hearing aids also fall into the category of traditional BTEs. What are often termed eyeglass hearing aids are simply a BTE that is integrated into the temple (or bow) of eyeglasses. This style reached the height of its popularity in the 1960s, particularly in the VA/Military health care system. In some respects, the notion was logical—most people who used hearing aids also used eyeglasses, so why not have an all-in-one

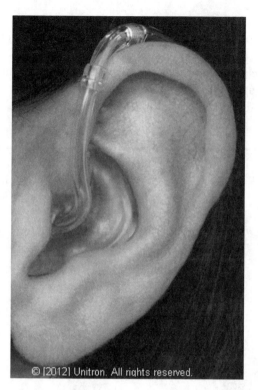

Figure 7–16. Example of a traditional BTE hearing instrument fitted on an ear (Photo © [2012] Unitron. All rights reserved).

product? Some even saw this as a cosmetic advantage, as it was more accepted to wear glasses than hearing aids. There were problems with this style from the beginning, however. These products were heavy and uncomfortable, and did not stay adjusted. Many people needed to keep their glasses on to see well enough to change the battery. Maintenance also was a big problem, as patients would be missing their eyeglasses while their hearing aids were repaired—people did not own several pairs of glasses in the 1960s as they do now.

The BTE/eyeglass style is rarely recommended today. Reduced use of eyeglasses because of increases in contact lenses and vision surgery, changes in popular eyeglass styles leading to very thin temples, and the general miniaturization of other styles of hearing aids have further contributed to the decline of the eyeglass style. A few models of eyeglass hearing aids are still available, however. This style continues to be sometimes suggested for provision of contralateral routing of signal (CROS) amplification (described later in this chapter) and as a way to provide a directional microphone array (along the temple of the eyeglasses) that can improve speech recognition in noise performance (as described in the directional microphone chapter of Book Two of this series). Allowing for such microphone arrays provides one potential advantage for eyeglass style hearing aids over any of the other styles. Furthermore, miniaturization has led to modern eyeglass hearing aids that are much more compact than their counterparts of the 1960s.

Mini-BTEs

A more recent incarnation of the traditional BTE instrument is the mini-BTE hearing aid. As the name suggests, these hearing aids are significantly smaller than traditional BTEs but do fit behind the ear. Mini-BTEs can be fitted in several different ways but fall into two general categories:

- RITA: These products are configured like a traditional BTE, except that the case is smaller, meaning that a smaller battery also is necessary (shorter battery life, probably less power). These products use a very thin tubing to transmit the signal to the ear, unlike the standard #13 tubing used by most traditional BTEs. There is no earhook; the tubing is attached directly to the BTE case. The ear canal coupling often is a stock eartip (many different sizes available), although a custom earmold or eartip also can be used. An example of a mini-BTE RITA product is shown in the bottom portion of Figure 7–17.
- RIC: As the name indicates, this is a small BTE case (usually even smaller than the RITA), which is coupled to a thin wire that attaches to a small external receiver that is placed in the ear canal. This receiver is then coupled to the ear using a custom or non-custom eartip. The advantage of the RIC over the RITA is that because the receiver is removed from the case, the case can be made somewhat smaller, and more unique designs can be implemented. Also, larger receivers can be coupled to the hearing aid to provide more power than usually available with a mini-RITA. Examples of RIC products are

shown in the top portion of Figure 7–17 and in Figure 7–18 and a close up of the wire with the receiver attached in shown in Figure 7–19.

The mini-BTE styles share all the potential feedback versus occlusion compromises with all other

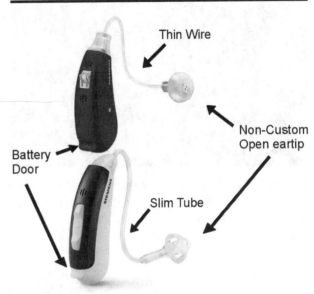

Figure 7–17. Two examples of mini-BTE hearing aids. The upper instrument is a RIC, and the lower instrument is a RITA configuration.

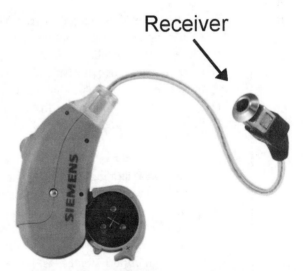

Figure 7–18. A mini-BTE RIC hearing aid. The fitting tip has been removed to show the receiver.

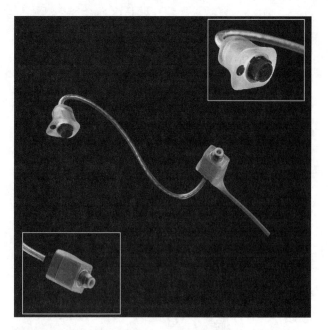

Figure 7–19. Detailed view of RIC receiver and hearing aid coupling (Photo courtesy of Siemens Hearing Instruments, Inc. All rights reserved).

traditional BTE hearing aids. When the RIC was first introduced, some suggested that this product would be less prone to feedback, as the receiver was separated from the microphone by a much greater distance. Although this might impact mechanical feedback, this has no effect on acoustic feedback, which is what we are nearly always concerned with. The feedback path is the same whether the sound is delivered in the ear canal via the receiver, or if it travels through a tube and is then delivered into the ear canal. Mueller and Ricketts (2006) compared two different mini-BTE products from the same manufacturer; one was a RIC and the other a RITA. The hearing aids had the same core processing, were programmed the same, and were fitted with the same level of *tightness* in the real ear. There was no difference in the maximum-gain-before-feedback for the two instruments.

Although we usually think that with hearing aids, small is good, some patients have trouble handling these mini-BTEs. The small size of the case also presents some problems regarding what controls can be included.

POINTS TO PONDER: RIC VERSUS RITA?

There is a general perception among audiologists that when fitting a mini-BTE, RIC is better than RITA. Why is this? Maybe it is because they typically are more expensive (from the manufacturer), but are there real acoustic benefits? We have listed some *potential* advantages of RIC, which have been mentioned in marketing literature.

- Smaller case: This is certainly true. This has allowed for smaller and more interesting case designs, not possible with RITA.
- More output flexibility: This is true. The same product can be fitted with different receivers (if they fit in the patient's ear canal), which can provide significant differences in gain (e.g., the same product could be fitted with receivers of 45, 55, or 65 dB).
- Extended high frequencies: In theory this is true, although some manufacturers have more high frequencies in the 3000 to 4000 Hz range with their RITA than their RIC. For extended high frequencies (above 5000 Hz), RIC would appear to be the best choice because the thin tube will provide attenuation to the high frequencies—although these extended highs are unlikely to matter for most patients, as gain will not be great enough for audibility.
- Smoother frequency response: There are some resonances of the RITA thin tube that are not present when the tube is eliminated with the RIC. These are mostly smoothed by the processing, however, and some of them are at higher frequencies that are not important for most fittings. Probably not a significant factor.

Many products do not have a volume control. Also, there is not room for a strong telecoil, and it is not possible to include some wireless features. If the RIC style is used, there are additional problems related to placing a large receiver in patients with small ear canals (particularly when high levels of amplification are required).

Another limitation reported for both mini-BTE styles from at least some manufactures relates to durability of the connection between the case and the very thin wire or tube. In the case of the RITA, a breakdown of this connection can allow leakage of the acoustic signal greatly increasing susceptibility of feedback. In the case of the RIC this can cause a loss of electronic connection to the receiver resulting in the hearing aid cutting out intermittently. In both cases, the problem can often be resolved by a simple and quick replacement of the tube or wire and receiver. In some cases however, a more significant repair is required. Regardless, this issue can certainly contribute to higher repair rates for mini-BTE than some other styles.

Finally, with the RIC product, there is a tendency for the receivers to become plugged with cerumen. Although patients possibly could repair this themselves at home (if they were given replacement receivers), this event usually prompts a clinic visit—patients simply notice that the aid is dead. This of course is not unique to the mini-BTE; the same problem would occur if we used a RIC coupling with a larger BTE, except that usually is not done. The plugged receiver problem is not a minor issue. Audiologists fitting a large percent of RIC products report a big increase in their walk-in patients needing repairs—so much so that some have gone back to mostly RITA products. It is important to note that the thin tube of the RITA also can become very easily clogged with cerumen, and this style may show more problems related to debris and occluded tubing than any other style. Fortunately, however, there is a very simple fix for this problem; the patient can insert a small plastic wire down the tube to clean it. Both the tube and wire are quite small, however, and the patient must have sufficient vision and dexterity to accomplish this task. For this reason, patients who demonstrate significant issues with cerumen may prefer the RITA style if they have good vision and dexterity, but may prefer the RIC if they do not.

Despite these limitations, the mini-BTE RIC and RITA styles continue to be very popular because of three main advantages when compared with traditional BTEs. First and foremost, there is a clear cosmetic advantage. Second, the smaller lighter case, coupled with placement of the receiver within a custom eartip within the ear canal, can lead to greater comfort and better retention. That is the smaller lighter case is less likely to flop off the pinna than the larger, heavier, traditional BTE case. The final advantage is a convenience issue. The mini-BTEs come with fitting kits that include stock non-custom earmold tips, which allows for a same day fitting.

Marketing experts believed these mini-BTE products will attract a younger hearing aid user, and this appears to be somewhat true. As we discussed in Chapter 2, given the same degree of hearing loss, market penetration for younger individuals is only about one-quarter of what it is for older individuals. There is a general movement to make these smaller hearing aids more fun and less old looking. To assist in attracting the younger generation (e.g., baby boomers), these hearing aids come in a wide range of designs and colors. Some manufacturers have replaced the traditional BTE color names of tan, beige, and brown with names like crème brûlée, snow blade, flower power, and pinot noir!

In a recent study, Kochkin (2011) examined the impact that mini-BTEs have had on the market over the past several years:

- Mini-BTE hearing aids are expansionary (e.g., new users), influencing more affluent and more active elderly consumer segments to come forward for a solution for their hearing loss; they also tapped into segments of people with milder hearing losses.
- Most important, when the degree of hearing loss was controlled, mini-BTE hearing aids provided significant improvements in overall satisfaction, cosmetics, sound quality, and multiple environmental listening utility.
- But, contrary to what was predicted, mini-BTE hearing aids *did not* tap into younger segments of people with hearing loss. They also did not improve consumer perceptions of fit and comfort, benefit, value, or impact reductions of hearing aids not being worn; nor did they generate more positive word-of-mouth advertising or develop greater hearing aid brand loyalty.

TECHNICAL TIPS: YES, THE TERMINOLOGY IS CONFUSING

We have been talking about RIC and RITA hearing aids, as these are the terms we prefer, but it is important to point out that several other terms also are used to describe these products, or similar products. RICs, for example, are sometimes referred to as RITEs (receiver in the ear). But when you think of it, neither RIC *nor* RITE is very descriptive. A custom hearing aid that is a CIC also is a RIC, as the receiver is indeed in the canal (except we do not call it a RIC). And all custom products would be RITEs, as the receiver is somewhere *in the ear* (but we do not call them RITEs). RITA does not really mean much either, as traditional BTEs and most all custom products are all RITAs (unless they are a BTE-RIC). Some audiologists and manufacturers call mini-BTE products *thin tube* hearing aids. They indeed do have a thin tube. But wait, the wire of the RIC is encased in a thin tube, but a RIC usually is not called a thin tube. And, you can take the thin tube of the mini-BTE and connect it to a traditional BTE. Is that then a thin tube product? It gets even more confusing when you start determining if the fitting is closed or open. Here is a quick review, hopefully to clarify, not confuse:

- A mini-BTE RITA has a thin tube but so does a RIC (with a wire inside), and you can put a mini-BTE RITA thin tube on a standard size BTE (which also is a RITA).
- Both a RITA and a RIC are commonly fitted open, but they also are commonly fitted closed (or partially closed).
- An open fitting commonly is conducted with a mini-BTE RITA or RIC, but larger BTEs and even custom instruments also can be used for an open fitting.

Traditional Custom Instruments

As advances in electronic circuitry continued, manufacturers were able to reduce further the size of the hearing aid and began developing custom hearing aids such as the ITE and a more recessed version called the ITC. For simplicity, we are going to call them traditional customs (TC). The TC actually includes several sizes between and including ITE and ITC, as shown in Figure 7–20. Functionally, most ITE and ITC styles are similar enough for our purposes, to fit into the TC category, although there are clear size and cosmetic differences. Although ITEs were developed in the 1960s, these early instruments were generally of poor quality. As a result of improved miniaturization, however, the quality of these instruments is now essentially identical to their larger siblings, and currently, many of the physical components and processing used in BTEs and TCs are the same.

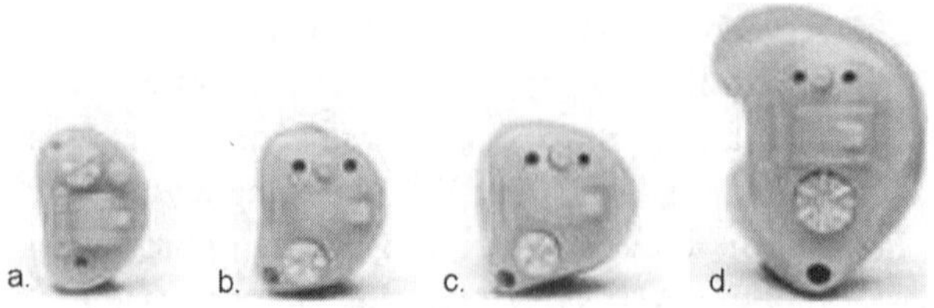

During the 1980s, the percentage of people purchasing all styles of custom hearing aids, including TC and those described in the following sections, quickly grew from 34% in 1980 to approximately 80% of total hearing aid sales by 1990. Improved cosmetics in comparison with the BTE style is the most often cited reason for this rapid increase in popularity. It was not just cosmetics, however; but rather, the custom product was considered to be the *modern* hearing aid, and anything behind the ear was old-fashioned. In recent times, however, the dominance of custom hearing aids has eroded with the introduction and increasing popularity of mini-BTE products, which we just discussed in the preceding section—strangely enough, the standard custom product is now considered old-fashioned. As a result,

Figure 7–20. Four examples of traditional custom hearing aids ranging in size from ITC to full-sized ITE.

at present in the United States, all custom hearing aid styles represent less than 30% of total hearing aid sales (Strom, 2013).

Like the BTE style, all the TC hearing aid electronics are contained within a plastic case. However, with TC instruments, the plastic case is small enough that it can be placed in the ear, usually within an earshell that is fabricated from an impression made of the individual patient's ear and covered with a faceplate that provides access to the battery and any user controls, as shown in Figure 7–21. With traditional custom hearing aids, the microphone port opening is on the instruments faceplate near the position of the natural ear canal opening. This placement gives the user the additional benefits over the BTE style related to the normal acoustics provided by the pinna, including increased high frequency gain. Pinna acoustics are also important in providing sound localization cues and some natural directional effect as discussed in detail in the next section. Most full-concha instruments employ, or at least allow for, the option of using directional technology by using two omnidirectional microphones, and as a result, there are two microphone ports, as shown on Figure 7–21.

The receiver output terminates in a short tube in the end of the case within the listeners ear canal. This termination is similar to the position provided by the earmold of BTE instruments. As is the case for BTE earmolds, TC instruments can be manufactured with varying canal lengths; however, the canal portion generally extends no more than 10 to 15 mm into the cartilaginous portion of the ear canal. Longer canal portions usually are avoided because this can lead to discomfort when wearing the hearing aid as well as increase the difficulty a patient has with insertion and removal.

ITCs in this TC category differentiate from ITEs in that they are smaller and generally fill little of the concha bowl. The larger ITE fits entirely in the outer ear, filling the concha, shown in Figure 7–22, left panel. The smaller ITC model fits mostly in the ear canal and generally does not extend beyond the tragus, shown in Figure 7–22, right panel. The technology for manufacturing ITE shells continues to improve as does miniaturization and sound processing technology. For these reasons, current TC hearing aids are appropriate for patients with hearing loss ranging from mild through severe. When combined with modern feedback suppression technologies, in some cases ITEs may even be appropriate for some listeners with severe-to-profound hearing loss. The maximum hearing loss that is appropriate, however, depends somewhat on ear geometry. In addition, the maximum severity of loss that can be appropriately fit decreases with progressively smaller instruments (i.e., ITE to ITC) because higher power instruments require larger batteries and larger receivers.

Microphone Ports

Battery Door

User Toggle Switch

External Vent Opening

Volume Control

Figure 7–21. External features of a full-concha ITE hearing aid (Photo courtesy of Siemens Hearing Instruments, Inc. All rights reserved).

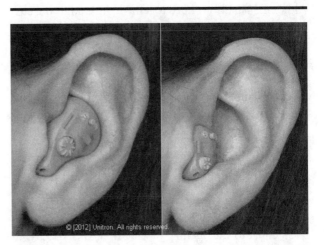

Figure 7–22. Example of full-shell ITE (*Left Panel*) and ITC (*Right Panel*) configurations of the TC hearing aid (Photos © [2012] Unitron. All rights reserved).

Given that these styles do not extend deeply into the canal portion, one potential problem with the TC style is that a tighter fit may lead to more problems with the occlusion effect. Although the occlusion effect can be reduced or eliminated by increased venting, this will also increase the hearing aid's susceptibility to feedback. Because of the close proximity of the microphone and receiver, the traditional ITC is usually not appropriate for patients with severe hearing loss, unless the products' digital feedback suppression (DFS) is particularly effective. Even then, power is limited in half-shell ITEs and ITCs because of the use of smaller receivers and smaller batteries.

Although smaller than the BTE, the ITE and ITC styles are still large enough to accommodate directional microphones, wireless streaming technologies, and telecoils; however, DAI usually is not possible. Further, because of size constraints, the telecoils in these smaller instruments are often weaker than those in BTEs, or not positioned to maximize effectiveness (see Book Two in this series for further explanation). Finally, because of their smaller size, patients with dexterity problems may have more difficulty changing batteries and operating the controls on ITEs—especially ITCs, when compared with traditional BTEs.

Traditional Custom Instruments with Recessed Faceplate

Although usually grouped together with traditional custom instruments, some hearing aids differ from the TC style by recessing the hearing aid faceplate and microphone deeper in the concha, traditional custom instruments with recessed faceplate (TCR). The amount of recess distance can be small, as is the case of the *Low profile ITE*, or slightly more pronounced, as is the case with some deep fitting ITC instruments. Clearly, the largest effects are seen with CIC instruments. In the case of the CIC, the microphone opening, as well as the entire hearing aid case, will be recessed into the ear canal, shown in Figure 7–23. In fact, by definition, to be a CIC, the faceplate must be recessed in the ear canal, or at the least, equal to the opening of the ear canal. The CIC in Figure 7–24 is somewhat smaller than the one shown in Figure 7–23 and would most probably be recessed. Depending on the specific manufacturer, the recessed

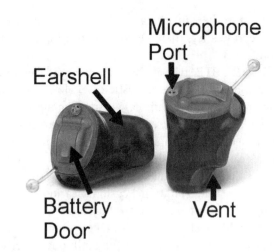

Figure 7–23. External features of a CIC hearing aid (Photo courtesy of Phonak).

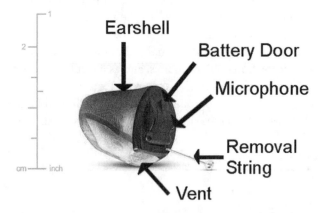

Figure 7–24. Latest generation of smaller CIC hearing aid.

ITC or the CIC are the physically smallest instruments made—in Figure 7–25, it might be debatable if the fitting on the left is truly a CIC, but note that for the one on the right, from this viewing angle, the hearing aid is not visible. In some cases the CICs are actually slightly larger (when viewed in your hand, not in the patient's ear) because they may be made to extend deeper into the ear canal as described in the next section.

The popularity of the CIC product grew rapidly in the early 1990s, as more and more manufacturers offered this model. As you might imagine, trade journals were filled with articles and advertisements extolling the many benefits of this hearing aid style. In a

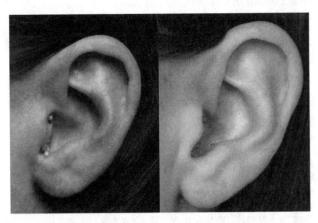

Figure 7–25. CIC hearing aids placed in ear. Note that for the Right Panel example, from this view, the hearing aid is not visible (Photos © [2012] Unitron. All rights reserved).

special issue of *The Hearing Journal*, Mueller (1994a, 1994b) reviewed 16 difference potential benefits of the CIC instrument, which he had gleaned from articles or marketing materials. We have revisited those potential benefits in Table 7–1 and added our opinions regarding the *real benefit* that was derived from CIC fittings of this era. As you can observe from our comments, many of the potential benefits were directly linked to the deepness and tightness of the fit; something that seemed ideal from a theoretical aspect, but was not well received by most patients. In the early days, it generally was assumed that a CIC would be deeply fitted, but manufacturers soon became proficient at producing smaller hearing aids that indeed were recessed in the ear canal but were not fitted much deeper than the standard ITE.

POINTS-TO-PONDER: WHAT IS A CIC?

- In the 1980s, very small ITCs with recessed faceplates were developed and marketed. These invisible hearing aids were prized because of their excellent cosmetics but had considerable limitations related to limited power and susceptibility to occlusion and feedback.

- In the early 1990s, CICs became quite popular. One of the earliest models was the Philips XP Peritympanic deep canal CIC. Peritympanic instruments were fitted very closely to the tympanic membrane, and for a period of time, some manufacturers required special training prior to dispensing these instruments.

- This style only lasted for a brief period of time and gave way to a CIC that was not as deeply fitted, but still extended into (or close to) the bony portion of the ear canal reducing or eliminating problems with the occlusion effect.

- Because of the importance of good cosmetics to marketing, there was a push to make hearing aids as small as possible. This was a problem for some early CIC hearing aids because although they were difficult to see when fitted to the ear, the fact that they were deeply inserted made many of them larger in your hand than some ITCs. Because of patient comfort issues, however, the longer CIC canals became the exception (unless specified by the audiologist ordering the instrument).

- Current manufacturers have chosen to market their instruments in different ways. The smallest recessed instruments that do not extend down to the bony portion (called ITCs in the 1980s) are referred to as ITCs by some manufacturers and CICs by other manufacturers. Those manufacturers that refer to these instruments as CICs usually differentiate them from deep fitting CICs. In other words, one manufacturer's CIC may be another's ITC. And, if your patient has a smaller-than-average ear canal, you may order a CIC, but when the patient puts it in his or her ear, it will be an ITC.

- Our thoughts are that it is not a CIC unless the faceplate is equal with, or recessed into the ear canal.

Table 7–1. The benefit of CIC hearing aids: What 20 years of experience has revealed.

Purported CIC Benefit (circa 1994)	True Benefit in Day-To-Day Fittings
Cosmetics: Recessed faceplate will make hearing aid nearly invisible	**Mostly True:** It was soon learned however, that many patients did not have an ear canal small enough to recess the faceplate.
Increased gain: High frequency input to the microphone is increased because of pinna and concha effects.	**Mostly True:** This is less important today as current products have more high frequency gain.
Increased output: The deep fitting would reduce the residual ear canal volume, increasing the output.	**Mostly False:** The fittings were generally not deep enough to make this factor significant.
Reduced distortion: Because of the reduced ear canal volume, less amplifier gain would be needed, which would reduce saturation-introduced distortion (peak-clipping).	**Mostly False:** The fittings were generally not deep enough to make this factor significant. This is less of a factor today due to the routine use of AGCo.
Reduction of the occlusion effect: A secure deep fitting of the hearing aid shell reduces vibrations of the cartilaginous portion of the ear canal.	**Mostly False:** The fittings were generally not deep enough to make this factor significant.
Reduction of acoustic feedback: A receiver output closer to the eardrum and a tight fitting reduces leakage.	**Mostly False:** The fittings were generally not deep enough or tight enough to make this factor significant
Ease of Removal: A rigid removal string makes the CIC easier to remove than other custom products.	**True:** The success with the CIC removal string has led to this feature being added to other custom products when necessary.
Improved localization: Placing the microphone at the opening of the ear canal allows for more natural pinna effects.	**True:** If faceplate placement is recessed and the hearing loss is not too severe, localization can be near that of people with normal hearing.
Reduced wind noise: With the microphone recessed, it is less affected by wind, due to shadowing by the pinna.	**True:** Especially for wind originating from the front of the user.
Comfort: A more comfortable fit due to smaller size, and fitting only in ear canal.	**Toss-Up:** For some patients, this is definitely true. For other patients, especially those with sharp turns in their ear canal, this is false.
Fewer receiver wax problems: Because the receiver extends beyond the area of wax production, there is less chance of plugging.	**False:** The fittings were generally not deep enough for this logic to apply, but even if they were, wax accumulated during insertion.
No volume-control wheel: Early CICs did not have a VC, and this was promoted as an advantage.	**Mostly False:** Even when the fitting was carefully verified (most weren't), the majority of hearing aid users wanted to be able to adjust he volume.
Telephone use: Because of the deep fit and recessed fitting, less feedback. And, the recessed fitting would help with comfort.	**Mostly True:** If fitted tightly, some improvement with feedback, and more comfortable when phone was placed to ear than when compared to a traditional ITE.
Using headsets: Professional and recreational headsets can be used with less feedback. Maybe allow for stethoscope use.	**Mostly True:** If fitted tightly, some improvement with feedback, and more comfortable when compared to a traditional ITE.
Security of fit: Deeper fit allows for security for use in strenuous work or recreational activity.	**Mostly True:** Especially when compared to BTEs. If not deeply fit, and the patient has relatively straight canals, CICs would "work out" of ear for some patients.
Use during sleep: Because of recessed fit and comfort, can be used during sleep to allow hearing warning signal and important environmental sounds.	**Toss-Up:** Seems reasonable, but not a topic that received much research interest.

Regardless of whether the tip of the CIC is made to extend deep into the canal or not, the fact that the faceplate is intended to be recessed inside the ear canal can make the CIC the most cosmetically appealing of all the styles. In fact, in some fittings, these instruments are difficult to see without looking into the ear canal. Because of this, there is some debate as to whether the faceplate of the CIC should be skin-colored to blend in with the concha, or colored to blend with the shadow of the ear canal. The close proximity of the microphone to receiver has negative connotations with regards to feedback. Therefore, the smallest of the recessed faceplate instruments (CIC/ITC) are usually not appropriate for patients with hearing loss falling above the moderately severe range unless highly effective digital feedback suppression is used.

The primary functional advantage provided by the ITC/CIC style relates to the more natural listening position of the microphone. Why might this provide an advantage? Actually there are a couple of reasons, namely advantages related to localization and natural directional sensitivity. Browse through the "Things To Remember: Auditory Localization" presented earlier in this chapter if you are unfamiliar with human localization.

The filtering properties related to microphone position, commonly referred to as microphone location

effects (MLE), can act to change the frequency shape of sounds entering the hearing aid (MLE is explained in detail in Book Two of this series). Simplistically, we can think of the MLE of instruments with recessed faceplates as providing *free gain*. That is, the greater the boost provided by the pinna, the less that is needed by the hearing aid amplifier. For the open ear, the average concha effect is around 5 dB at 3000 Hz with a peak at 4250 of around 10 dB (Shaw, 1966). The differences in the MLE among hearing aid styles, therefore, also are predominately in the high frequencies, as the concha is the main player influencing these differences. This is illustrated in Figure 7–26. Notice in this figure that the benefit of the deeper microphone placement begins at about 1000 Hz, and the CIC advantage (compared with the ITE) is 5 to 10 dB above 2000 Hz. We have mentioned that CICs are not recessed too much more than many ITCs, and this is reflected in the MLE data in Figure 7–26; the CIC, however, does have a 2 to 4 dB MLE increase in the 4000 Hz region.

By moving the place where sound is sampled normally (the tympanic membrane) outward to a less natural position, the change in filtering can limit or even destroy localization in the vertical plane and remove a cue that is also used in horizontal localization. For example, consider the disadvantages of placing a microphone on top of the pinna. Conversely, a microphone

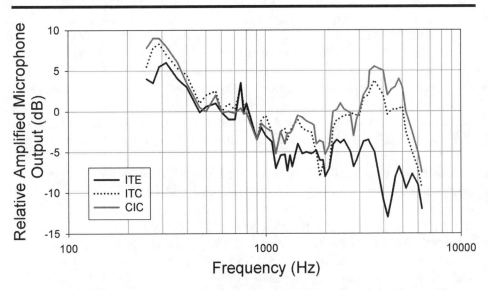

Figure 7–26. Relative MLEs (for microphone location effects) for three different custom instruments. (Modified from Fortune and Preves, 1994.)

placed inside the ear canal can provide nearly normal filtering cues that are especially important for localization in the vertical plane. As reviewed by Mueller and Ebinger (1997), when mean minimum audible angles for vertical localization were compared for the same subjects (with mild-moderate high frequency hearing loss) fitted with ITEs and CICs, there was a significant advantage for CICs over ITEs, and aided CIC localization was not significantly worse than the open ear findings. There was not a CIC advantage, however, for horizontal localization, compared with traditional ITEs.

In addition to being important for localization, the natural filtering for this style has the (usually) desirable property of providing less sensitivity to sounds arriving from behind the user in comparison with sounds arriving in front (especially in the high frequencies). This natural directional sensitivity can help us in noisy situations like restaurants by essentially turning down the level of noise and other sounds behind us a little bit relative to the level of sounds arriving from in front. By moving the microphone outward, or in the case of a traditional BTE above the ear, we change this natural directional sensitivity. This can result in sounds

being the most sensitive from the sides and even arriving from behind! The *Directivity Index* (DI; see related Key Concept for more explanation) measured across three hearing aid styles using standard omnidirectional microphones and the unaided ear are shown in Figure 7–27.

Two things are especially of note in Figure 7–27. First, the traditional BTE style is much less directional (lower DI values) than all other styles *and* the unaided ear (especially in the high frequencies). Consequently, if you took someone with normal hearing, or even a mild hearing loss, and placed them in a noisy room, we might expect the speech understanding to become worse if the individual was wearing a traditional omnidirectional BTE hearing aid (assuming they were listening to someone directly in front of them). The second, more subtle point of interest is that the CIC style is slightly more directional in the highest frequencies than the ITE and is very similar to the directivity of the unaided open ear. This is partially related to the MLE values shown earlier in Figure 7–26, combined with greater pinna shadow for sounds from the back. This illustrates that the deeper the microphone placement, the more normal the direc-

---

KEY CONCEPT:
A BRIEF EXPLANATION OF THE DIRECTIVITY INDEX (DI)

■ One way we can look at sound sensitivity in a directional manner is the DI (for Directivity Index). The DI is a calculation that gives us the output for a sound input that originates from all possible angles and elevations of arrival at the same time (diffuse sound), relative to the output for the same sound (same total acoustic power) arriving only from directly in front of the listener (0° angle and elevation).

■ Truly omnidirectional microphones are equally sensitive to sounds arriving from all angles and have a DI = 0 dB. However, primarily because of head shadow and pinna diffraction, when an omnidirectional microphone is placed in a hearing aid shell and then placed on a head, it is no longer truly omnidirectional, and the DI may be different than 0 dB (better or worse).

■ Positive DI values indicate that the microphone output for sounds directly in front are greater than that for sound integrated across all other angles and elevations. For example, if the output of the sound from 0° was 80 dB SPL, and the output from a diffuse sound arriving from all around the listener was 76 dB SPL, this would be a DI of +4 dB.

■ Although there is not a one-to-one relationship, you can roughly think of a positive DI as being an equal improvement in the SNR if the hearing aid user was listening to speech at 0° and was surrounded by noise.]

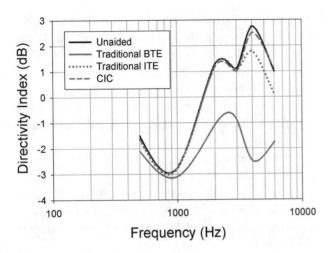

Figure 7–27. Plotting of the frequency-specific DI (for directivity index) for the open ear and three different hearing aid configurations.

tional sensitivity. Notice, however, that there is not a directional effect with these omnidirectional hearing aids in the lower frequencies—this is why directional technology (providing a DI of 4 to 5 dB or higher with a closed fitting) is nearly always the preferred fitting for listening in background noise when the listener is facing a single talker of interest.

In addition to these DI and localization advantages, the deep faceplate placement can lead to a reduction in wind noise. The wind noise advantage varies considerably depending on the origin of the wind. This was studied extensively by Fortune and Preves (1994), who compared the wind noise from a CIC to that generated by an ITC and an ITE. When averaged across several wind source azimuths, the CIC provided a 7 dB advantage compared with the ITE and was 4 dB superior (less noise) than the ITC. Most impressive, however, was when the wind originated from directly in front of the listener. For this condition, the CIC microphone location reduced wind noise by 23 dB compared with the ITE. As we discuss in Book Two of this series, modern hearing aids have wind noise cancellation algorithms, but these algorithms are not nearly as effective as simply having a deep placement of the microphone.

Finally, if these instruments are fitted tightly enough and with low enough gain settings (and/or a strong digital feedback suppression algorithm is activated), effective acoustic telephone use without feedback may be possible. Telephone use typically exacerbates feedback because bringing any surface close to the hearing aid microphone can cause sound leaking out of the ear canal to reflect back toward the microphone. This increased sound reflection, also common in many of situations such as hugging, scratching your ear, etc., greatly increases the likelihood of feedback.

Despite the positives, there are also a few potential disadvantages of the TCR style for some patients. Most notable are problems for patients without good dexterity as the instruments become smaller and insertion depth increases. Changing the smaller batteries, especially in the case of the recessed ITC and CIC styles, can be quite challenging both for those with limited dexterity or poor vision. In addition, the instruments can be more difficult to insert and remove, although this difficulty is somewhat alleviated in the CIC style through the use of a plastic handle that can be seen peeking out of the ear in Figure 7–25. These handles also can be ordered for the ITC product if necessary.

The very small size of this style and their rounded shape can also be confusing to many patients. It is not unusual for patients to try to force them into their ears sideways or upside-down or even confuse the right and left instruments before they have enough training and practice. We even know of a situation when a CIC that had been laid on a table during an intense card game was mistaken for a peanut, which then required both hearing aid and dental repair.

Differentiating between instruments made for the right and left ears can be made easier through the use of colored ink or other markers that are often added during the manufacturing process. Some manufacturers make the entire earshells different colors (commonly red and blue) while matching the faceplate to the users' skin color and tone.

In addition to the previously stated limitations, ITCs and CICs are generally not large enough and/or are in the wrong position to implement directional microphones. This technology requires that sounds arriving from the front and the back can be differentiated. This is very difficult if the microphone ports are recessed inside the ear, as sound will hit the ports after bouncing around on the surface of the pinna and ear canal. Space limitations also prevent the effective use of telecoils, FM coupling, or DAI.

Deep Canal CIC Hearing Aids

As we described earlier in this chapter, fitting hearing aids deeply into the external ear canal has the advantage of reducing or eliminating the occlusion effect. In addition, deep canal fittings lead to an overall increase in sound pressure level (especially in the high frequencies) for the same amplifier setting (the Boyle's law principle discussed earlier). More specifically, the residual ear canal volume associated with a traditional custom instrument is about 0.7 cm^3. However a deep canal CIC (CIC-DC) instrument will have a residual ear canal volume of only about 0.25 cm^3. This can result in increased output of 4 dB in the low frequencies and 8 to 10 dB at 4000 Hz (Kuk, 1994). This is an advantage in that a less powerful amplifier is needed, and because the amplifier gain is less, there is the potential for a reduction in feedback. Although almost any hearing aid type can be fitted deeply in the canal, the most commonly fitted is the CIC-DC. Most recently, the receivers of RIC instruments have also been increasingly fitted deeply in the canal for specific patients as described below. This deep fitting is usually accomplished with custom eartips and is particularly beneficial for listeners with more severe hearing loss.

The CIC-DC has all the advantages and limitations of the recessed CIC; however, the deep, tight fit has the additional advantages of alleviation of occlusion and reduction of susceptibility to feedback. Although many clinicians had high hopes for the deep fit CIC style in the 1990s, the deep, tight fit is uncomfortable for many patients, particularly for CICs with hard exterior shells (which encompasses the majority of CICs). This discomfort results both from heightened sensitivity to touch exhibited by some patients and, more important, the fact that the majority of patients demonstrate significant changes in ear canal shape and volume with jaw movement resulting in increased pressure on the ear canal from the hearing aid (e.g., Darkner, Larsen, & Paulsen, 2007). Deep canal CIC fittings are therefore not that common because many patients will not tolerate them because of discomfort. Some clinicians try to counteract these complaints by ordering them slightly shorter, but this can eliminate the advantage of the deep fittings. These shortcomings clearly remain a problem because surveys suggest that many clinicians fitting the CIC-DCs have reported problems with feedback, occlusion, and the hearing aid working itself out of the ear. Otoscopy can be a useful tool when considering whether patients may be a candidate for a deep canal style.

Because they can use a softer custom or non-custom eartip, some clinicians choose to fit mini-BTE instruments deeply in the canal. These instruments share some of the cosmetic and most of the acoustic benefits of the deep fit CIC other than the fact that the microphone position (above the ear) is slightly less optimal from the standpoint of normal localization and directivity. The use of a BTE case, however, allows for the implementation of directional microphones and

---

**TECHNICAL TIP:
HEARING AID SELECTION CONSIDERATIONS DURING OTOSCOPY**

It is important and useful to consider hearing aid styles when performing routine otoscopy:

- Look for cerumen, even small hard pockets of cerumen can be uncomfortable when pressed on by an earmold/earshell. Depending on the position, walls or shelves of cerumen can increase feedback problems. Ask the patient if they have cerumen problems. How often do they have to have their ears cleaned?
- Ask the patient to open their mouth, talk, and simulate chewing. Does their ear canal move a lot, does it completely change shape? If so, a deeper and or tighter fitting may not be possible without discomfort.
- How does the patient react to the otoscope tip? If the otoscope tip is uncomfortable, or if he or she seems jumpy, a tight shell probably will be bothersome too!

telecoils, as well as high levels of gain and a softer eartip, providing potential advantages over CICs.

For the rare patient with large, straight ear canals, little ear canal movement associated with jaw movement, and ear canals that are relatively insensitive to pain, the CIC-DC fitting can be used to fit up through severe hearing losses. Although certainly not for everyone, more success fitting severe hearing loss is expected for the deep canal placement when using flexible, soft tips with RICs in comparison with more traditional hard shell CICs.

Several attempts have been made to try to make deep fitted CICs more comfortable by using a softer earshell. The softer earshell has sometimes been problematic, however, because the internal components can be damaged during insertion and removal as there is not a hard shell to protect them. At least one manufacturer has attempted to circumvent this problem by making a deep fitting CIC that is intended to be professionally placed in listeners with less than severe hearing loss and left in the ear for an extended wear period (reportedly up to 120 days). According to the manufacturer, this extended wear time is made possible through the use of soft antibacterial seals and a proprietary mechanical and coating technology developed to protect the device from moisture and ear wax. Although not waterproof (swimming is not recommended), the manufacturers claim the instruments are water-resistant enough to allow the patient to shower.

In addition to the possibility of discomfort, placing the receiver increasingly closer to the ear canal and close to the medial tip of the earshell or eartip can create another difficulty. This proximity to the outer ear environment, which can be moist and cerumen-filled, increases the chances that the receiver will become clogged with debris. A number of *wax-guard* designs are currently in use, many of which are expected to help with this problem, but it certainly is not solved (the guards themselves become clogged).

Open Canal (OC) Fittings

Recall that we mentioned earlier that we would be categorizing the different hearing aid styles relative to their *function*. This clearly applies for OC (for open canal) fittings, as the style could be traditional BTE, mini-BTE, or a variety of types of custom instruments. As the name implies, OC hearing aids are functionally differentiated from other styles because they leave the ear canal mostly open, which then results in the absence of the objective or subjective occlusion effect when they are fitted. In general, the occlusion effect is eliminated when the hearing aid has a vent of 4-mm or larger (e.g., Kiessling, Brenner, Thunber-Jespersen, Groth, & Jensen, 2005). Because such a large vent is needed, most OC fittings use a BTE case (usually the mini-BTE, as the gain from the larger model is not needed); however, there are some

---

TECHNICAL TIP: WAX GUARDS

■ Most manufacturers have a variety of wax guards, and because there is no magical wax guard, designs continually change. The goal of these devices is to protect the receiver from being impacted with wax. Instead the wax guard will become clogged, and it can be changed rather than requiring a receiver repair or replacement. You can think of it as a trap, as well as a guard. In some cases, the patient is instructed to replace wax guards at home, which works fine for those patients with good vision, dexterity, and dilligence.

■ Wax guards differ in how effective they are. If we consider wax guards from a single manufacturer, those that protect the receiver very well tend to clog more easily and, therefore, require more frequent changing. Those that provide less protection also tend to clog less often. This of course also interacts with the consistency of the individual patient's cerumen. Therefore, the choice of wax guard is an individualized decision that requires weighing convenience and protection while considering individual patient differences.

POINTS-TO-PONDER: A LITTLE OC HISTORY

There is little documentation of the first OC fittings, but we know they received considerable attention immediately after the CROS-type hearing aids described in the next section were introduced. It was quickly discovered that the non-occluding earpieces used for the CROS hearing aid (or tubing only) also could be used for ipsilateral high-frequency amplification (hence, the term IROS [ipsilateral routing of signals], referring to a large vent).

In the late 1960s, researchers showed that OC fittings could provide useful high-frequency amplification (Green, 1969). In the early 1980s, OC fittings were attempted with *horn tubing*, with some success. Over the years, clinicians more or less lost interest in OC fittings because feedback problems precluded their use for all but the mildest high frequency hearing losses. This lack of interest persisted until key technological and cosmetic factors came together to greatly increase the popularity of OC fittings:

- Feedback suppression algorithms became more common and more effective.
- Miniaturization allowed for production of cosmetically appealing mini-BTEs.
- The mini-BTEs were coupled to the ear using a thin cosmetically appealing tube or wire.
- Non-custom eartips were developed that were comfortable and non-occluding.

It is fair to say that this culmination of factors had a huge impact on the entire hearing aid market in the mid to late 2000s, and rather quickly a large portion of custom hearing aid sales moved to the category of BTE. Specifically, BTE sales comprised only about 20% in 2004, were up to approximately 50% by 2007, and exceeded 70% in 2012. We do not really know what percent of these BTE sales were indeed for open fittings, but it probably was the majority. Mueller (2009) reported on a dispenser survey that revealed that approximately 25% of dispensers stated that at least 70% of their sales were mini-BTE open fittings. We wonder if some of these actually ended up being somewhat closed when feedback problems emerged, but nevertheless, they were using the mini-BTE style rather than custom.

methods that use custom instruments and also keep the ear canal mostly open.

The OC style typically includes a mini-BTE case that directs sound to the ear through a thin (approximately 0.9 mm) tube or a thin wire that attaches to a small external receiver that is placed in the ear canal. Recall from our earlier discussion that these configurations are referred to as RITA and RIC, respectively—see Figures 7–28 and 7–29. The success of modern OC instruments has been made possible through the advent and refinement of modern hearing aid sound processing algorithms that act to suppress or filter out feedback. These digital feedback suppression algorithms are discussed in more detail in Book Two of this series.

Because nearly all OC fitting are implemented using mini-BTE hearing aids, we include some of these

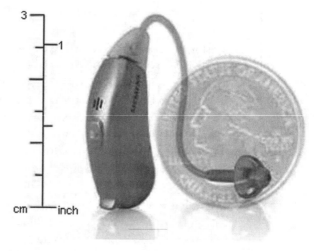

Figure 7–28. Example of a mini-BTE RITA hearing aid.

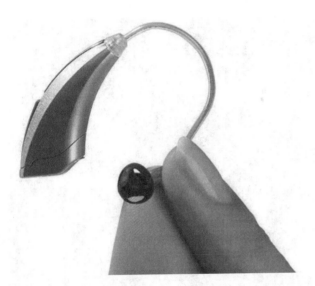

Figure 7–29. Example of a mini-BTE RIC hearing aid (Photo courtesy of Starkey).

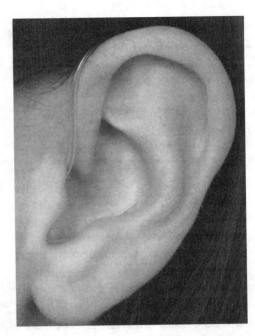

Figure 7–30. Example of a mini-BTE RITA fitted to the ear—from this view all that is visible is the thin tubing (Photo © [2012] Unitron. All rights reserved).

features in our discussion (see earlier section on mini-BTEs for more details). The physical design of this fitting provides many potential advantages including relief from occlusion, a light and expectedly comfortable fit over the ear, although also potentially providing greater physical comfort through the use of a comfortable non-occluding eartip. The non-occluding tips usually fit comfortably into the ear canal, and as a consequence, when on the ear, all that is noticeable is the thin tube, shown in Figure 7–30. The non-occluding eartips can be either non-custom or custom-made for an individual's ear to improve retention. Several styles of non-custom, non-occluding eartips are shown in Figure 7–31 and discussed in detail in Chapter 8. In addition to the elimination of occlusion and all of its negative consequences as reviewed earlier, the open eartip also allows natural, low-frequency sounds to leak in, which is expected to improve sound quality for patients with low frequency hearing thresholds at or near the normal range (Cox & Alexander, 1983).

The advantages of OC hearing aids and mini-BTE instruments in both open and more closed configurations are clearly supported in current sales numbers as mentioned previously. Patients also appear to show a strong preference for this style. A recent study within the VA health system demonstrated that after trials with mini-BTE OC instruments and traditional custom instruments, approximately 85% of the 288 patients evaluated reported a preference for the OC style .

TECHNICAL TIP: OC FITTINGS—IT IS THE *RESULT* NOT THE *INTENT*

The style category of OC fittings is somewhat different from the other styles we have discussed, as what is important is the result of the fitting, not the intent. We explain. If you were fitting a patient with a pair of CICs, and when you put the hearing aids in the ear you saw that the faceplates were recessed into the ear canal, you indeed would know that you fitted the CIC style. But an OC fitting is only an OC fitting if the ear canal is left open (which easily can be determined by conducting probe-microphone REOR measures, but often difficult to determine doing a visual inspection). The point being, simply using mini-BTEs, thin tubes, and stock eartips that are labeled open does not mean that the result will be an open fitting. Conversely, some eartips that are labeled closed result in so much slit leak venting in some ear canals, the resultant fitting is essentially open. The final result, of course, impacts the benefit of OC fittings that we have discussed here.

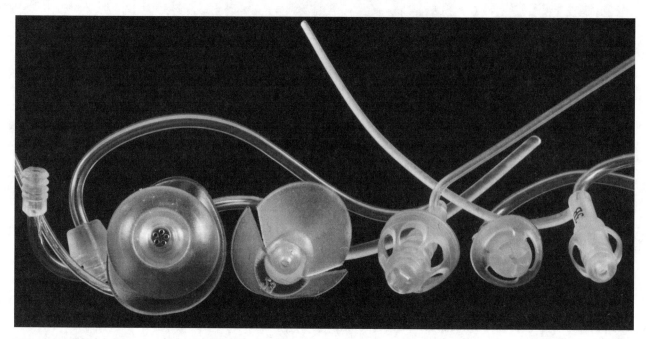

Figure 7–31. Five examples of non-custom eartips attached to either thin tubing or a thin wire, for use with OC hearing aids.

TECHNICAL TIP: EARTIPS FOR OC FITTINGS

We review the different eartips that are available in Chapter 8. But, because we are talking about OC fittings at this time, here are some bonus points to remember:

- Because no earmold impression is needed, non-custom eartips have a clear advantage in time, cost savings, and time efficiency. They typically also are comfortable, as they fit quite loosely.
- There are several limitations to non-custom eartips though, including:
  - Limited retention, especially in ear canals with unusual shapes.
  - Many non-custom eartips have extremely limited durability and may require changing as often as every 3 to 6 months.
  - It may be more difficult to direct the sound outlet away from an ear canal wall leading to greater susceptibility to feedback in some patients.
  - Many patients may have difficulty consistently placing the non-custom tip in the same place. This can affect the frequency response, sound level, and susceptibility to feedback. That is, the hearing aid may work better on some days than others simply depending on how well the patient is able to insert it.

While many clinicians fit the majority of mini-BTEs on patients with non-custom eartips, some clinician's we have spoken with have switched back to using custom eartips, even when fitting with an open venting configuration because of these limitations. These custom eartips are expected to allow for better retention, better ability to direct the sound outlet away from the ear canal wall reducing susceptibility to feedback, and better durability of the eartip.

As discussed previously, one larger limitation that can affect a large number of potential patients relates to one of the mini-BTE instruments' primary advantages, its diminutive size and the challenges that it presents to those with limited dexterity or poor vision. In some cases, simply using a larger BTE with the thin tubing will make enough difference, and then the OC fitting is still possible.

Another limitation to an OC fitting is that the large vent allows a great deal of the amplified low frequencies to leak out. Consequently, a very high amount of low frequency amplifier gain is needed to provide any amplification at the patient's tympanic membrane. Due in part to the negative affect high amplifier gain has on battery life and amplification of circuit noise, as well as the need for a larger receiver, many manufacturers choose to forgo this low frequency amplifier gain altogether and target patients with hearing loss limited to the higher frequencies (above 1000 Hz or even 2000 Hz).

This of course can be a problem when a closed mold is added to provide additional gain at 500 Hz. As an alternative, as we mentioned earlier, manufacturers of RIC instruments will sometimes have multiple receivers available for the same model, so clinicians may select the receiver with adequate power for the patient, while still considering that the receiver and eartip must be small enough to fit in the patient's ear canal. Clearly clinicians must be careful to select instruments with adequate low frequency gain available when fitting patients with low frequency hearing loss. Furthermore, because of artifacts including an echo type effect and hearing a talker's voice emanating from the listeners ear, the magnitude of low-frequency amplification provided by the OC style is generally limited. One simple fix for patients with more low frequency loss, however, is to fit a mini-BTE instrument but simply select a tighter fitting eartip.

The lack of low frequency gain also has other implications. Although presented as a limitation, the ability to

POINTS TO PONDER: OPEN OR CLOSED FOR HIGH FREQUENCY GAIN?

Regarding high frequency gain, consider that with an OC fitting that is truly open, the patient retains all or most of the natural ear canal resonance (with a closed fitting this is not the case). This of course primarily is in the 2000 to 3000 Hz range—the very frequency range where we usually are struggling to obtain desired gain. See Figure 7–32 for an example of the average residual ear canal resonance when an open tip is placed in the ear (Mueller & Ricketts, 2006). The remaining average ear canal resonance is around 15 dB or so, so is this a *free* 15 dB of gain for our patients? Sound too good to be true? It is. Remember the advantages of a deep fitting that we discussed earlier—the increased SPL when we make the residual ear canal smaller? With an OC fitting, we do not obtain this advantage, which can amount to 10 dB or more, depending on how deep the earmold goes into the ear canal.

So what is the true gain advantage of leaving the ear canal open? This was studied by Mueller and Ricketts (2006) and is displayed in Figure 7–33. By conducting probe-microphone measures on real ears and changing only the earmold (open versus closed), they were able to identify the true advantage of leaving the ear canal open. This figure represents a difference curve; above the 0 dB line indicates an advantage for the OC fitting. Observe that on average, this advantage is about 5 dB in the region of the ear canal resonance. There are individual variations depending on the patient's open ear resonance (how much do they have to lose?) and the size of the ear canal (smaller ear canals will be impacted more by a closed earmold). As expected, the closed earmold made a large difference in the average gain in the lower frequencies, especially for hearing aid A; hearing aid B did not have amplifier gain for the very low frequencies. This shows just how much gain really is leaking out with the OC fitting. Normally, this leakage is not a concern, as we would not be conducting an OC fitting if the patient needed low frequency gain.

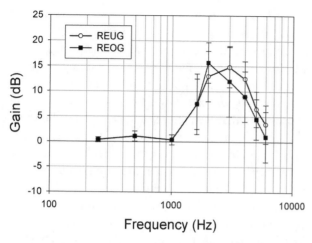

Figure 7–32. Average REUR and REOR for 14 individuals, fitted with non-custom stock open eartips for the REOR measures. (Adapted from Mueller and Ricketts, 2006.)

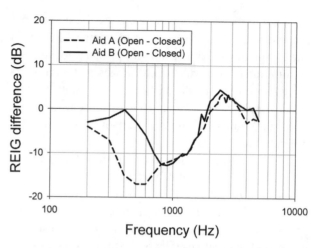

Figure 7–33. Difference in average insertion gain for two mini-BTE hearing aids measured using an open and closed fitting tip. Earmold tubing and hearing aid settings were unchanged. (Adapted from Mueller and Ricketts, 2006.)

provide only high frequency gain can also be seen as an advantage for many patients. Specifically, the OC style is ideal for patients with normal or near-normal hearing in the low frequencies, but requiring substantial high-frequency amplification because of the presence of mild to moderately severe high frequency hearing loss. This steeply sloping hearing loss configuration was quite difficult to fit prior to the introduction of OC instruments and now may be fitted quite easily.

It is important to point out, that even in patients without low frequency hearing loss for which no gain is required, the lack of low frequency gain will have an effect on the function of specific features. That is, certain features such as digital noise reduction and directional microphone technology only will be effective in OC instruments in the high frequency range for which significant gain is provided. These features likely will be less noticeable by the patient in an OC fitting. A detailed discussion of this topic is presented in Book Two of this series, illustrated using probe-microphones measures in Book Three.

Although the amount of low frequency gain may be affected by manufacturers' design decisions, the amount of high frequency peak gain (i.e., in the 2000 to 3500 Hz range) before the introduction of audible feedback is commonly limited by the effectiveness of the feedback suppression algorithm. Although such sys-

tems are constantly improving, current OC hearing aids are generally limited to patients with less than severe high frequency thresholds, assuming that audibility in these high frequencies is desired. In addition, large and clear differences in the effectiveness of feedback suppression continue to be exhibited across manufacturers and models. Consider that if there is a 10 dB difference between the gain-before-feedback between hearing aid models (and there is), this could affect the fitting range by 20 dB or more. These differences again highlight the importance of a clinician's knowledge related to the operation and limitations of the specific models they choose to fit. The effectiveness of the different feedback systems is very easy to assess on real patients using your probe-microphone equipment.

Although the vast majority of OC hearing aids use a thin tube or thin wire and are designed for BTE placement of the case, at least two companies have introduced unique case placements such as those designed to fit in the fossa of the helix, shown in Figure 7–34, and those that place the microphone in the fossa of the helix or in the ear canal, shown in Figure 7–35. Some of these designs are quite unique and are aimed at improving the naturalness of the microphone placement and/or targeted to individuals who wish to integrate their hearing aid into their personal sense of fashion. This target audience is assumed because some configurations

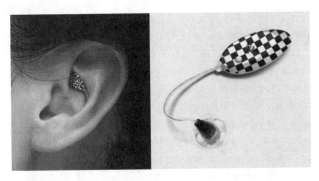

Figure 7–34. Unique RIC product with hearing aid case designed to fit in the fossa of the helix (Photo courtesy of Siemens Hearing Instruments, Inc.).

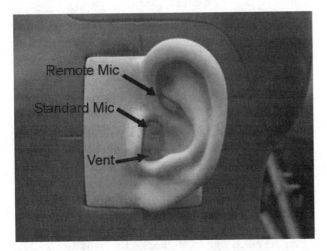

Figure 7–35. Hearing aid designed with detachable microphone (Photo courtesy of GN ReSound).

are available with a wide range of interchangeable case covers, which use a variety of color schemes (including checkerboard, leopard skin, etc.). Although there are some potential benefits, these designs all typically result in closer spacing between the receiver and microphone that can greatly limit available gain before feedback and are therefore primarily aimed at individuals with mild-moderate high frequency hearing loss.

Hearing Aid Style: Mini-Summary

■ Selection of hearing aid style is a complex process. Although some styles can be ruled out based on the degree of hearing loss alone,

many styles may be appropriate for a single hearing loss configuration.

■ Style decisions can be highly impacted by cosmetics; however, the cosmetics in the hand do not always relate to the cosmetics on the head. Hair style, choice of color and material, and the exact instrument chosen can all affect the final cosmetics on the head.

■ In addition to cosmetics and degree of hearing loss, the desired features should always be an important consideration because not all features are available in all styles. Size and movement of the ear canal should also be considered, especially when considering a tight and/or deep fit.

■ Finally, regardless of what *you believe* is the best style, it is important to involve the patient in this selection process. Fitting a pair of full-concha ITEs to a patient who really wants CICs, so that an extra 3 dB directional advantage can be added, is only a good move if the patient wears the hearing aids.

Special Designs and Styles

The styles we have talked about so far are all quite common in clinical use. Although the distinction is somewhat artificial, we will now talk about some styles and designs that are either less common or aimed at specific populations. This distinction is especially artificial because one could argue that few hearing aid styles we have discussed so far are really appropriate for all populations and hearing loss configurations, and certainly no hearing aid style discussed so far is optimal for all populations and hearing loss configurations. Despite this artificial distinction, it is common for new clinicians to have significantly less experience with the following hearing aid styles that include CROS/BiCROS, those that deliver sound through bone conduction (both traditional and implantable) and middle ear implants. Rather than an in-depth treatment of these options, they are only briefly introduced here for completeness and to highlight the importance of considering all possible styles as well as hearing assistive technologies when making fitting decisions. To aid in selection decisions, we have summarized all the hearing aid styles presented in a single table at the end of this chapter (Table 7–2).

Contralateral Routing of Signal (CROS) and BiCROS Hearing Aids

The CROS (for contralateral routing of signal) hearing aid is designed for patients with no usable hearing in one ear, and normal hearing or a minimal hearing loss in the other ear (Harford & Barry, 1965; Harford & Dodds, 1966; Matkin & Thomas, 1972). This configuration of hearing loss is commonly referred to as *single-sided deafness*. The goal is to give the patient two-sided hearing, when true bilateral hearing is not possible. Recall that one of the requirements for bilateral amplification is aidable hearing in both ears; the CROS is an alternative to a traditional unilateral fitting for these patients.

Consider this scenario. Your Monday morning patient is a 40-year-old woman who just lost her hearing in her right ear three months ago, as a result of surgery to remove an acoustic neuroma. She is bothered by not hearing in this ear, is having some problems at work, and is eager to try whatever is available that might help. You really have five different CROS choices:

- A pair of hearing aids that are connected by wire (probably routed behind the head).
- A pair of hearing aids with the sound conducted wirelessly from the bad side to the good side.
- A single hearing aid: A transcranial CROS with an air conduction receiver in the bad ear.
- A single hearing aid: A transcranial CROS with a bone conduction receiver in the bad ear.
- An implantable bone conduction hearing aid on the bad side.

Traditional Air Conduction

In the traditional CROS system, the microphone and amplification stages are contained within either a BTE or ITE case that is located on the impaired side. Early versions of the CROS often used a wire, sometimes routed through eyeglasses or a headband. The receiver is located on the side with better (normal) hearing within a BTE or ITE case. The microphone and receiver may be coupled by a wire that runs around the back of the neck, through the frame of eyeglass BTEs, or the signal may be transmitted wirelessly. The wired BTE style used to account for the majority of CROS hearing aids

(circa 1980 and before). Current CROS fittings, however, are commonly achieved through the use of wireless transmission that is usually in BTE, mini-BTE or ITE cases—the appearance is more or less the same as we discussed earlier for these styles. Currently, it is common for wireless streaming from one hearing aid to the other to be completed by near field induction or one of a number of radio wave protocols. Although the newest protocols allow for wireless streaming in a much greater range of styles, including mini-BTE, and can sometimes have much less interference, they may also be limited by very short battery life (in some cases less than a full day). We expect this to be a short-term problem however, as these protocols will continue to improve both in terms of quality and battery consumption.

The clearest advantage for the CROS fitting is that the user can use the good ear to hear signals from the impaired side that are otherwise attenuated by head shadow. For all of these type of fittings, when there is normal hearing in the better ear, sound from the receiver is usually directed into the ear using as much venting as possible, so that the normal sound pathway for the better ear is not blocked. As a result of the large amount of venting, it is typical for only higher frequency signals to reach the ear with normal hearing, leading to complaints of a tinny sound quality. By convention, it is usual to refer to the device as a left CROS when the aided signal is routed to the left ear and a right CROS when the aided signal is routed to the right ear.

Clearly, CROS hearing aids are more successful in some instances than others (e.g., Gelfand, 1979; Upfold, 1980). It is our experience, however, that overall the success rate of this style for patients with single-sided deafness (normal hearing in the better ear) is relatively low. The inconvenience of using two devices, poor sound quality, audible circuit noise, and poor cosmetics are often cited as reasons for rejection of CROS amplification. Successful users often report a critical communication need in an environment in which they are surrounded by important speakers and are highly motivated to hear sounds arriving from both sides equally. Recent reports suggest that the modern CROS hearing aid is more readily accepted than earlier models (e.g., Hill, Marcus, Digges, Gillman, & Silverstein, 2006). This probably is because they are less bulky and have a more appropriate and adjustable frequency response. Despite these data, acceptance rates for CROS hearing aids in the literature generally are between 20% and

---

THINGS-TO-REMEMBER: HEARING AIDS AND HEAD SHADOW

Listening conditions change throughout the day, and input from the side without hearing can be useful for people who cannot always control the direction of the sound reaching their ears. People in the business world, for example, seem to notice the greatest handicap from single-sided deafness, as they are frequently in meetings, luncheons, etc, where the talker of interest often is located on their "bad side."

■ The benefit from placing a microphone on the side without usable hearing mainly relates to offsetting audibility and SNR difficulties related to head shadow. Specifically, for unaided listening, when a talker is on the impaired side, the signal will reach the good ear after the level has been reduced by head shadow.

■ The amount of attenuation from head shadow is essentially zero in the low frequencies but can reach more than 15 dB in the higher frequencies (see Figure 7–2).

■ If noise happens to be present on the good side, the attenuation provided by head shadow can be especially detrimental because of the decreased SNR.

■ Conversely, if noise is on the bad side and speech is on the good side, head shadow can work to the patient's advantage. That is, the CROS configuration in this case can *decrease* speech recognition in noise in comparison with unaided listening.

50%. Due in part to the lack of acceptance of CROS hearing aids, a variety of device types that stimulate the cochlea through bone conduction have been advocated for treatment of single-sided deafness. These devices are discussed in the next section of this chapter. As you might guess, very few CROS hearing aids are dispensed, and for this reason, many manufacturers do not even offer this style.

BiCROS Applications. Patients with SSD who also have some hearing impairment in the better ear are often more successful candidates than those with normal hearing, partly because they entered the fitting with more communication problems. In cases in which amplification is provided to the better ear in addition to the contralateral routing of signals, the instruments are referred to as BiCROS (e.g., there also is a microphone for the instrument on the side of the "better" ear; two microphones sending signals to one amplifier/receiver). The higher success rates in patients with hearing loss in their better ear has been partially attributed to the reduced annoyance because of audibility of circuit noise,

and the decreased venting typically used (to provide low-frequency amplification) improves the sound quality of signals arriving from both sides (Del Dot, Hickson, & O'Connell, 1992; Hill et al., 2006). The general rule of thumb is that if you look at the good ear in isolation, and you consider that ear in need of amplification, then the BiCROS rather than the CROS would be selected. These products are also switchable, so that the patient can turn on or off either microphone for specific listening situations—if noise is present from the side of the bad ear, this microphone could be turned off.

Verification. Finally, we want to mention that traditional CROS and BiCROS hearing aids need to be fitted just like all other hearing aids. That is, probe-microphone testing is required to assure that the frequency response and output is appropriate. This is sometimes overlooked, as the setup is somewhat different than with a standard fitting. We discuss the protocol for CROS verification in detail in Book Three of this series; Pumford (2005) also has written a useful review on this procedure.

Transcranial CROS

As the name indicates, in this type of fitting we are referring to sending the signal through the skull (via bone conduction). *Transcranial CROS* fittings have been proposed as a way to alleviate some of the complaints related to CROS amplification (e.g., Valente, Potts, Valente, & Goebel, 1995). The goal of this type of CROS fitting is to place an air-conducted signal in the bad ear that is loud enough that it crosses over via bone conduction to the good ear. This intervention usually implements a single deep canal instrument (usually a CIC or BTE style with deep fitted earmold), which is fitted to the ear without hearing. In true transcranial CROS implementation, the deep fit allows for mechanical coupling between the hearing aid shell and the bony portion of the ear canal. The mechanical coupling, when combined with high levels of hearing aid output, allows for transmission of sound to the contralateral cochlea through both bone conduction and air conduction (traveling around the head). In the usually less successful *quasi transcranial CROS*, the instrument is not placed tight and/or deep enough to achieve mechanical coupling. The transcranial CROS has the advantage of using only a single instrument on the impaired side and the fact that little, if any, circuit noise will be transmitted to the better ear. We talk about clinical methods to assess the potential success of a transcranial fitting in probe-microphone section of Book Three of this series. Valente et al. (1995) has published a useful review on this topic.

Fitting Considerations. The patient's hearing for bone conduction in the good ear and their interaural attenuation will determine what output levels are needed for this type of a transcranial CROS to be successful. We believe that it is important to first develop *fitting targets*. By using probe-microphone equipment to measure ear canal SPL in the bad ear, it is possible to determine what output in this ear will crossover to the good ear. Frequency-specific, pure-tone signals are delivered from the audiometer, and the transducer used *does* matter. It is best to use an insert receiver, placed at approximately the depth of the hearing aid, using a tip that has a hardness that is similar to the hearing aid. Hard rubber immittance tips coupled to an insert earphone is one option. When the patient says they hear the tones in the good ear, the real-ear SPL in the bad ear is measured for each frequency. In general, we would like to

place speech at least 15 to 20 dB SL in the good ear, so adding 20 dB or so to the measured values will provide the ear canal SPL targets for the hearing aid fitting. For example, if the 2000 Hz signal is heard in the good ear at 80 dB RESPL (real-ear SPL), then the ear canal SPL target at 2000 Hz for an average-level speech-shaped signal would be 100 dB RESPL for this frequency. The mechanical vibrations of an actual hearing aid (which, as we mentioned will greatly influence the transmission) are different than those of the insert used for testing, so these targets still are not as precise as we would like.

Other than probe-microphone testing, it is difficult to verify the effectiveness of the transcranial CROS fitting in the office or clinic. However, it is probable that benefit only will occur when:

- The bone-conducted signal originating from the bad ear exceeds the air-conducted signal arriving at the good ear.
- The bone-conducted signal originating from the bad ear exceeds the background noise level at the good ear.

Because we know that the transcranial bone-conducted signal at the cochlea of the good ear probably will not be more than 30 to 40 dB SPL, for the above two conditions to occur, the patient would need to be listening to soft speech in quiet, with the speech delivered from the side of the bad ear. (Because of head shadow, the amplified bone-conducted high frequencies of speech now will be louder in the good ear than the air-conducted signals traveling around the head.) If this listening situation occurs frequently in the patient's everyday life and the patient considers this listening situation important, then the patient just might become a regular transcranial CROS user.

Despite the potential advantages, most patients are not appropriate candidates for this type of transcranial CROS because they find the required deep fitting uncomfortable or even painful. As a consequence, appropriate screening to determine if the patient will tolerate a deep tight fit is critical prior to trying this fitting. This screening can be done by having the patient try a deep fitting earplug made of a harder plastic material.

Alternative Transcranial Choices. As we have discussed, one problem with the traditional transcranial attempts is generating a strong enough, bone-conducted signal. For this reason, a number of bone conduction devices also have been introduced over the years, which include those that stimulate in a number of different ways. In general, these devices have been aimed at patients with single-sided deafness who are looking for an alternative CROS application but are not interested in surgical options (which we describe in the next section). One method that has been used for many years, originally designed for individuals with conductive hearing losses, is a bone conduction eyeglass hearing aid. Historically, these have not been successful, for all the reasons we mentioned earlier in this chapter regarding why eyeglass hearing aids in general are usually not successful. Additionally, we now have a hearing aid that is even heavier and more cumbersome to use—the vibrator in the temple needs to be positioned firmly on the mastoid. There are two other bone conduction devices, however, that are fairly new to the market: the TransEar and the SoundBite.

TransEar. The TransEar was introduced in 2004 by United Hearing Systems and is now manufactured by Ear Technology Corp and has been specifically marketed as a solution for single-sided deafness. With this device, the microphone and processing are contained within a BTE case that connects to a piece in the ear using a small wire. The configuration of this part of the device is essentially identical to that used in receiver in the ear mini-BTE devices, so we could call this a RIC hearing aid. The difference, however, is that with the TransEar the wire terminates in a small bone conduction vibrator encased in an earmold placed in the ear canal of the poorer ear, rather than in a typical receiver, shown in Figure 7–36. As with other transcranial approaches, the patient must be willing to accept a hard shell that is fitted fairly deeply into the ear canal. The device has modern features such as digital noise reduction and directional technology. And as with other devices, acoustic feedback can be an issue.

SoundBite. Another interesting way of delivering bone-conducted signals to the cochlea is demonstrated by the SoundBite,™ which also has been marketed as a solution for single-sided deafness and conductive hearing loss. It is not considered a "hearing aid" and has been labeled as a *prosthetic device* by the FDA. The manufacturer, Sonitus Medical, therefore, refers to the SoundBite as a prosthetic hearing device, which can cause some

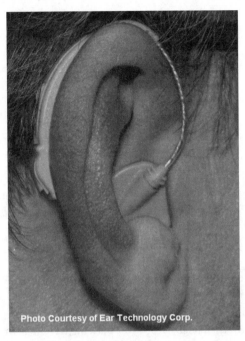

Photo Courtesy of Ear Technology Corp.

Figure 7–36. Example of a BTE hearing aid with a bone conduction receiver fitted in the ear (Photo courtesy of Ear Technology Corp.)

confusion. In this device, the microphone and processing are housed in a mini-BTE case, and then the signal is wirelessly routed to a vibrating transducer that is worn on the upper back teeth, shown in Figure 7–37.[46] And yes indeed, the manufacturer of the product refer to it as an In-the- Mouth (ITM) device. There are no replaceable batteries for either device; a system charger is used for both. Although there is little research with this product, one early study with single-sided deafness (SSD) participants reported significant improvement in laboratory speech and noise testing, and also for real-world ratings of speech-in-noise understanding (Murray, Popelka, & Miller, et al., 2011). They also reported no audiologic, medical, or dental complications (based on a 30-day and 6 month clinical trial).

Implantable Bone Conduction Stimulation

Our final solution for single-sided deafness is an implantable bone conduction device. These instruments were initially designed for individuals with conductive

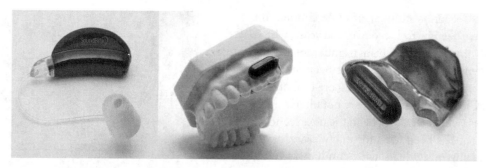

Figure 7–37. BTE microphone and ITM bone conduction receiver of the SoundBite hearing aid (Photo courtesy of Sonitus Medical.)

hearing losses, so we review their clinician applications in general, including to the patient with single-sided deafness.

Many hearing impaired patients have hearing loss that is primarily conductive in nature. Although conductive and mixed hearing loss often can be habilitated with traditional air conduction hearing aids, these aids are sometimes not appropriate because of problems with retention or other issues. For example, a patient may have physical malformation of the pinna and/or an external ear canal that makes retention a problem—see Figure 7–38 for an example. In some cases, the external ear malformation (e.g., stenosis) may preclude placement of a hearing aid because of space limitations, the lack of an external ear canal, or other factors. Still other patients may find that a hearing aid or earmold placed in the ear may exacerbate an existing ear problem or result in the recurrence of a pathologic condition. It is important to reiterate that for many patients with conductive and mixed hearing loss, air conduction hearing aids may be a reasonable or even the optimal solution. The potential advantage for air conduction instruments for conductive hearing losses relates to the fact that they generally are able to provide a broader frequency response. However, when air conduction hearing aids are problematic, stimulation of the inner ear through bone conduction may be a reasonable alternative.

With traditional bone conduction hearing aids, a bone conduction receiver is placed on the mastoid and held in position by a headband, shown in Figure 7–39, or using eyeglasses. With these traditional bone conduction hearing aids, the cochlea is stimulated in the same way as it is during bone conduction threshold

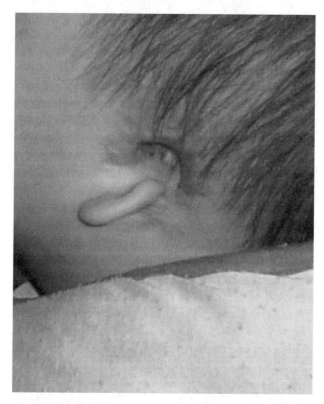

Figure 7–38. Example of pinna and ear canal malformation precluding the use of a traditional air conduction hearing aid.

assessments. Some patients may need stronger vibrations because of unusually thick or dense skin and/or fat deposits under the skin at the stimulation site (Laitakari, Löppönen, Salmivalli, & Sorri, 1995). Therefore,

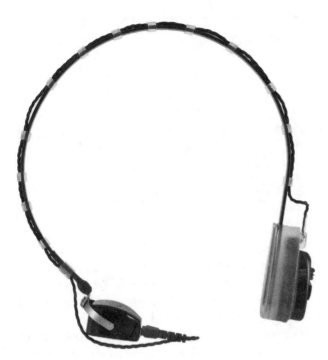

Figure 7–39. Example of a traditional bone conduction hearing aid.

although bone conduction hearing aids can be used for any degree of conductive component, only a mild-to-moderate sensorineural component may be present before providing appropriate audibility becomes difficult or impossible.

Despite the fact that some patients enjoy success with traditional bone conduction hearing aids, they have been criticized by others because of the often large, sometimes cumbersome, sometimes physically uncomfortable, and not particularly cosmetically appealing nature of their retention systems. In response to these complaints, many methods have been investigated for coupling a bone conduction vibrator to the head. To date, the most successful alternative method for patients who experience unilateral or bilateral conductive or mixed losses has been to surgically implant a titanium screw and abutment assembly into the skull that allow for the snapping on of a bone vibrator. The first such device that received FDA (for U.S. Department of Food and Drug Administration) approval in the United States is known as the Baha (e.g., Hol, Bosman, Snik, Mylanus, & Cremers, 2004; Wazen et al., 1998; Westerkull, 2002). The Baha was approved for use in the United States by the FDA for patients with bilateral conductive hearing loss in January, 1999 (FDA, 1999). Its original manufacturer, Entific Medical Systems, was purchased by Cochlear Corporation in 2005. In recent times, Oticon Medical received FDA approval to market its devices known as the Ponto in 2011. Currently, both Baha (Baha 3) and Ponto (Ponto Pro) ear-level devices are available. Each model has a *family*; the primary differences within each family relate to the amount of power available.

In all cases, these are percutaneous (through the skin) devices, and all the hearing aid components including a bone conduction vibrator are inside a plastic

---

KEY CONCEPT: HEARING THROUGH BONE CONDUCTION

- The bones of the skull can be stimulated directly by vibrations that are then carried through the skull to both cochleas with little attenuation. It is interesting to note that bone conduction has been used as a way to stimulate the cochlea in patients with conductive hearing loss since at least the seventeenth century (Berger, 1976a).

- Unfortunately however, a fair amount of vibration energy is required to stimulate the ear by bone conduction, due in part to the attenuation provided by the skin.

- Stimulation is only needed in one spot to stimulate both cochleas, because the transcranial attenuation for bone conduction is usually low.

- Despite what you may have learned at one time or another, interaural attenuation for bone-conducted signals is not always 0 dB. There are individual patient differences, and there is usually significant attenuation above 5 kHz in most listeners.

POINTS TO PONDER: BAHA AND Baha

In this section we talk about the "Baha." A rather strange name, unless you think it's a botched spelling of Baja, California. Here's the story. In a former life, Baha was BAHA, which was an acronym for Bone-Anchored Hearing Aid. When Cochlear acquired the device in the mid-2000s, it was officially renamed an "osseointegrated cochlear stimulator"—a term more acceptable to insurance companies that do not reimburse for hearing aids. So today, we don't have a BAHA, but still do have a Baha, which is the name of specific products, not a class of products or amplification approach.

---

case that is coupled to a titanium screw that is usually implanted in the upper mastoid region of the temporal bone via a titanium abutment screw that protrudes through the skin, shown in Figure 7–40.

Depending on the version, additional features including directional microphones and DAI are commonly available. A number of advanced processing features common in air conduction hearing aids including multichannel directivity, multichannel gain processing, and digital feedback suppression have also been introduced in some implantable bone stimulating devices. Data have shown that implantable bone stimulating devices can lead to a significant decrease in handicap, as well as an enhanced perception of general well-being and disease specific quality of life when compared with pretreatment across a range of conductive hearing loss etiologies (e.g., Laitakari et al., 1995; Lustig et al., 2001). More recently, bilateral implantable bone stimulating devices have also been advocated for use in patients with bilateral mixed or conductive hearing loss. Data as to the effectiveness of this intervention, however, is still limited.

As with all hearing aid styles, there are also a few limitations to implantable bone stimulating devices. First, the lower power versions are primarily effective for patients with conductive hearing loss (no sensorineural component). However, according to the manufacturers, the power versions can be used with mixed hearing losses having sensorineural components of up to 50 dB HL (bone conduction average of 500, 1000, and 2000 Hz). In addition to hearing loss considerations, surgical care must be taken to ensure optimal placement on the side of the head, especially if a directional microphone is used. Finally, a limited percentage of patients will experience a few medical complications (Wade, 2002). Most com-

mon complications are unresolvable irritation around the abutment because of rejection of the percutaneous device or uncontrollable skin growth. We even know of a few patients for which the abutment was completely covered by new skin growth during the healing period before initial fitting was possible. Most interesting, some clinicians choose to implement the stimulating processor portion of implantable bone stimulating devices using a softband, or headband, avoiding surgery. This appears to be particularly common for children and is required in children younger than five years. Although the softband implementation removes the need for surgery, because the device is not directly coupled to the bone, less power will be transferred and the amount of power transfer will vary more across patients.

Because bone conduction is able to provide stimulation to both cochleas at the same time, as we mentioned at the beginning of the section, these devices can also be used to treat single-sided deafness (Wazen et al., 2003). The Baha was FDA-approved to treat single-sided deafness in 2002, and data support these devices over traditional CROS in this population with regard to patient preference (Hol et al., 2004; Niparko, Cox, & Lustig, 2003). The relative benefits for implantable bone stimulating devices and traditional CROS interventions for single-sided deafness are expected to be similar and mainly related to alleviation of some of the negative effects of head shadow.

As with other CROS applications, clinical verification is essential (see Dickinson [2010] for review). Implantable bone stimulating devices may reduce or eliminate a number of complaints associated with traditional CROS. Specifically addressed are complaints of having to use two devices, the lack of low-frequency amplification reducing sound quality, and retention

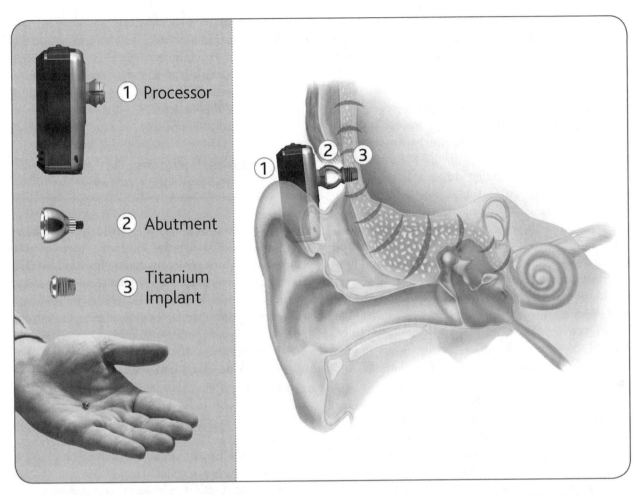

Figure 7–40. Schematic of the Baha osseointegrated hearing device that stimulates the cochlea via bone conduction (Photo courtesy of Cochlear Americas).

problems/discomfort from the retention mechanism associated, which are all associated with the traditional CROS. An obvious disadvantage to this surgical solution is that with a traditional CROS or the transcranial CROS options we discussed earlier, if the expected benefit is not present after 30 days, the patient can return the instrument. This is somewhat more difficult when there is an implanted titanium abutment.

Middle Ear Implants

Middle ear implants (MEI) were developed for patients who have sensorineural hearing loss and are usually thought of as candidates for traditional air conduc-

tion hearing aids (Chasin, 2002). The use of MEIs for listeners with sensorineural hearing loss in lieu of conventional amplification stems from manufacturers' claims of improved fidelity and the elimination of feedback, and the occlusion effect in listeners fit with these devices (Arthur, 2002; Bankaitis & Fredrickson, 2002; Kroll, Grant, & Javel, 2002; Luetje et al., 2002; Uziel et al., 2003). Results of studies investigating these claims have been mixed. It should be noted that some of the most popular MEI devices use essentially the exact same sound processing algorithms that are used in commercial air conduction hearing aids. The continued advancement of feedback suppression technologies and the OC style appears to further limit the potential advantages of this style over conventional air conduction hearing aids in listeners with mild to moderate hearing loss. The fact that these devices require surgical implantation must also be weighed against the strength of any advantages over air conduction hearing aids. The requirement of surgical implantation also precludes any usual trial period as removal also requires surgery.

In contrast, consistent patient preference has been shown for MEI devices in patients who have more severe hearing loss, particularly those that have rejected traditional air conduction hearing aids (Luetje et al., 2002; Uziel et al., 2003). The cosmetic appeal of this style would at first seem assured because of their implantable nature. Some of these devices are not fully implanted, however, and usually retain a small plastic case on the side of the head that houses the microphone and processing, shown in Figure 7–41. Regardless, these devices appear to be a reasonable alternative for some patients who are not satisfied with traditional air conduction hearing aids, have too much hearing loss to be fitted with OC instruments but desire a cosmetically appealing instrument with no occlusion effect and requiring limited care.

A final potential benefit of a MEI over conventional amplification is comfort (at least after surgery) because nothing is placed in the ear canal. Current MEIs use piezoelectric, electromagnetic, or electrodynamics principles. The least common of these schemes uses a piezoelectric crystal that bends in response to electrical charge. The low power consumption and other factors in this design have led to the design of a device that is fully implantable. The more common methods are either to mount a very small vibrator (about the size of a grain of rice) on the ossicular chain or place a very small magnet on the ossicular chain and *drive* it (force it to vibrate) with an oscillating magnetic field. As of this writing, at least two middle ear implant have received full FDA approval for implantation in adults, and in some cases, it is possible to get third-party payment of implantation of this device.

Knobs, Switches, Buttons, and Remote Controls

Another decision that must be considered in concert with hearing aids style is the selection of user controls. Some styles will be physically limited in size to such a degree that few user controls are possible. Some hearing aids in fact have no user control. The need for user control of the hearing aid primarily depends on five factors:

- How well the audiologist programmed the hearing aids. If both the gain and output are set appropriately for a large variety of input signals at the time of the fitting, the patient will not need to make as many changes during use.
- How well the patient *trained* the hearing aids. If the hearing aids are trainable, and the patient actively adjusts gain for different settings during the first few weeks of use, there should be less need for a volume control once training is completed (see the section on trainable hearing aids in Book Two of this series).

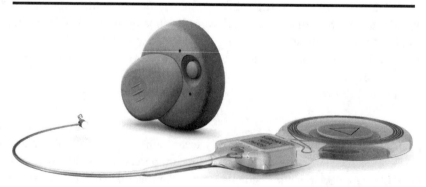

Figure 7–41. Schematic of a middle ear implant (Photo courtesy of Med-El.)

- The quality of the signal classification system and automatic functions of the hearing aids. For example, if the classifier correctly identifies speech in noise and switches to appropriate directional and noise reduction characteristics, there is less need for the patient to change gain or programs.
- Lifestyle of the patient. If the patient has a very active lifestyle and different telephone and wireless streaming applications are included in the fitting, this will require more active program changes by the patient.
- The patient's interest in controlling the acoustic environment. Some patients like to fiddle and make discrete volume control adjustments as the listening environment changes.

Common user controls include volume control (VC) wheels, *slider switches* (often used in BTE instruments to change user programs, activate telecoils, activate directional microphones, and turn the instrument on and off), and button/toggle switches (used in many styles to switch between programs or features by repeatedly pushing either the same button or two different buttons). For bilateral fittings, hearing aids often are paired using wireless communication. This allows for simultaneous volume control changes on both hearing aids by only pushing the button on one of them. As an alternative, hearing aids may be fitted so the button on one side changes the gain, and the button on the other side changes programs (memories).

User controls including volume control also can be placed on a separate remote control. Remote controls range from the extremely simple (a small magnet that can be used to activate a feature, change programs, or change volume using a magnetic sensor in the hearing aid) to quite sophisticated (individual controls for on and off, volume and hearing aid user memories, and even frequency response). Patient demand for remote controls has been fairly low since they were introduced in the 1980s. The low demand likely relates to complaints or concerns about keeping track of another device and cost, and/or the patient does not see any potential benefit. Also, audiologists do not seem to actively encourage the use of remote controls—they are not commonly included with the hearing aid purchase, as they would be if you bought a TV or CD player. Maybe this is because of the user problems we mentioned.

In a study we conducted in the early 1990s, we found the most commonly cited patient benefit was being able to discreetly turn the hearing aid on and off (Ricketts & Bentler, 1992). For some patients, especially those who use multiple programs and are technology savvy, a hearing aid remote control can be desirable. Current manufacturers have worked hard to make their remote controls more discrete. Currently, companies are making hearing aid remote controls as part of wristwatches, pens, and key chains—for example, see Figure 7–42.

In recent times, there has been a minor resurgence in remote control technology. This resurgence stems in part from their use as a *bridge* that can allow for streaming of audio from external sources through the remote wirelessly to the hearing aid (e.g., cell phone, television, etc.). Other more modern uses include using the remote as an external microphone or microphone array that allows wireless streaming of sound from the remote to the hearing aid or to activate sophisticated processing such as directional steering algorithms. These technologies are discussed in more detail in Book Two of this series.

Over the last few decades, the routine use of amplitude compression processing has decreased the need for a patient control of hearing aid volume (level). The logic is that if the gain is programmed so that soft sounds are audible, average input levels are comfortable, and loud sounds are loud but not too loud, why does the gain

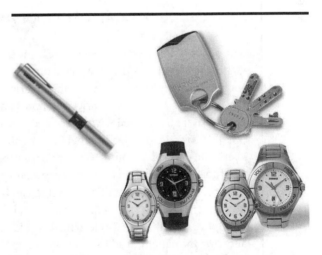

Figure 7–42. Three commercially available hearing aid remote controls. (Photos courtesy of Phonak and Siemens Hearing Instruments, Inc.)

need to be changed? Many patients, therefore, are perfectly happy to never have to adjust their hearing aid level using a VC. More recently, automatic systems have become increasingly sophisticated in their attempts to make accurate switching decisions for activation of hearing aid features. That is, until recently, some features such as telecoils, different amplification characteristics for different environments (multiuser memories), and directional microphones required user input for activation. Although automatic switching systems are certainly not perfect, some patients are happy with them. Other patients who may or may not be happy with automatic systems are either unwilling or unable to switch features off and on manually because of physical limitations, inconvenience, or a host of other factors.

In contrast, some patients are willing, able, and interested in manipulating their acoustic environment. Such patients may be unhappy with automatic features and a lack of volume control. In fact, about half of patients if given a choice, will prefer to have a VC (Dillion & Storey, 1998; Harnack-Knebel & Bentler, 1998; Lunner, Hellgren, Arlinger, & Elberling, 1997; Surr, Cord, & Walden, 2001; Valente, Fabry, Potts, & Sandlin, 1998), and approximately one-third of hearing aid users without a VC desire one.

Whether or not a hearing aid has a VC may be key to the ultimate success of the end user. According to MarkeTrak surveys carried out over a 10-year period by Kochkin (2002), the difference in overall satisfaction ratings between consumers who need a VC and those who do not need a VC is almost 40%, and over three-fourths (75%) of hearing aid users rate the VC as highly desirable. In addition, 72% of U.S. consumers report wanting hearing aids that are easier to regulate. These data have been supported by more recent data suggesting that 77% of experienced hearing aid users wanted to have a VC, no matter how infrequently they used it. For fitting success, most manufacturers have provided VCs that can be engaged or disengaged, depending upon the ultimate wishes of the consumer. The dB range of the VC also is programmable. It is important to assess each individual patient's needs relative to user controls by probing a few specific areas. Some questions that you might consider:

- Does the patient need features that need to be controlled by a switch?
- Has the patient used a VC in the past?
- Does the patient report frequently adjusting the volume of music and/or the television based on their mood or other factors?
- Is the style under consideration too small for user switches and/or a VC? How many switches/controls are possible?
- Is the patient physically able to manipulate small controls?

TECHNICAL TIP: MODERN HEARING AIDS AND VCS

The surveys we have reviewed were conducted before hearing aids had the sophisticated switching capacitates that they have today, and also before the use of trainable hearing aids. As we review in Book Two, trainable hearing aids allow the user to train the hearing aid to their desired use gain for a variety of inputs and environments. This is accomplished by storing the user's adjustments when he or she is in a given listening situation. For example, it is possible to train gain independently for soft, average, and loud inputs for speech-in-quiet, speech-in-noise, and music. Once this training has been accomplished, we would expect the need for a VC to decrease. This is especially useful for the very small products that do not have room for a VC, where the training can be conducted using a remote. It is important to note that it has been shown that fitting to validated prescriptive targets prior to training is just as important with these modern hearing aids. That is, simply starting with minimal gain and allowing the patient to adjust the volume up to their preferred level does not lead to optimal outcomes, so appropriate verification is still critical!

Obviously, the basic purpose of a VC is to provide patient control of amplification level. Although this seems like a good idea, it can also create problems. If the patient has dexterity problems or the VC is very small/sensitive, it may be accidentally adjusted during insertion, removal, or even through inadvertent movements. Some patients will have trouble getting the level adjusted just right or achieving a level balance between two hearing aids. In some hearing aids, these problems can be exacerbated because of the relationship between position of the VC and amplification level (called a *taper curve* when shown graphically), especially in older hearing aids. That is, the optimal level may be half of the total amount of amplification for one patient. Rather than being *half-way* up on the VC, however—shown in HA1 in Figure 7–43—this level may occur too close to the minimum VC position (e.g., HA3 in Figure 7–42), or too near the maximum position. Sometimes VCs are made in this nonlinear fashion on purpose. That is, it may be desirable to reach a level near that which is deemed optimal for a patient (often 60 to 75% of maximum level) for a VC position near the minimum, so the majority of the VC travel can be used for fine adjustments around that optimal level (e.g., HA2 in Figure 7–43).

Fortunately, many modern hearing aids have greatly enhanced the old-fashioned hearing aid VC. These enhancements might include: the ability to link the VC of two hearing aids together (changing the volume on

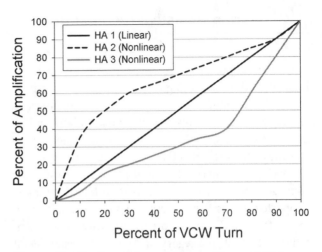

Figure 7–43. Examples of three different VC taper curves for hearing aid gain.

one hearing aid changes both), clinician control of volume range and/or step size (e.g., volume range could be as small as 4 to 6 dB or as large as 16 dB or more), and digital control allowing for linear or nonlinear taper curves. Finally, for small children or others who may not be able to appropriately adjust level, but for which a VC is still desired, a screw-set VC may be used. This is simply a VC that must be set with a small screwdriver.

TECHNICAL TIP: USING MEMORIES AS VC

One other method that can be very useful for patients who have poor dexterity but who desire some control over the hearing aid level is to use a program switch. That is, most hearing aids have three or four (or more) user memories that can be programmed to different VC settings. The level can then be adjusted by pressing a memory button on the hearing aid (most often a single button that toggles between available user memories) or on a remote control. We find this technique most useful if there are three to four user memories available. Two levels may not give the patient enough control (although this is fine for a few patients), and more than four levels can become confusing and/or difficult to manipulate. The audiologist will need to work with the patient to determine exactly what gain alterations are programmed, but often one memory might have gain 3 to 5 dB louder, another 3 to 5 dB softer, and if the patient has considerable low frequency gain for the primary fitting, maybe a program that cuts some of the gain in this region. This technique, however, may not be possible if the user memories are already being used to activate other features (e.g., telecoil, wireless connectivity).

Hearing Assistive Technology

One very important, but unfortunately often overlooked portion of hearing assessment for the purpose of (re)habilitation, is consideration of hearing assistive technology (HAT). This category includes any and all devices that are specifically used to assist patients with hearing difficulties other than the primary interventions of hearing aids and cochlear implants. A common, older term used to describe HAT that is still used by many people today is assistive listening device (ALD). We prefer the term HAT, as it is more descriptive and representative of the entire category of devices. For example, it seems odd to us to refer to a vibrating alarm clock as a listening device because this device has nothing to do with listening.

We think it is important to generally address HATs whenever considering hearing aid selection. HATs differ from hearing aids and cochlear implants in that they usually are aimed at addressing a small range of needs, rather than general hearing problems. Therefore, HATs often fill a useful supplementary roll to hearing aids, and in some cases, more than one different type of HAT may be appropriate for the same patient. That is, some patients may benefit from two, three, or even several HAT devices. For some patients, however, the benefit provided by a HAT may not be large enough to warrant the cost and/or inconvenience. Trial periods may be used, but it is clear that not all patients are candidates for HAT. For still other patients, one or more HATs may be appropriate even when a hearing aid is not.

We had one such patient many years ago whose case still stands to remind us of this fact. This patient had few remaining family members, and a terminal illness was expected to provide him little remaining life. He desperately wanted, however, to see the Summer Olympics on television one more time before he died (something he and his deceased wife had enjoyed doing together). We set him up with a television amplifier that could also be used to amplify other voices in the room through a microphone when people came to visit. Although we are sure we did not achieve a perfect fit, the patient was able to understand the television announcer. The time and inconvenience to obtain the device was minimal on his part, and the device was quite inexpensive compared with a hearing aid. We had the satisfaction of knowing that we had enhanced his quality of life for the short time he had left.

This has just been a brief introduction to HAT, as it is something to think about while hearing aid style is selected. We devote a chapter in Book Two of this series to this topic, where you find a complete description of all the options available.

TECHNICAL TIPS: COMMON USES FOR HAT

- Near-sound personal listening devices aimed at increasing the level of sounds near the listener (e.g., personal amplifiers, amplified stethoscopes, etc.).
- Far-sound personal listening devices aimed at bringing sounds far from the listener effectively *nearer* (e.g., note-takers, speech-to-text systems, FM systems, room loops, infrared systems, wireless routing from microphones (e.g. spouse microphone) and other devices that route signals of interest to the hearing aid or listener).
- Alerting and warning devices (e.g., flashing and vibrating alarm clocks, smoke alarms, door bells, telephone ringers, and amplified telephone ringers and smoke alarms).
- Telephone assistance (e.g., amplified telephones, teletypewriters, instant messaging translation services).
- Television and radio assistance (e.g., closed captioning, television amplifiers—many personal listening devices can assist with television and radio listening).

Mini-Summary

- Many patients (as many as half) will be happier if they are given a VC, even if they have properly fitted compression. Most past VC users will want to have one in their new hearing aids. Modern hearing aids have several adjustments that can make a VC easier to use.
- Automatic systems will make more mistakes than a person manually switching. A patient's desire to control their listening environment must be weighed against their willingness to use controls when assessing manual versus automatic controls.
- HAT devices should always be in the back of your mind when assessing a hearing loss for the purposes of selecting hearing aids. Depending on the patient, HATs may not be needed, may be a useful addition to the hearing aid, or may be selected even if a hearing aid is not!

Table 7–2. Summary of the benefits and limitations of different hearing aid styles.

Style	Main Advantages	Main Limitations
Body	Least susceptible to feedback, fit any degree of hearing loss through profound, user controls are the easiest to see and manipulate.	Unnatural microphone placement, bilateral fittings difficult, does not have sophisticated circuitry of other models, poor cosmetics.
Traditional BTE	Little susceptibility to feedback, fit any degree of hearing loss through profound, excellent venting flexibility, separation of receiver from the ear canal increases durability, good control of acoustics through plumbing, allows for directional microphone, telecoil, FM, DAI, most appropriate for children as the earmold can be remade to account for growth.	Cosmetics somewhat of a problem, considered the "old fashioned" hearing aid, tubing changes are required for maintenance.
Mini-BTE	Improved cosmetics because of size of instrument and slim tubing/wire. Use of RIC technology has potential for improved acoustics, and allows for unique sizes and shapes. Easily used for open fittings with stock eartips.	May not be large enough to accommodate all desired features, has less gain and output than traditional BTEs. Manipulation of these instruments can be quite challenging for patients with dexterity/vision problems.
Traditional Custom (ITE, ITC)	The largest sizes will be appropriate for most degrees of hearing loss, particularly when used with Digital Feedback Suppression though more susceptible to feedback than BTEs. Many allow for directional microphone and telecoil. Reducing size (ITE to ITC) may lead to improved cosmetics.	Smaller size may increase problems with manipulation for patients with dexterity problems as well as increasing problems with feedback and/or occlusion. The traditional ITC is mainly appropriate for patients with mild to moderate hearing loss.
Recessed Custom	Expected improvement of localization in the vertical plane and improved directivity in comparison to traditional custom instruments. Smallest sizes lead to improved cosmetics. May also lead to reduced wind noise and may allow more normal telephone use without feedback.	Increasingly smaller size may increase problems with manipulation for patients with dexterity/vision problems as well as increasing problems with feedback and/or occlusion. The recessed ITC is mainly appropriate for patients with mild to moderate hearing loss. Directional microphones and telecoils are not likely to be possible or available in the CIC or smaller ITC models.

continues

Table 7–2. *continued*

Style	Main Advantages	Main Limitations
Deep Canal CIC	The smaller residual ear canal volume allows for a less powerful amplifier. The DC CIC has all the advantages of the recessed CIC, but also can lead to a reduction or elimination of occlusion.	Many patients will not tolerate the deep tight fit because of discomfort. Discomfort can be minimized by using a softer tip but the subsequent "slit-leak" venting may result in feedback. Manipulation of these instruments can be quite challenging for patients with dexterity/vision problems. The DC CIC has most of the limitations of the recessed CIC, but may be fitted to patients with up-to moderately severe hearing loss if very tight.
Open-Canal Fitting	Lack of occlusion leads to a more natural sound of own voice and elimination of other problems related to occlusion, high cosmetic appeal, light and comfortable over the ear, natural sound quality for low frequency external sounds for patients with near normal low frequency hearing, often can be fit without using a custom earmold.	More prone to feedback. When mini-BTE RITA and RIC models are used, the thin tube in the RITA style can result in problems with cerumen clogging the tip. The RIC style can lead to increased problems with debris clogging the receiver as in the CIC style. The directional and noise reduction benefits will be more limited than in a closed earmold style. Limited gain makes them inappropriate for patients with severe hearing losses. Many models are only appropriate for patients with near normal low frequency thresholds.
CROS (Traditional CROS, BiCROS, Transcranial CROS)	Only for patients with profound hearing loss in one ear and either normal (CROS, TransCranial CROS) or mild/moderate hearing thresholds in the other ear. Can overcome hearing and SNR difficulties due to head shadow effects.	Benefit limited to very specific situations. Inconvenience of using two devices when there is mainly only hearing loss in one ear (CROS), poor sound quality (CROS, Transcranial CROS), physical discomfort (transcranial CROS), audible circuit noise (CROS) and poor cosmetics (CROS, BiCROS).
Bone Conduction	Directly stimulate both cochlea through bone conduction bypassing the middle and outer ears. This sound transmission path can be useful both for patients with primarily conductive hearing loss as well as patients with single sided deafness. For patients with single sided deafness fewer negatives are associated with the Baha device than with CROS or transcranical CROS (mainly related to sound quality, use of two devices and cosmetics).	As with CROS, benefit for patients with single-sided deafness limited to very specific situations. For patients with conductive hearing loss fewer negatives are associated with the Baha device than with traditional bone-conduction hearing aids (mainly related to comfort and the retention system). Surgery and appropriate placement are required for the Baha.
Middle Ear Implants	Potentially improved comfort and cosmetics compared to air conduction hearing aids for listeners with moderately severe (or better) sensorineural hearing loss. Advantages are particularly apparent in comparison to traditional, occluding custom hearing aids.	Requires surgical implantation. Benefits may be much more limited compared to some modern styles such as OC (studies still need to be done however). Much higher cost than traditional air conduction hearing aids (though patients out of pocket cost may be less due to third-party payment issues).

8

Ear Impressions, Earmolds, and Associated Plumbing

In the previous chapter, we discussed how the choice of hearing aid style not only affects cosmetics and available features, but also can have important acoustic implications. More specifically, we know that hearing aid style can have considerable implications for amount of gain, potential feedback problems, and issues related to the *occlusion effect*. Although the general choice of hearing aid style will impact these factors, how tightly and deeply an instrument is fitted in the ear canal can also have a significant effect. That is, two different products that are both full-concha ITEs can have very different fit properties. The physical fit matters in no small part because it can affect the amount of venting (as detailed later in this chapter), as well as the overall wearing comfort for the patient. If the hearing aids are not comfortable, it is unlikely the patient will wear them.

For the majority of hearing aid styles, other than the OC (for open canal) mini-BTEs, which are often fitted with non-custom coupling systems, the quality of the ear impression greatly affects how well a hearing aid shell or earmold physically fits an individual patient's ear. Therefore, we begin this chapter by discussing the process of taking ear impressions, followed by a discussion of physical hearing aid design factors affecting the acoustics of the sounds reaching the patient's tympanic membrane. Although the physical fit can affect comfort and acoustics, the earmold or earshell is just one component of the overall sound delivery system, which also includes earhooks and/or tubing in BTE instruments, as well as damping, venting, receiver tubing, and a variety of other factors.

The sound delivered to the patient's ear(s) from the hearing aid can be significantly altered by the sound delivery system in a number of ways. We generally refer to this delivery system and the resulting physical changes as hearing aid *plumbing*, a term we think fits well, and that has been made popular in the 1970s by the publications of Samuel Lybarger and Mead Killion to refer to physical changes affecting earmold acoustics.

Ear Impressions

An ear impression is a physical or virtual cast of the outer ear and ear canal space. These impressions are used to make a negative cast of the outer ear (essentially trying to mimic the surface of the outer ear and ear canal in three dimensions), which is in turn used to make earmolds and earshells for custom instruments. A well fitted earmold or earshell is highly dependent on the quality of the ear impression. A poor impression-making technique can lead to custom hearing aids or earmolds that are consistently too loose or too tight, or that have uncomfortable pressure points.

The tools and techniques used to make ear impressions have changed over the years, and the technology for making these impressions, like all technology related to hearing aids, has experienced incremental improvements.[47]Because of the different materials and techniques available, it is important to follow each individual manufacturer's instructions to ensure the best impressions possible. There are, however, some general techniques that we discuss here, that apply to all ear impression making. All methods are similar in that they require the same general steps:

- A thorough otoscopic examination of the ear and ear canal to assure that there are no conditions that would adversely affect the procedure (e.g., a large collection of cerumen, or sometimes even impacted cerumen is the most common).
- Placement of the ear dam (oto-dam).
- Preparation or mixing of the impression materials.
- Insertion of the materials into the ear using an impression syringe or impression gun.
- Allowance for curing time.
- Careful removal and reinspection of the ear.

Syringe or Gun?

Impression material is commonly premixed and inserted in the ear using an impression syringe or automatically mixed using premeasured cartridges and mixing tips, shown in Figure 8–1. These are used with a manual or electric impression gun, sometimes called an impression pistol. Common impression syringes and impression guns are shown in Figure 8–2. Whether a syringe or gun is chosen depends on several factors, including the clinician's preference and the type of impression material. For example, extremely stiff impression material may require premixing and the use of an impression syringe. This is because the gun injectors may not be strong enough to extrude a very stiff material through

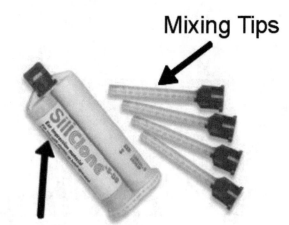

Figure 8–1. Example of one brand of premeasured cartridges and mixing tips used with impression guns. The mixing tip is attached to the end of the premeasured cartridge and then the entire assembly is attached to the impression gun as shown in the right-hand portion of Figure 8-2. Reprinted with permission from Westone.

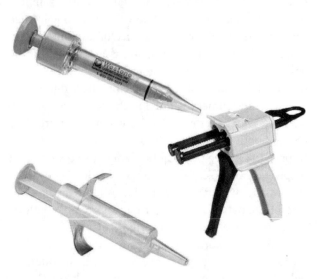

Figure 8–2. Examples of two different impression syringes (*left-hand side*) and a manual impression gun (*right-hand side*). Please note these are not to scale and the impression gun is much larger than the impression syringes. Reprinted with permission from Westone.

the mixing tip. Cartridge guns are sometimes regarded as superior to syringes because there is an assumption that the material flows more freely into the ear canal with this tool. However, currently available cartridge materials are designed specifically so that they do not flow freely. Regardless, we believe it is the injection technique, rather than the simple choice of material, that is most important for obtaining an optimal impression.

THINGS TO REMEMBER: IMPORTANT IMPRESSION MATERIAL TERMS

Viscosity: A material's viscosity refers to its consistency. With regard to impression materials, this term applies to the consistency before the material hardens. In general, impression materials are often categorized as having low, medium, or high viscosity. A low viscosity material is soft and/or *runny* and flows easily; a higher viscosity silicone is often denser, firmer, thicker, and/or stickier.

- Lower viscosity materials are generally recommended as the default because they will lead to the tightest fit and will produce an impression that most accurately mimics the shape of the ear canal. Some low viscosity materials require particular care, however, because of concerns during the shipping process as described below.
- A higher viscosity material is sometimes better to use on patients having a large amount of hair in their ears. This denser material will press down the hair whereas low viscosity materials may flow through the hair, which can make the impression painful to remove and leave holes and flaws on the impression surface.

Shore Value: After-cure hardness is commonly quantified using the hardness scale referred to as *Shore Value*, this is of little importance other than its relationship to damage during the shipping process. The after-cure hardness does not relate to viscosity.[48]

- There is also less of a relationship between the cured impression hardness and the ease of extraction from the patient's ear than might be expected. That is, in addition to the general hardness, the *slipperiness* of the cured impression material, which is often caused by an added material release agent, also has a large effect on the ease of impression extraction.

Contraction Ratio: The contraction ratio describes how much an impression shrinks over time. Shrinkage of less than 3% is often considered acceptable; however, changing the recommended mixing ratio can result in shrinkage exceeding 20% (e.g., Pirzanski, 2003). Therefore, changing the mixing ratio in an attempt to soften the material to minimize the stretching of the ear tissue should clearly be avoided.

Stress relaxation: This is related to after-cure hardness and describes how well the impression returns to its original shape after being bent or stretched. It is clearly important that the impression does not change shape as a result of its removal from the patient's ear or during shipping or in-lab processing.

Impression Materials

There are three primary families of impression materials including ethyl methacrylate (powder and liquid), addition-cure silicone, and two-part vinylpolysiloxane, and each require slightly different preparation techniques. These general material types as well as the specific products within them also differ with regards to the specific properties of viscosity, stress relaxation, contraction ratio, after-cure hardness, and effectiveness of the release agent.

Powder and Liquid Material

The powder and liquid impression material has been available for several decades and produces a highly accurate impression if you follow a few basic rules (adapted from http://www.westone.com):

■ A slight change in the ratio of liquid to powder can produce an impression that either sags because it is not stiff enough or expands in the ear canal because it is too dry. These problems can be minimized by using premeasured materials.

■ Put the powder in after the liquid for easier mixing, and use a glass mixing bowl and metal spatula rather than wooden mixing spoons or other tools that may absorb liquid.

■ Quickly mix the material and load the impression syringe; the curing process starts as soon as the powder and liquid come into contact.

Impressions taken with powder and liquid can prove superior to impressions taken with some of the lighter silicones described below that are applied using a gun-cartridge. This is related to the fact that mixed powder and liquid is more viscous compared with a light silicone, but will expand the ear canal, enhancing acoustic seal and ensuring a secure fit for the earmold. Although generally more viscous than light silicones, the powder and liquid materials do not have a fixed viscosity; rather, they begin to increase in viscosity immediately after mixing. In addition, the powder and liquid materials have a very long shelf life compared with the silicone materials.

Although potentially yielding accurate impressions, there is a major limitation to powder and liquid materials that is significant enough that some manufacturers refuse to accept them. Namely, they produce impressions that have a low after-cure hardness and poor stress relaxation. Therefore, they are susceptible to damage during shipping or even removal from the ear canal if proper care is not taken. Shipping damage may be caused by physical trauma or heat. Further, the magnitude of volume shrinkage is approximately 3% in seven days, so timely shipping is critical.

Earmold and hearing aid manufacturers suggest securing powder and liquid-based impressions to the bottom of the shipping box with an adhesive, such as household cement (e.g., Elmers glue). In addition, nothing should be placed in the same box space with the impression to minimize distortion. However, even taking these steps does not ensure there will be no distortion during shipping, particularly in the hot summer months.

Concern with damage during shipping is likely the reason for a decreased use of the powder and liquid impression materials. We believe, however, that given the high accuracy and low cost, these materials may see a comeback given that newer technologies allow for three-dimensional scanning of the finished impression. An electronic copy of the digital impression, which will not distort during shipping, can then be sent in lieu of a physical impression (see our section on scanning ear impressions). That is, if the impression is simply scanned immediately after it has been taken, many of the down sides of this material have been eliminated.

Condensation-Cure Silicone

This impression material is commonly distributed in two parts: a large container containing silicon that requires use of a manufacturer-supplied measuring scoop and a tube of catalyst. Less commonly this material may be found in cartridge form for use with an impression gun. Condensation-cure, hand-mixed silicones are either medium or higher viscosity when compared with all available materials. In contrast, the lighter cartridge system materials typically exhibit low to medium viscosity. With the powder-and-liquid materials, condensation-cure silicone maintains a fixed viscosity for a brief period of time, typically less than one or two minutes, depending on the specific material.

The clinician should always follow the specific manufacturer's instructions for preparation. In general, these instructions are similar to the following:

- Prepare the material by first flattening out a recommended measurement of impression material on a mixing surface.
- Then *draw* a line of catalyst (using the manufacturer-recommended amount) on top and mix.
- Mixing can be done in your hand, but a metal mixing blade and hard mixing surface is recommended for hygienic reasons—so your skin does not need to contact the material.
- The material needs to be mixed quickly until it reaches a consistent color and loaded into the impression syringe. Mixing needs to be done in 20 to 30 seconds, or the material will become too hard before completing insertion of the impression material.
- Using a little extra catalyst to speed things up, or a little less to slow things down, is usually not recommended because the material may harden too quickly or reach an inappropriate final consistency. It should be noted, however, that adjustment in the amount of catalyst used is sometimes necessary, as the effectiveness of some catalysts decreases with age. (Although, it is probably best to just throw the old catalyst away and buy new.)

The relatively limited hardening time, limited shelf life, and imprecise method for obtaining the proper mixture ratio (especially obtaining the correct amount of the catalyst) have likely all led to the limited popularity of the condensation-cure silicone materials.

Addition-Cure Vinylpolysiloxane

This material, which is also commonly referred to as silicone, is the most popular impression material in use. It is commonly available in bulk containers, individual portion packs, or in cartridges for use in an impression gun. Addition-cure, hand-mixed silicones are either medium or higher viscosity when compared with all available materials. In contrast, the less dense (light) cartridge system materials typically exhibit low to medium viscosity. Addition-cure silicone maintains a fixed viscosity for a brief period of time. For cartridge silicones, this time ranges from one to two minutes; for hand mixed silicones, it is typically two to four minutes. After this brief period of approximately stable viscosity ends, the viscosity increases rapidly to its final cured level (sometimes referred to as the *snap* effect).

The components for all hand-mixed silicones are supplied in contrasting colors to provide means of indicating when a uniform (streak-free) mix is achieved. Addition-cure silicone has several desirable attributes that have led to its popularity. For example, these materials typically exhibit an excellent contraction ratio, shrinking from 0.1% to 0.7% in seven days, and exhibit good stress relaxation properties, with a 99.4% [±0.5%] return to original shape after application of stress (e.g., Pirzanski, 2003). As a consequence, silicone impressions do not generally need to be glued to the shipping box. These materials do have a limited shelf life of approximately one year, however.

Making a Good Ear Impression

Now that we have discussed the different impression materials and their preparation, let us get down to the *technique* of making a good ear impression. You know the old saying, "You only have one chance to make a first impression"—so let us see if we can help you get your first one right by using this step-by-step procedure.

Step One: Before beginning the impression-making process, it is important that appropriate hand washing and other infection control procedures are followed.

Step Two: The patient's ear must first be thoroughly examined. We assume that an otoscopic examination was completed at the beginning of the assessment and that you are already familiar with these techniques from your hearing evaluation coursework. Regardless, it is important to reinspect the ear just prior to making an impression to become familiar with the shape, angle, and depth of the individual patient's ear canal, and to determine if there are any impression contraindications. Contraindications include, but are not limited to, impacted earwax, foreign objects (should be removed prior to taking the impression), active fluid discharge, perforated eardrum, and inflammatory conditions such as swimmer's ear—which should be medically resolved prior to taking the impression. In addition, there are a host of other things you might see that may require increased care or surgical intervention prior to taking the impression (e.g., bony growths/exostosis, collapsed canal, enlarged canal, thick hair growth, cauliflower ear, mastoidectomy, or other surgical deformation). Some of these conditions can be overlooked, as they will be irresolvable, but may lead to a poor impression and may need to be discussed with the manufacturer constructing the earmold or custom hearing instrument.

Step Three: Once all contraindications are accounted for, an appropriate ear dam needs to be selected based on the otoscopic examination. An ear dam is a manufactured block that is intended to stop impression material from traveling too far into the ear canal or making contact with the tympanic membrane. Yes, we have had personal experience viewing an audiologist who forgot to use an ear dam and painfully (for both the patient *and* the audiologist) extracted the patient's tympanic membrane and ossicles along with the ear impression. This is a mistake you do not want to make, and avoiding it is worth the trouble of carrying around this disturbing mental image. This also can happen when the ear dam is too small, as the material will go around the dam and reach the eardrum. This is referred to as *blow-by* —again, something to avoid.

Ear dams should be selected to be slightly larger than the ear canal. This way it is compressed by the canal walls, which act to create a better barrier and hold it in place against the force of the impression material. Care must be taken, however, to make sure that an ear dam that is too large is not selected because it can lead to discomfort or stretching of the ear canal, and it can prevent you from obtaining a deep enough impression. Ear dams commonly consist of a rounded block of foam or cotton that is connected to a string or tube that aids in removal of the ear dam if it does not come out with the impression material, shown in Figure 8–3. When a very tight impression is needed, or a material is chosen that does not have an effective release agent, there may be discomfort when removing the impression because of suction. In addition to using a proper impression removal technique (described below), this discomfort also can be alleviated using vented ear dams. In a vented ear dam, the removal string is replaced with a thin pressure release tube that allows for pressure equalization during removal (see Figure 8–3).

Step Four: Once the proper size ear dam has been selected, it is placed in the ear with an ear light, shown in Figure 8–4. Then, an otoscope is used to verify that the dam is placed properly. The ear dam should be placed beyond the second bend in the ear canal. This is the case even if a shorter canal portion is being ordered, so that the receiver can be properly angled. A receiver wrongly *pointed* at an ear canal wall can greatly increase the susceptibility to feedback. As with an otoscope, it is important to properly brace the ear light by making contact with the patient's head with at least one finger of the hand holding the ear light. This is critical because children can wiggle, and even adults can experience a cough or gag reflex when you touch their ear canal.[49] To get the ear dam in place appropriately, it is often best to gently work it into place by pushing around the edges of the ear dam with the ear light. This ensures that it does not tumble sideways, as can often happen when it is simply pushed straight in.

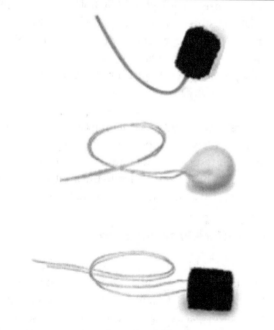

Figure 8–3. Three examples of common ear dams including: (1) Vented foam block with pressure release tube (top), (2) Cotton material with string (middle), (3) Foam block with string (bottom). Reprinted with permission from Westone.

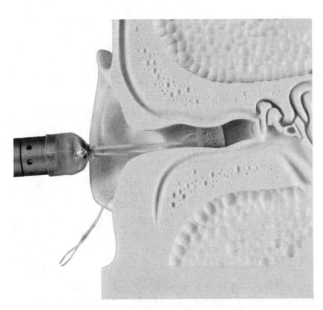

Figure 8–4. Example of proper placement of an ear dam using an ear light. The tip of the ear light is used to press around the edges of the ear dam so that it goes in straight without rolling into the ear canal.

■ Brace the syringe using your little finger and place the end of the syringe approximately 0.25 inches inside the ear canal opening. Gently squeeze the material into the ear canal, allowing it to flow back over the syringe tip. Once the material starts to flow past the tip, start backing the tip out of the ear canal. However, the tip should always remain embedded in the impression material.

■ As the tip leaves the ear canal, fill all the spaces, cracks, and crevices of the ear. We suggest you start with the concha bowl, move up into the antihelix crevice, then follow the contour of the ear, finishing at the center of the concha, as seen in Figure 8–5. This of course is not as critical for a CIC as for a full concha earmold or custom instrument, but it is best to have a full impression (a potential CIC fitting may turn into a full-concha fitting).

■ Once completed, it is recommended that you leave the impression material untouched while hardening. After the impression material hardens for the manufacturer-specified hardening time, check to see if the impression has cured by pressing a plastic card or fingernail gently into the material to see if an indentation remains.

Step Five: After placing the ear dam as described previously, mix the materials and put them in the impression syringe or gun. If the materials are mixed before placing the ear block, they should be thrown away and the process started over. The cost of the impression material is simply not worth a potentially bad fit because the material was too firm on insertion. The patient should be seated, with his or her head tilted slightly away from you.

Step Six: To remove the impression, gently pull the patient's pinna up and back to break the seal. It may require a little wiggling and a couple tries. Remove the

---

TECHNICAL TIP: OPEN OR CLOSED JAW?

There has been a lot of debate regarding what patients should do with their jaw while the impression is being taken. This debate results from data that clearly show that patients' ear canal size and shape can be dramatically altered by jaw position (e.g., Darkner et al., 2007; Oliveira, 1997). Our experience leads us to believe that for most impressions, it is best to have the patient open and close the mouth and move the jaw around during the impression. For a tighter fit, however, the patient should be required to keep their mouth open using a bite block. In fact, many experts recommend the bite block procedure as a default, because it will lead to the best possible seal in the resultant earmold or earshell. Like others (e.g., Pirzanski, 1998), we have had the least amount of success with closed-mouth impressions and, therefore, do not recommend them.

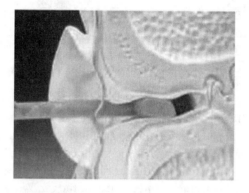

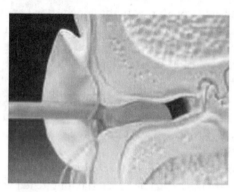

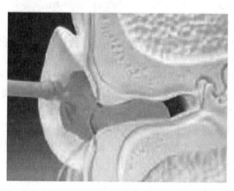

Figure 8–5. Step-by-step example of the insertion of impression material. Notice how the tip of the syringe remains embedded in the material throughout the filling process. Reprinted with permission from Westone.

impression from the antihelix area and gently rotate forward and out. The removal string or vent tube can be used to remove the ear dam if it remains in the ear canal.

Step Seven: Finally, after removal, check the ear canal with your otoscope to assure that it is free from any material remaining from the impression process. Some slight redness may be evident and is normal.

**TECHNICAL TIP:
MARKING EAR IMPRESSIONS FOR
MICROPHONE PORT OPENINGS**

As we discussed in Chapter 7, the case or shell of custom hearing aids have one or two microphone port openings. When microphones are used to obtain a *directional effect*, which is the design of the majority of custom hearing aids today, there will be two port openings. The distance between these ports, relative to the horizontal plane of the hearing aids when they are placed on the ear, is important for obtaining the desired directional effect. When custom instruments are ordered, therefore, it is important that the manufacturer knows the horizontal plane, as this will determine how the faceplate is attached. This cannot be determined very accurately once the ear impression has been removed from the ear. The directional effect can be reduced for relatively small deviations—anything >15 degrees. For this reason, when ordering custom instruments with directional technology, we recommend *scoring* (marking) the horizontal plane on the ear impression while the impression is still in the patient's ear. This can be accomplished with a marking card, furnished by most manufacturers (most any rigid card will work). Some audiologists simply affix a plastic paper clip in the material at the desired angle. Do not use a pen marker, as this may rub off.

After making an impression, it should be inspected to make sure that the necessary canal length and all anatomical landmarks are present. If not, another impression should be taken. A bad impression results in a bad earmold or custom hearing aid shell, and this is not something our patients are content just living with. If you make a bad impression, simply let the patient know it is important to get the impression perfect for a good fit, and it sometimes requires more than one try.

Scanning Ear Impressions

After it has been determined that the impression is adequate, it is commonly mailed to an earmold or hearing aid manufacturer so that an earmold or custom product can be ordered. As we have discussed, there is some concern that the important fine details of the impression can be altered through this mailing process (e.g., shrinkage, damage from excessive heat, squashing, etc.). For this reason, technologies that can perform three-dimensional scans of earmolds in the clinician's office and store the earmold as a digital image have been introduced. The first such device designed to do so was the iScan, which was introduced by Siemens in 2005. This technique of creating a *virtual earmold*, as seen in Figure 8–6, has the benefits of avoiding any shipping related deformation of the ear impression and providing a nonshrinking, permanent impression that can be easily stored and used for making additional earshells or earmolds.

The scanning devices that are commonly used are about the size of a computer printer and use three-dimensional technology with color-coded triangulation. The ear impression is affixed to a rotating platform where a projector illuminates it with colored light stripes from different angles. The light stripes conform to the object's surface in line with its geometry. This is simultaneously captured with a camera. The process takes about two minutes. Changes, markings, or comments to assist in the fabrication can be made by the audiologist directly on the digital scan. The resulting scan can then be e-mailed to the earmold lab or the manufacturer. The reported benefits of using the scanner include:

- Reduced shrinkage and damage during shipping.
- Digital record of impression is available, which can be used for remakes (e.g., lost or damaged earmolds/hearing aids).
- Provides electronic method to indicate where changes need to be made on remakes (the audiologist can draw and write on the scan).
- Reduced turnaround time.
- Reduced cost of impression material and shipping expenses.

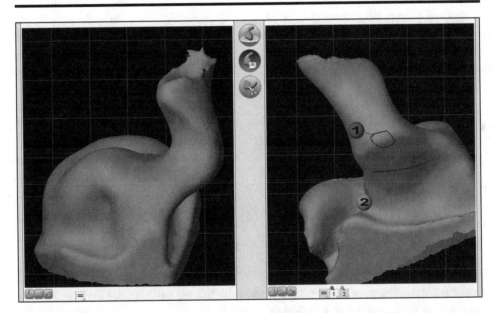

Figure 8–6. Example of a left and right scanned ear impression. These scans are three-dimensional and can be rotated so that the entire impression can be viewed. See numbering and marks on the right scan. An advantage of this procedure is that the audiologist can digitally mark the impression at specific points and make notes to the manufacturer regarding what needs to be done for these areas. Where to cut the canal is a common instruction. In this case, the previous earmold was causing irritation in the area of #1, and extra smoothing was therefore requested. (Photo courtesy of Siemens Hearing Instruments, Inc.)

■ Convenience: Impressions do not have to be boxed-up, and orders can be placed at any time, night or day.

One manufacturer, who has had the option of electronic earmold scanning available for several years, reports that about 60% of their customers have the earmold scanning equipment, and those that have the equipment use scans for about 70 to 80% of their orders. In the past, unfortunately, the scanners have been linked to specific hearing aid and earmold manufacturers, limiting utility and the choice of product when ordering. This has recently changed, in that at least one scanner, the iScan, uses an open data format so audiologists can transfer electronic impressions independent of the manufacturer. It is reasonable to assume that this technology will soon become more available and will be common place.

It should be acknowledged that the effectiveness of such technology is still limited by the fact that if the ear impression is poor to begin with, the scan will simply reflect this. The true gold standard will be three-dimensional imaging of the outer ear and ear canal. We have little doubt that this technology will someday be available for hearing aids as it already exists in other fields. However, currently it is not nearly cost-effective enough for clinical use.

Selecting Earmold Material and Styles

We discussed the selection of hearing aid style in Chapter 7; however, if the BTE style is selected (including both traditional and mini-BTE instruments), and if the manufacturer's modular eartips are not used, there is a secondary process of selecting the earmold. The choice of earmold will depend on several factors, some of which are similar to the factors considered when choosing a hearing aid style. They include: the degree of hearing loss, how *open* you want the fit to be (based on hearing loss configuration and quality of the feedback suppression algorithm you are ordering), shape and size of the external ear, texture and sensitivity of the patient's skin, stiffness of the patient's external ear, and potentially other factors. Because all of these factors are important, how the choice of earmold material and earmold style might interact with the patient and the fit

must be considered at every step in this process. Let us start by considering earmold materials.

Earmold Materials

There are three primary families of earmold materials including acrylic/lucite, polyvinyl chloride (vinyl/PVC), and silicone, each of which has potential benefits and limitations. A fourth material type, polyethylene, is used less often. It is similar in advantages and disadvantages to acrylic; however, it is slightly more prone to feedback, but the most hypoallergenic of all the materials. It is also sometimes criticized for its plasticy appearance.

Acrylic/Lucite

This material may be regular or body temperature reactive, which gets slightly softer when warm.

■ Positives: Because it is very hard, it is possible to make thin ridges, keeps its shape without shrinking, is very durable, and is easy to modify. The hard slick surface also makes earmolds made of this material easier to insert and remove. It is fairly hypoallergenic and the best material for many older patients.

■ Negatives: Because of the hardness, it will not bend or compress to get past narrow openings on insertion, and it may be more prone to feedback. However, studies suggest a good seal can be obtained with this material as well as softer materials. Not usually recommended for children for fear of ear injury if struck in the earmold.

Polyvinyl Chloride

This material is often available in softer (recommended for children) and harder varieties.

■ Positives: Softer and more comfortable than acrylic. Softness makes it appropriate for children and for hearing losses in the moderate to severe range. Although not as slick as acrylic, it is also not as tacky (sticky) as silicone, making it reasonably easy to remove and insert.

■ Negatives: Not very durable, lasting from 4 months to 2 years depending on body chemistry. Soft nature makes them much more difficult to modify than acrylic. More prone to discolor after time. Problematic for patients with vinyl allergies.

Silicone

This material is often available in tacky/low pressure cured (recommended for greater hearing loss) and high pressure cured varieties.

■ Positives: Soft and tacky nature makes this material appropriate for children and ideal for severe to profound hearing loss, and it is fairly hypoallergenic.

■ Negatives: Soft nature makes it much more difficult to modify than acrylic. Soft and tacky nature makes it the most difficult to insert and remove (especially difficult for floppy ears) and can cause skin abrasions in patients with fragile skin. Tubing adhesive does not bond well with some versions, leading to the need for a mechanical tubing lock.

THINGS TO REMEMBER: MINI-SUMMARY

■ There is no one best viscosity. Rather than using a single type of impression-making material for all patients, it is sometimes useful to choose a type that better addresses a patient's specific situation. For example, a higher-than-usual viscosity may be chosen for a patient with particularly hairy ear canals, whereas a lower-than-usual viscosity may be chosen when a particularly tight fit is desired.

■ In all earmold impression materials, it is desirable to have an effective release agent. A contraction ratio of less than 3% over the time period between making the impression and their use by manufacturers. Low stress relaxation are important, particularly if the impression is being mailed.

■ Acrylic earmolds have the advantages of being long lasting and easy to modify, but generally are not recommended for children. In contrast, polyvinyl chloride earmolds are softer, still reasonably easy to remove and insert, but are generally not very durable. Finally, silicone earmolds are soft and fairly hypoallergenic, but they may require a tubing lock and their tacky (sticky) nature can make them more difficult to insert and remove, and they are generally not recommended for individuals with fragile skin.

POINTS TO PONDER: DECISIONS, DECISIONS

We have provided a relatively simplified listing of the earmold materials available—limiting it to the three general categories. On the day of the order, however, consider that it might be a bit more complicated. The following is the list of the *20 material options* for just one earmold style from just one of the major manufacturers: Acrylic, Acrylic with Flex Canal, Acrylic with hard or soft e-Compound canal, Acrylic DisappEar, FIT, Formula II, Formula II Clear, Rx, Superflex, Neon Colors, Vinyl Marble, Mediflex, Mediflex with e-Compound, Frosted Flex, Frosted Flex with e-Compound, OtoBlast, OtoBlast DisappEar, and Cat Eyes. Once comfortable with a manufacturer, the clinician can learn the subtleties of a particular manufacturer's material potions to best select the materials for every patient.

Earmold Styles

Now that we have considered earmold materials, let us discuss earmold styles. One of the things that makes selection challenging is that there are so many different styles, and many manufacturers use different naming schemes. Even within the same manufacturer, naming schemes are often either nondescriptive (e.g., based on numbers or letters) or inconsistent (e.g., depending on the earmold, descriptive names, inventor names, application names, and function names are used).

It is very important, therefore, that you really get to know the earmold manufacturer(s) whom you decide to use most often. Given the large number of names and the fact that we recommend you get to know individual manufacturers, we only provide a few general categories. First, let us talk about a few earmold landmarks. The earmold landmarks generally either correspond to a particular shape or landmark on the pinna or the external ear canal. Although you have probably heard all these terms before, we will revisit the pinna landmarks that are commonly used with earmolds in Figure 8–7 as a reminder. Given this Figure, it should then be possible to match where specific portions of the earmold shown in Figure 8–8 fit in the ear. One other common earmold term not shown on this figure is *canal lock*. A canal lock is a small section encompassing only the *heel* and *antitragus* portions. There is not a complete concha portion when using an earmold with a canal lock.

With this terminology in mind, let us examine a few general categories of earmold style, shown in Figure 8–9.

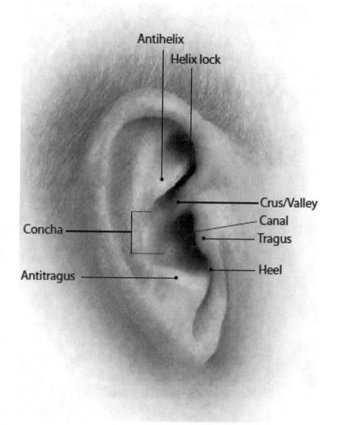

Figure 8–7. Common Pinna landmarks corresponding to earmold landmarks. One can see how the earmold fits into the ear by comparing to the labeled landmarks in Figure 8–8. Reprinted with permission from Westone.

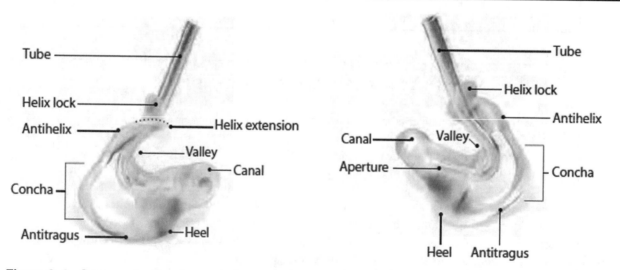

Figure 8–8. Common landmarks used when ordering and naming earmolds. These are useful when describing where problem areas are or where modifications need to be made. Reprinted with permission from Westone.

Full Shell

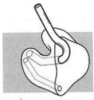

- Often used for more severe to profound hearing losses and younger children
- Canal portion can be made thicker (better seal), thinner (for better cosmetics), fitted with a snap ring instead of tubing (for body aid, powered stethoscopes, etc.), or the top portion of the canal can be removed (half shell).
- Can be difficult to insert if tight fitting.

Skeleton

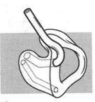

- One of the more common styles used with traditional BTE hearing aids.
- Can be used with a wide range of hearing loss.
- Sometimes modified to remove the middle portion of the "ring" that fills the concha bowl (semi-skeleton).

Canal

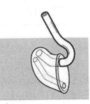

- Not usually fit as tight, so it is more suitable for mild-moderate loss. Appropriate for some patients with severe hearing loss using soft materials. Retention can be a problem, though easier insertion than many styles.
- Can be modified with a "concha lock" or by hollowing out the canal (sometimes combined with soft material for a comfort fit for patients with large changes in earcanal size with jaw movement).

Custom Open

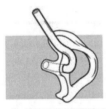

- Many styles with various combinations and configurations of the heel, concha and helix lock portions.
- Can be used for CROS style, open fits with BTE style or with the OC style for better retention than non-custom open.

Non-Custom Mini-BTE

- Usually manufacturer specific and using tubing with a very narrow inner diameter.
- Both RITA (tube) and RIC styles available.
- Can have some problems with retention for which a custom solution is suggested.

Custom Mini-BTE

- Similar to the standard canal, but intended to be used with specific models of deep canal (occluding) RIC fittings. Manufacturers often supply non-custom versions, but custom versions are often available from earmold companies when better retention is desired.
- Usually made using soft materials.

Figure 8–9. Advantages and limitations to a few common earmolds. This information is particularly useful when deciding on an earmold style within the constraints of individual patient differences, cosmetics, and gain requirements.

Depending on your patient population, the earmold manufacturer(s) you choose, and the types of hearing aids you fit, you will likely learn many clinical tricks and shortcuts that improve your clinical skills with earmolds. We offer a few tips here that we have found to be useful over the years:

- Although seemingly logical, it is not the case that bulkier earmolds guarantee more gain before feedback. The accuracy of the earmold impression is often more important than the style of the earmold when concerned about maximum amplification.

- A variety of canal lengths are possible in nearly all custom earmold styles; longer canals are generally associated with less feedback if they fit tightly, but more feedback is possible if they terminate facing a canal wall.

- Tapering the end of the canal can make insertion easier and may add comfort, but it may increase chances of feedback.

- Canal locks do not always help as much as one might think with retention. A small *wire retention adapter* (a thin stiff plastic line or

plastic coated wire) can sometimes help with retention.

- Avoid tacky earmold materials for older patients with thin skin to prevent insertion abrasions.

- Buffing and grinding works well for major and minor modifications of acrylic. But, use of a scalpel or razor blade (and a steady hand) is needed for softer materials, and major modifications usually are not possible in these softer earmolds.

Modular Earmold Plumbing

As we have mentioned, today's mini-BTE products come with an assortment of modular/semi-disposable earmold fittings. Originally, the mini-BTE products were designed to be fitted in an open manner, so a small supply of non-custom open tips was provided. As the fitting ranges have expanded, so has the selection of plumbing options. There is a large array of products from all manufacturers. An example of the variety of fitting tips for just one product is shown in Figure 8–10. Moreover, the mini-BTE hearing aids can be RITA or RIC, which means that different fitting kits are needed depending on

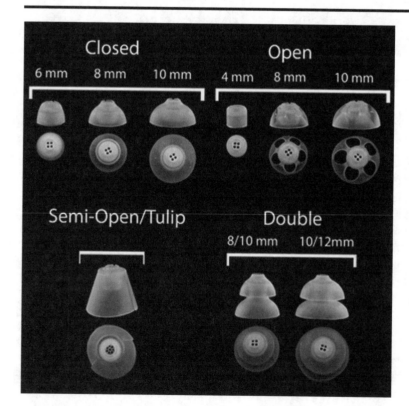

Figure 8–10. Example of eartip choices available when using modular earmolds for fitting mini-BTE products. Reprinted with Permission from Siemens Hearing Instruments, Inc.

the location of the receiver. The RITA also has the thin tubing, which replaces the standard tone hook/tubing that comes in different lengths. There also is a screw-on version of the thin tubing, which can be used with traditional BTEs. The RIC also has different wire lengths, as well as different size receivers (e.g., required for different maximum gain levels, such as 45 dB, 55 dB, and 65 dB).

Manufacturers provide kits that include all the tips and tubing that are used for these modular fittings. The fitting kits also often include tube shapers, measuring gauges, wax guards, and cleaning wires. It can be confusing, however, as a #2 tip from one manufacturer can be quite different than a #2 tip from another. Some tips are even negative numbers. Some manufacturers call the tips, tips; some call them domes; and some call them tips for some products and domes for others. Some tubing/tip combinations are named after a specific hearing aid, but they also work with other hearing aids. An example of the variety that is available is shown in Table 8–1. Consider that from just one manufacturer, for a RIC product, there are 3 different receiver power choices, 4 different wire length choices, and 8 different dome choices—96 different combinations for your Monday morning patient!

Audiologists seem to be somewhat divided regarding the use of these modular fittings. The thin tube can be fitted into a custom mold, and the RIC wire/receiver also can be fitted to a custom mold, so the issue surrounds the use of the modular tips and domes versus taking an impression and ordering a custom earmold. Here are some of the commonly cited pros and cons.

Reasons Why Modular Fittings Are a Good Choice

- Openness: The open fitting tips are indeed open (see Figure 7–31 from Chapter 7). It is not uncommon that the REOR (for real ear occluded response) is essentially identical to the REUR (for real ear unaided response). Not only does this eliminate the occlusion effect, but it provides some *free gain*, as the ear canal resonance is still in play.

Table 8–1. Sample of different earmold plumbing available from three major manufacturers.

	Oticon	Siemens	Widex
Slim tubing for RITAs	Called "Corda²" Available in lengths 0-0.9, 1-0.9, 2-0.9, and 3-0.9.	"Life Tube" Available in lengths of 1, 2, 3, 4, 5, and 6.	Called "é-tips" and "m-tips" for élan fittings or micro fittings, respectively
		"S tube" Available in lengths of 1, 2, 3, and 4.	Available in lengths of 1, 2, 3, 4, and 5.
Tips/Domes for RITAs	Available in sizes small (6 mm), medium (8 mm), large (10 mm) and Plus domes.	Available in Open Domes sizes 4 mm, 6 mm, 8 mm and 10 mm; Closed Domes size 8 mm; Double Domes sizes 8/10 mm and 10/12 mm.	Available in sizes 1L, 2L, 1S, and 2S 1 and 2 denote small and large diameters, respectively. L and S denote long and short insertion depths, respectively
RIC receiver attachments	Available in lengths of 1, 2 3, and 4. Also in receiver powers S (Standard), M (Medium), and P (Power).	Available in lengths of 0, 1, 2, and 3. Also in receiver powers of S (45 dB Gain), M (55 dB Gain), and P (65 dB Gain)	Available in lengths of -2, -1, 0, 1, 2, 3, 4, and 5 Also in receiver powers of S, M, P, and SP
Tips/Domes for RICs	Available in sizes small (6 mm), medium (8 mm), large (10 mm) and Plus domes.	Available in Open Click Domes sizes 4 mm, 8 mm and 10 mm; Closed Click Domes sizes 6 mm, 8 mm, and 10 mm; Double Domes sizes 8/10 mm and 10/12 mm; Semi-Open Domes; Tulip Domes	Available in Open Domes sizes S and L; Double Dome sizes S, M, and L; Gum Drop sizes 8, 9, 10 and 11; Tulip Domes.

■ Efficiency: The modular tips allow for same-day service. The patient can walk in the door with an appointment for a diagnostic and leave a couple hours later owning a pair of hearing aids. Assuming that these hearing aids will provide benefit for the patient, which is almost always true, this is a good thing. It also saved a patient visit, which is important for people who need to travel large distances or are required to fight traffic and parking issues coming to the clinic.

■ Reduced procrastination: Related to efficiency, there is the old adage, "strike while the iron is hot." Although not blacksmiths, audiologists dispensing hearing aids know well that when a patient says, "You know, I think I'll go home, talk to my wife about this, and get back to you," you very well might not see that patient again for five years, if ever. Or, the patient goes home, starts price shopping, and returns a week later with a bulging folder of competitive offers and Internet printouts.

■ Comfort: Most of the modular tips and domes, especially the open ones, fit rather loosely and are more comfortable than a custom earmold.

■ Cosmetics: The modular tip is typically less noticeable than a custom earmold.

■ Cost: The patient does not have the $75 to $100 extra cost of the custom earmold. Many manufacturers provide the tips and domes free-of-charge to the audiologists.

■ Maintenance: If the patient has good dexterity and is attentive, they can replace the tips when they become plugged or discolored. With RITAs, the tubing usually becomes stretched (because the patient uses it to take off the hearing aids), and this easily can be replaced by the patient also.

Reasons Why Modular Fittings May *Not* Be a Good Choice

■ Feedback: If a patient needs considerable gain, it is difficult to find a non-custom tip or dome that will fit tight enough.

■ Ear geography: If the patient has a sharp turn in their ear canal, there may be problems with the tip bumping against the canal wall. There is not the flexibility of going deeper or shallower, like one would have with custom earmolds.

■ Insertion: Because the tip is so small and light, some people with poor dexterity have trouble knowing when it is in the ear canal.

■ Retention: It is fairly common for modular tips to work out of the ear when the person talks or chews. Because they are light and fit loosely, the patient sometimes does not even know that the tip is not in the ear canal.

■ Maintenance: In general, the tips need more maintenance (changing) than a standard custom earmold. A common problem is the plugging of the RIC receiver. This occurs more frequently when a modular tip is used, than when the receiver is cased in a custom earmold.

■ Overall product impression: A pair of hearing aids is the most expensive electronic devices most people purchase. Fitting them to the ear with a 50-cent disposable eartip may not seem consistent with the purported high level of technology.

The Acoustics of Hearing Aid Plumbing

We start this section by acknowledging the pioneering work conducted by Samuel Lybarger in the area of ear-mold acoustics.[50] As early as the mid-1950s, Lybarger wrote the germinal Pamphlet for Radioear Corporation titled: "The Earmold as Part of the Receiver Acoustic System." At the time, he was writing about earmolds for body aid receivers, but many of the same principles apply today. Many audiologists cut their *earmold acoustics teeth* reading the chapters that Lybarger wrote for the different editions of the Katz Clinical Audiology Handbooks.

Although there may be some argument among clinicians about the importance of hearing aid plumbing considerations in modern hearing aids, there is little doubt that changes in plumbing can have a significant effect on the sound reaching the patients ears. The range of effects was clearly demonstrated by Killion (1980) and

> ## ON THE SOAP BOX:
> ## UNDERSTANDING EARMOLD ACOUSTICS
>
> In the modern digital age of hearing aids, it is sometimes tempting to think that earmold and earshell acoustics do not matter anymore. After all, why should we go to all the effort of learning a topic as complex as earmold acoustics when we can just fine tune the hearing aid digitally? Although it is certainly the case that modern hearing aids are much more adjustable than their counterparts of the past, we think the argument against spending time on earmold and earshell acoustics is flawed for at least two reasons. First, it is still the case that not all hearing aids are as acoustically flexible as we might wish they would be. A dip or peak in amplitude in the wrong place can sometimes be easily remedied with simple physical changes affecting the acoustics of the plumbing. Second, and more important, we sometimes need to make adjustments to the earmold or earshell such as changing tubing size or changing vent size for a number of reasons other than acoustics (e.g., cosmetics, comfort). In such instances, it is important to know what effect these changes will have on sound delivered to the patient's ears. For these and other reasons, we will spend some time here discussing earmold and earshell acoustics, but we will focus on areas we think are of the most utility in the clinic on a routine basis.

is reprinted in Figure 8–11. It is important to note that all changes you see were made using different plumbing configurations, without any changes in the frequency-specific gain or output of the hearing aid. Incredibly, we

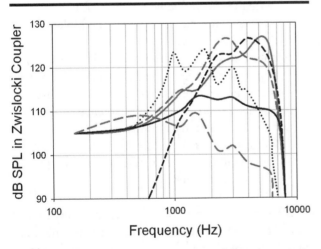

Figure 8–11. Affect of various plumbing configurations applied to the same BTE hearing aid (Adapted from Killion, 1980). This figure demonstrates how much change in amplification can be applied through physical changes in the earmold plumbing including, venting, tubing, horns, constrictions, damping, and other modifications.

can see differences in high-frequency hearing aid output exceeding 40 dB.

To review, the individual curves in Figure 8–11 are commonly referred to as hearing aid frequency response curves. The frequency response is a display of the frequency-specific level measured at the output of the hearing aid in dB SPL. Another common figure we can use is the hearing aid *gain* response, which displays the amount of amplification (gain) and/or attenuation provided at each frequency. To understand how hearing aid plumbing can affect the frequency response in hearing aids, we need to first review the acoustic behavior of air volumes and acoustic resonance:

■ As you likely remember from your study of acoustics, sound is propagated through air as a series of condensations and rarefactions. Propagation of sound in response to a vibratory force occurs as a longitudinal wave of energy that oscillates molecules of air in an expanding sphere. In a closed space, the mass of the air molecules is dependent on the volume assuming the air is uncompressed.

■ We can think of the sound pathway in a hearing aid as a series of tubes and cavities extending from the diaphragm of the receiver to the tympanic membrane.

- The volume of air in a tube is not compressed by low-frequency vibration, and the waveform is propagated through the volume of air in response to vibratory force. In such a volume (commonly referred to as an acoustic mass), the total impedance to sound energy increases with increases in frequency because there is compression of the air molecules at higher frequencies. Total impedance in an acoustic mass increases with increasing length and decreasing cross-sectional area of the tube.

- Unlike an acoustic mass, the volume of air in small hard-walled cavities oscillates as a unit, undergoing compression and expansion at the frequency of the vibratory force. In such a volume (commonly referred to as an acoustic compliance), the total impedance to sound energy decreases with increases in volume of the cavity and frequency, because it is increasingly difficult to compress air molecules as volume increases.

- In addition to the reactant (energy storage) properties of acoustic mass and acoustic compliance, acoustic resistance (conversion of acoustic energy to heat) is present in the system. Additional acoustic resistance can be intentionally introduced by narrowing the tubing or introducing an object that impedes flow (e.g., a mesh screen). However, this is somewhat complicated by the fact that unlike mesh screens (pure resistors), narrowing the tubing (constriction) will also increase compliant reactance.

In addition to reactance and resistance, it is also important to consider resonance. The following is a review of how acoustic resonance interrelates with hearing aid plumbing:

- At some frequency or frequencies, reactance in an acoustic system will be minimized leaving only resistance to impede the flow of sound energy. These are called resonance frequencies and are seen as peaks in the hearing aid frequency response. Resonance can occur because reactance is minimized in one component (e.g., the tubing), or it is minimized by the combination of adjacent components (e.g., the residual ear canal volume and the vent volume).

- When one component (e.g., volume of air), which acts as an acoustic mass, and a second component, which acts as an acoustic compliance, are adjacent to each other, a Helmholtz resonance will occur. This occurs at the frequency in which reactance of the acoustic mass and the acoustic compliance are equal to each other and cancel because they are out of phase. (Recall the magnitude of reactance is proportional to frequency in an acoustic mass and inversely proportional to frequency in an acoustic compliance.)

- When a component in an acoustic system has either a very high or very low impedance at the beginning and/or end (compared with the middle) such as a tube open at both ends, a wavelength resonance will occur. The fundamental frequency of the wavelength resonance will depend on the effective length of the tube.

- Tubes (or sections of tubes), which have either high impedance or low impedance at both ends, are referred to as half wave resonators and generate fundamental resonant frequencies that have a wavelength that is twice the effective length of the tube and additional resonances at integer multiples of this fundamental.

- Tubes (or sections of tubes), which have high impedance at one end and low impedance at the other end, are referred to as quarter wave resonators and generate fundamental resonant frequencies that have a wavelength that is four times the effective length of the tube and additional resonances at odd integer multiples of this fundamental.

The previous sections were intended only to provide very brief reviews, and those of you unfamiliar with these topics are encouraged to study them in more depth. With a general understanding of acoustics as they relate to volumes of air, we can then consider differences in the various portions of the acoustic system such as the residual ear canal volume, tubes, vents, screens, and cavities in the custom hearing aid or earmold/earhook affect the frequency response of hearing aids.

> ## KEY CONCEPT: HELMHOLTZ RESONATOR
>
> The common method for explaining the effect of a Helmholtz resonator is to use the example of air flowing over the neck of a bottle. Most of us have tried this at one time or another. The resonance will be a result of the velocity of the air, the diameter and length of the neck, and the volume of the cavity. You may recall that when applying this *scientific experiment* with a bottle containing one of your favorite beverages, if you consume some of the liquid, the volume of the cavity will become larger and the resonance then will be altered (a decrease in the resonant frequency will result). Regarding earmold plumbing, this is very similar to what happens when a closed earmold has a vent (similar to the neck of the bottle) that extends and opens to the residual volume of the ear canal (the cavity). When applied to the real ear, the Helmholtz resonator can be activated in one of three ways: external sounds going through the vent, amplified sounds from the hearing aid, or vibrations from the canal walls when the person speaks (refer to the section on the occlusion effect in Chapter 7). In the section on venting later in this chapter, we show you how alterations of the vent size and the residual cavity change the hearing aid's frequency response, all related to the Helmholtz resonance.[51]

In hearing aid systems, simple resonances as well as combinations of these resonances occur, and the effects of length and impedance of various components, and combinations of components is not always intuitive. For example, hearing aid receivers generally present high input impedance to the tubing that they are attached, but this is not always the case. These issues present a challenge to engineers designing hearing aid systems given the common goal of a broad, smooth frequency response that is relatively free of resonant peaks and unwanted dips. From a clinical standpoint, the job of the audiologist, fortunately, is to solve somewhat simpler acoustic problems. More specific, we need only to focus on physical changes to the plumbing that have acoustic implications. These physical changes may be applied for nonacoustic reasons such as cosmetics or comfort (e.g., venting, tubing diameter) or to purposely effect the hearing aid frequency response, especially when the desired acoustic changes may be difficult to apply electronically (e.g., additional high frequency gain).

Although very intricate effects are possible with hearing aid plumbing, these effects generally are the largest in specific frequency regions. It is useful to keep these regions in mind when making specific changes.

In the following, we consider a few specific hearing aid plumbing factors, which are expected to affect acoustics of the sound reaching the patient's ears that we think are the most important for everyday clinical practice. These include:

- Differences in the BTE earhooks (these most often include specific sound bore configurations and damping materials).
- Differences in the sound bore (sound pathway from the diaphragm of the receiver to the tympanic membrane)—most important, the BTE earmold tubing—including internal diameter, tube thickness, and internal diameter change effects.
- Differences in venting across all hearing aid styles—these include both intentional venting and venting differences resulting from how tightly the earmold or earshell fits in the ear.

We should point out that we do not intend to cover every possible commercially available plumbing system. Instead it is our goal to provide a basic foundation of knowledge that can be applied to any current or future plumbing system. Our thought is that commercial products come and go, but basic acoustic principles are always important, so consider each one of these three general areas.

THINGS TO REMEMBER: EARMOLD PLUMBING AND FREQUENCY RESPONSE RANGE

Residual Ear Canal Volume: How much an earshell or earmold fills up the ear canal directly affects the magnitude of the residual ear canal volume. The smaller the residual volume (the deeper the fit), the more gain that will be produced in the ear canal for the same amplifier setting (e.g., related to Boyle's law of gasses, published in 1662). This affects all frequencies but has the greatest effect for the higher frequencies.

Venting: Vents primarily affect low frequency gain, especially frequencies below 1500 Hz—the lower the frequency, the greater the effect. Increasing vent size decreases low frequency gain. One specific deviation of common venting rules relates to truly open fittings. The natural ear canal resonance of an open ear gives listeners not wearing hearing aids a boost in high frequencies (particularly around 2500 to 3000 Hz). This resonance typically is eliminated for this frequency region when an earmold or earshell is placed in the ear canal. If a highly vented (non-occluding earmold) is used, however, the hearing aid user may retain some or all of this natural ear canal resonance. Indirectly then, venting *increases* high frequency gain (see the discussion of open versus closed fittings in Chapter 7).

Damping: Dampers primarily affect frequencies between 750 and 3000 Hz, although some smaller effects may also be seen in the higher frequencies. Damping acts to reduce resonant peaks, so the exact frequency of the effect depends in part on the frequency of the resonant peaks. These peaks are usually lower frequency in BTEs than in custom instruments.

Sound bore shape and size: The overall size of the sound bore can affect all frequencies, especially those above 500 Hz. Horn-shaped tubing/sound bore and reverse-horn changes to the sound bore primarily affect gain above 2000 Hz.

Earhooks and Damping Effects

A BTE earhook (sometimes called an elbow or tone hook) has two primary functions: it directs sound from the hearing aid to the earmold tubing and it helps with hearing aid retention. Although retention does not directly impact acoustics, it is often the primary concern when selecting an earhook. Although retention is usually a greater issue with children than adults, it is always important to select the size of earhook that provides the best retention, and the best overall fit of the instrument. In addition to the size of the tone hook, some pediatric earhooks are made of a malleable material, so they can be bent for better retention on smaller and unusually

TECHNICAL TIP: DAMPED EARHOOKS

Hearing aid manufacturers commonly ship hearing aids with earhooks attached that have been acoustically modified (most commonly dampers have been added). There may be other earhooks available, however, that fit the instrument. It is important to replace earhooks with an identical match unless a change in frequency response is desired. Replacement with the wrong earhook or removal of clogged damping elements without replacement is an easy way to create an unhappy patient who is disturbed by the change in the hearing aid after it was fixed. Although the first choice would be to obtain a match, it is possible to *retune* the fitting through programming, especially if a real-ear output of the previous fitting is available.

shaped ears. If we were writing this text ten years ago, we may have spent several pages discussing acoustics related to earhooks. However, current technology has limited the need for some of these considerations; in particular, many of the smaller mini-BTEs, both RICs and RITAs (see Chapter 7) do not use earhooks. Despite these changes, one factor that should still be considered is damping.

Damping must be considered because resonant peaks are commonly present in the hearing aid frequency response. These resonant peaks are due, at least in part, to wavelength resonances. For example, the typical 75-mm sound bore associated with traditional BTE instruments will result in one-half-wave resonances at approximately 2300, 4600, and 6900 Hz; and, one-quarter-wave resonances at approximately 1100, 3300, and 5500 Hz (Cox, 1979; Walker, 1979). Examples of peaky and smoothed hearing aid frequency responses are shown in Figure 8–12.

Frequency responses of modern hearing aids are generally smoother (less peaky) than those of old because precise digital filtering can be used to smooth the response. However, the use of dampers can still be important to limit remaining peaks. Some general points to remember:

- Many modern digital hearing aids use a precise digital filter to smooth out the wavelength resonances introduced by the earhook or tubing.

- In some cases, the clinician may want to change the length of tubing for retention or other purposes. In such cases, it may be necessary to reprogram the hearing aid if this occurs, because the exact frequency and magnitude of resonant peaks will be affected by tubing length.

- If a nonstandard length is used, some undesirable resonances may remain that may be reduced through damping.

It is important to note that some research suggests that the frequency response associated with damping is preferred by hearing aid users (Davis & Davidson, 1996). Further, limiting the *peakiness* of the response can also lead to higher overall output levels without narrow bandwidth, high-level, peaks of sound exceeding the patient's threshold of discomfort (Bryne, Christen, & Dillon, 1981). That is, the hearing aid may have a peak around 1500 Hz, which exceeds the patient's LDL (for loudness discomfort level). If this peak were damped and reduced by, say 10 dB, it may be possible to raise the overall MPO of the hearing aid across all the other frequencies considerably, improving headroom for the peaks of speech, yet not exceeding the patient's LDL.

Dampers are commonly screens or other materials that act to provide resistance to acoustic energy. For example, before today's machined dampers were available, it was common for audiologists to use lambswool as a damper.[52] Prepackaged dampers are available in a range of sizes, with the largest sizes usually surrounded by a metal can. Several investigations have reported the specific effects of different types of damping (e.g., Cox & Gilmore, 1986; Davis & Davidson, 1996; Studebaker, 1974). It is important to note that because dampers provide acoustic resistance, dampers act to reduce the level (provide attenuation) of peaks in the hearing aids frequency response. This point is important because the maximum effect provided by any specific damper will not always occur at the same frequency but will rather be determined in part, by the frequencies of the resonant peaks in the specific hearing aid prior to damping.

In addition to the frequency at which the resonant peaks naturally occur in a hearing aid, the effect damping has on the existing resonant peaks primarily depends on two factors: (1) the impedance of the damper (measured in ohms) and (2) the placement of

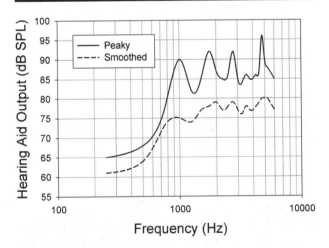

Figure 8–12. Examples of peaky and smoothed frequency responses. The smoothed frequency response was obtained by introducing a highly resistive damper near the sound outlet.

the damper. Generally the higher the impedance, the more attenuation. As for placement, the greatest attenuation will occur for most frequencies when the damper is placed nearest the sound outlet. For example, there will be greater damping for a placement near the tip of an earhook than near the receiver—see Figures 8–13 and 8–14 for the effects on a typical traditional BTE with resonant peaks near 1100 and 3300 Hz. In addition to BTE earhooks, dampers can be placed in the receiver tubing of custom hearing aids as well as in the earmold tubing.

With today's products, the clinician's work with dampers likely will be limited. For those who have the interest, dampers can still be obtained from hearing aid

supply stores such as Hal-Hen, who carry the Knowles fused-mesh damper. [53] These dampers consist of a metal ferrule that contains a finely woven plastic acoustic resistance screen and are designed to fit snugly into #13 gauge tubing. These dampers are color-coded and come in five impedances.

In addition to damping, we should also mention the availability of special purpose earhooks, which can be very useful for certain patients. Special purpose earhooks, such as those available from some hearing aid manufacturers and companies like Etymotic Research, work well for unusual hearing loss configurations such as patient's with cookie-bite, reverse cookie bite, and reverse slope audiograms.[54]

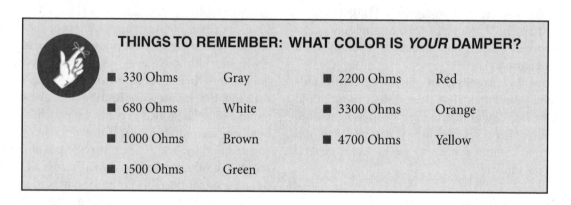

THINGS TO REMEMBER: WHAT COLOR IS *YOUR* DAMPER?

■ 330 Ohms	Gray	■ 2200 Ohms	Red
■ 680 Ohms	White	■ 3300 Ohms	Orange
■ 1000 Ohms	Brown	■ 4700 Ohms	Yellow
■ 1500 Ohms	Green		

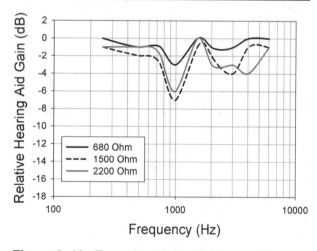

Figure 8–13. Examples of the attenuation that may be provided by various dampers for a BTE instrument with the damper placed in the earhook very near the receiver.

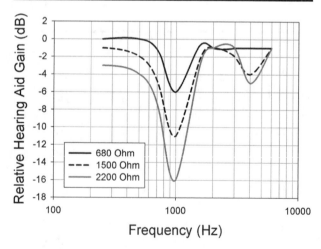

Figure 8–14. Examples of the attenuation that may be provided by various dampers for a BTE instrument with the damper place in the tip of the earhook adjacent to the earmold tubing. Note how much greater the effect is when compared to Figure 8–13.

TECHNICAL TIP: DAMPING IN CUSTOM PRODUCTS

Although we normally think about dampers in the earhook of BTE products, or sometimes inserted in earmold tubing, it is also possible to use dampers with custom instruments:

- By extending the tubing slightly from the receiver (10 mm is common), dampers can be placed in custom products. The effect is usually no larger than 5 to 9 dB at the resonant peak (commonly near 2000 Hz).
- As is the case with BTE instruments, placement nearest the sound outlet will commonly provide the greatest amount of smoothing for a *peaky* response. Unfortunately, however, this placement will likely lead to the need for regular replacement because of blockage by moisture and debris from the ear canal. The extended tubing also can be uncomfortable for patients if their ear canal has a turn in this area, and if/when the tube becomes hardened, there can be scratching during insertion.

KEY CONCEPT: COMMON CLINICAL SLANG

Some of you may be unfamiliar with some of the clinical slang used when referring to different hearing loss configurations. For the uninitiated:

- Ski-Slope: A downward sloping hearing loss, usually one that is particularly precipitious—often associated with the need for an open fitting.
- Reverse slope: This is used to refer to patients with significant hearing loss in the low frequencies, sloping upward to normal or near-normal high frequency thresholds.
- Cookie bite: This is used to refer to patients with significant hearing loss in the middle frequencies (750 to 2000 Hz) and near-normal hearing in the high and low frequencies.
- Reverse cookie-bite: This is used to refer to patents with significant hearing loss in the lower and higher frequencies and near-normal thresholds in the middle frequencies. Unfortunately, some clinicians and even manufacturers have reversed our definitions related to cookie bite so make sure to note the exact configuration when ordering special purpose earhooks and other acoustic accessories.
- Corner audiogram: Refers to a patient who only has measureable hearing in the lower frequencies.

Sound Bore and Tubing Effects

In a BTE instrument, tubing serves the purpose of directing sound from the reciever to the ear canal and helps with retention by anchoring the hearing aid to the earmold or eartip. In traditional BTE instruments, the tubing is usually pushed into a hole in the earmold drilled just for the tube (typically referred to as the earmold tubing bore). The excess tubing beyond the earmold canal is trimmed off, and then the tubing is glued in place or held in place with a physical tubing lock (a small plastic or metal ring aroud the tubing). It is common to trim the tubing so that it is recessed inside the tip of the earmold. Acoustic changes resulting from tubing changes primarily relate to the internal diameter of the tubing (including changes in internal diameter over the length of the tubing).

In 1979, the National Association of Earmold Laboratories (NAEL) reached an agreement on a naming convention for tubing based on internal diameter that is still intact today—see Table 8–2. Today, the most common tubing internal diameters include the fixed bore #13 tubing, typically referred to as *standard* tubing for traditional BTE instruments and the thin tube (typically 0.9 to 0.95 internal diameter) commonly used with RITA instruments. We talk about hearing aid verification in Book Three of this series; however, an interesting clinical aside is that the standard 2-cc couplers aimed at BTE verification do not mimic standard #13 tubing, but rather, a 4 mm horn tubing that we describe later in this chapter.

Bore Diameter

Reducing tubing diameter increases the effective acoustic mass and overall impedance. Although this can affect the overall frequency response, the most notable effect of decreasing tubing diameter is that the frequency of the resonant peaks resulting from wavelength resonances are slightly lowered, see Figure 8–15. Note that the effect of changing tubing size on the resonant peaks is relative;

Table 8–2. NAEL Standard Sizes for Earmold Tubing. (Blue, 1979)

NAEL Size	Internal Diameter (mm)	External Diameter (mm)
No. 9	3.00	4.01
No. 12	2.16	3.18
No. 13	1.93	2.95
No. 14	1.68	2.95
No. 15	1.5	2.95
No. 16	1.35	2.95
Add for "thick wall" (No. 13)		0.35
Add for "double wall" (No. 13)		0.66
Add for "medium" (No. 13)		0.15
Subtract for "thin" (No. 16)		0.79
Non-NAEL Size		
Thin Tube	0.75 to 0.95	1.0 to 1.2

the exact frequencies that are affected will depend on where the resonant peaks are to begin with. It is interesting to note that these relatively small effects can actually be accentuated in modern hearing aids. Let us assume

---

TECHNICAL TIP: GETTING THE TUBING LENGTH RIGHT

■ Tubing length directly affects how the hearing aid case is positioned on the ear. Long tubing will result in an instrument that hangs behind the pinna. Shorter tubing may cause the hearing aid to sit on top the pinna. This choice directly affects patient comfort as well as cosmetics.

■ We suggest inserting the earmold, placing the hearing aid on the ear, and adjusting for optimal position, then cutting the tubing to the appropriate length. Like carpentry, it is good to remember the motto "measure twice, cut once." Cutting the tubing too short means you will need to retube the earmold.

■ As we discussed earlier, several predetermined lengths of tubing are typically available in the fitting kit for mini-BTE hearing aids. Because these instruments often do not use a custom earmold, correct selection of length is particularly important for retention purposes (this is also true for selection of the length of wire in RIC instruments). The fitting kits usually provide a device that might assist with sizing. Better retention and reduced feedback may also require bending the thin tube to best fit an individual ear. Application of heat can sometimes aid in this process.

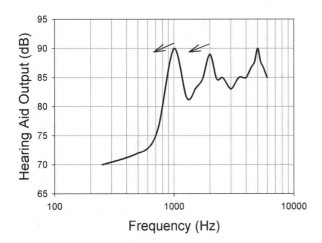

Figure 8–15. General affect of decreasing internal tubing diameter on the resonant peaks of the hearing aid frequency response. That is, the magnitude of peaks is decreased in frequency and amplitude as internal diameter is decreased.

a manufacturer implements a group of *notch* filters that act to reduce gain over the narrow frequency ranges for which wavelength resonance peaks are expected. This filter will be designed for a specific internal diameter.

If however, a significantly different internal diameter of tubing is used, the frequency response could have both *dips* from the notch filter set as at the old resonant frequencies as well as *bumps* at the adjacent new resonant frequencies (see associated "Points to Ponder"). As noted previously, this can be an even greater problem if the length of the tubing is changed.

In addition to frequency lowering of the resonant peaks, reducing the tubing internal diameter can also lower the magnitude of the resonant peaks (dampening). However, the magnitude of the dampening of the resonant peaks is clearly most effective with the smallest tubing diameters. Figure 8–16 shows the deviation in frequency response from a typical BTE using standard #13 tubing. The largest deviation is clearly evident for a very thin tube, such as is commonly used with the mini-BTE OC style of hearing aid described in Chapter 7. For the thin tube, there is a slight 6 to 7 dB boost in the low frequencies and up to 20 dB of attenuation in the middle and high frequencies when compared with standard #13 tubing. Note that the effects will be slightly different from those shown depending on the original magnitude and frequency of the resonant peaks of the instrument in the presence of #13 tubing as well as acoustic properties of the earhook used. Also, it should be pointed out that

---

POINTS TO PONDER: PLUMBING AND MODERN HEARING AIDS

As we described, some hearing aids will employ notch filtering to reduce the *expected* and unwanted effects of resonances of the earmold plumbing. If you change the plumbing and introduce a different set of resonances, an undesirable fitting may result. Here is a typical example of when this might happen: You fit a patient with a larger BTE instrument that has the standard earhook and the #13 tubing. After a few weeks of use, the patient is concerned that this plumbing is bulky and much more noticeable than the plumbing used with the mini-BTEs that the patient's friend wears. You realize that an option is for you to remove the standard earhook and use a thin-tube screw-on adapter (which will also require a new earmold for the thin-tube fitting). This indeed will be a noticeable cosmetic improvement for the patient. But what if the hearing aids fitted employ filtering to reduce the large resonant peak around 1500 Hz that would be expected for the standard hook/tubing? What you will likely see with the new fitting is a large dip in this frequency range in the real-ear output, which will need to be accounted for with a substantial amount of added gain. But what if someone simply changed the plumbing and did not repeat probe-microphone verification? How would they know that outcome? To correct this mistake it will be necessary to change the tubing configuration in the manufacturers fitting software and then refit the hearing aid using your prescriptive gain targets of choice and probe microphone verification.

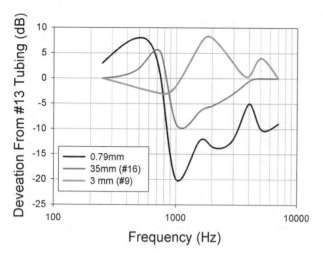

Figure 8–16. Deviation in frequency response for the same BTE hearing aid when changed from #13 (standard) tubing. It is important to note that although this provides a view of the general effect of changing tubing length, the specific changes shown here result from the specific instrument evaluated. Instruments with different resonant peaks will show different specific effects.

these differences assume that you have the same coupling to the ear. Clinical fitting of the same instrument using thin tubes (RITA) versus traditional tubing and an earhook will often result in even larger differences than shown in Figure 8–16, particularly in the low frequencies, because different earmolds/eartips with different amounts of venting are usually paired with each type.

Unlike internal diameter, a tube's external diameter is not expected to affect the hearing aid frequency response. However, unintentional changes related to constriction of the tubing can occur, as described in the next section. The choice of external tubing diameter is usually based on how much amplification is needed (based on the degree of hearing loss) and cosmetic factors. The more amplification, the more likely it is to create vibration in the earmold tubing. This vibration can in turn set the hearing aid case and surrounding air into vibration providing pathways that increase the likelihood of acoustic and mechanical feedback. Therefore, thicker walled tubing is sometimes recommended for patients with severe-to-profound hearing loss. Although sometimes necessary to prevent feedback, this thicker

tubing is a little harder to shape and work with, so it is only used when necessary.

Horn Effects

The majority of patients that we fit with hearing aids have downward sloping losses, and obtaining the desired amount of gain in the higher frequencies often is challenging. In some cases, you find that you need a little more amplification at 3000 Hz, and you already increased gain as much as the programming software will allow. This can occur despite the fact that the patient appeared to be within the manufacturer's fitting range for the hearing aid you ordered. We do not want to underfit the patient, but yet we do not want to send the patient home to sit and wait while we reorder a different hearing aid. What can we do?

One method that has been used for many years, and is effective in changing the magnitude of amplification only in the high frequencies, is a change in the bore diameter of the transmission system from the receiver to the sound outlet at the medial tip of the canal portion of the earmold or hearing aid shell. Such increases in the bore diameter can result in a boost in high frequency gain and are generally referred to as *acoustic horns* (e.g., Killion, 1979, 1993, 1998, 2003; Libby, 1982a, 1982b; Lybarger, 1985). In contrast, decreases in the bore diameter lead to decreases in gain and are generally referred to as reverse horns or constrictions (Cox, 1979). A change in bore diameter can be achieved in a large number of ways, shown in Figure 8–17, leading to a variety of changes in the hearing aid frequency response, shown in Figure 8–18. Fortunately however, acoustic horns do follow a few general rules that allow for prediction of how they will work:

- All horns have a cutoff frequency that can be mathematically derived. Little or no change in amplification level (horn effect) occurs below this cutoff frequency.
- The magnitude of the horn effect exponentially increases from the cutoff frequency to reach a maximum dB level increase (approximately 20 log [outlet diameter/inlet diameter]) at a frequency one octave above the cutoff frequency. This peak occurs at approximately the frequency where

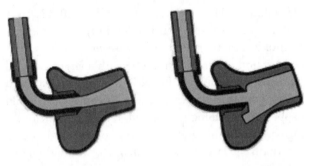

Figure 8–17. Change in sound bore diameter can be achieved in a large number of ways. This figure displays two types of CFA horns including a smoothed bore (*left-hand portion*) and stepped horn (*right-hand portion*).

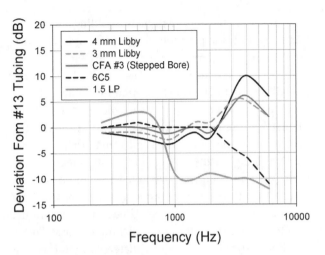

Figure 8–18. Deviation in frequency response for the same BTE hearing aid when changing from #13 (standard) tubing to one of the several available horns or constrictions. (Adapted from data presented by Dillon, 1985, 1991 and Killion, 1981.)

a quarter wavelength equals the distance between the change in the tubing diameter and the medial tip of the earmold.

- The cutoff frequency in a smooth horn is calculated by (Beranek, 1954):

$$Horn\ Cutoff\ Frequency =$$
$$\frac{Speed\ of\ Sound \times natural\ log(\frac{outlet\ diameter}{inlet\ diameter})}{2\pi \times length\ of\ Horn}$$

- In other words, the shorter the effective horn length, the higher the cutoff frequency. For example, one of the most effective horns is a 4-mm Libby horn (22 mm long) that has a cutoff frequency of about 1700 Hz and reaches its maximum horn effect (around 5 to 10 dB) at around 3400 Hz (see Figure 8–18).
- In contrast, the same inlet and outlet diameters in a 10-mm long horn, as might be available in a belled canal of a custom instrument, move the cutoff frequency to near 4000 Hz (with a maximum not reached until almost 8000 Hz), rendering them of little use in most common hearing aids.
- Stepped horns will have a shorter effective length than smooth bores, because the change in diameter occurs closer to the medial tip.

These rules clearly show that although the change in bore diameter is important regarding the magnitude

of the horn effect, having a horn with a long, effective length is critical to providing an increase in amplification that is low enough in frequency to be useful in most modern hearing aids, other than those providing extended high-frequency amplification (greater than 4 to 6 kHz). We should note, however, that sometimes the introduction of a belled canal, or pulling the tubing back from the medial tip of the earmold, can provide a larger than expected level increase in the high frequencies. However, this unexpectedly large level increase usually occurs because a constriction was removed, rather than being due to the horn effect as explained later in this chapter.

Based on his work with Knowles Electronics, Killion (1979) introduced the idea of abutting tubes of differing internal diameter together in a *stepped horn* for hearing aids. The procedure provided the desired boost in the high frequencies very effectively, but when this new horn earmold style was rolled out for routine patient use, some practical problems emerged. The dampers that had been strategically placed in the tubing for fine tuning became plugged, and after continuous use, the glued pieces of tubing would come apart (many patients use the tubing to pull the earmold out of the ear, which most probably contributed to this problem). Entrepreneur E. Robert "Cy" Libby (1982a) modified the horn acoustic concept of Killion by molding and manufacturing a plastic tube into a one-piece smooth horn with a stepped-internal diameter.[55] This earmold style quickly became known as *The Libby Horn*. These horns are still in use today, which commonly are available in 3 mm and 4 mm configurations (denoting the internal diameter at the medial end of the horn). Although the best boost will be found with the 4-mm horn, this diameter is too big for the ear canal of most patients. Many clinicians and scientists have noted a small horn effect can be introduced by inserting standard earmold tubing only partially into the earmold. Although still a minimal effect compared with the other methods discussed here, this horn effect can be slightly increased by increasing the diameter of the sound bore at the medial end of the earmold or custom earshell, commonly referred to as a belled canal. It is unlikely that the belled canal approach will provide a significant high-frequency boost, simply because of the short distance of the horn length. More recently, approaches that attach a hard plastic elbow directly to the earmold or by using a snap ring have been introduced. These approaches, such as the Continuous Flow Adaptor (CFA) allow for easy attachment of tubing between the hearing aid and earmold and a variety of horn and reverse-horn configurations.

In contrast with the acoustic horns designed to *increase* high frequencies, constrictions and reverse horns act to decrease the magnitude of high-frequency energy. Although horns are least effective when they are placed nearest the sound outlet (medial tip of the earmold or earshell), constrictions are most effective in this position. Clinically, reverse horns are rarely intentionally used because it is fairly uncommon to desire a reduction in high-frequency output, because the majority of hearing loss configurations are sloping (greatest loss in the high frequencies). In addition, the majority of modern hearing aids are flexible enough to reduce gain electronically or digitally. Despite these facts, we still feel it is necessary to discuss constrictions for two reasons: (1) the rare case of an inflexible (usually relatively inexpensive) hearing aid that does not allow for enough high frequency gain reduction in the presence of needed gain in the lower frequencies and, perhaps more important, (2) the inadvertent constriction of standard, constant diameter tubing.

Inadvertent and typically unwanted constrictions can happen across a variety of instrument styles with patients who have very narrow ear canals. For example, Killion (1988) reported a loss of 5 to 10 dB in the high frequencies from constriction in typical children's earmolds. Another common cause of an inadvertent constriction occurs when a tube with a larger external diameter is mistakenly forced into a smaller earmold tubing bore than for which it was intended. This could happen when tubing is replaced, if a thick-walled tubing was mistakenly grabbed instead of standard tubing. Alternatively, larger external diameter tubing may be forced into an earmold tubing bore drilled for smaller external diameter to try to keep the tubing from being pulled out. This is not recommended, because tubing that is too large for the sound bore can cause the internal diameter of the tubing to be squeezed by the earmold sound bore. These inadvertent constrictions can significantly reduce the amplified sound level in the high frequencies in a similar manner to the intentional constriction affects shown in Figure 8–18. The 6C5 and 1.5 LP tubing configurations shown in this figure are available from Etymotic Research. The 6C5 consists of #13 tubing (1.93 mm internal diameter) that is partially inserted in the earmold, followed by a small 3 mm cavity with 14 mm of #16 tubing (1.35 mm internal diameter) in the medial tip of the earmold. The 1.5 LP tubing configuration is #15 tubing (1.5 mm internal diameter) that is stepped down to a 0.9 mm internal diameter for the last 12 mm of the medial tip of the earmold.

Venting Effects

Venting is a term that simply refers to opening up an air/sound transmission pathway from the tympanic membrane to the environment outside the head. Venting is the most common alteration made to earmold plumbing by audiologists. The effects of venting can make a substantial change to low frequency gain and output. Venting is used with hearing aid fittings for several reasons, including the following (from Mueller & Hall, 1998):

■ To allow amplified low-frequency signals to escape: In some cases, the gain of the instrument in the lower frequencies is greater than necessary, or what is desired by the patient. Although this usually can be adjusted with the fitting software, venting can provide an additional release of amplified low-frequency output.

■ To allow low-frequency signals generated in the ear canal to escape: As discussed in Chapter 7, when a person talks, his or her voice is transmitted from the throat via bone conduction along the mandible to the condyle, which is adjacent to the ear canal. This vibrates the cartilaginous portion of the ear canal, which creates low-frequency, air-conducted energy within the cavity. If this energy cannot escape (e.g., entrance is plugged with an earmold or hearing aid), it can distort the person's own voice (e.g., sounds hollow, echo, etc.), and cause annoyance and sometimes hearing aid rejection. This is referred to as the occlusion effect. The most effective treatment of the occlusion effect is venting—allowing the low-frequency energy to escape (see Chapter 7 for complete review).

■ To allow unamplified signals to pass unobstructed to the eardrum: When a person has normal hearing for a given frequency range (usually the lows), it often is desirable to allow speech and environmental sounds to pass naturally to the eardrum and not be attenuated by an earmold/hearing aid shell. This may improve localization, make sounds more natural, and improve the overall quality of the signal. This is easy to verify using the REOR (for real ear occluded response) measure with your probe-microphone equipment.

■ To allow pressure relief: When earmolds or hearing aid shells are fitted tightly, there can be a buildup of pressure in the residual ear canal, and the patient will report a sensation of *fullness*. Some patients can sense this pressure increasing as the daily hearing aid use continues. A small vent can relieve this pressure, and in fact, these small vents often are called *pressure vents*.

■ To allow aerations of the ear canal and/or middle ear: In some cases, when external or middle ear pathology exists, the pathology is aggravated when the normal ventilation of the ear is altered. For these patients, venting is used for medical rather than acoustic reasons, and there may need to be some compromise in the applied low frequency gain (e.g., less than desired) to allow for the necessary aeration.

Venting can be contrasted with a *fully occluded* situation in which a sealed cavity is formed between the tympanic membrane and the medial portion of the hearing aid or earmold upon insertion. This distinction between vented and occluded is generally theoretical, however, because almost no earmold or hearing aid will entirely seal the ear canal regardless of the earmold material used. Such a fit would prove to be uncomfortably tight for most people, not to mention the problems caused relative to insertion and removal. Instead, almost all hearing aids include some magnitude of slit leak venting, which allows sound and air to pass between the residual ear canal cavity and the outside world. It is no surprise to note that the magnitude of slit leak venting is affected by the tightness of fit, the earmold or hearing

---

KEY CONCEPT: FIVE IMPORTANT FACTORS FOR VENTING

Not all vents are created equal, and vents that are equal can have a different effect for different fittings or for different people. When thinking about the effects that a given vent may have on the amplified signal, there are five general areas to consider:

■ The length of the vent
■ The diameter of the vent
■ The leakage of the fitting not directly associated with the vent
■ The residual ear canal volume
■ The middle ear impedance

---

aid material, the depth of the earmold/shell in the ear canal, and the degree that the earmold shell fills up the concha—ITCs will generally have more slit leak venting than ITEs and BTE earmolds. The magnitude of slit leak venting will affect the maximum available gain before feedback and will limit the use of some smaller styles with greater magnitudes of hearing loss. Fortunately, the advent of modern feedback suppression technology has extended the fitting range (available gain before feedback) of all hearing aid styles.

Although slit leak venting is certainly a consideration, particularly when selecting the hearing aid style, the term venting is most commonly used to refer to intentional air pathways that are opened between the residual outer ear canal cavity and the outside environment. Intentional venting also acts to limit the maximum gain available before feedback. This limitation is primarily found in the 2000 to 4000 Hz range—the frequencies most prone to feedback because this is where there is the largest difference between the environmental SPL and the amplified real-ear signal. Gain in the lower and higher frequencies is more typically limited by the physical output limits of the hearing aid amplifier and receiver. The maximum available gain measured in patient's ears at 2000 and 3000 Hz across a range of hearing aid styles and venting configurations and in the *absence* of feedback suppression technology is shown in Figure 8–19. Keep in mind, however, that although these are average values, individual patients may exhibit feedback at acoustic gain values that are 5 to 10 dB less than shown here (others may receive up to 5 to 10 dB more gain before feedback). As might be expected, the magnitude of available gain decreases with increasing vent size and across styles as the microphone and receiver outlet are more closely spaced (from BTE to

ITE to ITC). If you are unfamiliar with the term, *real ear insertion gain*, you can simply assume it to refer to the amount of amplification provided by the hearing aid.

Hearing aid vents are available in a variety of different shapes and sizes. In one common configuration, a cylindrical hole is drilled from the lateral to the medial surfaces of the custom hearing aid or earmold in paral-

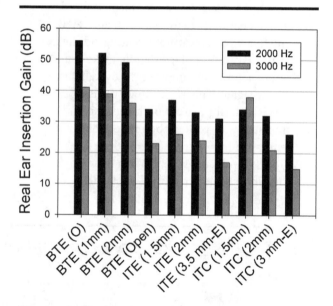

Figure 8–19. Maximum Real Ear Insertion Gain available for 2000 and 3000 Hz for various venting configurations and hearing aid styles, when not using digital feedback suppression technology. (O) refers to a fully occluded fitting, whereas (-E) makes reference to the effective vent size resulting from the combination of slit leak and intentional venting. (Derived from Dillon, 1991; Egolf, Howell, Weaver, and Barker, 1985; and Kuk, 1994.)

lel to the sound bore. This is referred to as a *parallel vent*, shown in Figure 8–20. The smallest vents are the approximately 0.5 to 0.8 mm diameter *pressure relief vents*. Parallel vents as large as 3.5 to 4 mm may be possible in some earmolds if the patient has a large enough diameter ear canal. A completely non-occluding fit is also possible through several methods including (1) an open earmold, sometimes referred to as IROS,[56] (2) inserting tubing with a simple *concha lock* consisting of a flexible wire or thin plastic arm that presses slightly against the concha to hold the tube in place, or (3) one of the many custom and modular eartip styles available with OC hearing aids as described in Chapter 7 and earlier in this chapter.

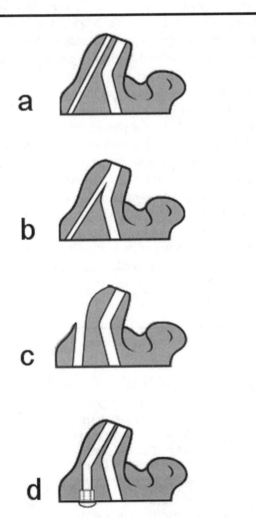

Figure 8–20. Examples of (**A**) parallel, (**B**) side branch, (**C**) trough vent, and (**D**) SAV vent configurations. Reprinted with permission from Westone.

Because of space limitations, parallel vents are usually limited to a diameter of 2.5 mm or less in ITEs and 2 mm in ITCs. When space is particularly limited, or active drainage or other problems routinely clog the vent, a *trough vent*, sometimes referred to as an *external vent*, is used. This consists of a channel ground into the canal and concha bowl portion of the hearing aid or earmold (see Figure 8–20).

Sometimes a vent is started as a trough vent on the canal portion and then is transitioned into a parallel vent. Trough vents effectively increase the magnitude of slit-leak venting and typically behave acoustically in the exact same way as parallel vents of the same size. Trough vents are less desirable for some patients, however, as the consistency of the patient's skin and tissue can lead to the trough being *filled up* to various degrees leading to a less controlled vent size. In some cases of extreme space constraints, it may be tempting to use a side-branch vent (also referred to as a Y-vent, angle vent, or diagonal vent). In this configuration, the tubing is only minimally inserted into the earmold, and then a vent is drilled from the lateral surface of the earmold to the earmold sound bore (see Figure 8–20). That is, the medial sound bore opening also serves as the medial opening for the vent. Although certainly tempting from a space conservation standpoint, we agree with many other authors (e.g., Cox, 1979) in stating that side-branch vents should not be used unless there is no other alternative, or the patient has minimum need for high-frequency amplification. This recommendation is based on two negative acoustic consequences of side-branch vents: (1) The magnitude of high-frequency amplification is decreased, and (2) The likelihood of feedback is increased.

To review, venting serves several purposes and increasing the magnitude of venting will have several potential consequences:

- Increases the susceptibility to feedback.
- Decreases the occlusion effect.
- Reduces low frequency gain by allowing low-frequency amplified sound to leak out, shown in Figure 8–21.
- Allows unamplified low-frequency sound from the environment to leak in.

Because of the acoustic consequences of increased vent size, for decades clinicians have needed to balance comfort and occlusion reduction with a loss of low frequency gain and increased susceptibility. Because of slit leak venting and differences in ear geometry, it is commonly quite difficult to know *a priori* how large of a vent can be used for any individual patient. As a consequence, it is common to drill out a larger vent bore and then provide a means for blocking part of the vent (either with a small tube or valve). Commercially available versions known by names such as Select-a-Vent

(SAV) and Positive Venting Valve (PVV) come in a variety of sizes and allow for easy office modifications to the vent size without drilling. However, as explained below, it is not uncommon for the effect of changing an SAV plug on the venting effect to be more limited than might be expected. An example of different SAV options is shown in Figure 8–22. In addition to the more limited range of venting effects, another downside of the SAV is that it is a bit more noticeable than a single drilled vent.

Although the balancing problem of feedback versus occlusion exists today, the introduction of digital feedback suppression technology has moved the fulcrum of this clinical teeter-totter. Specifically, feedback suppression processing allows for more gain and more venting before feedback and has increased the available maximum gain before feedback by as much as 10 to 18 dB (e.g., Ricketts & Johnson, 2008). If the patient has a significant hearing loss, this balancing problem remains, however, and peak high frequency gain in an open configuration is still limited to approximately 35 dB SPL of insertion gain for a truly open fitting.

With all of these different vent configurations, you might wonder how it is possible to quantify vent size and the meaning of equivalent vent size. Does the smallest constriction in the vent bore determine the acoustic properties of the vent? An important question given the common use of SAV style plug interchange products. It turns out that short constrictions, relative to the total length of the vent, have little impact on venting. Instead, the acoustic properties of venting and their measured effect on occlusion and feedback are based on the acoustic mass of the vent.

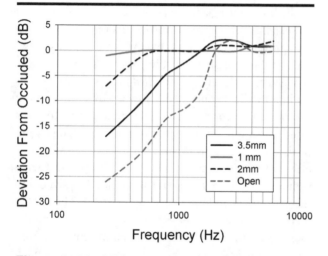

Figure 8–21. Affect of venting on the hearing aid frequency response in comparison with a tight fitting BTE earmold without intentional venting. Note both an increase in magnitude of gain reduction and an increase in the frequency at which the gain reduction begins with increasing vent size. (Adapted from Dillon, 1985.)

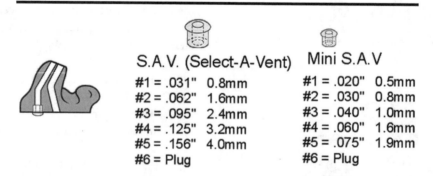

S.A.V. (Select-A-Vent)
#1 = .031" 0.8mm
#2 = .062" 1.6mm
#3 = .095" 2.4mm
#4 = .125" 3.2mm
#5 = .156" 4.0mm
#6 = Plug

Mini S.A.V
#1 = .020" 0.5mm
#2 = .030" 0.8mm
#3 = .040" 1.0mm
#4 = .060" 1.6mm
#5 = .075" 1.9mm
#6 = Plug

Figure 8–22. Two examples of SAV options from one manufacturer. These are both limited in length compared to vent tubes which can have a much greater relative effect on the change in total acoustic mass. Reprinted with permission from Westone.

THINGS TO REMEMBER: CALCULATING ACOUSTIC MASS

For understanding acoustic mass, we can go back to the work of Beranek in 1954.

■ Acoustic Mass = 1.18 (Air Density) × (Effective Length [m]/Cross-Sectional Area [m²]). Where cross-sectional area = π × radius²

■ Effective Length = Length of the Vent × (0.4 × Vent Diameter at the Medial Tip)

More specific, the greater the acoustic mass, the smaller the vent effect. From the formula shown on this page, we can see that the smaller the cross-sectional area of the vent and the longer the vent bore, the greater the acoustic mass. That is, short wide vents will provide more venting than long narrow ones.

The concept of acoustic mass as related to vents has at least three important applications. First, it is important for understanding the effect of vent diameter. Moving from a 1-mm to 2-mm constant diameter vent of the same length will quadruple the cross-sectional area leading to an acoustic mass that is nearly one-quarter as large. (Note: It is *nearly*, rather than *exactly* one-quarter because the change in diameter also changes the effective length of the vent as shown in the second formula above.) In contrast, moving from a 2-mm to 3-mm constant diameter vent reduces acoustic mass by only about one-half.

A second important consideration is how acoustic mass and venting affects our understanding of SAV plugs. When a vent channel is made up of different cross-sectional areas (e.g., a small diameter short plug in the end of a large diameter long vent bore), the total acoustic mass is the sum of the mass in each section. Therefore, if the rest of the vent has high acoustic mass (i.e., is long and thin) or the combination of the rest of the vent and slit leak venting has very low acoustic mass (i.e., loose-fit or wide and short vent), the effect of placing a short plug in one end of the vent on the overall acoustic mass will be minimal. Further, similar vent plug sizes may yield nearly identical venting effects, because the change in overall acoustic mass of the entire vent will be small.

Finally, acoustic mass is also important related to vent shape. For example, you might wonder if it is possible to put an effective vent in a CIC or ITC that is recessed in the ear. In this case, the faceplate area is lim-

ited by the diameter of the ear canal, and the diameter of the vent will be limited by the battery door. This may only allow a 1-mm (or smaller) vent opening on the lateral portion of the hearing aid. However, if the ear canal is wide enough, there may be room for a wider opening on the medial tip; in many cases, this wider opening is accomplished with a trough vent. This configuration is commonly referred to as a reverse-horn vent. In the example we present here, if we can half the overall acoustic mass by using a reverse-horn vent, the effective vent size will grow to about 1.5 mm assuming a 1-mm vent opening in the faceplate.

In Closing

In this chapter, we have taken a close look at earmold plumbing, and we hope you have gained some insight regarding how this can impact the success of the fitting. A hearing aid with the best technology on the market may be rejected if the plumbing is not right.

It all starts with a good ear impression. Although we reviewed many acoustic concerns, comfort also is very important. This ear impression is even more critical for custom instruments, as fixing the problem could mean a complete remake of the hearing aid. Indeed, the modular earmolds that have become common with mini-BTEs have several advantages, but custom earmolds are still necessary in many cases. We reviewed three different general categories when considering changes in earmold acoustics. A brief review is as follows:

■ Damping with commercial dampers, or other products, acts to smooth the peaks in the hearing aid frequency response. The closer the damper is to the sound outlet, the more effective it will be. Damping primarily reduces resonant peaks in the middle frequencies.

■ Widening the sound bore/tubing over the course of its length creates an acoustic horn. The horn effect increases the sound level in the high frequencies (generally above 2500 Hz or higher). The frequency at which the level increase begins will be increasingly lower with longer horns.

■ Increasing the vent size increases the susceptibility to feedback, decreases the occlusion effect, reduces low frequency gain, allows unamplified low-frequency sound from the environment to leak in, and allows an air exchange pathway that will decrease the buildup of moisture and increase comfort.

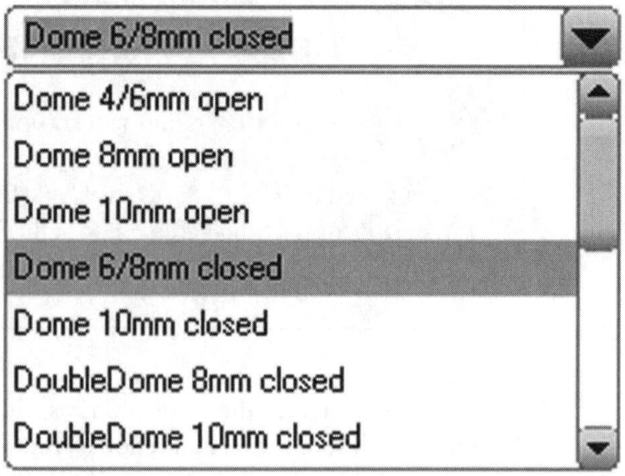

Figure 8–23. Acoustic parameter selection.

A Final Case Study

We close this chapter with a case study that illustrates how the understanding of venting can play an important role in the everyday fitting of hearing aids. This patient was a 72-year-old male with a mild-to-moderate downward sloping hearing loss (approximately 30 dB in the lows dropping to 60 to 65 dB in the 3000 to 4000 Hz region) who was fitted with a mini-BTE RIC, using a modular fitting tip. Because of the degree of hearing loss in the low frequencies, the audiologist selected a dome labeled *closed* from the manufacturer's fitting kit. As part of the pre-fitting process, therefore, she also selected closed from the pull-down menu in the fitting software. Figure 8–23 shows the menu options. Note that for this manufacturer, and for this particular product, there are seven choices if the modular dome is used.

In general, manufacturers do their best to make their automated fittings close to what is desired by the audiologist, particularly when the audiologist is using a standard fitting formula. In this case, the audiologist was programming the hearing aid to the NAL prescriptive targets. The fitting software then takes into account the effects of the earmold (a dome modular tip in this case) and alters the hearing aid gain accordingly using earmold correction factors similar to those contained in the figures, charts, and tables that we have shown throughout this chapter.

Shown in Figure 8–24 (Panel A, Output A) is the output that resulted for this fitting (output is the aver-

age of real-ear SPL for a real speech shaped signal of 55 dB SPL). The goal of the fitting was to match these average speech values to the target values. Notice that we are below our desired NAL prescriptive target output by as much as 15 to 20 dB in the 500 to 1000 Hz range and do not approach desired target until above 1500 Hz. It is unlikely this would be a successful fitting. So what happened? Because this patient's ear canal was larger than average and the fact that modular ear domes rarely fit truly closed (the kind of closed that is used in correction tables), this patient actually had a fairly open fit, although the software did not know it. To further illustrate, we went back into the software, selected the earmold setting of "open" and reprogrammed the hearing aid. The output that resulted from this adjustment is labeled Output B in Figure 8–24, Panel A. Although still not a perfect fit in the lower frequencies, note that the software has added considerable gain for the 500 to 1000 Hz region, because of this earmold selection change.

To further illustrate this relationship between software adjustment, earmold fit and resulting real-ear output, we refit this patient with a modular dome that actually *did* fit tight (labeled *double dome*) and repeated our probe-microphone speechmapping measure. These results are shown in Panel B of Figure 8–24. Note that we now have a fairly good fit to the NAL targets for all frequencies. It appears, therefore, that the manufacturer's software works, but only when the audiologist enters the correct information!

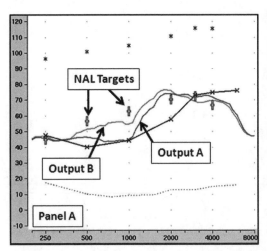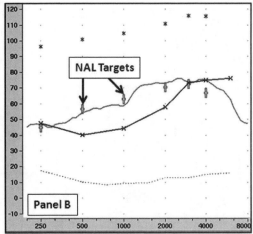

Figure 8–24. Example of the relationship between modular eartip selection in the fitting software and the resulting changes in real-ear output (55 dB SPL real-speech input). *Panel A, Output A:* Closed tip selected in software, tip fitted loosely in ear canal. *Panel A, Output B:* Open tip selected in fitting software, tip fitted loosely in ear canal. *Panel B:* Closed tip selected in software, tip fitted moderately tight in ear canal.

Now, you might say that because we are verifying the fit by conducting probe-microphone measures, the knowledge of the earmold tightness and venting effects does not matter so much, and that the software does not really have to know what is going on in the ear canal, as our mistakes will be obvious in the real-ear output. Eventually, we will make the needed corrections to overall gain to bring us back to the desired output (e.g., match to target values). This is true, although we would have saved considerable time if we had selected the correct earmold fitting to begin with. But more importantly, what if there are audiologists who do not conduct probe-microphone verification? How would they know?

Endnotes

Chapter 1

1. Leland A. Watson originally worked for the Sonotone hearing aid company in Minneapolis, but in 1937, he set out to manufacture audiometers and established the Medical Acoustics Tools Corporation (later changed to the acronym MAICO; the word tools was probably changed to instruments). The Maico D5 was the first audiometer established by the American Medical Association (AMA) and the Nationwide Bureau of Standards. Maico began manufacturing hearing aids in 1938 and perhaps are best known for introducing the first directional microphone hearing aid to the United States in 1971 (their partner company Wilco introduced the product in Germany in 1968). The pioneering work of Watson helped establish Minneapolis as the *hearing aid manufacturing capital* of the United States. Since 1995, Maico has been owned by Danish firm William Demant Holding, which also owns Oticon. Today, the Maico brand manufactures primarily hearing test equipment. (Adapted from Wayne's World @ Hearing Health and Technology Matters.)

2. In the late 1930s, the New York-based John Kirby Sextet was known as the Biggest Little Band in the Land. The group also went by the name John Kirby and His Onyx Club Boys or John Kirby and His Orchestra. Kirby tended toward a lighter, classically influenced style of jazz, often referred to as chamber jazz. Most of his music was recorded between 1938 and 1941, and one of his original songs that you might be interested in was something called "Audiology." Could it be that Carhart, Canfield, or Davis listened to a little John Kirby before naming this new profession a few years later?

3. We started to see *digitally programmable hearing aids* in the late 1980s. These hearing aids did not have the common external screw-sets to change the potentiometers, but rather these changes were made electronically, usually with a dedicated handheld programmer. The term *digital* referred to the programmer, not the hearing aids, which were still analog at this time. Both manufacturers and dispensers, however, were eager to use the term digital in their marketing, so considerable confusion existed among consumers. Researchers questioned if these new products were really better, or if a better fitting would be obtained. Because these products replaced the time-honored screwdriver potentiometers, the term *electronic screwdriver* often was used to describe these early programmable products.

4. Our discussion here relates to the selling of hearing aids. But interesting, during this same time period (1960–1970), audiologists who worked for hearing aid manufacturers were also considered to be unethical (or close to it) and were often referred to as *traitors* by their friends and colleagues. There were six or seven brave souls who tested the waters and went to work for hearing aid manufacturers, and a couple of them managed to maintain their ASHA membership. They were closely monitored at ASHA conventions, however, to assure that they were not present in the manufacturer's exhibit booth, hotel suite, or at any event sponsored by the manufacturer. As far as we know, it was never really clear if this rigid policy was from the ASHA Ethical Practice Board, or if it came directly from Kenneth O. Johnson, the Executive Director of the ASHA (from 1958 to 1980), who had strong beliefs regarding this issue. Fast forward to today—in

just the United States, over 500 audiologists work for hearing aid manufacturers; one company alone employs 130 audiologists. Things do change.

5. As we mentioned, dispensing hearing aids in the 1950s and 1960s was much different than it is today. This excerpt, taken from the October, 1956, *Time Magazine*, summarizes the situation and discusses the early efforts of John Victoreen, founder of Vicon hearing aids:

> Many doctors with limited testing devices in their offices wind up saying simply: "Try a hearing aid." After that, the patient is lost among at least 117 types of aids made by 40 companies all pushing their products with vigorous sales promotion. If the confused patient gets the right type of aid, it is often just plain luck. Last week an energetic Colorado inventor named John Victoreen was trying to replace reliance on luck with a higher degree of certainty. No MD, but a self-educated physicist who has made a fortune in X-rays and nucleonics, Victoreen "retired" from business six years ago to work longer hours than ever in his own research laboratory in Colorado Springs. The real controversy is over Victoreen's determination to keep his hearing aid out of the hands of dealers. He has set up a special company to handle the Vicon, insists that he will sell it only on prescription, and will not advertise to the public. He wants doctors, not dealers, to distribute it (at $200 plus whatever fee the doctor chooses to add). So far, Colorado otologists have balked at the idea of acting as distributors because they do not want to be responsible for servicing instruments. "I can't take calls at 2 o'clock in the morning from patients who want a hearing aid adjusted," objected one doctor. Victoreen retorts that under his system, a lot of people will hear a lot better.

6. There is a reason they call it *politics*, and some licensure laws have interesting histories. In the late 1980s, the Colorado state sunset legislation reviewed the licensure of several disciplines, and in a budget saving move, *sun-setted* the license for audiology and hearing aid dispensing. As you might expect, this quickly led to unscrupulous hearing aid sales practices. Most notably, hearing tests and ear impressions taken in the back of vans parked on main streets of small Colorado towns, payment accepted for special-order, custom instruments to be delivered later, and the dealer was never seen again. The Colorado Academy of Audiology was formed in 1992, and

this group quickly hired a lobbyist and began the arduous task of getting licensure reinstated. The political climate at that time was that if a profession does little or nor harm, there is no reason that they should be licensed. After several months of hunting for bad audiologists (and not finding any), it was pointed out that the only way the licensure would go through would be if nonaudiologist hearing aid dispensers were included. It was reinstated.

7. Regarding the 1967 ASHA reports, it is interesting to note that a section of the report addressed the issue of audiologists dispensing hearing aids. In general, their recommendations were that audiologists be permitted to dispense hearing aids under the ASHA's ethical guidelines, and they laid out a nine-step procedure regarding how this could be handled, including this statement:

> The present restriction preventing all audiologists from dispensing hearing aids was established solely by ASHA. It is possible, therefore, for ASHA to eliminate these restrictions at any time.

Twelve years passed before the restriction was changed!

8. The Stark Law is related to, but not the same as, the federal antikickback law. It is named after California Congressman Fortney Hillman "Pete" Stark, who sponsored the initial bill. This bill included a provision in the Omnibus Budget Reconciliation Act of 1989, which barred self-referrals for clinical laboratory services under the Medicare program, effective January 1, 1992. This provision was known as *Stark I*. In 1993, it expanded the restriction to a range of additional health services and applied it to both Medicare and Medicaid; this legislation, known as *Stark II*. There have been additional modifications since then.

9. As we mentioned, PSAPs are starting to look more like hearing aids every day. According to the FDA, a hearing aid is a wearable sound-amplifying device intended to compensate for impaired hearing. As such, hearing aids are subject to different types of premarket review requirements. In recent years, well-known names such as Bell & Howell, Panasonic, and RCA have entered the PSAP market. For several months, PSAPs that very closely resembled hearing aids were sold at Best Buy, although at this writing, they have been pulled. Supposedly, PSAPs are designed to be used by non-hearing impaired

consumers, but, most marketing efforts clearly are geared toward the hearing impaired. Stay tuned.

Chapter 2

10. One of the most provocative elements of the 1984 MarkeTrak was the use of the so-called PRIZM segmentation of the potential hearing aid market. The resulting cluster analyses included some jaunty descriptions used to define the different groups: *Shotguns and Pickups*, *Norma Rae-ville*, and *Furs and Station Wagons*.

11. The Kübler-Ross model, commonly known as The Five Stages of Grief, was first introduced by Elisabeth Kübler-Ross in her 1969 book, *On Death and Dying*. Included in the book was a model, The Model of Coping with Dying, which she based on research and interviews with more than 500 dying patients. In the late 1970s, Kübler-Ross became interested in out-of-body experiences, mediumship, spiritualism, and in other ways attempting to contact the dead.

12. Dr. Francis Peabody (1881–1927) was a noted internal medicine physician and a founder of the *Journal of Clinical Investigation*. Peabody was a member of a prominent New England family and trained at Harvard. His influence as a physician, researcher, teacher, and person was subsequently felt far and wide. He attended Harvard Medical School and interned at the Massachusetts General Hospital. At the age of 45, he became incurably ill, and after being a patient himself, he gave a series of talks about what it really means to be a physician. His words apply equally well to the profession of audiology: "Medicine is not a trade to be learned but a profession to be entered. The treatment of a disease may be entirely impersonal, but the care of a patient must be completely personal. The secret of the care of the patient is in caring for the patient."

Chapter 3

13. There were many early researchers who studied the characteristics of conversational speech, but the article you see referenced the most is written by Dunn and White (1940), "Statistical Measurements on Conversational Speech," in the *Journal of the Acoustical Society of America*.

14. The Rainbow Passage is from Grant Fairbanks' *Voice and Articulation Drillbook* and is probably the most famous reading passage in the English language. Our crack research team could not confirm if it was in the first edition, but it is on page 127 of the 1960 2nd edition. The passage is only missing two phonemes. It is commonly used for studying articulation, speech production, accents, reading comprehension, and even for testing speech recognition software.

15. It is difficult to document how long this phrase has been used in acoustic research, but its use at Bell Labs goes back to at least the 1920s. The phrase was even discussed in a February 1, 1936, article in the *New Yorker* magazine! In this article, the author who visited Bell and interviewed John Mills comments, "nobody remembers who invented the shoebench."

16. The articulation index has an interesting history, which began with research in the early 1900s at Western Electric Research, later named Bell Telephone Laboratories (or just Bell Labs). The most notable scientist from this group was Harvey Fletcher, who was employed from 1916 to 1948. If you are interested in the development and history of the AI over the years (and frankly, who isn't?), we recommend the summary provided by Christine Rankovic, PhD, at her website, http://www.articulation.com. She provides an excellent review of the early work of Crandell, Fletcher's mentor at Bell Labs, Fletcher's 1921 report, the 1950 finely tuned Fletcher and Galt publication, the work of French and Steinberg, ANSI S3.5 1969, and S3.5 1997, along with more recent comparative studies. All good reading!

17. A simplified version of the STI has been developed for practical application for measuring the efficiency of public address systems in airports and railway stations. It is referred to as the Speech Transmission Index for Public Address systems, or STIPA. STIPA employs a special amplitude modulation scheme to generate its test signal. The depth of modulation of the received signal is measured and compared with that of the test signal in each of a number of frequency bands. Reductions in the modulation depth are associated with loss of intelligibility.

18. The life and work of Harvey Fletcher are nicely documented in a series of video interviews

conducted in 1963 by Bruce Bogert at Bell Labs. These can be viewed at www.auditorymodels. org (see the heading "Fantastic Fletcher" video). It is interesting to note that in the portion of the interview titled "Retirement," Dr. Fletcher discusses his past reluctance to retire—his computations were that the average Bell Lab employee only lived four more years after retirement. At the age of 79, he did state in this 1963 interview, however, that indeed he was finally retiring. He lived another 18 years! Although the work of Dr. Fletcher in speech acoustics is widely known, it is not as commonly known that in 1907, while a student at BYU, he was involved in the design of the "Y" on the mountainside overlooking Provo, Utah.

Chapter 4

19. We are reminded of a telephone conversation from a few years ago that went something like this: "I need to schedule an appointment for my husband," said the elderly lady who had just called the audiologist's office. "He needs to come in and buy hearing aids for each ear." "Okay, okay," said the audiologist, controlling his enthusiasm. "Do you know that he has a hearing loss?" "Oh, most definitely," said the woman. "You tested him a year or so ago." "And he's having some problems?," asked the audiologist. "Most definitely," the woman replied. "He's only hearing 8 dots with his left ear and 12 dots with his right." I wish my referral sources understood the importance of audibility this well, thought the audiologist.

20. As we have mentioned, one unfortunate but sometimes necessary solution to handling the *loud sounds too loud* problem is for the patient to turn down hearing aid gain, which may make soft sounds inaudible. When Mead Killion introduced the K-AMP, he was quick to point out that this new wide dynamic range compression (WDRC) system was not like the linear processing of old, as the gain would be turned down automatically. To facilitate his teaching point, he coined the acronym *DHTTDGTLWI* and even provided us with a guide of how to pronounce it: *Dit-ta-dug-attle-we*. This acronym represents, "Doesn't Have To Turn Down Gain To Live With It." Although this Killion acronym did not sur-

vive, nearly all hearing aids today employ WDRC that is much like the early K-AMP, and with hope, our patient DHTTDGTLWI.

21. The loudness anchors used by David Hawkins had nine categories; anchors #1 through #7 are the same as the Cox anchors. Hawkins had #8: Extremely Uncomfortable and #9: Painfully Loud. We agree with the elimination of these two categories for two reasons: (1) Because we are only concerned with when the sound first becomes uncomfortable (the #7 rating), they really are not needed and (2) When patients see the words *Painfully Loud* on the chart, they sometimes become a little apprehensive and alter their ratings to ensure that this level never is reached.

22. As we have mentioned, there have been a wide variety of instructions used regarding defining a patient's LDL. Many were searching for a point well above "First Uncomfortable." Some instructions used phrases such as "what you can tolerate for ten minutes." One of the most intriguing set of instructions comes from a hearing aid fitting protocol published by Wallenfels in 1967: "As soon as you see the muscles around his eyes start twitching, you have your measurement."

23. In the classic publication regarding hearing aids dubbed, "The Harvard Report," senior authored by Hallowell Davis in 1946, the hearing aid with the lowest MPO was referred to as *Beginners*, suggesting that one could move on the higher output after some experience. In 1947, Silverman encouraged tolerance training by exposing patients to sounds just below their LDL for several minutes a day, over three- to four-week intervals.

24. In 2004, Van Summers of Walter Reed Army Medical Center published an interesting article related to cochlear dead regions and hearing aid fitting. Eleven clinical audiologists were given audiograms (all downward sloping) of six individuals with confirmed dead regions and asked to identify at what frequency they would likely give up trying to provide audibility. Then, the findings were compared with a larger group of individuals with and without dead regions. In general, he found that experienced clinicians tended to use a *90 dB rule*, and their clinical judgments, based solely on the audiogram, were essentially the same as what would be recommended using Brian Moore's *1.7 × edge* rule based on dead region testing. It is interesting

that the five audiologists with less experience who participated in the study tended to use a higher cutoff value (i.e., go after greater hearing loss).

Chapter 5

25. A couple things about terminology. For many years, monosyllabic speech testing was referred to as a measurement of *discrimination*. In fact, it was not uncommon for an audiologist to say something like "That last patient really had bad 'discrim!'" It was around the late 1970s that opinion leaders on speech audiometry such as Fred Bess began pointing out that we really were not measuring discrimination, as the patient was not required to discriminate between two or more words, but simply repeat the word that they heard, which is a *recognition* task. So the term has been recognition for the past 30 years or so. Many of the word lists that we use are still either phonetically balanced, or phonemically balanced—in both cases this gives us the abbreviation PB, so we still hear that term used on occasion—for example, finding *PB-Max* or a *PI/PB function.*

26. The use of *cocktail party noise* often is to provide face validity, as we have heard about *the cocktail party effect*, which if you did not know, is a scientific term! In the early 1950s, much of the early work in this area was related to the problems faced by air traffic controllers. At that time, controllers received messages from pilots over loudspeakers in the control tower. Hearing the intermixed voices of many pilots over a single loudspeaker made the controller's task very difficult. The effect was first defined and named the *cocktail party problem* by Colin Cherry in 1953.

27. If you were an audiology student, hanging around the Northwestern audiology department in the 1950s and 1960s must have been much like being a writer in Paris in the 1920s. The talented audiologists and germinal research that emerged during this time frame has never been equaled. But, it was not all work and no play. Each day over the lunch hour, in a smoke-filled room, professors and *select* students matched wits in a card game, the same game played every day. And what card game was it? Sheepshead—a game that originated in Central Europe in the late eighteenth century under the German name

Schafkopf. It is mostly popular in Wisconsin, and the national championship games are still held there each year. Could it be that James Jerger, a native of Milwaukee, brought the game to Northwestern?

28. Audiologists who routinely use the NU#6 list might smile when they read the phrase *high degree of familiarity* as we all know the typical patient response for the word *laud*—which maybe was commonly used when Lehiste-Peterson selected it in 1959, but not so much now. The frequent comments from audiologists regarding the word laud prompted AudiologyOnline to run this April Fools (2011), "Say Goodbye to Laud" news update:

> **April 1, 2011. Scottsdale AZ**—The International Committee of Speech Recognition Measures (ICSRM) held their annual meeting March 4th, 2011, in conjunction with the American Auditory Society Scientific and Audiology meeting. In an unprecedented move, this prestigious group of researchers resolved to remove the word "laud" from the Northwestern University List #6. ICSRM President Richard Wilson stated: "Although we all have a certain fondness for 'laud,' its usefulness has run its course. At this point, it may be best to move on. The intent of speech recognition testing is not to trick the subject using archaic or unfamiliar test items."
>
> Following this action, a sub-group was formed, which led to the recommendation of adding the replacement word "broad" as this new item would closely maintain the phonemic balance of the list. This was opposed, however, by some group members, in that broad is not "gender-neutral" and could be deemed offensive to females. This issue was forwarded to the ICSRM Word Review working group, who also continue to study the appropriateness of the word "but." Until a suitable replacement for laud is approved, the ICSRM recommends that clinicians conduct testing with 49 rather than 50 word lists, and use the multiplier of 2.041 to calculate percent correct scores.
>
> The ICSRM is seeking input on this issue from the audiology community and the general public. Comments and feedback can be submitted at www.icsrm.org.

Many readers missed the April Fools point of the article, as an outpouring of support rolled in. On the other hand, a *Save the Word Laud* website quickly was established. Who knew monosyllabic speech testing was this exciting?

29. Since the 1970s, whenever the discussion occurred regarding the need for a recorded speech test, the first response has always been "Call Bill." Today of course, most people "Email Bill." The *Bill* we are talking about is William Carver, founder and CEO of Auditec. Bill *is* Auditec—a reliable friend in need for anyone needing recorded speech materals or special CDs for audiometric testing constructed. A brief history of Auditec goes like this. After moving to St. Louis to head the hearing clinic at Washington University School of Medicine, Dr. Carver met a new friend who had a recording studio in his basement. Bill suggested they collaborate in a business adventure to create and market speech testing materials on tape. The company was called *Auditec of St. Louis*. Working one night a week for several months, Bill and his partner recorded four lists each of NU-6, W-22, and PBK-50, plus a list of spondee words. Their first sale was to a local audiometer dealer, and the word soon spread that tape recordings were available. After a few years and the slow addition of additional tests, the partners disagreed on marketing methods, resulting in the dissolution of the partnership with Bill becoming sole owner. Over the 43 years that Auditec has now been in business, the company has expanded its catalog of tests to include nearly all of the clinical auditory tests in use today.

30. Research in the mid-2000s, conducted at Iowa University and the University of Pittsburgh by prominent researchers, used the HINT to demonstrate the benefit of a new 3-microphone directional hearing aid. As usual, the directional performance was compared with omnidirectional, and a very significant 5 dB SNR advantage was observed. The researchers also compared the aided performance of these hearing impaired listeners to *unaided performance* of young normal hearing individuals. Somewhat a surprise, there was no difference—that is, when using these new hearing aids, the hearing impaired subjects were understanding speech in noise as well as normal. As you might guess, this was sweet news to the marketing department of the manufacturer, and a "Hear Young Again" campaign was launched. What caused considerable buzz among audiologists was when the editor of a major trade journal changed the news release slightly, so when published, the marketing claim read "*FEEL* Young Again." A rather bold statement based solely on HINT results—a retraction was in the next issue!

31. Although you might think that when you order a CD version of an audiology speech test, what would arrive in the mail would be a neatly packaged CD, much the same as if you had ordered a CD by one of your favorite artists from Amazon. This is usually true, but it certainly was not true during the years that the HINT was licensed and distributed by Starkey Laboratories. What was included with the CD, all contained in a large display box, was the 34-page HINT manual, a separate manual on Binaural Hearing, an instruction VCR tape, a quick reference guide, score sheets, a cardboard protractor (for audiologists who have trouble with the concept of 90 degrees), a pocket calculator, and yes . . . even a tape measure, complete with the HINT logo!

32. In case you are not aware, the National Institutes of Health (NIH) has a toolbox. In fact, they may have more than one, but the one we are referring to is the Assessment of Neurological and Behavioral Function. A subcategory of this toolbox is the Sensation Domain, which includes Audition. The toolbox describes audition as "the processing of sound in the environment. It is necessary for navigating in the environment and communicating with others." What you might find interesting, is that the primary test that the toolbox recommends for measuring audition is not pure-tone thresholds but the WIN. They do mention that pure-tone audiometry may be preferred in some instances.

33. On the campus of the University of Tennessee in Knoxville, you will find Neyland Stadium, home of the Volunteers, a perennial college football powerhouse. With a seating capacity of over 102,000, it is one of the largest sports stadiums in the world. You may have seen the orange-clad capacity crowd *in* the stands, but what is happening *under* the stands? Sure, you will find the usual hot dog and souvenir shops, but you will also find the UT Department of Audiology and Speech Pathology, which has its own distinguished pedigree.

34. As we mentioned, Doreen Kimura was a pioneer in dichotic speech testing. Dr. Kimura grew up in a small town near the Qu'Appelle Valley in southern Saskatchewan. By the age of 17, she was teaching in a one-room, rural schoolhouse

in northern Manitoba. She went on to attend McGill University in Montreal, where she eventually obtained her PhD and studied with the noted neuropsychologists Donald Hebb and Brenda Milner. In 1967, she became professor in psychology at the University of Western Ontario, where she stayed for over 30 years. Whereas the audiology world knows Dr. Kimura for her work relating to auditory processing, the rest of the world probably knows her best for her research regarding gender and cognition. Her book *Sex and Cognition* is widely acclaimed, and Dr. Kimura is one of the leading authorities in this sometimes controversial area of research. Kimura has this to say about her early test material:

> Our first dichotic task was made on a reel-to-reel stereophonic tape recorder and was far from high-tech. Since we knew the tape moved at 7½ inches per second, we marked with a felt pen on the tape a sequence of three points one second apart, for three successive dichotic pairs of digits, with six digits in a set. There were 32 such sets. I first spoke all of the words for one ear into one channel via a microphone, using the pen marks as guide, then rewound the tape and recorded the other channel in the same way. The simultaneity of the word pairs was not as exact as we wished, and there was some noise arising from the felt pen marks . . . but the imperfections were apparently not a disadvantage, as we did find that patients with left temporal-lobe pathology reported fewer digits correctly than did those with right temporal damage.

35. The father of the DSI is the Synthetic Sentence Identification (SSI) test, first reported by Speaks and Jerger in 1965, and still in use today. As the name indicates, this test uses sentence material, which are third-order approximations of English sentences, most containing seven words. The SSI in not dichotic but can be presented using a contralateral competing message (CCM) or an ipsilateral competing message (ICM). The SSI-ICM is the most commonly used. The SSI uses 10 sentences, six of which are used in the DSI (Sentences 1, 2, 3, 8, 9, and 10). The SSI is known for its unique competing message, which is a story about Davy Crockett, composed and recorded by Dr. James Jerger. For those of you with a keen interest in competing messages used in audiologic practice (or an interest in Davy Crockett), the complete story is printed in the Mueller and Hall Audiologists' Desk Reference, Volume II (pp. 872–878). Related to the SSI, in discussing the need for a greater use of sentence material for speech testing, we have this often cited 1980 quote from Dr. Jerger:

> We are, at the moment, becalmed in a windless sea of monosyllables. We can sail farther only on the fresh winds of imagination.

Chapter 6

36. As most of you know, the HHIE was developed by Barbara Weinstein and Ira Ventry in the early 1980s, with the seminal article published in 1982. Dr. Weinstein, who did most of the psychometric analysis, believed at the time that it was a strong instrument and had great potential. She tells us that in 1981, she had just finished her doctorate, and Dr. Ventry hired her to teach at Columbia University. She relates that she very matter-of-factly stated that they needed to copyright the scale. He emphatically replied: "There is no need for that, it will never gain widespread acceptance." The rest is history.

37. An excellent article, published to coincide with the twentieth anniversary of the IHAFF, was published in *Audiology Today* (2011), written by Dennis VanVliet. There is no reason for us to repeat all that history here, but we do want to highlight a couple of IHAFF items. First, there is an IHAFF song; lyrics and the music of the IHAFF chorus are available at http://www.earTunes.com. Second, in case you do not know who the 12 IHAFF players were (are), here is a summary from Mueller and Hall's Desk Reference, presented in the style of famous television sports personality Chris "Boomer" Berman: Babe Ruth Bentler, Lapel-Mike Valente, Nightin-Gail Gudmundsen, Dave Fabry-Cate, David Toma-Hawkins, Aspara-Gus Mueller, Mead Over-Killion, Larry Revit-Ting, Lu-Minary Beck, Rockin-Robin Cox, Dennis Moving Van Vliet, and Michael Maid Marion. The unofficial consultants were Richard Going Deep Seewald and Margo Mule Skinner Blues.

38. Ruth Bentler and colleagues at the University of Iowa conducted an interesting study a few years ago that indirectly relates to hearing aid expectations (and to some extent, supports the notion

that high expectations regarding amplification are okay). The research was conducted around the time that digital hearing aids were being introduced. There of course was considerable hype surrounding these new products, widely promulgated by manufacturers and audiologists alike. The purpose of the Bentler study was to determine whether the label attached to the hearing aid (i.e., *digital*) would bias hearing aid outcome measures. Outcome measures used consisted of a number of behavioral speech perception tasks and self-report measures, each completed at the onset and after one month use with the hearing aids. Subjects wore the same digital hearing aids for two months but were told that one of the months they were wearing *digital* hearing aids and one of the months they were wearing *conventional* hearing aids. Although objective speech testing showed no labeling effects, self-report measures significantly favored the digital labeling. When asked to choose between the two hearing aids (which were really the same hearing aids), the subjects overwhelmingly selected the product labeled digital.

39. If you are reading through the hearing aid literature, you find that there are (or at least there *were*) two HASPs in the world of hearing aid fitting. In addition to the one we are talking about here, in the 1990s, fitting software was produced and distributed by the National Acoustic Laboratories (NAL), which was called the Hearing Aid Selection Program (HASP). This software was used with the NAL-R prescriptive fitting method and provided a variety of fitting targets, including real-ear insertion gain and full-on coupler gain.

40. In troubleshooting patient complaints during post-fitting visits, it is common to discuss the patient's loudness perceptions of various environmental sounds. Often, hearing aid adjustments are made based on the patient's specific comments. When a scale is developed, however, there needs to be *norms* that can be used in the interpretation of the data for a wide range of patients. Many sounds have different loudness perceptions for different people. For example, background research during the development of the PAL revealed that the loudness rating for *clinking of glasses* (based on the Cox anchors) was pretty evenly divided between the ratings of #2 to #6. So, what is the *right* answer? How would you know if you should turn the gain

up or down? It also was discovered that young people and older people do not agree on the loudness of such common everyday sounds as: the hum of a refrigerator, TV commercials, and noise at a cocktail party. Finally, it is interesting to note that of the 95 sounds from the PAL pilot study, the one that received the best test-retest and tightest rating cluster (making it an ideal item) was *galloping horses*—consistently rated #6 on the Cox Loudness Anchors by nearly every one of all age groups! Apparently, for some unknown reason, Palmer and Mueller did not believe this sound would be commonly experienced by hearing aid users during their first few weeks of hearing aid use, and therefore it was not included on the final PAL scale.

Chapter 7

41. Regarding counseling for bilateral fittings, here is a quick report of a study conducted at Letterman Army Medical Center in the late 1980s, the results of which were presented at the first meeting of the Academy of Audiology at Kiawa Island. All subjects (*n* = 96) were male retired military, who were provided hearing aids free of charge. They all had symmetric downward sloping sensorineural hearing losses, and audiometrically, were candidates for bilateral amplification. When the patients reported for their hearing aid evaluation, they were asked if they would like to use one or two hearing aids. Approximately 1/2 chose two, and 1/2 chose one. All were fitted with two, however. Following the fitting, all patients received 30 minutes of informational counseling from the same staff audiologist. Each group (those who wanted two and those who wanted one) was randomly split in half, with each half receiving different counseling. One half of each group was instructed on all the benefits of bilateral, and told that this was the best solution for them. The other half of each group was told that some people prefer two, and some people prefer one. It was up to each of them to try two versus one and decide the arrangement that worked best for them.

Six months later, the patients completed a self-assessment questionnaire regarding hearing aid use, bilateral use, benefit and satisfaction. So did counseling matter? The same pattern emerged among groups for bilateral use, benefit and satisfaction. As you might guess, the "stars" were the people who wanted two hearing aids, and were given the "two is best" counseling. And the group that had significantly less use, benefit and satisfaction, was the group who only wanted one hearing aid, and received the "lukewarm" counseling. Most interestingly, however, is that there was no difference between the group who wanted only one, and received the "two is best" counseling and the group who wanted two, but received the "lukewarm" counseling.

42. So what is the history of the study of the *occlusion effect*? As you probably recall, it was because of this effect that Albert Bing and Friedrich Weber had moderate success with their tuning fork tests back in the 1800s. And, of course we all know how the occlusion effect complicates bone conduction testing and masking procedures. In fact, most research on the occlusion effect relates to using a bone-conduction oscillator to present the stimulus. Regarding hearing aids, we suspect that the occlusion effect has been a problem as long as earmolds have been used. Who knows, maybe it even occurred for a tightly fitting ear trumpet! It is surprising to note that there really wasn't much written about the *hearing aid* occlusion effect until the 1980s. A 1980 report by Macrae from the National Acoustic Laboratories in Australia is one of the first we recall on the topic. It is interesting to note, however, von Bekesy indirectly talked about the hearing aid occlusion in his 1960 book, *Experiments in Hearing,* where he states, "For maximally useful hearing, it is important to reduce not only the sounds of vocalization but also noises produced by chewing, swallowing, and the like. Even walking produces vibrations of the body that can be heard if the auditory meatus is closed."

43. Back in 1988, an article by Mead Killion, Laura Wilber, and Gail Gudmundsen caught our eye. It was titled "Zwislocki Was Right . . . " Prior to seeing this title, it never had occurred to us that Zwislocki *might be* wrong, so we were hooked. The reference to Zwislocki related to an article he published in 1953 in the *Journal of the Acoustical Society of America*, in which he illustrated that placing an earplug deep in the ear canal significantly reduced the occlusion effect. This was some of the first research supporting one of the benefits of today's insert earphones and of course, also relates to one of the benefits of

deep fitting CICs. Perhaps the most interesting aspect of this article, however, was the finding that when noted audiologist Laura Wilber chewed nacho-flavored Doritos, the SPL in her occluded ear canal was nearly 80 dB in the 200 Hz region.

44. Although sound localization certainly is important for humans, it can be even more important for some animals, as it is critical for their survival. One animal that has been studied extensively relative to sound localization is the barn owl. What makes the barn owl unique is that the ears are asymmetric. Ear asymmetry allows for sound originating from below the eye level to sound louder in the left ear, while sound originating from above the eye level to sound louder in the right ear. Asymmetric ear placement also causes ILDs for high frequencies (between 4 kHz and 8 kHz) to vary systematically with elevation, converting ILDs into a map of elevation. Barn owls can locate prey in total darkness using only the sense of hearing. The error in both the vertical and horizontal planes is no more than one to three degrees. And in case you're curious, neither the screech owl nor the great horned owl can locate prey in total darkness—they do not have asymmetric ears!

45. It was common in the 1940s to stress *durability* as a way to market body-type hearing aids. Perhaps the extreme of this was a full page ad from Paravox titled, "Airplane Tested." The text of the ad reads:

> On March 8th, 1949, four PARAVOX VERI-small Hearing Aids, complete with batteries, cord and receiver were dropped 600 feet from an airplane traveling 90 miles an hour. All four operated after the fall, an amazing demonstration of endurance and resistance to shock. Without question, the PARAVOX is the only hearing aid in the world that has ever survived this type of test. Now, you can understand why—PARAVOX IS BEST BY TEST!

46. The efficiency of hearing via bone conduction has prompted numerous attempts to use this transmission means in hearing aids. The teeth are good transducers, and the SoundBite is not the first attempt to use "dental hearing." In the 1880s we had the patented "Dentaphone," which was said to provide 30 dB of gain, assuming the user was willing to bite down hard on a wooden fan. Some say that this approach was invented by Beethoven, who reportedly had a rod attached

to his piano. Not to be confused with Thomas Edison, who designed a concrete piano in an effort to combat his hearing loss.

Chapter 8

47. Ear impressions and earmolds certainly have changed over the years. Here is a personal story from noted audiologist Mark Ross, PhD, who was issued his first hearing aid at Walter Reed Hospital in the 1950s:

> I well remember the first ear impressions taken of my ears over 50 years ago. After inserting a protective tab in my ear canal (a small cotton ball tied with dental floss), the technician would coat the inside of the ear and his hands with mineral oil and proceed to hand insert a mixture of plaster of Paris into my ear. When the mixture got warm enough to be uncomfortable, that meant the impression had hardened and could be removed. Thank goodness for the coating of mineral oil, otherwise he'd be taking some of my skin out with the impression! Later when I began working as an audiologist, this was how I made my first ear impressions also.

Yes, as recent as the 1950s, ear impressions were taken with plaster of Paris. Records indicate that the first patent for a custom earmold was granted in 1933 to Hugo Lieber of the Sonotone Corporation. The earmold, made out of soft rubber material, came in one color—black!

48. The durometer is a testing procedure for determining the hardness of a variety of things, particularly elastomers and plastics, including the material used for making ear impressions. It is derived from the Latin word *duro* meaning hard or tough. Albert F. Shore, who founded Shore Instruments in New York City, produced the first durometer in 1915. He was succeeded by his son Fred, who developed the first round-style durometer in 1941. This style is similar to what is still commonly used today (although a digital version is now available). Although the Shore Instrument Company no longer exists, Shore durometers are still manufactured, and hence, the term *Shore values* remains in common usage.

49. The cough reflex, sometimes experienced when the otoblock is placed deeply in the ear canal, occurs because the path of the auricular branch of the vagus cranial nerve travels in this area. The vagus has nerve fibers extending into the pharynx. The auricular branch is referred to as Alderman's nerve or more commonly Arnold's nerve, named after Friedrich Arnold, of Heidelberg, Germany, who reportedly was the first to describe this reflex in the mid-1800s. For this reason, the common cough reflex is sometimes referred to as *Arnold's Reflex*.

50. Although we mention the contributions that Sam Lybarger has made in the area of earmold acoustics, he has many other accomplishments that are even more noteworthy. Among the many devises that Lybarger designed or invented were a high-output audiometer, vacuum tube hearing aids with crystal microphones, a wearable vacuum tube hearing aid with a magnetic microphone, an induction telephone pickup for a hearing aid (the industry standard for many years), and the B-70 and B-71 bone conduction vibrators. In the early 1950s, he was one of the first to begin work on transistor hearing aids.

On the lighter side, Sam also was known for his definition of a hearing aid. His parent company, RadioEar, had his definition printed, and it was distributed nationally, often seen hanging in the offices of audiologists and dispensers. His one-sentence, 84-word definition went like this:

> A hearing aid is an ultra-small electroacoustic device that is always too large, that has to faithfully amplify speech a million times without bringing in any noise, that has to work without failure—in a flood of perspiration or a cloud of talcum powder, that one usually puts off buying for 10 years after he needs it because he doesn't want anyone to know he is hard-of-hearing, but which he can't do without for 30 minutes when it needs to be serviced.

This definition was written nearly 60 years ago. If we substituted the words *hair spray* for *talcum powder*, you may have thought it was written yesterday. Some things do not change much.

51. As you would guess, *Helmholtz resonance* is named after the German scientist Hermann von Helmholtz. You might think that this is because he simply was the first to explain this phenomenon, but in fact, he actually built a device that was used to demonstrate it (called the Helmholtz resonator; a bulb-shaped device with a short neck). Helmholtz was particularly interested in the resonances of musical instruments—both the

guitar and violin have a primary resonance from what we now call the Helmholtz resonance. The Helmholtz resonance theory also can be used to reduce unwanted sounds, and often is used in architectural acoustics (reducing low-frequency standing waves) and even for reducing the noise level of aircraft engines.

52. Yes indeed, a common damping element for many years has been lambswool (one word, not *lamb's wool* as you might think). As the name indicates, the wool is from the first shearing of a young sheep, usually around the age of 6 to 8 months. It is desirable as a damping element as it is soft and elastic and, therefore, easy to work with in small pieces that fit into tubing—you simply grab a small piece with a tweezers. Although less than scientific, most audiologists of the 1960s and 1970s who were fitting hearing aids were quite skillful in using just the right dab of lambswool to improve the sound quality of hearing aids, or fix aided loudness discomfort issues. Lambswool also was often placed in vents when feedback was an issue. We are not sure how often lambswool is used today, but it still can be purchased from hearing aid supply stores such as Hal-Hen (see the following Endnote).

53. Most all audiologists have heard of the company Hal-Hen, and have probably ordered something from them at one time or another. The background of the company is quite interesting. The name Hal-Hen comes from the first names of the two founders, Harold Spar and Henry Meltsner, who were childhood friends from the Bronx. In January of 1946, they had just returned from serving in the U.S. Navy, and decided to use the technical knowledge they acquired in the Navy and form a company to manufacture colored light bulbs. Shortly after they started their business, the American Earphone Company asked them to assemble a receiver cord for a hearing aid they were manufacturing. As they say, the rest is history. Today, Hal-Hen offers hundreds of products for both audiologists and the hearing aid user, many of them designed and produced exclusively by Hal-Hen's technical craftspeople.

54. As we mentioned, there have been some special tone hooks developed over the years. One of these was the KBASS, described in an article by Mead Killion, Chuck Berlin, and Linda Hood, which originally was a hook/earmold combination, but was later modified so just the hook

could be used. As the acronym suggests, when coupled with a high-power BTE, this was an attempt to provide substantial gain in the low frequencies for people with upward sloping hearing losses (a special interest of Dr. Berlin at the time). In case you are wondering what the acronym stands for: K = Killion-Berlin (neither Chuck or Linda got their own letter), B = Bass, A = Amplified, S = unobStructed (a stretch we think), and S = Sound.

55. Perhaps the most unique person associated with earmold acoustics is E. Robert "Cy" Libby. Trained as an optometrist, he started to dispense hearing aids as part of his optometry practice in 1943. He soon also became involved in audiologic instrumentation distribution, and he was the president of Associated Hearing Instruments for over 60 years. He was one of the first to distribute impedance, ABR, and probe-mirophone equipment in the United States. In fact, it was his early work with probe-microphone measures in his own private practice that prompted him to publish a prescriptive fitting rationale (most commonly known as the *Libby one-third gain* formula). As associate editor of the trade journal *Hearing Instruments*, Cy was always tuned in to the latest developments in the area of hearing aids. As a long-time proponent of bilateral fittings, he published a two-volume collection of articles on this topic in 1980. It was his interest in the work of Mead Killion's special earmolds in the late 1970s, which led him to manufacture the single-piece horn tubing in 1982—which of course soon became known as *The Libby Horn*.

56. If you are new to earmold acoustics, the acronym IROS (pronounced *eye-ross*) does not have much meaning. Even if you know that the acronym stands for Ipsilateral Routing of Signal, it still does not have much meaning. After all, aren't nearly all earmolds involved with an ipsilateral routing of the signal? The history of the IROS term goes back to the mid-1960s development of CROS amplification. Because the CROS fitting usually channeled the signal to an ear with normal or near-normal hearing (which is still true today), it was desirable to use an open earmold so that signals directly presented to that ear could pass freely to the eardrum. This was new to hearing aid fittings at the time, so this new open earmold design simply was referred to as a CROS mold. As years went by, audiologists tried

using the CROS earmold with a standard BTE fitting. As the frequency responses of BTE instruments became smoother, this approach became more and more successful. Because it was no longer a CROS fitting, the earmold became an IROS, and today the term IROS is more or less synonymous with *big vent* and *open earmold*.

References

Aazh, H., & Moore, B. C. (2007). Dead regions in the cochlea at 4 kHz in elderly adults: Relation to absolute threshold, steepness of audiogram, and pure-tone average. *Journal of the American Academy of Audiology*, *18*(2), 97–106.

Abrams, H. B., & Doyle, P. J. (2000). Functioning, disability, and quality of life in the adult with hearing impairment. In *Rehabilitation research and development service merit review*. Washington, DC: Department of Veterans Affairs.

Academy of Doctors of Audiology. (2012). *HIPAA*. Retrieved from http://www.audiologist.org/practice-management/federal-regulations/ hipaa.html

American Academy of Audiology. (2003). *Ethical practice guidelines on financial incentives from hearing instrument manufacturers*. Retrieved from http://www.audiology.org/resources/documentlibrary/Documents/financialinfinancia.pdf

American Academy of Audiology. (2004). *Scope of practice*. Retrieved from http://www.audiology.org/resources/documentlibrary/Pages/ScopeofPractice.aspx

American Academy of Audiology. (2006). *Guideline for audiologic management of the adult patient*. Retrieved from http://www.audiology.org/resources/documentlibrary/documents/ haguidelines.pdf

American National Standards Institute. (1994). *Acoustical terminology* (ANSI S1.1-1994). New York, NY.

American National Standards Institute. (1997). *The calculation of the speech intelligibility index* (ANSI S3.5-1997). New York, NY.

American National Standards Institute. (2004). *Specification for audiometers* (S3. 6-2004). New York, NY.

American Speech-Language Hearing Association. (1997). *Guidelines for audiologic screening*. Retrieved from http://www.asha.org/docs/html/GL1997-00199.html

American Speech-Language Hearing Association. (1998). Guidelines for hearing aid fitting for adults. *American Journal of Audiology*, *7*, 5–13.

American Speech-Language-Hearing Association. (2006). *Preferred practice patterns for the profession of audiology [Preferred practice patterns]*. Retrieved from http://www.asha.org/ policy.

Amlani, A. M. (2001). Efficacy of directional microphone hearing aids: A meta-analytic perspective. *Journal of the American Academy of Audiology*, *12*(4), 202–214.

Arehart, K. H., Kates, J. M., & Anderson, M. C. (2010). Effects of noise, nonlinear processing, and linear filtering on perceived speech quality. *Ear and Hearing*, *31*(3), 420–436.

Arthur, D. (2002). The Vibrant Soundbridge. *Trends in Amplification*, *8*(2), 67–72.

Baer, T., Moore, B. C. J., & Kluk, K. (2002). Effects of low-pass filtering on the intelligibility of speech in noise for people with and without dead regions at high frequencies. *Journal of the Acoustical Society of America*, *112*(3), 1133–1144.

Baguley, D. (2003). Hyperacusis. *Journal of the Royal Society of Medicine*, *96*(12), 582–585.

Balfour, P. B., & Hawkins, D. B. (1992). A comparison of sound quality judgments for monaural and binaural hearing aid processed stimuli. *Ear and Hearing*, *13*(5), 331–339.

Bankaitis, A. U., & Fredrickson, J. M. (2002). Otologics middle ear transducer (MET) implantable hearing device: Rationale, technology, and design strategies. *Trends in Amplification*, *6*(2), 53–60.

Bench, J., Kowal, Å., & Bamford, J. (1979). The BKB (Bamford-Kowal-Bench) sentence lists for partially-hearing children. *British Journal of Audiology*, *13*(3), 108–112.

Bentler, R. A. (2000). List equivalency and test-retest reliability of the speech in noise test. *American Journal of Audiology*, *9*(2), 84–100.

Bentler, R., & Cooley, L. (2001). An examination of several characteristics that affect the prediction of OSPL90. *Ear and Hearing*, *22*(1), 3–20.

Bentler, R. A., Niebuhr, D. P., Getta, J. P., & Anderson, C. V. (1993) Longitudinal study of hearing aid effectiveness: Objective measures. *Journal of Speech, Language, and Hearing Research, 36*(4), 820–831.

Beranek, L. L. (1954). *McGraw-Hill electrical and engineering series: Acoustics.* New York, NY: McGraw-Hill.

Berger, K. W. (1976a). Genealogy of the words of audiology and audiologist. *Journal of the American Audiological Society, 2*(2), 38–44.

Berger, K. W. (1976b). Prescription of hearing aids: A rationale. *Ear and Hearing, 2*(3), 71–78.

Bergman, M. (2002). On the origins of audiology: American wartime military audiology [Monograph]. *Audiology Today, 1,* 1–28.

Bess, F. (*1983*). Clinical assessment of speech recognition. In D. Konkle & W. Rintelmann (Eds.), *Principles of speech audiometry* (pp. 127–201). Baltimore, MD: University Park Press.

Better Hearing Institute. (n.d.). *Prevalence of hearing loss.* Retrieved from http://betterhearing. org/hearing_loss/ prevalence_of_hearing_ loss/index.cfm

Bilger, R. C. (1984). *Manual for the clinical use of the revised SPIN test.* Champaign, IL: University of Illinois Press.

Bilger, R. C., Neutzel, J. M., Rabinowitz, W. M., & Rzeczkowski, C. (1984). Standardization of a test of speech perception in noise. *Journal of Speech and Hearing Research, 27*(1), 32–48.

Bird, J., & Cohen-Cole, S. A. (1990). The three-function model medical interview: An educational device. *Advances in Psychosomatic Medicine, 20,* 65–88.

Bistafa, S. R., & Bradley, J. S. (2000). Reverberation time and maximum background-noise level for classrooms from a comparative study of speech intelligibility metrics. *Journal of the Acoustical Society of America, 107*(2), 861–875.

Blamey, P. J., & Martin, L. F. (2009). Loudness and satisfaction ratings for hearing aid users. *Journal of the American Academy of Audiology, 20*(4), 272–282.

Blue, V. J. (1979). NAEL—An important part of the team. *Hearing Instruments, 30,* 16.

Boike, K. T., & Souza, P. E. (2000). Effect of compression ratio on speech recognition and speech-quality ratings with wide dynamic range compression amplification. *Journal of Speech, Language, and Hearing Research, 43*(2), 456–468.

Bradley, J. S., Reich, R. D., & Norcross, S. G. (1999). On the combined effects of signal-to-noise ratio and room acoustics on speech intelligibility. *Journal of the Acoustical Society of America, 106*(4), 1820–1828.

Bratt, G. W., Rosenfeld, M. A. L., Poek, B. F., Kang, J., Williams, D. W., & Larson, V. (2002). Coupler and real-ear measurement of hearing aid gain and output in the NIDCD/VA hearing aid clinical trial. *Ear and Hearing, 23*(4), 308–324.

Byrne, D., Christen, R., & Dillon, H. (1981). Effects of peaks in hearing aid frequency response curves on comfortable listening levels of normal hearing subjects. *Australian Journal of Audiology, 3,* 42–46.

Byrne, D., Dillon, H., Tran, K., Arlinger, S., Wilbraham, K., Cox, R., . . . Ludvigsen, C. (1994). An international comparison of long-term average speech spectra. *Journal of the Acoustical Society of America, 96,* 2108–2120.

Carhart, R. (1946a). Selection of hearing aids. *Archives of Otolaryngology-Head and Neck Surgery, 44,* 1–18.

Carhart, R. (1946b). Tests for selection of hearing aids. *Laryngoscope, 56,* 780–794.

Carhart, R. (1946c). Volume control adjustment in hearing aid selection. *Laryngoscope, 56*(9), 510–526.

Carhart, R., & Tillman, T. W. (1970). Interaction of competing speech signals with hearing losses. *Archives of Otolaryngology-Head and Neck Surgery, 91*(3), 273–279.

Carney, E., & Schlauch, R. S. (2007). Critical difference table for word recognition testing derived using computer simulation. *Journal of Speech, Language, and Hearing Research, 50*(5), 1203–1209.

Causey, G. D., Hood, L. J., Hermanson, C. L., & Bowling, L. S. (1984).The Maryland CNC test: Normative studies. *International Journal of Audiology, 23*(6), 552–568.

Cavanaugh, W., Farrell, W., Hirtle, P., & Waters, B. (1962). Speech privacy in buildings. *Journal of the Acoustical Society of America, 34*(4), 475–483.

Chasin, M. (2002). Bone anchored middle ear implants. *Trends in Amplification, 6*(2), 33–38.

Ching, T. Y., Dillon, H., & Byrne, D. (1998). Speech recognition of hearing-impaired listeners: Predications from audibility and the limited role of high-frequency amplification. *Journal of the Acoustical Society of America, 103*(2), 1128–1140.

Ching, T. Y., Dillon, H., Katsch, R., & Byrne, D. (2001). Maximizing effective audibility in hearing aid fitting. *Ear and Hearing, 22*(3), 212–224.

Chmiel, R., & Jerger, J. (1996). Hearing aid use, central auditory disorder, and hearing handicap in elderly persons. *Journal of the American Academy of Audiology, 7*(3), 190–202.

Cienkowski, K. M., & Speaks, C. (2000). Subjective vs. objective intelligibility of sentences in listeners with hearing loss. *Journal of Speech, Language, and Hearing Research, 43*(5), 1205–1210.

Clark, J. G., & English, K. M. (2003). *Counseling in audiologic practice: Helping patients and families adjust to hearing loss.* Boston, MA: Pearson Education.

Clarke, C. M. (2000). Lexical neighborhood properties of the original and revised speech perception in noise

(SPIN) tests. *Research on spoken language processing* (Progress Report No. 24), 305–320.

Cooper, J. C., & Cutts, B. P. (1971). Speech discrimination in noise. *Journal of Speech and Hearing Research, 14,* 332–337.

Cord, M. T., Walden, B. E., & Atack, R. M. (1992). *Speech recognition in noise test (SPRINT) for H-3 profiles.* Unpublished report, Audiology and Speech Center, Walter Reed Army Medical Center, Washington, DC.

Cox, R. M. (1979). Acoustic aspects of hearing aid ear canal coupling systems. In *Monograph in contemporary audiology.* Minneapolis, MN: Maico Hearing Instruments.

Cox, R. M. (1982). Combined effects of earmold vents and suboscilatory feedback on hearing aid frequency response. *Ear and Hearing, 3*(1), 12–17.

Cox, R. M. (1995). Using loudness data for hearing aid selection: The IHAFF approach. *Hearing Journal, 48*(2), 10–16.

Cox, R. M. (1997). Administration and application of the APHAB. *Hearing Journal, 50*(4), 32–48.

Cox, R. M. (2004). Waiting for evidence based practice for your hearing aid fittings? It's here. *Hearing Journal, 57*(8), 10–17.

Cox, R. M., & Alexander, G. C. (1983). Acoustic versus electronic modifications of hearing aid low-frequency output. *Ear and Hearing, 4*(4), 190–196.

Cox, R. M., & Alexander, G. C. (1995).The abbreviated profile of hearing aid benefit. *Ear and Hearing, 16*(2), 176–186.

Cox, R. M., & Alexander, G. C. (1999). Measuring satisfaction with amplification in daily life: The SADL scale. *Ear and Hearing, 20*(4), 306–320.

Cox, R. M., & Alexander, G. C. (2000). Expectations about hearing aids and their relationship to fitting outcome. *Journal of the American Academy of Audiology, 11*(7), 368–382.

Cox, R., Alexander, G., & Gilmore, C. (1987). Development of the connected speech test (CST). *Ear and Hearing, 8*(5s), 119s–126s.

Cox, R., Alexander, G., Gilmore, C., & Pusakulich, K. (1988). Use of the connected speech test (CST) with hearing-impaired listeners. *Ear and Hearing, 9*(4), 198–207.

Cox, R. M., Alexander, G. C., & Gray, G. A. (1999). Personality and the subjective assessment of hearing aids. *Journal of the American Academy of Audiology, 10*(1), 1–13.

Cox, R. M., Alexander, G. C., & Gray, G. A. (2003). Audiometric correlates of the unaided APHAB. *Journal of the American Academy of Audiology, 14*(7), 361–371.

Cox, R. M., Alexander, G. C., & Rivera, I. M. (1991). Comparison of objective and subjective measures of speech intelligibility in elderly hearing-impaired listeners. *Journal of Speech and Hearing Research, 34*(4), 904–915.

Cox, R. M., Alexander, G. C., Taylor, I. M, & Gray, G. A. (1997). The contour test of loudness perception. *Ear and Hearing, 18*(5), 388–400.

Cox, R. M., & Gilmore, C. (1986). Damping the hearing aid frequency response: Effects on speech clarity and preferred listening level. *Journal of Speech and Hearing Research, 29*(3), 357–365.

Cox, R. M., & Gilmore, C. (1990). Development of the profile of hearing aid performance (PHAP). *Journal of Speech and Hearing Research, 33,* 343–357.

Cox, R. M., Gilmore, C., & Alexander, G. C. (1991). Comparison of two questionnaires for patient-assessed hearing aid benefit. *Journal of the American Academy of Audiology, 2*(3), 134–145.

Cox, R. M., Johnson, J. A., & Alexander, G. C. (2012). Implications of high-frequency cochlear dead regions for fitting hearing aids to adults with mild to moderately severe hearing loss. *Ear and Hearing, 33*(5), 573–587.

Cox, R. M., & McDaniel, D. M. (1989). Development of the speech intelligibility rating (SIR) test for hearing aid comparisons. *Journal of Speech and Hearing Research, 32*(2), 347–352.

Cox, R. M., Schwartz, K. S., Noe, C. M., & Alexander, G. C. (2011). Preference for one or two hearing aids among adult patients. *Ear and Hearing, 32*(2), 181–197.

Crandell, C., & Smaldino, J. (2000). Classroom acoustics and amplification. In M. Valente, R. Roeser, & H. Hosford-Dunn (Eds.), *Audiology: Treatment* (Vol. 2). New York, NY: Thieme Medical.

Darkner, S., Larsen, R., & Paulsen, R. (2007). Analysis of deformation of the human ear and canal caused by mandibular movement. In N. Ayache, S. Ourselin, & A. Maeder (Eds.), *MICCAI 2007, Part II.* (LNCS, Vol. 4792, pp. 801–808). Heidelberg, Germany: Springer-Verlag.

Darkner, S., Larsen, R., & Paulsen, R. R. (2007). Analysis of deformation of the human ear and canal caused by mandibular movement. *Medical Image Computing and Computer-Assisted Intervention, 4792,* 801–808.

Davis, H., & Silverman, S. R. (1960). *Hearing and deafness.* New York, NY: Holt Reinhart and Winston.

Davis, L. A., & Davidson, S. A. (1996). Preference for and performance with damped and undamped hearing aids by listeners with sensorineural hearing loss. *Journal of Speech and Hearing Research, 39*(3), 483–93.

Del Dot, J., Hickson, L. M., & O'Connell, B. (1992). Speech perception in noise with BiCROS hearing aids. *Scandinavian Audiology, 21*(4), 261–264.

Demorest, M., Wark, D., & Erdman, S. (2011). Development of the screening test for hearing problems. *American Journal of Audiology, 20,* 100–110.

Dickinson, W. W. (2010). Verification of baha fitting for single-sided deafness: How, what, where and why do we measure? *Seminars in Hearing, 31*(4), 350–365.

Dillon, H. (1982a). A quantitative examination of the sources of speech discrimination test score variability. *Ear and Hearing, 3*(2), 51–58.

Dillon, H. (1982b). The sources of speech discrimination test score variability: A reply to Thornton and Raffin. *Ear and Hearing, 3*(6), 340–341.

Dillon, H. (1985). Earmolds and high frequency response modification. *Hearing Instruments, 36*(12), 8–12.

Dillon, H. (1991). Allowing for real ear venting effects when selecting the coupler gain for hearing aids. *Ear and Hearing, 12*(6), 406–416.

Dillon, H. (2001). *Hearing aids.* Turramurra, Australia: Boomerang Press.

Dillon, H., James, A., & Ginis, J. (1997). Client oriented scale of improvement (COSI) and its relationship to several other measures of benefit and satisfaction provided by hearing aids. *Journal of the American Academy of Audiology, 8*(1), 27–43.

Dillon, H., Koritschoner, E., Battaglia, J., Lovegrove, R., Ginis, J., Mavrias, G., . . . Macaskill, F. (1991). Rehabilitation effectiveness I: Assessing the needs of clients entering a national hearing rehabilitation program. *Australian Journal of Audiology, 13*(2), 55–65.

Dillon, H., & Storey, L. (1998). The national acoustics laboratories' procedure for selecting the saturation sound pressure level of hearing aids: Theoretical derivation. *Ear and Hearing, 19*(4), 255–266.

Dirks, D. D., Kamm, C. A., Dubno, J. R., & Velde, T. M. (1981). Speech recognition performance at loudness discomfort level. *Scandinavian Audiology, 10*(4), 239–246.

Dirks, D. D., Morgan, D. E., & Dubno, J. R. (1982). A procedure for quantifying the effects of noise on speech recognition. *Journal of Speech and Hearing Disorders, 47*(2), 114–123.

Donaldson, G. S., Chisolm, T. H., Blasco, G. P., Shinnick, L. J., Ketter, K. J., & Krause, J. C. (2009). BKB-SIN and ANL predict perceived communication ability in cochlear implant users. *Ear and Hearing, 30*(4), 401.

Drennan, W. R., Gatehouse, S., Howell, P., Van Tasell, D., & Lund, S. (2005). Localization and speech-identification ability of hearing-impaired listeners using phase-preserving amplification. *Ear and Hearing, 26*(5), 461–472.

Dreschler, W. A., Verschuure, H., Ludvigsen, C., & Westerman, S. (2001). ICRA noises: Artificial noise signals with speech-like spectral and temporal properties for hearing instrument assessment. *International Collegium for Rehabilitative Audiology, 40*(3), 148–157.

Dubno, J. R., Lee, F. S., Klein, A. J., Matthews, L. J., & Lam, C. F. (1995). Confidence limits for maximum word-recognition scores. *Journal of Speech, Language and Hearing Research, 38*(2), 490–502.

Dubno, J. R., Lee, F. S., Matthews, L. J., & Mills, J. H. (1997). Age-related and gender-related changes in speech recognition. *Journal of Speech, Language, and Hearing Research, 40*(2), 444–452.

Duncan, K. R., & Aarts, N. L. (2006). A comparison of the HINT and quick SIN tests. *Journal of Speech Language Pathology and Audiology, 30*(2), 86–94.

Egan, M. D. (1988). *Architectural acoustics.* New York, NY: McGraw-Hill.

Egolf, D. P., Howell, H. C., Weaver, K. A., & Barker, D. S. (1985). The hearing aid feedback path: Mathematical simulations and experimental verification. *Journal of the Acoustical Society of America, 78*(5), 1578–1587.

Eisenberg, L. S., Dirks, D. D., Takayanagi, S., & Martinez, A. S. (1998). Subjective judgments of clarity and intelligibility for filtered stimuli with equivalent speech intelligibility index predictions. *Journal of Speech, Language, and Hearing Research, 41*(2), 327–339.

Eisenthal, S., & Lazare, A. (1977). Evaluation of the initial interview in a walk-in clinic: The clinician's perspective on a negotiated approach. *Journal of Nervous and Mental Disease, 164*(1), 30–35.

Elliott, L. L. (1979). Performance of children aged 9 to 17 years on a test of speech intelligibility in noise using sentence material with controlled word predictability. *Journal of the Acoustical Society of America, 66*(3), 651–653.

Erdman, S. A. (2009). Audiologic counseling: A biopsychosocial approach. In J. J. Montano & J. B. Spitzer (Eds.), *Adult audiologic rehabilitation: Advanced practices* (pp. 171–215). San Diego, CA: Plural.

Etymotic Research. (2005). BKB-SIN: Speech-in-Noise Test (Version 1.03) [Computer software CD]. Elk Grove Village, IL: Etymotic Research.

Etymotic Research. (2006). QuickSIN: Speech-in-Noise Test (Version 1.3) [Computer software CD]. Elk Grove Village, IL: Etymotic Research.

Fallon, M., Trehub, S. E., & Schneider, B. A. (2000). Children's perception of speech in multitalker babble. *Journal of the Acoustical Society of America, 108*(6), 3023–3029.

Fifer, R. C., Jerger, J. F., Berlin, C. I., Tobey, E. A., & Campbell, J. C. (1983). Development of a dichotic sentence identification test for hearing impaired adults. *Ear and Hearing, 4*(6), 300–305.

Flamme, G. A., Mudipalli, V. R., Reynolds, S. J., Kelly, K. M., Stromquist, A. M., Zwerling, C., . . . Merchant, J. A. (2005). Prevalence of hearing impairment in a rural midwestern cohort: Estimates from the Keokuk county rural health study, 1994–1998. *Ear and Hearing, 26*(3), 350–360.

Fletcher, H., & Galt, R. H. (1950). The perception of speech and its relation to telephony. *Journal of the Acoustical Society of America, 22*(2), 89–151.

Food and Drug Administration . (1999). *Summary of safety and effectiveness* [Bilateral fitting] (K984162-[June 28, 1999]). Retrieved from http://www.accessdata.fda.gov/cdrh_docs/ pdf/k984162.pdf

Fortune, T. W., & Preves, D. (1994). Effects of CIC, ITC, and ITE microphone placement on the amplification of wind noise. *Hearing Journal, 47*(9), 23–27.

Frankel, R., & Stein, T. (1999). Getting the most out of the clinical encounter: The four habits model. *Journal of Medical Practice Management, 16*(4), 184–191.

Frankel, R. M., & Stein, T. (1999). Getting the most out of the clinical encounter: The four habits model. *Permenente Journal, 3*(3), 79–83.

French, N. R., & Steinberg, J. C. (1947). Factors governing the intelligibility of speech sounds. *Journal of the Acoustical Society of America, 19*(1), 90–119.

Freyaldenhoven, M.C., Nabelek, A.K., Burchfield, S.B., & Thelin, J.W. (2005). Acceptable noise level (ANL) as a measure of directional benefit. *Journal of the American Academy of Audiology 16*(4), 228–236.

Freyaldenhoven, M. C. (2007). Acceptable noise level (ANL): Research and current application. *Audiology Online,* Retrieved from http://www.audiologyonline.com/articles/acceptable-noise-level-anl-research-956

Freyaldenhoven, M. C., Nabelek, A. K., & Tampas, J. W. (2008). Relationship between acceptable noise level and the abbreviated profile of hearing aid benefit. *Journal of Speech, Language, and Hearing Research, 51*(1), 136–146.

Federal Trade Commission, Office of the Federal Register, National Archives and Records Service, General Services Administration. (1975). Hearing aid industry: Proposed trade regulation rules. *Federal Register,* 26650.

Gagné, J-P., Southall, K., & Jennings, M. B. (2009). The psychological effects of social stigma: Applications to people with acquired hearing loss. In J. Montano & J. B. Spitzer (Eds.), *Advanced practice in adult audiologic rehabilitation: International perspective* (pp. 63–92). New York, NY: Plural.

Gatehouse, S. (1994). Components and determinants of hearing aid benefit. *Ear and Hearing, 15*(1), 30–49.

Gates, G. A., Murphy, M., Rees, T. S., & Fraher, A. (2003). Screening for handicapping hearing loss in the elderly. *Journal of Family Practice, 52*(1), 56–62.

Gelfand, S. A. (1979). Usage of CROS hearing aids by unilaterally deaf patients. *Archives of Otolaryngology-Head and Neck Surgery, 105*(6), 328–332.

Glaser, R., & Traynor, R. (2007). *Strategic practice management: A patient-centric approach.* San Diego, CA: Plural.

Grande, D., Frosch, D., Perkins, A., Barbara, E., & Kahn, B. (2009). Effect of exposure to small pharmaceutical promotional items on treatment preferences. *Archives of Internal Medicine, 169*(9), 887–893.

Grayson, A. W., & Liang, B. (2000). Interview with Bryan Liang, M.D., Ph.D., J.D. and Arthur W. Grayson professor of law and medicine, Southern Illinois University schools of law and medicine. *AudiologyOnline,* Retrieved from http://www.audiologyonline.com/interviews/interview-with-bryan-liang-m-1822

Green, D. S. (1969). Non-occluding earmolds with CROS and IROS hearing aids. *Archives of Otolaryngology-Head and Neck Surgery, 89*(3), 512–522.

Groen, J. J. (1969). Social hearing handicap: Its measurement by speech audiometry in noise. *International Journal of Audiology, 8*(1), 82–183.

Guenette, L. A. (2006). How to administer the dichotic digit test. *Hearing Journal, 59*(2), 50.

Guthrie, L. A., & Mackersie, C. L. (2009). A comparison of presentation levels to maximize word recognition scores. *Journal of the American Academy of Audiology, 20*(6), 381–390.

Hall, J. W. (2013). 20Q: Treating patients with hyperacusis and other forms of decreased sound tolerance. *Audiology Online,* Retrieved from http://www.audiologyonline.com/content/preview/11679/83f6a091a358dbc608

Halpin, C. (2002). The tuning curve in clinical audiology. *American Journal of Audiology, 11*(2), 56–64.

Hamilton, A. M., & Munro, K. J. (2010). Uncomfortable loudness levels in experienced unilateral and bilateral hearing aid users: Evidence of adaptive plasticity following asymmetrical sensory input. *International Journal of Audiology, 49*(9), 667–671.

Hanks, W. D., & Johnson, G. D. (1998). HINT list equivalency using older listeners. *Journal of Speech, Language, and Hearing Research, 41*(6), 1335–1340.

Harford, E. R. (2000). Professional education in audiology. In H. Hosford-Dunn, R. Roeser, & M. Valente (Eds.), *Audiology practice management* (pp. 17–40). New York, NY: Thieme Medical.

Harford, E., & Barry, J. (1965). A rehabilitative approach to the problem of unilateral hearing impairment: The contralateral routing of signals (CROS). *Journal of the Speech Language Hearing Association, 30,* 121–138.

Harford, E., & Dodds, E. (1966). The clinical application of CROS. *Archives of Otolaryngology-Head and Neck Surgery, 83*(5), 455–464.

Harnack Knebel, S. B., & Bentler, R. A. (1998). Comparison of two digital hearing aids. *Ear and Hearing, 19*(4), 280–287.

Hawkins, D. B., Beck, L. B., Bratt, G. W., Fabry, D. A., Mueller, H. G., & Stelmachowicz, P. G. (1991). Vanderbilt/

VA hearing aid conference 1990 consensus statement. Recommended components of a hearing aid selection procedure for adults. *Journal of the American Speech-Language Hearing Association, 33*(4), 37–38.

Hawkins, D. B., Hamill, T., & Kukula, J. (2006). Ethical issues in hearing. *Audiology Today, 18*(4), 22–29.

Hawkins, D. B., Hamill, T., Van Vleet, D., & Freeman, B. (2002). Potential conflicts of interest as viewed by the audiologist and the hearing-impaired consumer. *Audiology Today, 14*(5), 27–33.

Hawkins, D. B., Walden, B. E., Montgomery, A., & Prosek, R. A. (1987). Description and validation of the LDL procedure designed to select SSPL90. *Ear and Hearing, 8*(3), 162–169.

Haynes, B. (1999). Can it work? Does it work? Is it worth it?: The testing of healthcare intervention is evolving. *British Medical Journal, 319*(7211), 652–653.

Hearing Industries Association. (1984). *Market survey: A summary of findings and business implications for the U.S. hearing aid industry*. Washington, DC: Author.

Hétu, R. (1996). The stigma attached to hearing impairment. *Scandinavian Audiology, 25*(Suppl. 43), 12–24.

Hill, S. L. III, Marcus, A., Digges, E. N., Gillman, N., & Silverstein, H. (2006). Assessment of patient satisfaction with various configurations of digital CROS and BiCROS hearing aids. *Ear Nose and Throat Journal, 85*(7), 427–430, 442.

Hol, M. K. S., Bosman, A. J., Snik, A. F. M., Mylanus, E. A. M., & Cremers, C. W. R. J. (2004). Bone-anchored hearing aid in unilateral inner ear deafness: A study of 20 patients. *Audiology and Neurotology, 9*, 274–281.

Hornsby, B. W. Y., & Dundas, J. A. (2009). Factors affecting outcomes on the TEN (SPL) test in adults with hearing loss. *Journal of the American Academy of Audiology, 20*(4), 251–263.

Hornsby, B. W. Y., Johnson, E. E., & Picou, E. (2011). Effects of degree and configuration of hearing loss on the contribution of high-and low-frequency speech information to bilateral speech understanding. *Ear and Hearing, 32*(5), 543–555.

Hornsby, B. W., & Ricketts, T. A. (2003). The effects of hearing loss on the contribution of high- and low-frequency speech information to speech understanding. *Journal of the Acoustical Society of America, 113*(3), 1706–1717.

Hornsby, B. W., & Ricketts, T. A. (2006). The effects of hearing loss on the contribution of high-and low-frequency speech information to speech understanding. II. Sloping hearing loss. *Journal of the Acoustical Society of America, 119*(3), 1752–1763.

Hornsby, B. W. Y., Ricketts, T. A., & Johnson, E. E. (2006). The effects of speech and speechlike maskers on unaided and aided speech recognition in persons with hearing loss. *Journal of the American Academy of Audiology, 17*(6), 432–447.

Houtgast, T. (1981). The effect of noise on speech intelligibility in classrooms. *Applied Acoustics, 14*(1), 15–25.

Houtgast, T., & Steeneken, H. J. M. (1971). Evaluation of speech transmission channels by using artificial signals. *Acustica, 25*, 355–367.

Houtgast, T., & Steeneken, H. J. M. (1973). The modulation transfer function in room acoustic as a predictor of speech intelligibility. *Acustica, 28*(1), 66–73.

Houtgast, T., & Steeneken, H. J. M. (1985). A review of the MTF concept in room acoustics and its use for estimating speech intelligibility in auditoria. *Journal of the Acoustical Society of America, 77*(3), 1069–1077.

Houtgast, T., Steeneken, H. J. M., & Plomp, R. (1980). Predicting speech intelligibility in rooms from the modulation transfer function: I. General room acoustics. *Acustica, 46*(1), 60–72.

Humes, L. E. (1991). Understanding the speech-understanding problems of the hearing impaired. *Journal of the American Academy of Audiology, 2*, 59–69.

Humes, L. E. (2002). Factors underlying the speech-recognition performance of elderly hearing-aid wearers. *Journal of the Acoustical Society of America, 112*(3), 1112–1132.

Humes, L. E. (2003). Modeling and predicting hearing aid outcome. *Trends in Amplification, 7*(2), 41–75.

Humes, L. E., Dirks, D. D., Bell, T. S., Ahlstrom, C., & Kincaid, G. E. (1986). Application of the articulation index and the speech transmission index to the recognition of speech by normal-hearing and hearing-impaired listeners. *Journal of Speech and Hearing Research, 29*(4), 447–462.

Hurley, R. M. (1999). Onset of auditory deprivation. *Journal of the American Academy of Audiology, 10*(10), 529–534.

Hurley, R. M., & Sells, J. P. (2003). An abbreviated word recognition protocol based on item difficulty. *Ear and Hearing, 24*(2), 111–118.

Hutcherson, R. W., Dirks, D. D., & Morgan, D. E. (1979). Evaluation of the speech perception in noise (SPIN) test. *Otolaryngology-Head and Neck Surgery, 87*(2), 239–245.

IEEE. (1969). *IEEE recommended practice for speech quality measurements. Appendix C*. Boulder, CO: Global Engineering Documents.

Jacobson, G. P., Newman, C. W., Fabry, D. A., & Sandridge, S. A. (2001). Development of the three-clinic hearing aid selection profile (HASP). *Journal of the American Academy of Audiology, 12*(3), 128–141.

Jacobson, G. P., Newman, C. W., Sandridge, S. A., & McCaslin, D. L. (2002). Using the hearing aid selection profile to identify factors in hearing aid returns. *Hearing Journal, 55*(3), 30–33.

Jenstad, L. M., Van Tasell, D., & Ewert, C. (2003). Hearing aid troubleshooting base on patients' descriptions. *Journal of the American Academy of Audiology*, 14(7), 347–360.

Jerger, J. (Ed.). (1969). *Modern developments in audiology*. New York, NY: Academic.

Jerger, J. F. (2006). Informational masking. *Journal of the American Academy of Audiology*, 17(6), 1.

Jerger, J. F. (2009). *Audiology in the USA*. San Diego, CA: Plural.

Jerger, J., Chmiel, R., Allen, J., & Wilson, A. (1994). Effects of age and gender on dichotic sentence identification. *Ear and Hearing*, 15(4), 274–286.

Jerger, J., Stach, B., Johnson, K., Loiselle, L., & Jerger, S. (1990). Patterns of abnormality in dichotic listening. In J. Jensen (Ed.), *Presbyacusis and other age related aspects*. Copenhagen, Denmark: Stougaard Jensen.

Johnson, J., & Cox, R. M. (2009, March). *QuicksSin™ HFE and LP lists: Learning effect, equivalence and sensitivity*. Paper presented at the annual meeting of the American Auditory Society, Scottsdale, AZ.

Johnson, J. A., Cox, R. M., & Alexander, G. C. (2010). Development of APHAB norms for WDRC hearing aids and comparisons with original norms. *Ear and Hearing*, 31(1), 47–55.

Johnson, E. E., Mueller, H. G., & Ricketts, T. A. (2009). Statistically derived factors of varied importance to audiologists when making a hearing aid brand decision. *Journal of the American Academy of Audiology*, 20(1), 40–48.

Kalikow, D. N., Stevens, K. N., & Elliott, L. L. (1977). Development of a test of speech intelligibility in noise using sentence materials with controlled word predictability. *Journal of the Acoustical Society of America*, 61(5), 1337–1351.

Kamm, C. A., Morgan, D. E., & Dirks, D. D. (1983). Accuracy of adaptive procedure estimates of PF-max level. *Journal of Speech and Hearing Disorders*, 48(2), 202–209.

Keidser, G., Yeend, I., O'Brien, A., & Hartley, L. (2011). Using in-situ audiometry more effectively: How low-frequency can affect prescribed gain and prescription. *Hearing Review*, 18(3), 12–16.

Kiessling, J., Brenner, B., Thunberg Jespersen, C., Groth, J., & Jensen, O. D. (2005). Occlusion effect of earmolds with different venting systems. *Journal of the American Academy of Audiology*, 16(4), 237–249.

Killion, M. C. (1979). *Design and evaluation of high-fidelity hearing aids* (Unpublished doctoral dissertation). Northwestern University, Evanston, IL.

Killion, M. C. (1980). Problems in the application of broadband hearing aid earphones. In G. A. Studebaker & I. Hochberg (Eds.), *Acoustic factors affecting hearing aid performance*. Baltimore, MD: University Park Press.

Killion, M. C. (1981). Earmold options for wideband hearing aids. *Journal of Speech and Hearing Disorders*, 46, 10–20.

Killion, M. C. (1988). Earmold design: Theory and practice. In J. Jensen (Ed.), *Hearing aid fitting: Theoretical and practical views* (pp. 155–174). Copenhagen, Denmark: Stougaard Jensen.

Killion, M. C. (1993). Transducers and acoustic couplings. In G. A. Studebaker & I. Hochberg (Eds.), *Acoustical factors affecting hearing aid performance* (2nd ed., pp. 31–50). Boston, MA: Allyn & Bacon.

Killion, M. C. (1997). SNR loss: I can hear what people say, but I can't understand them. *Hearing Review*, 4(12), 8–14.

Killion, M. C. (2003). Earmold acoustics. *Seminars in Hearing*, 24(4), 299–312.

Killion, M. C., & Mueller, H. G. (2010). Twenty years later: A new count-the-dots method. *Hearing Journal*, 63(1), 10–17.

Killion, M. C., Mueller, H. G., Pavlovic, C. V., & Humes, L. E. (1993). A is for audibility. *Hearing Journal*, 46(4), 29.

Killion, M. C., & Niquette, P. A. (2000). What can the pure-tone audiogram tell us about a patient's SNR loss. *Hearing Journal*, 53(3), 46–53.

Killion, M. C., Niquette, P. A., Gudmundsen, G. I., Revit, L. J., & Banerjee, S. (2004). Development of a quick speech-in-noise test for measuring signal-to-noise ratio loss in normal-hearing and hearing-impaired listeners. *Journal of the Acoustical Society of America*, 116(4), 2395–2405.

Killion, M. C., & Villchur, E. (1993). Kessler was right—partly: But SIN test shows some aids improve hearing in noise. *Hearing Journal*, 46(9), 31–35.

Killion, M. C., Wilber, L., & Gudmundsen, G. I. (1988). Zwislocki was right. *Hearing Instruments*, 39(1), 14–18.

Kimura, D. (1961a). Cerebral dominance and the perception of verbal stimuli. *Canadian Journal of Psychology*, 15, 166–171.

Kimura, D. (1961b). Some effects of temporal lobe damage on auditory perception. *Canadian Journal of Psychology*, 15, 156–165.

Koch, D. B, Nilsson, M. J., & Soli, S. D. (2004). Using the HINT test on compact disk. House Ear Institute—Qsound. Licensed by Starkey Laboratories.

Kochkin, S. (1990). One more time . . . what did the 1984 HIA market survey say? *Hearing Instruments*, 42, 11–13.

Kochkin, S. (1991). MarkeTrak II: More MDs give hearing tests, yet hearing aid sales remain flat. *Hearing Journal*, 44(2), 24–35.

Kochkin, S. (1995). Customer satisfaction and benefit with CIC hearing aids. *Hearing Review*, 2(4), 16–26.

Kochkin, S. (1997). What is the viable market for hearing aids? *Hearing Journal, 50*(1), 31–38.

Kochkin, S. (2001). MarkeTrack VI: The VA and direct mail sales spark growth in hearing-aid market. *Hearing Review, 8*(12), 16–24, 63–65.

Kochkin, S. (2002). 10-year customer satisfaction trends in the U.S. hearing instrument market. *Hearing Review, 10*(9), 14–26.

Kochkin, S. (2007). MarkeTrak VII: Obstacles to adult non-user adoption of hearing aids. *Hearing Journal, 60*(4), 27–43.

Kochkin, S. (2010). MarkeTrak VIII: Customer satisfaction with hearing aids is slowly increasing. *Hearing Journal, 63*(1), 11–19.

Kochkin, S. (2011). Mini-BTEs tap new market, users more satisfied. *Hearing Journal, 24*(3), 17–24.

Kochkin, S. (2012, July 9). 20Q: More highlights from MarkeTrak. *AudiologyOnline,* Retrieved from http://www.audiologyonline.com/articles/more-highlights-from-marketrak-6830

Kochkin, S., Beck, D. L., Christensen, L. A., Compton-Conley, C., Fligor, B. J., Kricos, P. B., . . . Turner, R. G. (2010). MarkeTrak VIII: The impact of the hearing healthcare professional on hearing aid user success. *Hearing Review, 17*(4), 12–34.

Kringlebotn, M. (1999). A graphical method for calculating the speech intelligibility index and measuring hearing disability from audiograms. *Scandinavian Audiology, 28*(3), 151–160.

Kroll, K., Grant, I. L., & Javel, E. (2002). The Envoy totally implantable hearing system, St. Croix Medical. *Trends in Amplification, 6*(2), 73–80.

Kuk, F. K. (1994). Maximum usable real-ear insertion gain with ten earmold designs. *Journal of the American Academy of Audiology, 5*(1), 44–51.

Kuk, F. (2003). reconsidering the concept of aided of the aided threshold for nonlinear hearing aids. *Trends in Amplification, 7*(3), 77–97.

Kuk, F., Keenan, D., Lau, C. C., Dinulescu, N., Cortez, R., & Keogh, P. (2005). Real-world performance of a reverse-horn vent. *Journal of the American Academy of Audiology, 16*(9), 653–661.

Laitakari, K., Löppönen, H., Salmivalli, A., & Sorri, M. (1995). Brief communication: Objective real ear measures of bone conduction hearing aid performance. *Scandinavian Audiology, 24*(1), 53–56.

Lehiste, I., & Peterson, G. E. (1959). Linguisitic considerations in study of speech intelligibility. *Journal of the Acoustical Society of America, 31*(3), 280–286.

Libby, E. R. (1982a). A new acoustic horn for small ear canals. *Hearing Instruments, 33*(9), 48.

Libby, E. R. (1982b). In search of transparent insertion gain hearing aid responses. In G. A. Studebaker & F. H. Bess (Eds.), *The Vanderbilt hearing aid report* (pp. 112–123). Upper Darby, PA.

Lichtenstein, M., Bess, F., & Logan, S. (1988). Validation of screening tools for identifying hearing-impaired elderly in primary care. *Journal of the American Medical Association, 259*(19), 2875–2878.

Lindley, G. A., Palmer, C. V., Durrant, J., & Pratt, S. (2000). Adaptation to loudness and environmental stimuli in three newly fitted hearing aid users. *Journal of the American Academy of Audiology, 11*(6), 316–322.

Luce, P. A. (1986). *Neighborhoods of words in the mental lexicon. Research on speech perception* (Technical Report No. 6).

Luce, P. A., & Pisoni, D. B. (1998). Recognizing spoken words: The neighborhood activation model. *Ear and Hearing, 19*(1), 1–36.

Luetje, C. M., Brackmann, D., Balkany, T. J., Maw, J., Baker, R. S., Kelsall, D., . . . Arts, A. (2002). Phase III clinical trial resuls with the Vibrant® Soundbridge implantable middle ear hearing device: A prospective controlled multicenter study. *Otolaryngology-Head and Neck Surgery, 126*(2), 97–107.

Lundeen, C. (1996). Letter to the editor. *American Journal of Audiology, 5*, 57–58.

Lunner, T., Hellgren, J., Arlinger, S., & Elberling, C. (1997). A digital filterbank hearing aid: Three digital signal processing algorithms—User preference and performance. *Ear and Hearing, 18*(5), 373–387.

Lustig, L. R., Arts, H. A., Brackmann, D. E., Francis, H. F., Molony, T, Megerian, C. A., . . . Niparko, J. K. (2001). Hearing rehabilitation using the BAHA bone-anchored hearing aid: Results in 40 patients. *Otology and Neurotology, 22*(3), 328–334.

Lybarger, S. (1985). Earmolds. In J. Katz (Ed.), *Handbook of clinical audiology* (3rd ed., pp. 885–910). Baltimore, MD: Lippincott Williams & Wilkins.

Lyregaard, P. (1982). Frequency selectivity and speech intelligibility in noise. *Scandinavian Audiology, 15*(Suppl.), 113–122.

MacKenzie, D. J. (2006). Open-canal fittings and the hearing aid occlusion effect. *Hearing Journal, 59*(11), 50–56.

Mackersie, C. L., Crocker, T. L., & Davis, R. A. (2004). Limiting high frequency hearing aid gain in listeners with and without suspected cochlear dead regions. *Journal of the American Academy of Audiology, 15*(7), 498–507.

Margolis, R. H. (2004). Boosting memory with informational counseling: Helping patients understand the nature of disorders and how to manage them. *ASHA Leader, 28*, 10–11.

Matkin, N., & Thomas, J. (1972). The utilization of CROS hearing aids by children. *Maico Audiological Library Series, 10.*

McArdle, R. A., Killion, M. C., Mennite, M. A., & Chisolm, T. H. (2012). Are two ears not better than one? *Journal of the American Academy of Audiology, 23*(3), 171–181.

McArdle, R. A., & Wilson, R. H. (2006). Homogeneity of the 18 QuickSIN lists. *Journal of the American Academy of Audiology, 17*(3), 157–167.

McArdle, R. A., Wilson, R. H., & Burks, C. A. (2005). Speech recognition in multitalker babble using digits, words, and sentences. *Journal of the American Academy of Audiology, 16*(9), 726–739.

Mid-Atlantic Addiction Technology Transfer Center. *Motivational interviewing.* Retrieved from http://motivational interview.org/

Miller, W. R., & Rollnick, S. (2002). *Motivational interviewing: Preparing people for change* (2nd ed.). New York, NY: Guilford Press.

Moncur, J. P., & Dirks, D. (1967). Binaural and monaural speech intelligibility in reverberation. *Journal of Speech and Hearing Research, 10*(2), 186–195.

Moore, B. C. (1989). *An introduction to the psychology of hearing.* London, UK: Academic Press.

Moore, B. C. J. (2010). Testing for cochlear dead regions: Audiometer implementation of the TEN (HL) test. *Hearing Review, 17*(1), 10–16, 48.

Moore, B. C. J., Creeke, S., Glasberg, B. R., Stone, M. A., & Sek, A. (2012). A version of the TEN test for use with the ER-3A insert earphones. *Ear and Hearing, 33*(4), 554–557.

Moore, B. C. J., Glasberg, B. R., & Stone, M. A. (2004). New version of the TEN test with calibrations in dB HL. *Ear and Hearing, 25*(5), 478–487.

Moore, B. C. J., Huss, M., Vickers, D. A., Glasberg, B. R., & Alcántara, J. I. (2000). A test for the diagnosis of dead regions in the cochlea. *British Journal of Audiology, 34*(4), 205–224.

Mormer, E., & Palmer, C. V. (2001). *Reliability of hearing aid expectation responses.* Paper presented at the annual meeting of the American Academy of Audiology.

Mueller, H. G. (1985). Evaluation of central auditory function: Monosyllabic procedures. In J. Katz (Ed.), *Handbook of clinical audiology* (3rd ed., pp. 355–382). Baltimore, MD: Lippincott Williams & Wilkins.

Mueller, H. G. (1994a). CIC hearing aids: What is their impact on the occlusion effect? *Hearing Journal, 47*(11), 20–35.

Mueller, H. G. (1994b). Getting ready for the IHAFF protocol. *Hearing Journal, 47*(6), 10, 46–48.

Mueller, H. G. (1994c). Small can be good too! *Hearing Journal, 47*(11), 11–12.

Mueller, H. G. (2003a). Fitting test protocols. *Hearing Journal, 56*(10), 19–26.

Mueller, H. G. (2003b). There's less talking in barrels, but the occlusion effect is still with us. *Hearing Journal, 56*(1), 10–18.

Mueller, H. G. (2009). A candid round table discussion on open-canal fittings. *Hearing Journal, 62*(4), 19–26.

Mueller, H. G. (2010). Three pre-tests: What they do and why experts say you should use them more. *Hearing Journal, 63*(4), 17–23.

Mueller, H. G., & Bentler, R. A. (1994). Measurements of TD: How loud is allowed? *Hearing Journal, 47*(1), 10, 42–46.

Mueller, H. G., & Bentler, R. A. (2002). How loud is allowed? *Hearing Journal, 52*(1), 10–17.

Mueller, H. G., & Bentler, R. A. (2005). Fitting hearing aids using clinical measures of loudness discomfort levels: An evidence-based review of effectiveness. *Journal of the American Academy of Audiology, 16*(7), 461–472.

Mueller, H. G., & Bentler, R. A. (2008). How loud is allowed? It's a three-peat! *Hearing Journal, 61*(4), 10–15.

Mueller, H. G., Bentler, R. A., & Wu, Y. H. (2008). Prescribing maximum hearing aid output: Differences among manufacturers found. *Hearing Journal, 61*(3), 30–36.

Mueller, H. G., & Bright, K. E. (1994). Selection and verification of maximum output. In M. Valente (Ed.), *Strategies for selecting and verifying hearing aid fittings.* New York, NY: Thieme Medical.

Mueller, H. G., Bright, K. E., & Northern, J. L. (1996). Studies of the hearing aid occlusion effect. *Seminars in Hearing, 17*(1), 21–32.

Mueller, H. G., & Ebinger, K. A. (1996). CIC hearing aids: Potential benefits and fitting strategies. *Seminars in hearing, 17*(1), 29–35.

Mueller, H. G., & Ebinger, K. A. (1997). Verification of the performance of CIC hearing aids. In M. Chasin (Ed.), *CIC handbook* (pp. 101–126). San Diego, CA: Singular.

Mueller, H. G., & Hall, J. W. (1998). *Audiologists' desk reference.* San Diego, CA: Singular.

Mueller, H. G., & Hawkins, D. B. (1992). Assessment of fitting arrangements, special circuitry, and features. In H. G. Mueller, D. B. Hawkins, & J. L. Northern (Eds.), *Probe microphone measurements* (pp. 201–226). San Diego, CA: Singular.

Mueller, H. G., & Hornsby, B. (2002). Selection, verification and validation of maximum output. In M. Valente (Ed.), *Strategies for selecting and verifying hearing aid fittings* (pp. 23–66). New York, NY: Thieme Medical.

Mueller, H. G., & Johnson, E. E. (2013). Hearing aids. In S. Kramer (Ed.), *Audiology: Science to practice* (2nd ed., pp. 287–320). San Diego, CA: Plural.

Mueller, H. G., Johnson, E. E., & Weber, J. (2010). *Fitting hearing aids: A comparison of three pre-fitting speech tests* (Article 2332). Retrieved from http://www. audiologyonline.com

Mueller, H. G., & Killion, M. C. (1990). An easy method for calculation the articulation index. *Hearing Journal, 43*(9), 14–17.

Mueller, H. G., & Palmer, C. V. (1998). The profile of aided loudness: A new "PAL" for '98. *Hearing Journal, 51*(1), 10–19.

Mueller, H. G., & Ricketts, T. A. (2006). Open-canal fittings: Ten take-home tips. *Hearing Journal, 59*(11), 24–39.

Mueller, H. G., Weber, J., & Hornsby, B. (2006). The effects of digital noise reduction on acceptance of background noise. *Trends in Amplification, 10*(2), 83–93.

Munro, K. J., & Davis, J. (2003). Deriving the real-ear SPL of audiometric data using the "coupler to dial difference" and the "real ear to coupler difference." *Ear and Hearing, 24*(2), 100–110.

Munro, K. J, & Millward, K. E. (2006). The influence of the RECD transducer when deriving the real-ear sound pressure level. *Ear and Hearing, 27*(4), 409–423.

Munro, K. J., & Patel, R. (1998). Are clinical measurements of uncomfortable loudness levels a valid indicator of real-world auditory discomfort? *British Journal of Audiology, 32*(5), 287–293.

Murray, M., Popelka, G. R., & Miller, R. (2011). Efficacy and safety of an in-the-mouth bone conduction device for single-sided deafness. *Otology and Neurology, 32*(3), 437–443.

Musiek, F. E. (1983). Assessment of central auditory dysfunction: The dichotic digit test revisited. *Ear and Hearing, 4*(2), 79–83.

Nabelek, A. K., Freyaldenhoven, M. C., Tampas, J. W., Burchfield, S. B., & Muenchen, R. A. (2006). Acceptable noise level as a predictor of hearing aid use. *Journal of the American Academy of Audiology, 17*(9), 626–639.

Nabelek, A. K., Tampas, J. W., & Burchfield, S. B. (2004). Comparison of speech perception in background noise with acceptance of background in aided and unaided conditions. *Journal of Speech, Language, and Hearing Research, 47*(5), 1001–1011.

Nabelek, A. K., Tucker, F. M., & Letowski, T. R. (1991). Toleration of background noises: Relationship with patterns of hearing aid use by elderly persons. *Journal of Speech and Hearing Research, 34*(3), 679–685.

Newman, C. W., Jacobson, G. P., Hug, G. A., & Sandridge, S. A. (1997). Perceived hearing handicap of patients with unilateral or mild hearing loss. *Annals of Otology, Rhinology, and Laryngology, 106*(3), 210–214.

Newman, C. W., & Weinstein, B. E. (1986). Judgments of perceived hearing handicap by hearing-impaired elderly men and their spouses. *Journal of the Academy of Rehabilitative Audiology, 19*, 109–115.

Newman, C. W., Weinstein, B. E., Jacobson, G. P., & Hug, G. A. (1990). The Hearing Handicap Inventory for Adults: Psychometric adequacy and audiometric correlates. *Ear and Hearing, 11*(6), 430–433.

Newman, C. W., Weinstein, B. E., Jacobson, G. P., & Hug, G. A. (1991). Test-retest reliability of the Hearing Handicap Inventory for Adults. *Ear and Hearing, 12*(5), 355–357.

Nilsson, M. J., & Soli, S. D. (1994). Norms for a headphone simulation of the hearing in noise test: Comparison of physical and simulated spatial separation of sound sources. *Journal of the Acoustical Society of America, 95*(5), 2994.

Nilsson, M., Soli, S. D., & Sullivan, J. A. (1994). Development of the hearing in noise test for the measurement of speech reception thresholds in quiet and noise. *Journal of the Acoustical Society of America, 95*(2), 1085–1099.

Niparko, J. K., Cox, K. M., Lustig, L. R. (2003). Comparison of the bone anchored hearing aid implantable hearing device with contralateral routing of signal of offside signal amplification in the rehabilitation of unilateral deafness. *Otology and Neurotology, 24*(1), 73–78.

O'Brien, A., Keidser, G., Yeend, I., Hartley, L., & Dillon, H. (2010). Valitdity and reliability of in-situ air conduction thresholds measures through hearing aids coupled to closed and open instant-fit tips. *International Journal of Audiology, 49*(12), 868–876.

Oliveira, R. J. (1997). The active earcanal. *Journal of the American Academy of Audiology, 8*(6), 401–410.

Owen, J. H. (1981). Influence of acoustical and linguistic factors on the SPIN test difference score. *Journal of the Acoustical Society of America, 70*(3), 678–682.

Painton, S. W. (1993). Objective measure of low-frequency amplification reduction in canal hearing aids with adaptive circuitry. *Journal of the American Academy of Audiology, 4*(3), 152–156.

Palmer, C. V. (2009). Best practice: It's a matter of ethics. *Audiology Today, 21*(5), 31–35.

Palmer, C. P., & Lindley, G. (1998) Reliability of the contour test in a population of adults with hearing loss. *Journal of the American Academy of Audiology, 9*(3), 209–215.

Palmer, C. V., & Mueller, H. G. (2000). Hearing aid selection and assessment. In J. G. Alpiner & P. A. McCarthy (Eds.), *Rehabilitative audiology, children and adults* (pp. 332–376). Baltimore, MD: Lippincott Williams & Wilkins.

Palmer, C. V., Mueller, H. G., & Moriarty, M. (1999). Profile of aided loudness: A validation procedure. *Hearing Journal, 52*(6), 34–42.

Palmer, C. V., Solodar, H. S., Hurley, W. R., Byrne, D. C., & Williams, K. O. (2009). Self-perception of hearing ability as a strong predictor of hearing aid purchase. *Journal of the American Academy of Audiology, 20*(6), 341–347.

Parbery-Clark, A., Strait, D. L., Anderson, S., Hittner, E., & Kraus, N. (2011). Musical experience and the aging auditory system: Implications for cognitive abilities and hearing speech in noise. *PLoS One, 6*(5), e18082.

Pascoe, D. P. (1980). Clinical implications of nonverbal methods of hearing aid selection and fitting. *Seminars in Hearing, 1*(3), 217–228.

Pascoe, D. P. (1988). Clinical measurements of the auditory range and their relation to formulas for hearing aid gain. In J. Jensen (Ed.), *Hearing aid fittings: Theoretical and practical views.* 13th Danavox Symposium. (pp. 129–152), Copenhagen, Denmark: Stongaard Jensen.

Pavlovic, C. V. (1984). Use of the articulation index for assessing residual auditory function in listeners with sensorineural hearing impairment. *Journal of the Acoustical Society of America, 75*(4), 1253–1258.

Pavlovic, C. V. (1987). Derivation of primary parameters and procedures for use in speech intelligibility predictions. *Journal of the Acoustical Society of America, 83*(2), 413–422.

Pavlovic, C. (1988). Articulation index predictions of speech intelligibility in hearing aid selection. *ASHA, 30*(6/7), 63–65.

Pavlovic, C. V. (1989). Speech spectrum considerations and speech intelligibility predictions in hearing aid evaluations. *Journal of Speech and Hearing Disorders, 54*(1), 3–8.

Pavlovic, C. (1991). Speech recognition and five articulation indexes. *Hearing Instruments, 42*(9), 20–24.

Pavlovic, C. V. (1993). Problems in the prediction of speech recognition performance of normal-hearing and hearing impaired individuals. In G. A. Studebaker & I. Hochberg (Eds.) *Acoustical factors affecting hearing aid performance* (2nd ed, pp. 221–234), Boston, MA: Allyn & Bacon.

Pavlovic, C. V., & Studebaker, G. A. (1984). An evaluation of some assumptions underlying the articulation index. *Journal of the Acoustical Society of America, 75*(5), 1606–1612.

Pavlovic, C. V., Studebaker, G. A., & Sherbecoe, R. (1986). An articulation index–based procedure for predicting the speech recognition performance of hearing-impaired individuals. *Journal of the Acoustical Society of America, 80*(1), 50–57.

Pearsons, K. S., Bennett, R. L., & Fidell, S. (1977). *Speech levels in various noise environments* (Report No. EPA-600/1-77-025). Washington, DC: U.S. Environmental Protection Agency.

Peterson, G. E., & Lehiste, I. (1962). Revised CNC lists for auditory tests. *Journal of Speech and Hearing Disorders, 27*(1), 62–70.

Peutz, V. (1971). Articulation loss of consonants as a criterion for speech transmission in a room. *Journal of the Audio Engineering Society, 19*(11), 915–919.

Picou, E. M., & Ricketts, T. A. (2011). Comparison of wireless and acoustic hearing aid-based telephone listening strategies. *Ear and Hearing, 32*(2), 209–220.

Pirzanski, C. (1998). The anatomy of a perfect ear impression. *Hearing Review, 5*(12), 2–24.

Pirzanski, C. Z. (2003). Issues in earmold fitting and troubleshooting. *Seminars in Hearing, 24*(4), 355–363.

Plomp, R. (1976). Binaural and monaural speech intelligibility of connected discourse in reverberation as a function of azimuth of a single competing sound source (speech or noise). *Acustica, 34*, 200–211.

Plomp, R. (1978). Auditory handicap of hearing impairment and the limited benefit of hearing aids. *Journal of the Acoustical Society of America, 63*(2), 533–549.

Plomp, R. (1986). A signal-to-noise ratio model for the speech-reception threshold of the hearing impaired. *Journal of Speech and Hearing Research, 29*(2), 146–154.

Plomp, R., & Mimpen, A. M. (1979). Speech-reception threshold for sentences as a function of age and noise level. *Journal of the Acoustical Society of America, 66*(5), 1333–1342.

Plyler, P. N. (2009). Acceptance of background noise: Recent developments. *Hearing Journal, 62*(4), 10–17.

Preminger, J. E., Carpenter, R., & Ziegler, C. H. (2005). A clinical perspective on cochlear dead regions: Intelligibility of speech and subjective hearing aid benefit. *Journal of the American Academy of Audiology, 16*(8), 600–613.

Pumford, J. (2005). Benefits of probe-mic measures with CROS/BiCROS fittings. *Hearing Journal, 58*(10), 34–40.

Rankovic, C. M. (1991). An application of the articulation index to hearing aid fitting. *Journal of Speech and Hearing Research, 34*(2), 391–402.

Revit, L. J. (1997). The circle of decibels: Relating the hearing test, to the hearing aid, to the real-ear response. *Hearing Review, 4*(11), 35–38.

Ricketts, T. A., & Bentler, R. A. (1992). Comparison of two digitally programmable hearing aids. *Journal of the American Academy of Audiology, 3*(2), 101–112.

Ricketts, T. A., & Bentler, R. A. (1996). The effect of test signal type and bandwidth on the categorical scaling of loudness. *Journal of the Acoustical Society of America, 99*(4), 2281–2287.

Ricketts, T. A., Johnson, E., & Federman, J. (2008). Individual differences within an across feedback suppression hearing aids. *Journal of the American Academy of Audiology, 19*(10), 748–757.

Sackett, D. L., Rosenberg, W. M. C., Gray, J. A. M., Haynes, R. B., & Richardson, W. S. (1996). Evidence-based medicine: What it is and what it isn't. *British Medical Journal, 312,* 71–72.

Sandridge, S. A., & Newman, C. W. (2006). *Improving the efficiency and accountability of the hearing aid selection process—Use of the COAT.* Retrieved from http://www.audiologyonline.com/articles/article_detail.asp?article_id=1541

Saunders, G. H. (2009). Understanding in noise: Perception vs. performance. *Hearing Journal, 62*(5), 10–16.

Saunders, G., & Forsline, A. (2006b). The performance-perceptual test (PPT) and its relationship to aided reported handicap and hearing aid satisfaction. *Ear and Hearing, 27*(3), 229–242.

Saunders, G., Forsline, A., & Fausti, S. (2004). The performance-perceptual test (PPT) and its relationship to unaided reported handicap. *Ear and Hearing, 25*(2), 117–126.

Saunders, G. H., & Morgan, D. E. (2003). Impact on hearing aid targets of measuring thresholds in dB HL versus dB SPL. *International Journal of Audiology, 4*(6), 319–326.

Schafer, E. C., Pogue, J., & Milrany, T. (2012). List equivalency of the AzBio sentence test in noise for listeners with normal-hearing sensitivity or cochlear implants. *Journal of the American Academy of Audiology, 23*(7), 501–509.

Schmitt, N. (2004). *National Acoustic Laboratories Research & Development annual report 2003/2004: A new speech test (BEST test). Practical training report.* Sydney, Australia: National Acoustics Laboratory.

Schum, D. (1996). Speech understanding in background noise. In M. Valente (Ed.), *Hearing aids: Standards, options, and limitations* (pp. 368–406). New York, NY: Thieme Medical.

Schum, D. J. (1999). Perceived hearing aid benefit in relation to perceived needs. *Journal of the American Academy of Audiology, 10*(1), 40–45.

Schwartz, K., & Cox, R. (2011, March). *Relationship between acceptable noise levels and hearing aid success.* Presented at the American Auditory Society Convention, Scottsdale, AZ.

Schwartz, K., & Cox, R. (2012, March). *Does acceptable noise level predict hearing aid success?* Presented at the American Auditory Society Convention, Scottsdale, AZ.

Shaw, E. A. G. (1966). Ear canal pressure generated by a free sound field. *Journal of the Acoustical Society of America, 39*(3), 465–470.

Sherbecoe, R. L., & Studebaker, G. A. (2002). Audibility-index functions for the connected speech test. *Ear and Hearing, 23*(5), 385–298.

Shi, L. F., Doherty, K. A., Kordas, T. M., & Pellegrino, J. T. (2007). Short-term and long-term hearing aid benefit and user satisfaction. *Journal of the American Academy of Audiology, 18*(6), 482–495.

Silman, S., Gelfand, S. A., & Silverman, C. A. (1984). Late-onset auditory deprivation: Effects of monaural versus binaural hearing aids. *Journal of the Acoustical Society of America, 76*(5), 1357–1362.

Simon, H. J. (2005). Bilateral amplification and sound localization: Then and now. *Journal of Rehabilitations Research and Development, 42*(4), 117–132.

Sindhusake, D., Mitchell, P., Smith, W., Golding, M., Newall, P., Hartley, D., & Rubin, G. (2001). Validation of self-reported hearing loss. The Blue Mountains Hearing Study. *International Journal of Epidemiology, 30*(6), 1371–1378.

Sjoblad, S., & Warren, B. W. (2011). Myth busters: Can you unbundle and stay in business? *Audiology Today, 23*(5), 37–45.

Skinner, M. W., Holden, L. K., Holden, T. A., Demorest, M. E., & Fourakis, M. S. (1997). Speech recognition at simulated soft, conversational, and raised-to-loud vocal efforts by adults with cochlear implants. *Journal of the Acoustical Society of America, 101*(6), 3766–3782.

Smith-Olinde, L., Nicholson, N., Chivers, C., Highley, P., & Williams, D. K. (2006). Test-retest reliability of in situ unaided thresholds in adults. *American Journal of Audiology, 15*(1), 75–80.

Souza, P. (2012). *20Q: Cognition measures—They might change the way you fit hearing aids!* Retrieved from http://www.audiologyonline.com/articles/august-20q-by-pamela-souza-6925

Spahr, A. J., & Dorman, M. F. (2004). Performance of subjects fit with the advanced bionics CII and nucleus 3G cochlear implant devices. *Archives of Otolaryngology-Head and Neck Surgery, 130*(5), 624–628.

Spahr, A. J., Dorman, M. F., Litvak, L. M., Van Wie, S., Gifford, R. H., Loizou, P. C., . . . Cook, S. (2012). Development and validation of the AzBio sentence lists. *Ear and Hearing, 33*(1), 112–117.

Sperry, J. L., Wiley, T. L., & Chial, M. R. (1997). Word recognition performance in various background competitors. *Journal of the American Academy of Audiology, 8*(2), 71–80.

Steeneken, H. J. M., & Houtgast, T. (1980). A physical method for measuring speech-transmission quality. *Journal of the Acoustical Society of America, 67*(1), 318–326.

Stelmachowicz, P. G., Mace, A. L., Kopun, J. G., & Carney, E. (1993). Long-term and short-term characteristics of speech: Implications for hearing aid selection for young children. *Journal of Speech Language Hearing Research, 36*(3), 609–620.

Stewart, M. A., Brown, J. B., & Weston, W. W. (1989). Patient-centered interviewing part III: Five provocative questions. *Canadian Family Physician, 35*, 159–161.

Strom, K. (2013). Hearing aid sales up 2.9% in '12. *Hearing Journal, 20*(2), 6.

Strouse, A., & Wilson, R. H. (1999). Recognition of one-, two-, and three-pair dichotic digits under free and directed recall. *Journal of the American Academy of Audiology, 10*(10), 557–571.

Studebaker, G. (1974). The acoustical effect of various factors on the frequency response of a hearing aid receiver. *Journal of the Audio Engineering Society, 22*, 329–334.

Studebaker, G. (1985). A "rationalized" arcsine transform. *Journal of Speech and Hearing Research, 28*(3), 455–462.

Summers, V., Molis, M. R., Müsch, H., Walden, B. E., Surr, R. K., & Cord, M. T. (2003). Identifying dead regions in the cochlea: Psychophysical tuning curves and tone detection in threshold-equalizing noise. *Ear and Hearing, 24*(2), 133–142.

Surr, R. K., Cord, M., & Walden, B. (2001) Response of hearing aid wearers to the absence of a user-operated volume control. *Hearing Journal, 54*(4), 32–36.

Sutter, A. H. (1985). Speech recognition in noise by individuals with mild hearing impairments. *Journal of the Acoustical Society, 78*(3), 887–900.

Taylor, B. (2007). *Predicting real world hearing aid benefit with speech audiometry: An evidence-based review.* Retrieved from http://www.audiologyonline.com/articles/predicting-real-world-hearing-aid-946

Taylor, B. (2008). The acceptable noise level test as a predictor of real-world hearing aid benefit. *Hearing Journal, 61*(9), 39–42.

Taylor, B., & Mueller, H. G. (2011). *Fitting and dispensing hearing aids.* San Diego, CA: Plural.

Thibodeau, L. (2007). Speech audiometry. In R. Roeser, M. Valente, & H. Hosford-Dunn (Eds.), *Audiology: Diagnosis* (pp. 281–309). New York, NY: Thieme.

Thornton, A. R., & Raffin, M. J. M. (1978). Speech discrimination scores modeled as a binomial variable. *Journal of Speech and Hearing Research, 21*(3), 507–518.

Thornton, A. R., & Raffin, M. J. M. (1982). Comment on "a quantative examination of the sources of speech discrimination test score variability. *Ear and Hearing, 3*(6), 340.

Tillman, T. W., Carhart, R., & Wilber, L. (1963). *A test for speech discrimination composed of CNC monosyllabic words.* (Northwestern University, Auditory Test No. 4). SAM-TDR-62.

Tillman, T. W., & Olsen, W. O. (1973). Speech audiometry. In J. Jerger (Ed.), *Modern developments in audiology* (2nd ed., pp. 37–74). New York, NY: Academic.

Tuckett, D., Boulton, M., Olson, C., & Williams, A. (1985). *Meetings between experts: An approach to sharing ideas in medical consultations.* London, UK: Tavistock.

Turner, C. W., & Cummings, K. J. (1999). Speech audibility for listeners with high-frequency hearing loss. *American Journal of Audiology, 8*(1), 47–56.

United States Department of Health and Human Services, Administration for Children and Families. (2003). Program announcement. *Federal Register, 68*(131).

Upfold, L. J. (1980). The evaluation of CROS aids with the unilateral listener. *Scandinavian Audiology, 9*(2), 85–88.

Uziel, A., Mondain, M., Hagen, P., Dejean, F., & Doucet, G. (2003). Rehabilitation for high-frequency sensorineural hearing impairment in adults with the Symphonix Vibrant Soundbridge: A comparative study. *Otology and Neurotology, 24*(5), 775–783.

Valente, M. (2006). *Guideline for audiologic management of the adult patient.* Retrieved from http://www.audiologyonline.com/articles/pf_article_detail.asp?article_id=1716

Valente, M., Fabry, D., Potts, L. G., & Sandlin, R. E. (1998). Comparing the performance of the Widex SENSO digital hearing aid with analog hearing aids. *Journal of the American Academy of Audiology, 9*(5), 342–360.

Valente, M., Potts, L. G., Valente, M., & Goebel, J. (1995). Wireless CROS versus transcranial CROS for unilateral hearing loss. *American Journal of Audiology, 4*, 52–59.

Valente, M., Potts, L. G., Valente, L. M., Vass, W., & Goebel, J. (1994). Intersubject variability of real-ear sound pressure level: Conventional and insert earphones. *Journal of the American Academy of Audiology, 5*(6), 390–398.

Valente, M., & Van Vleet, D. (1997). The independent hearing aid fitting forum (IHAFF) protocol. *Trends in Amplification, 2*(1), 6–35.

Ventry, I., & Weinstein, B. (1982). The Hearing Handicap Inventory for the Elderly: A new tool. *Ear and Hearing, 3*(3), 128–134.

Ventry, I. M., & Weinstein, B. E. (1983). Identification of elderly people with hearing problems. *Journal of the American Speech Language Hearing Association, 25*, 37–42.

Vermiglio, A. J. (2008). The American English hearing in noise test. *International Journal of Audiology, 47*(6), 386–387.

Vinay, & Moore, B. C. J. (2007). Prevalence of dead regions in subjects with sensorineural hearing loss. *Ear and Hearing, 28*(2), 231–241.

Vinay, Moore, B. C. J., & Baer, T. (2008). Speech recognition in noise as a function of highpass-filter cutoff frequency for people with and without low-frequency cochlear dead regions. *Journal of the Acoustical Society of America, 123*(2), 456–464.

Wade, P. S. (2002). Medical aspects of bone anchored hearing aids and middle ear implants. *Trends in Amplification, 6*(2), 39–44.

Walden, B. E. (1997). Toward a model clinical-trials protocol for substantiating hearing aid user-benefit claims. *American Journal of Audiology, 6*(2), 13–24.

Walden, B. E., & Walden, T. C. (2005). Unilateral versus bilateral amplification for adults with impaired hearing [Report]. *Journal of the American Academy of Audiology, 16*(8), 574–584.

Walden, T. C., & Walden, B. E. (2004). Predicting success with hearing aids in everyday living. *Journal of the American Academy of Audiology, 15*(5), 342–352.

Walker, G. (1979). Earphone termination and the response of behind-the-ear hearing aids. *British Journal of Audiology, 13*(2), 41–46.

Warnaar, B., & Dreschler, W. (2012). Agreement between psychophysical tuning curves and the threshold equalizing noise test in dead region identification. *International Journal of Audiology, 51*(6), 456–464.

Warner, R. L., & Bentler, R. A. (2002). Thresholds of discomfort for complex stimuli: Acoustic and sound quality predictors. *Journal of Speech, Language, and Hearing Research, 45*(2), 1016–1026.

Wazen, J. J., Caruso, M., & Tjellstrom, A. (1998). Long-term results with the titanium bone-anchored hearing aid: the US experience. *American Journal of Otology, 19*(6), 737.

Wazen, J. J., Spitzer, J. B., Ghossaini, S. N., Fayad, J. N., Niparko, J. K., Cox, K., . . . Soli, S. D. (2003). Transcranial contralateral cochlear stimulation in unilateral deafness. *Otolaryngology-Head and Neck Surgery, 129*(3), 248–254.

Weinstein, B. E. (1986). Validity of a screening protocol for identifying elderly people with hearing problems. *ASHA, 28*(5), 41–45.

Westerkull, P. (2002). BAHA®: The direct bone conductor. *Trends in Amplification, 6*(2), 45–52.

Wiley, T. L., Cruickshanks, K. J., Nondahl, D. M., & Tweed, T. S. (2000). Self-reported hearing handicap and audiometric measures in older adults. *Journal of the American Academy of Audiology, 11*(2), 67–75.

Wilson, F. (2009). *Graduate medical education: Issues and options.* New York, NY: Radcliffe Medical Press.

Wilson, R. H. (2003). Development of a speech in multitalker babble paradigm to assess word-recognition performance. *Journal of the American Academy of Audiology, 14*(9), 453–470.

Wilson, R. H. (2011). Clinical experience with the words-in-noise test on 3,430 veterans: Comparisons with pure-tone thresholds and word recognition in quiet. *Journal of the American Academy of Audiology, 27*(7), 405–423.

Wilson, R. H., Abrams, H. B., & Pillion, A. L. (2003). A word-recognition task in multitalker babble using a descending presentation mode from 24 dB to 0 dB signal to babble. *Journal of Rehabilitation Research and Development, 40*(4), 321–327.

Wilson, R., & Burks, C. (2005). Use of 35 words for evaluation of hearing loss in signal-to-babble ratio. A clinic protocol. *Journal of Rehabilitation Research and Development, 42*(6), 839–852.

Wilson, R. H., Carnell, C., & Cleghorn, A. L. (2007). The words-in-noise (WIN) test with multitalker babble and speech-spectrum noise maskers. *Journal of the American Academy of Audiology, 18*(6), 522–530.

Wilson, R. H, & Cates, W. B. (2008). A comparison of two word-recognition tasks in multitalker babble: Speech recognition in noise test (SPRINT) and words-in-noise test (WIN). *Journal of the American Academy of Audiology, 19*(7), 548–556.

Wilson, R. H., Coley, K. E., Haenel, J. L., & Browning, K. M. (1976). Northwestern University Auditory Test No. 6: Normative and comparative intelligibility functions. *Journal of the American Audiological Society, 1*(5), 221–228.

Wilson, R. H., Farmer, N. M., Gandhi, A., Shelburne, E., & Weaver, J. (2010). Normative data for the words-in-noise test for 6- to 12-year-old children. *Journal of Speech, Language, and Hearing Research, 53*(5), 1111–1121.

Wilson, R. H., & McArdle, R. (2008). A change is in the air. *The Hearing Review, 61*(10), 10–15.

Wilson, R. H., & McArdle, R. (2012). Speech-in-noise measures: Variable versus fixed speech and noise levels. *International Journal of Audiology, 51*(9), 708–712.

Wilson, R. H., McArdle, R. A., & Smith, S. L. (2007). An evaluation of the BKB-SIN, HINT, QuickSIN, and WIN materials on listeners with normal hearing and listeners with hearing loss. *Journal of Speech, Language, and Hearing Research, 50*(4), 844–856.

Wilson, R. H., McArdle, R., Watts, K. L., & Smith, S. L. (2012). The revised speech perception in noise test (R-SPIN) in a multiple signal-to-noise ratio paradigm. *Journal of the American Academy of Audiology, 23*(8), 590–605.

Wilson, R. H., & Watts, K. L. (2012). The words-in-noise test (WIN), list 3: A practice list. *Journal of the American Academy of Audiology, 23*(2), 92–96.

Wu, Y. H., & Bentler, R. A. (2010). Impact of visual cues on directional benefit and preference: Part I-Laboratory tests. *Ear and Hearing, 31*(1), 22–34.

Appendixes

Appendix A

AAA Scope of Practice

Updated January 2004

Introduction

Development of a Scope of Practice document began in 1990 with the work of an ad hoc committee on Scope of Practice, chaired by Alison Grimes. The document was put into final format by Robert W. Keith in 1992, and revised again in 1996 and 2004.

The Scope of Practice document describes the range of interests, capabilities and professional activities of audiologists. It defines audiologists as independent practitioners and provides examples of settings in which they are engaged. It is not intended to exclude the participation in activities outside of those delineated in the document. The overriding principle is that members of the Academy will provide only those services for which they are adequately prepared through their academic and clinical training and their experience, and that their practice is consistent with the Code of Ethics of the American Academy of Audiology.

As a dynamic and growing profession, the field of audiology will change over time as new information is acquired. This Scope of Practice document will receive regular review for consistency with current knowledge and practice.

Purpose

The purpose of this document is to define the profession of audiology by its scope of practice. This document outlines those activities that are within the expertise of members of the profession. This Scope of Practice statement is intended for use by audiologists, allied professionals, consumers of audiologic services, and the general public. It serves as a reference for issues of service delivery, third-party reimbursement, legislation, consumer education, regulatory action, state and professional licensure, and inter-professional relations. The document is not intended to be an exhaustive list of activities in which audiologists engage. Rather, it is a broad statement of professional practice. Periodic updating of any scope of practice statement is necessary as technologies and perspectives change.

Definition of an Audiologist

An audiologist is a person who, by virtue of academic degree, clinical training, and license to practice and/or professional credential, is uniquely qualified to provide a comprehensive array of professional services related to the prevention of hearing loss and the audiologic identification, assessment, diagnosis, and treatment of persons with impairment of auditory and vestibular function, and to the prevention of impairments associated with them. Audiologists serve in a number of roles including clinician, therapist, teacher, consultant, researcher and administrator. The supervising audiologist maintains legal and ethical responsibility for all assigned audiology activities provided by audiology assistants and audiology students.

The central focus of the profession of audiology is concerned with all auditory impairments and their relationship to disorders of communication. Audiologists identify, assess, diagnose, and treat individuals with impairment of either peripheral or central auditory and/or vestibular function, and strive to prevent such impairments.

Audiologists provide clinical and academic training to students in audiology. Audiologists teach physicians, medical students, residents, and fellows about the auditory and vestibular system. Specifically, they provide instruction about identification, assessment, diagnosis, prevention, and treatment of persons with hearing and/or vestibular impairment. They provide information and training on all aspects of hearing and balance to other professions including psychology, counseling, rehabilitation, and education. Audiologists provide information on hearing and balance, hearing loss and disability, prevention of hearing loss, and treatment to business and industry. They develop and oversee hearing conservation programs in industry. Furthermore, audiologists serve as expert witnesses within the boundaries of forensic audiology.

The audiologist is an independent practitioner who provides services in hospitals, clinics, schools, private practices and other settings in which audiologic services are relevant.

Scope of Practice

The scope of practice of audiologists is defined by the training and knowledge base of professionals who are licensed and/or credentialed to practice as audiologists. Areas of practice include the audiologic identification, assessment, diagnosis and treatment of individuals with impairment of auditory and vestibular function, prevention of hearing loss, and research in normal and disordered auditory and vestibular function. The practice of audiology includes:

Identification

Audiologists develop and oversee hearing screening programs for persons of all ages to detect individuals with hearing loss. Audiologists may perform speech or language screening, or other screening measures, for the purpose of initial identification and referral of persons with other communication disorders.

Assessment and Diagnosis

Assessment of hearing includes the administration and interpretation of behavioral, physioacoustic, and electrophysiologic measures of the peripheral and central auditory systems. Assessment of the vestibular system includes administration and interpretation of behavioral and electrophysiologic tests of equilibrium. Assessment is accomplished using standardized testing procedures and appropriately calibrated instrumentation and leads to the diagnosis of hearing and/or vestibular abnormality.

Treatment

The audiologist is the professional who provides the full range of audiologic treatment services for persons with impairment of hearing and vestibular function. The audiologist is responsible for the evaluation, fitting, and verification of amplification devices, including assistive listening devices. The audiologist determines the appropriateness of amplification systems for persons with hearing impairment, evaluates benefit, and provides counseling and training regarding their use. Audiologists conduct otoscopic examinations, clean ear canals and remove cerumen, take ear canal impressions, select, fit, evaluate, and dispense hearing aids and other amplification systems. Audiologists assess and provide audiologic treatment for persons with tinnitus using techniques that include, but are not limited to, biofeedback, masking, hearing aids, education, and counseling.

Audiologists also are involved in the treatment of persons with vestibular disorders. They participate as full members of balance treatment teams to recommend and carry out treatment and rehabilitation of impairments of vestibular function.

Audiologists provide audiologic treatment services for infants and children with hearing impairment and their families. These services may include clinical treatment, home intervention, family support, and case management.

The audiologist is the member of the implant team (e.g., cochlear implants, middle ear implantable hearing aids, fully implantable hearing aids, bone anchored hearing aids, and all other amplification/signal processing devices) who determines audiologic candidacy based on hearing and communication information. The audiologist provides pre and post surgical assessment, counseling, and all aspects of audiologic treatment including auditory training, rehabilitation, implant programming, and maintenance of implant hardware and software.

The audiologist provides audiologic treatment to persons with hearing impairment, and is a source of information for family members, other professionals and the general public. Counseling regarding hearing loss, the use of amplification systems and strategies for improving speech recognition is within the expertise of the audiologist. Additionally, the audiologist provides counseling regarding the effects of hearing loss on communication and psycho-social status in personal, social, and vocational arenas.

The audiologist administers audiologic identification, assessment, diagnosis, and treatment programs to children of all ages with hearing impairment from birth and preschool through school age. The audiologist is an integral part of the team within the school system that manages students with hearing impairments and students with central auditory processing disorders. The audiologist participates in the development of Individual Family Service Plans (IFSPs) and Individualized Educational Programs (IEPs), serves as a consultant in matters pertaining to classroom acoustics, assistive listening systems, hearing aids, communication, and psycho-social effects of hearing loss, and maintains both classroom assistive systems as well as students' personal hearing aids. The audiologist administers hearing screening programs in schools, and trains and supervises non audiologists performing hearing screening in the educational setting.

Hearing Conservation

The audiologist designs, implements and coordinates industrial and community hearing conservation programs. This includes identification and amelioration of noise-hazardous conditions, identification of hearing loss, recommendation and counseling on use of hearing protection, employee education, and the training and supervision of non audiologists performing hearing screening in the industrial setting.

Intraoperative Neurophysiologic Monitoring

Audiologists administer and interpret electrophysiologic measurements of neural function including, but not limited to, sensory and motor evoked potentials, tests of nerve conduction velocity, and electromyography. These measurements are used in differential diagnosis, pre- and postoperative evaluation of neural function, and neurophysiologic intraoperative monitoring of central nervous system, spinal cord, and cranial nerve function.

Research

Audiologists design, implement, analyze and interpret the results of research related to auditory and balance systems.

Additional Expertise

Some audiologists, by virtue of education, experience and personal choice choose to specialize in an area of practice not otherwise defined in this document. Nothing in this document shall be construed to limit individual freedom of choice in this regard provided that the activity is consistent with the American Academy of Audiology Code of Ethics.

This document will be reviewed, revised, and updated periodically in order to reflect changing clinical demands of audiologists and in order to keep pace with the changing scope of practice reflected by these changes and innovations in this specialty.

Appendix B

ASHA Scope of Practice in Audiology

Statement of Purpose

The purpose of this document is to define the scope of practice in audiology in order to (a) describe the services offered by qualified audiologists as primary service providers, case managers, and/or members of multidisciplinary and interdisciplinary teams; (b) serve as a reference for health care, education, and other professionals, and for consumers, members of the general public, and policy makers concerned with legislation, regulation, licensure, and third party reimbursement; and (c) inform members of ASHA, certificate holders, and students of the activities for which certification in audiology is required in accordance with the ASHA Code of Ethics.

Audiologists provide comprehensive diagnostic and treatment/rehabilitative services for auditory, vestibular, and related impairments. These services are provided to individuals across the entire age span from birth through adulthood; to individuals from diverse language, ethnic, cultural, and socioeconomic backgrounds; and to individuals who have multiple disabilities. This position statement is not intended to be exhaustive; however, the activities described reflect current practice within the profession. Practice activities related to emerging clinical, technological, and scientific developments are not precluded from consideration as part of the scope of practice of an audiologist. Such innovations and advances will result in the periodic revision and updating of this document. It is also recognized that specialty areas identified within the scope of practice will vary among the individual providers. ASHA also recognizes that credentialed professionals in related fields may have knowledge, skills, and experience that could be applied to some areas within the scope of audiology practice. Defining the scope of practice of audiologists is not meant to exclude other appropriately credentialed postgraduate professionals from rendering services in common practice areas.

Audiologists serve diverse populations. The patient/client population includes persons of different race, age, gender, religion, national origin, and sexual orientation. Audiologists' caseloads include individuals from diverse ethnic, cultural, or linguistic backgrounds, and persons with disabilities. Although audiologists are prohibited from discriminating in the provision of professional services based on these factors, in some cases such factors may be relevant to the development of an appropriate treatment plan. These factors may be considered in treatment plans only when firmly grounded in scientific and professional knowledge.

This scope of practice does not supersede existing state licensure laws or affect the interpretation or implementation of such laws. It may serve, however, as a model for the development or modification of licensure laws.

The schema in Figure 1 depicts the relationship of the scope of practice to ASHA's policy documents that address current and emerging audiology practice areas; that is, preferred practice patterns, guidelines, and position statements. ASHA members and ASHA-certified professionals are bound by the ASHA Code of Ethics to provide services that are consistent with the scope of their competence, education, and experience (ASHA, 2003). There are other existing legislative and regulatory bodies that govern the practice of audiology.

Framework for Practice

The practice of audiology includes both the prevention of and assessment of auditory, vestibular, and related

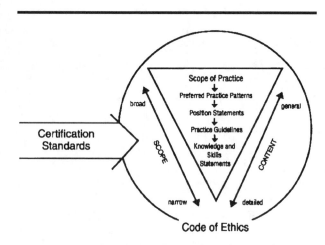

Figure 1. Conceptual Framework of ASHA Standards and Policy Statements.

impairments as well as the habilitation/rehabilitation and maintenance of persons with these impairments. The overall goal of the provision of audiology services should be to optimize and enhance the ability of an individual to hear, as well as to communicate in his/her everyday or natural environment. In addition, audiologists provide comprehensive services to individuals with normal hearing who interact with persons with a hearing impairment. The overall goal of audiologic services is to improve the quality of life for all of these individuals.

The World Health Organization (WHO) has developed a multipurpose health classification system known as the International Classification of Functioning, Disability, and Health (ICF) (WHO, 2001). The purpose of this classification system is to provide a standard language and framework for the description of functioning and health. The ICF framework is useful in describing the role of audiologists in the prevention, assessment, and habilitation/rehabilitation of auditory, vestibular, and other related impairments and restrictions or limitations of functioning.

The ICF is organized into two parts. The first part deals with Functioning and Disability while the second part deals with Contextual Factors. Each part has two components. The components of Functioning and Disability are:

- **Body Functions and Structures:** Body Functions are the physiological functions of body systems and Body Structures are the anatomical parts of the body and their components. Impairments are limitations or variations in Body Function or Structure such as a deviation or loss. An example of a Body Function that might be evaluated by an audiologist would be hearing sensitivity. The use of typanometry to access the mobility of the tympanic membrane is an example of a Body Structure that might be evaluated by an audiologist.
- **Activity/Participation:** In the ICF, Activity and Participation are realized as one list. Activity refers to the execution of a task or action by an individual. Participation is the involvement in a life situation. Activity limitations are difficulties an individual may experience while executing a given activity.

Participation restrictions are difficulties that may limit an individual's involvement in life situations. The Activity/Participation construct thus represents the effects that hearing, vestibular, and related impairments could have on the life of an individual. These effects could include the ability to hold conversations, participate in sports, attend religious services, understand a teacher in a classroom, and walk up and down stairs.

The components of Contextual Factors are:

- **Environmental Factors:** Environmental Factors make up the physical, social, and attitudinal environment in which people live and conduct their lives. Examples of Environmental Factors, as they relate to audiology, include the acoustical properties of a given space and any type of hearing assistive technology.
- **Personal Factors:** Personal Factors are the internal influences on an individual's functioning and disability and are not a part of the health condition. These factors may include but are not limited to age, gender, social background, and profession.

Functioning and Disability are interactive and evolutionary processes. Figure 2 illustrates the interaction of the various components of the ICF. Each component of the ICF can be expressed on a continuum of function. On one end of the continuum is intact functioning. At the opposite end of the continuum is completely compromised functioning. Contextual Factors (Environmental and Personal Factors) may interact with any of the components of functioning and disability. Environmental and Personal Factors may act as facilitators or barriers to functioning.

The scope of practice in audiology encompasses all of the components of the ICF. During the assessment phase, audiologists perform tests of Body Function and Structure. Examples of these types of tests include otoscopic examination, pure-tone audiometry, tympanometry, otoacoustic emissions measurements, and speech audiometry. Activity/Participation limitations and restrictions are sometimes addressed by audiologists through case history, interview, questionnaire, and

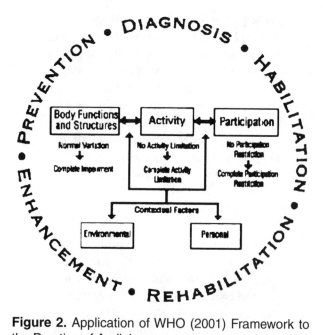

Figure 2. Application of WHO (2001) Framework to the Practice of Audiology.

counseling. For example, a question such as, "Do you have trouble understanding while on the telephone?" or "Can you describe the difficulties you experience when you participate in a conversation with someone who is not familiar to you?" would be considered an assessment of Activity/Participation limitation or restriction. Questionnaires that require clients to report the magnitude of difficulty that they experience in certain specified settings can sometimes be used to measure aspects of Activity/Participation. For example: "Because of my hearing problems, I have difficulty conversing with others in a restaurant." In addition, Environmental and Personal Factors also need to be taken into consideration by audiologists as they treat individuals with auditory, vestibular, and other related impairments. In the above question regarding conversation in a restaurant, if the factor of "noise" (i.e., a noisy restaurant) is added to the question, this represents an Environmental Factor. Examples of Personal Factors might include a person's background or culture that influences his or her reaction to the use of a hearing aid or cochlear implant. The use of the ICF framework (WHO, 2001) may help audiologists broaden their perspective concerning their role in evaluating a client's needs or when designing and providing comprehensive services to their clients. Overall,

audiologists work to improve quality of life by reducing impairments of body functions and structures, Activity limitations/Participation restrictions and Environmental barriers of the individuals they serve.

Definition of an Audiologist

Audiologists are professionals engaged in autonomous practice to promote healthy hearing, communication competency, and quality of life for persons of all ages through the prevention, identification, assessment, and rehabilitation of hearing, auditory function, balance, and other related systems. They facilitate prevention through the fitting of hearing protective devices, education programs for industry and the public, hearing screening/conservation programs, and research. The audiologist is the professional responsible for the identification of impairments and dysfunction of the auditory, balance, and other related systems. Their unique education and training provides them with the skills to assess and diagnose dysfunction in hearing, auditory function, balance, and related disorders. The delivery of audiologic (re)habilitation services includes not only the selecting, fitting, and dispensing of hearing aids and other hearing assistive devices, but also the assessment and follow-up services for persons with cochlear implants. The audiologist providing audiologic (re)habilitation does so through a comprehensive program of therapeutic services, devices, counseling, and other management strategies. Functional diagnosis of vestibular disorders and management of balance rehabilitation is another aspect of the professional responsibilities of the audiologist. Audiologists engage in research pertinent to all of these domains.

Audiologists currently hold a master's or doctoral degree in audiology from a program accredited by the Council on Academic Accreditation in Audiology and Speech-Language Pathology (CAA) of the American Speech-Language-Hearing Association. ASHA-certified audiologists complete a supervised postgraduate professional experience or a similar supervised professional experience during the completion of the doctoral degree as described in the ASHA certification standards. Beginning January 1, 2012, all applicants for the Certificate of Clinical Competence in Audiology must have a doctoral degree from a CAA-accredited university program. Demonstration of continued professional development is mandated for the maintenance of the Certificate of Clinical Competence in Audiology. Where required, audiologists are licensed or registered by the state in which they practice.

Professional Roles and Activities

Audiologists serve a diverse population and may function in one or more of a variety of activities. The practice of audiology includes:

A. Prevention
   1. Promotion of hearing wellness, as well as the prevention of hearing loss and protection of hearing function by designing, implementing, and coordinating occupational, school, and community hearing conservation and identification programs;
   2. Participation in noise measurements of the acoustic environment to improve accessibility and to promote hearing wellness.
B. Identification
   1. Activities that identify dysfunction in hearing, balance, and other auditory-related systems;
   2. Supervision, implementation, and follow-up of newborn and school hearing screening programs;
   3. Screening for speech, orofacial myofunctional disorders, language, cognitive communication disorders, and/or preferred communication modalities that may affect education, health, development or communication and may result in recommendations for rescreening or comprehensive speech-language pathology assessment or in referral for other examinations or services;
   4. Identification of populations and individuals with or at risk for hearing loss and other auditory dysfunction, balance impairments, tinnitus, and associated communication impairments as well as of those with normal hearing;
   5. In collaboration with speech-language pathologists, identification of populations and individuals at risk for developing speech-language impairments.

C. Assessment
   1. The conduct and interpretation of behavioral, electroacoustic, and/or electrophysiologic methods to assess hearing, auditory function, balance, and related systems;
   2. Measurement and interpretation of sensory and motor evoked potentials, electromyography, and other electrodiagnostic tests for purposes of neurophysiologic intraoperative monitoring and cranial nerve assessment;
   3. Evaluation and management of children and adults with auditory-related processing disorders;
   4. Performance of otoscopy for appropriate audiological management or to provide a basis for medical referral;
   5. Cerumen management to prevent obstruction of the external ear canal and of amplification devices;
   6. Preparation of a report including interpreting data, summarizing findings, generating recommendations and developing an audiologic treatment/management plan;
   7. Referrals to other professions, agencies, and/or consumer organizations.
D. Rehabilitation
   1. As part of the comprehensive audiologic (re)habilitation program, evaluates, selects, fits and dispenses hearing assistive technology devices to include hearing aids;
   2. Assessment of candidacy of persons with hearing loss for cochlear implants and provision of fitting, mapping, and audiologic rehabilitation to optimize device use;
   3. Development of a culturally appropriate, audiologic rehabilitative management plan including, when appropriate:
      a. Recommendations for fitting and dispensing, and educating the consumer and family/caregivers in the use of and adjustment to sensory aids, hearing assistive devices, alerting systems, and captioning devices;
      b. Availability of counseling relating to psycho social aspects of hearing loss, and other auditory dysfunction, and processes to enhance communication competence;

c. Skills training and consultation concerning environmental modifications to facilitate development of receptive and expressive communication;

d. Evaluation and modification of the audiologic management plan.

4. Provision of comprehensive audiologic rehabilitation services, including management procedures for speech and language habilitation and/or rehabilitation for persons with hearing loss or other auditory dysfunction, including but not exclusive to speechreading, auditory training, communication strategies, manual communication and counseling for psychosocial adjustment for persons with hearing loss or other auditory dysfunction and their families/caregivers;

5. Consultation and provision of vestibular and balance rehabilitation therapy to persons with vestibular and balance impairments;

6. Assessment and non-medical management of tinnitus using biofeedback, behavioral management, masking, hearing aids, education, and counseling;

7. Provision of training for professionals of related and/or allied services when needed;

8. Participation in the development of an Individual Education Program (IEP) for school-age children or an Individual Family Service Plan (IFSP) for children from birth to 36 months old;

9. Provision of in-service programs for school personnel, and advising school districts in planning educational programs and accessibility for students with hearing loss and other auditory dysfunction;

10. Measurement of noise levels and provision of recommendations for environmental modifications in order to reduce the noise level;

11. Management of the selection, purchase, installation, and evaluation of large-area amplification systems.

E. Advocacy/ Consultation

1. Advocacy for communication needs of all individuals that may include advocating for the rights/funding of services for those with hearing loss, auditory, or vestibular disorders;

2. Advocacy for issues (i.e., acoustic accessibility) that affect the rights of individuals with normal hearing;

3. Consultation with professionals of related and/or allied services when needed;

4. Consultation in development of an Individual Education Program (IEP) for school-age children or an Individual Family Service Plan (IFSP) for children from birth to 36 months old;

5. Consultation to educators as members of interdisciplinary teams about communication management, educational implications of hearing loss and other auditory dysfunction, educational programming, classroom acoustics, and large-area amplification systems for children with hearing loss and other auditory dysfunction;

6. Consultation about accessibility for persons with hearing loss and other auditory dysfunction in public and private buildings, programs, and services;

7. Consultation to individuals, public and private agencies, and governmental bodies, or as an expert witness regarding legal interpretations of audiology findings, effects of hearing loss and other auditory dysfunction, balance system impairments, and relevant noise-related considerations;

8. Case management and service as a liaison for the consumer, family, and agencies in order to monitor audiologic status and management and to make recommendations about educational and vocational programming;

9. Consultation to industry on the development of products and instrumentation related to the measurement and management of auditory or balance function.

F. Education/ Research/Administration

1. Education, supervision, and administration for audiology graduate and other professional education programs;

2. Measurement of functional outcomes, consumer satisfaction, efficacy, effectiveness, and efficiency of practices and programs

to maintain and improve the quality of audiologic services;

3. Design and conduct of basic and applied audiologic research to increase the knowledge base, to develop new methods and programs, and to determine the efficacy, effectiveness, and efficiency of assessment and treatment paradigms; disseminate research findings to other professionals and to the public;

4. Participation in the development of professional and technical standards;

5. Participation in quality improvement programs;

6. Program administration and supervision of professionals as well as support personnel.

Practice Settings

Audiologists provide services in private practice; medical settings such as hospitals and physicians' offices; community and university hearing and speech centers; managed care systems; industry; the military; various state agencies; home health, subacute rehabilitation, long-term care, and intermediate-care facilities; and school systems. Audiologists provide academic education to students and practitioners in universities, to medical and surgical students and residents, and to other related professionals. Such education pertains to the identification, functional diagnosis/assessment, and non-medical treatment/management of auditory, vestibular, balance, and related impairments.

References

American Speech-Language-Hearing Association. (1996, Spring). Scope of practice in audiology. *Asha, 38*(Suppl. 16), 12–15.

American Speech-Language-Hearing Association. (2003). Code of ethics (Revised). *ASHA Supplement, 23,* 13–15.

World Health Organization (WHO). (2001). *ICF: International classification of functioning, disability and health.* Geneva, Switzerland: Author.

Appendix C

FDA Regulations for Hearing Aid

(Original date: 1977; revisions of 2009)

[Code of Federal Regulations]
[Title 21, Volume 8]
[Revised as of April 1, 2009]
[CITE: 21CFR801.421]

TITLE 21—FOOD AND DRUGS
CHAPTER I—FOOD AND DRUG ADMINISTRATION
DEPARTMENT OF HEALTH AND HUMAN SERVICES
SUBCHAPTER H—MEDICAL DEVICES

PART 801 – LABELING

Subpart H—Special Requirements for Specific Devices

Sec. 801.421 Hearing aid devices; conditions for sale.

(a) *Medical evaluation requirements* –(1) *General.* Except as provided in paragraph (a) (2) of this section, a hearing aid dispenser shall not sell a hearing aid unless the prospective user has presented to the hearing aid dispenser a written statement signed by a licensed physician that states that the patient's hearing loss has been medically evaluated and the patient may be considered a candidate for a hearing aid. The medical evaluation must have taken place within the preceding 6 months.

(2) *Waiver to the medical evaluation requirements.* If the prospective hearing aid user is 18 years of age or older, the hearing aid dispenser may afford the prospective user an opportunity to waive the medical evaluation requirement of paragraph (a) (1) of this section provided that the hearing aid dispenser:

(i)   Informs the prospective user that the exercise of the waiver is not in the user's best health interest;

(ii)   Does not in any way actively encourage the prospective user to waive such a medical evaluation; and

(iii) Affords the prospective user the opportunity to sign the following statement:

I have been advised by _____ (Hearing aid dispenser's name) that the Food and Drug Administration has determined that my best health interest would be served if I had a medical evaluation by a licensed physician (preferably a physician who specializes in diseases of the ear) before purchasing a hearing aid. I do not wish a medical evaluation before purchasing a hearing aid.

(b) *Opportunity to review User Instructional Brochure.*
Before signing any statement under paragraph (a) (2) (iii) of this section and before the sale of a hearing aid to a prospective user, the hearing aid dispenser shall:

(1) Provide the prospective user a copy of the User Instructional Brochure for a hearing aid that has been, or may be selected for the prospective user;

(2) Review the content of the User Instructional Brochure with the prospective user orally, or in the predominate method of communication used during the sale;

(3) Afford the prospective user an opportunity to read the User Instructional Brochure.

(c) *Availability of User Instructional Brochure.* (1) Upon request by an individual who is considering purchase of a hearing aid, a dispenser shall, with respect to any hearing aid that he dispenses, provide a copy of the User Instructional Brochure for the hearing aid or the name and address of the manufacturer or distributor from whom a User Instructional Brochure for the hearing aid may be obtained.

(2) In addition to assuring that a User Instructional Brochure accompanies each hearing aid, a manufacturer or distributor shall with respect to any hearing aid that he manufactures or distributes:

(i)   Provide sufficient copies of the User Instructional Brochure to sellers for distribution to users and prospective users;

(ii) Provide a copy of the User Instructional Brochure to any hearing aid professional, user, or prospective user who requests a copy in writing.

(d) *Recordkeeping.* The dispenser shall retain for 3 years after the dispensing of a hearing aid a copy of any written statement from a physician required under paragraph (a) (1) of this section or any written statement waiving medical evaluation required under paragraph (a) (2) (iii) of this section.

(e) *Exemption for group auditory trainers.* Group auditory trainers, defined as a group amplification system purchased by a qualified school or institution for the purpose of communicating with and educating individuals with hearing impairments, are exempt from the requirements of this section.

[42 FR 9296, Feb. 15, 1977]

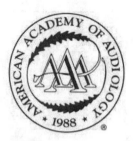

Ethical Practice Guidelines on Financial Incentives from Hearing Instrument Manufacturers

Ethical Guidelines

The following general guidelines have been accepted by the Board of Directors of the Academy of Dispensing Audiologists (ADA) and the American Academy of Audiology (AAA):

1. When potential for conflict of interest exists, the interests of the patient must come before those of the audiologist.

Any gifts accepted by the audiologist should primarily benefit the patient and should not be of substantial value. Gifts of minimal value ($100 or less) related to the audiologist's work (pens, earlights, notepads, etc.) are acceptable. Incentives or rewards based upon product purchases must not be accepted. This would include cash, gifts, incentive trips, merchandise, equipment, or credit towards such items. No "strings" should be attached to any accepted gift.

Audiologists should not participate in any industry-sponsored social function that may appear to bias professional judgment or practice. This would include accepting invitations to private convention parties, golf outings or accepting such items as theater tickets. Meals and social functions that are part of a legitimate educational program are acceptable. When social events occur in conjunction with educational meetings, the educational component must be the primary objective with the meal/social function ancillary to it.

2. Commercial interest in any product or service recommended must be disclosed to the patient.

This would include owning stock or serving as a paid consultant and then dispensing that product to a patient.

3. Travel expenses, registration fees, or compensation for time to attend meetings, conferences or seminars should not be accepted directly or indirectly from a manufacturer.

Trips sponsored by a manufacturer that are solely educational may be accepted, provided the cost of the trip is modest and acceptance of the trip does not reward the audiologist for past sales or commit the audiologist to future purchases. Faculty at meetings and consultants who provide service may receive reasonable compensation honoraria, and reimbursement of travel, lodging and meal expenses.

4. Free equipment or discounts for equipment, institutional support, or any form of remuneration from a vendor for research purposes should be fully disclosed and the results of research must be accurately reported.

All materials, presentations, or articles produced as a result of the investigation should also carry a disclosure of the funding source. Investigators should structure research agreements with industry to insure that the results are represented accurately, and presentation of findings is objective.

Frequently Asked Questions (FAQs)

Q. Why are AAA and ADA reviewing gift giving from manufacturers?

A. Gift giving from the hearing health care industry to audiologists has been a customary practice. Gifts serve two functions. First, they remind audiologists of the name of the product made by that company. Second, they help a company establish a relationship with the audiologist. However, if the decisions made by the professional are, or appear to be, influenced by an incentive or reward, or can be viewed as not being made objectively, then a conflict of interest may be present. The professional's belief that he or she is not personally influenced is not sufficient to avoid the appearance of a conflict of interest. Our organizations encourage manufacturer/audiologist interactions that serve to improve patient care. However, it is important that gifts do not have the potential to impact professional judgment.

Q. Why would audiologists want to adhere to these guidelines?

A. Audiologists must be committed to the principles of honesty, integrity, and fairness. The principle of putting patients' interests first is the basis of all healthcare professions. Adhering to these guidelines reflects positively on our profession. All healthcare profession licensure acts set limits on professional behavior. In return for a license, professionals are obliged to adhere to certain standards of conduct and have the obligation to self-regulate. Additionally, adhering to a uniform code of ethical conduct may prevent the audiologist from unintentionally violating federal and state regulations.

Q. If an audiologist accepts gifts, what are the potential legal consequences?

A. Acceptance of gifts may not only be construed as constituting a conflict of interest; it may also be illegal. Federal laws make it a criminal act for an audiologist who provides services to Medicare, TRICARE, Medicaid and VA patients to solicit or receive "any remuneration (including any...rebate) directly or indirectly, overtly or covertly, in case or in kind...in return for purchasing...or ordering any goods or services..." Medicare already indirectly covers hearing aids through some private Medicare HMO plans. The Office of the Inspector General has recently issued guidelines for gift-giving activities for the pharmaceutical industry and physicians that appear directly analogous to the issues covered for audiologists in this guideline.

Q. Are incentive trips, vacation packages, gift certificates, cruises, and credits toward equipment purchases or cash received from manufacturers allowed?

A. No. The acceptance of such gifts, whether related to previous purchases or future purchases, raises the question of whether the audiologist is, in fact, holding the patient's interests paramount. There can be no link between dispensing or referral patterns and gifts.

Q. What is the difference between acceptance of trips, lease arrangements, gifts, or receiving a larger discount level?

A. Establishing any type of savings plan with a specific manufacturer creates the appearance of a conflict of interest. Discount programs, however, are generally protected by the law if they have the potential for benefiting consumers. Discount programs are considered to present ethical issues only if they involve commitments by the audiologist that compromise professional judgment.

Q. Can an audiologist accept a trip to a manufacturing facility for the purpose of training?

A. Obviously, there are times when it is more economical and/or a better educational experience can be provided when audiologists are trained together regionally or at the manufacturer's facility. While it is preferable that audiologists pay their own travel expenses, there are circumstances where it is appropriate to accept tickets and/or hotel accommodations:
• The travel expenses should only be those strictly necessary.
• The conference or training must be the reason for the trip.
• Participation must not be tied to any commitment to manufacturers.
• The expense for a spouse or other travel companion may not be compensated by the manufacturer.

Q. Can an audiologist accept a lunch/dinner invitation from manufacturer's representative in order to learn about a new product?

A. Yes, modest business related meals are acceptable.

Q. What are the ethical considerations regarding attendance at sponsored social events at conventions or training seminars?

A. The following criteria should be considered before attending such events:
• The sponsorship of the event should be disclosed to, and open to, all registrants.

- The event should facilitate discussion among attendees.

- The educational component of the conference should account for a substantial amount of the total time spent at the convention.

Q. May an audiologist or a corporation obtain a loan from a manufacturer in order to purchase equipment and then repay a portion of the loan with every hearing aid purchased?

A. Audiologists are encouraged to obtain financing through recognized lending institutions or the equipment manufacturer to avoid potential conflict of interest. Repayment should include only repayment of the debt plus appropriate interest fees but with no additional considerations or obligations on the part of either party.

Q. May an audiologist "co-op" advertising costs with a manufacturer?

A. If the manufacturer wishes to share the cost of an advertisement that features both the manufacturer's name and the audiologist's name, this is acceptable as long as there are no strings attached.

Q. Is it acceptable for a manufacturer's representative to assist in seeing patients at an 'open house' at the audiologists' clinical facility?

A. Open houses are usually product or manufacturer specific with a manufacturer's representative in attendance. The consumer should be very much aware that the presentation would be focused on the purchase of hearing instruments from the featured manufacturer. However, the audiologist still has the responsibility to utilize the most appropriate instruments. The audiologist should consider the legal and ethical ramifications involved if a non-audiologist participates in the open house.

Q. Is there a potential conflict of interest if an audiologist joins a network or buying group?

A. Businesses and organizations are free to negotiate prices on products either directly with the manufacturer or by using the purchasing power of a buying group.

Q. If an audiologist is hired by a corporation that provides hearing aids or other related devices and is offered stock options, is there a cause for concern regarding conflict of interest?

A. If the stock is in the corporation the audiologist works for, there is no conflict of interest.

Q: Are there conflicts of interest implications for researchers?

A: One of the researcher's responsibilities is to fully disclose the funding of the research, whether it is in the form of direct grants, equipment grants or other forms of compensation such as a consultantship with a sponsor. This allows the consumer of the research to evaluate the potential for conflicts of interest. Additionally, researchers are ethically responsible for ensuring the rigor of the scientific design of the experiment and the accuracy and integrity of the interpretation.

Q. Will a similar document on ethical practice guidelines be written for audiologists involved in research and academia?

A. Yes. A set of guidelines is in development to address conflicts of interest in research.

Q. How will the ethical guidelines be enforced?

A. Given the increased enforcement of anti-kickback, fraud, and abuse laws, audiologists should stay abreast of changes in regulatory landscape, and establish procedures and protocols that will protect them in their employment settings and practices. These guidelines are not meant to address all possible interactions but are an effort to assist the audiologist in cases of ethical dilemmas. At this point, education of our members is our focus. However, any profession that fails to monitor misconduct and enforce its Code of Ethics invites the loss of autonomy and the loss of trust in the profession. When such activities exist, the profession must have appropriate disciplinary procedures in place.

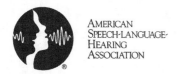

AMERICAN
SPEECH-LANGUAGE-
HEARING
ASSOCIATION

MODEL SUPERBILL
for AUDIOLOGY

The following is a model of a superbill which could be used by an audiology practice when billing private health plans. This sample is not meant to dictate which services should or should not be listed on the bill. Most billable codes are from the American Medical Association (AMA) *Current Procedural Terminology* (CPT)© 2011. Prosthetic and durable medical equipment codes, such as hearing aid codes, are published by the Centers for Medicare and Medicaid Services (CMS) as the *Healthcare Common Procedure Code System* (HCPCS).

The superbill is a standard form which health plans use to process claims. For the professional rendering services, it provides a time efficient means to document services, fees, codes, and other information required by insurance companies, (i.e., certification and licensure). The patient uses this form to file for health plan payment.

NOTE: This is only a model, therefore some procedures, codes, or other pertinent information may not be found on the following model. For a complete list of CPT and ICD-9 codes, the *ASHA Health Plan Coding & Claims Guide* is available through ASHA's Online Store or by calling ASHA's Product Sales at 1-888-498-6699.

MODEL AUDIOLOGY SUPERBILL

PATIENT:	INSURED:
REFERRING PHYSICIAN:	ADDRESS:
FILE:	INSURANCE PLAN:
DATE:	INSURANCE PLAN #:
DATE INITIAL SYMPTOM:	DATE FIRST CONSULTATION:

PLACE OF SERVICE: ☐ HOME ☐ OFFICE ☐ OTHER: _____

DIAGNOSIS:

PRIMARY (Audiology):	ICD-9 CODE:
SECONDARY (Medical):	ICD-9 CODE:
HEARING AID/EARMOLD DEFECT:	

SERVICES:

☑	PROCEDURE	CPT	CHARGE
	Audiological Assessment Procedures		
☐	Tympanometry and reflex threshold measurements	92550	
☐	Screening test, pure tone, air only	92551	
☐	Pure tone audiometry (threshold);air only	92552	
☐	Pure tone audiometry (threshold); air and bone	92553	
☐	Speech audiometry threshold	92555	
☐	Speech audiometry threshold; w/speech recognition	92556	
☐	Comprehensive audiometry threshold evaluation and speech recognition	92557	
☐	Audiometric testing of groups	92559	
☐	Bekesy audiometry; screening	92560	
☐	Bekesy audiometry; diagnostic	92561	
☐	Loudness balance test, alternate binaural or monaural	92562	
☐	Tone decay test	92563	
☐	Short increment sensitivity index (SISI)	92564	
☐	Stenger test, pure tone	92565	
☐	Tympanometry (impedance testing)	92567	
☐	Acoustic reflex testing, threshold	92568	
☐	Acoustic immittance testing, includes tympanometry (impedance testing), acoustic reflex threshold testing, and acoustic reflex decay testing	92570	
☐	Filtered speech test	92571	
☐	Staggered spondaic word test	92572	
☐	Sensorineural acuity level test	92575	
☐	Synthetic sentence identification test	92576	
☐	Stenger test, speech	92577	
☐	Visual reinforcement audiometry (VRA)	92579	
☐	Conditioning play audiometry	92582	
☐	Select picture audiometry	92583	
☐	Electrocochleography	92584	

☑	PROCEDURE	CPT	CHARGE
☐	Auditory evoked potentials, comprehensive	92585	
☐	Auditory evoked potentials, limited	92586	
☐	Evoked otoacoustic emissions, screening (qualitative measurement of distortion product or transient evoked otoacoustic emissions), automated analysis	92558	
☐	Distortion product evoked otoacoustic emissions; limited evaluation (to confirm the presence or absence of hearing disorder, 3-6 frequencies) or transient evoked otoacoustic emissions, with interpretation and report	92587	
☐	Distortion product evoked otoacoustic emissions; comprehensive diagnostic evaluation (quantitative analysis of outer hair cell function by cochlear mapping, minimum of 12 frequencies), with interpretation and report	92588	
☐	Evaluation of central auditory function, with report; initial 60 minutes	92620	
☐	each additional 15 minutes	92621	
☐	Assessment of tinnitus (includes pitch, loudness matching, and masking)	92625	
	Hearing Aid Assessment and Fitting Procedures		
☐	Hearing aid exam and selection; monaural	92590	
☐	Hearing aid exam and selection; binaural	92591	
☐	Hearing aid check; monaural	92592	
☐	Hearing aid check; binaural	92593	
☐	Electroacoustic evaluation for hearing aid; monoaural	92594	
☐	binaural	92595	
☐	Ear protector attenuation measurements	92596	
☐	Intraoperative nerve test add-on	95920	
☐	Somatosensory testing	95925	
☐	Visual evoked potential test	95930	
☐	H-reflex test, amplitude and latency study	95934	
☐	H-reflex test, not g/s muscle	95936	
☐	Neuromuscular junction test	95937	

368

☑	PROCEDURE	CPT	CHARGE

Vestibular and Balance System Assessment Procedures

☐	Spontaneous nystagmus, including gaze	92531	_____
☐	Positional nystagmus test	92532	_____
☐	Caloric vestibular test, each irrigation (binaural, bithermal stimulation constitutes 4 tests)	92533	_____
☐	Optokinetic nystagmus test	92534	_____
☐	Basic vestibular evaluation, incl. spontaneous nystagmus test w/eccentric gaze fixation nystagmus, w/recording, positional nystagmus test, min. of 4 positions, w/recording, optokinetic nystagmus test, bidirectional foveal & peripheral stimulation, w/recording, & oscillating tracking test, w/recording	92540	_____
☐	Spontaneous nystagmus test, incl. gaze and fixation nystagmus, with recording	92541	_____
☐	Positional nystagmus test, minimum of four positions	92542	_____
☐	Caloric vestibular test, each irrigation (binaural, bithermal stimulation constitutes four tests), with recording	92543	_____
☐	Optokinetic nystagmus test, bi-directional, foveal or peripheral stimulation, w/ recording	92544	_____
☐	Oscillating tracking test, with recording	92545	_____
☐	Sinusoidal vertical axis rotational testing	92546	_____
☐	Use of vertical electrodes in any or all of the above tests	92547	_____
☐	Computerized dynamic posturography	92548	_____

Vestibular and Balance Rehabilitation Services

| ☐ | Canalith repositioning procedure(s) (eg, Epley maneuver, Semont maneuver) per day. | 95992 | _____ |

Cerumen Management Services

| ☐ | Removal of impacted cerumen, one or both ears | 69210 | _____ |

Auditory Implant Services

☐	Cochlear implant follow-up exam <7 years of age	92601	_____
☐	Reprogram cochlear implant <7 years of age	92602	_____
☐	Cochlear implant follow-up exam >7 years of age	92603	_____
☐	Reprogram cochlear implant > 7 years of age	92604	_____
☐	Diagnostic analysis with programming of auditory brainstem implant, per hour	92640	_____

Habilitative and Rehabilitative Services

☐	Evaluation of speech, language, voice, communication, and/or auditory processing	92506	_____
☐	Treatment of speech, language, voice, communication, and/or auditory processing disorder; individual	92507	_____
☐	group, two or more individuals	92508	_____
☐	Evaluation of auditory rehabilitation status, 1st hour	92626	_____
☐	each additional 15 minutes	92627	_____
☐	Auditory rehabilitation; pre-lingual hearing loss	92630	_____
☐	Auditory rehabilitation; post-lingual hearing loss	92633	_____

Hearing Aids (HCPCS Level II Codes)

| ☐ | Assessment for Hearing Aid | V5010 | _____ |

☑	PROCEDURE	CPT	CHARGE
☐	Fitting/Orientation/Checking of Hearing Aid	V5011	_____
☐	Repair/Modification of a Hearing Aid	V5014	_____
☐	Conformity Evaluation	V5020	_____
☐	Hearing aid, Monaural, body worn, air conduction	V5030	_____
☐	bone conduction	V5040	_____
☐	Hearing Aid, Monaural, in the ear (ITE)	V5050	_____
☐	Hearing Aid, Monaural, behind the ear (BTE)	V5060	_____
☐	Glasses, air conduction	V5070	_____
☐	Glasses, bone conduction	V5080	_____
☐	Dispensing fee, Unspecified Hearing Aid	V5090	_____
☐	Hearing Aid, bilateral, body worn	V5100	_____
☐	Dispensing fee, bilateral	V5110	_____
☐	Binaural, body	V5120	_____
☐	Binaural, ITE	V5130	_____
☐	Binaural, BTE	V5140	_____
☐	Binaural, glasses	V5150	_____
☐	Dispensing fee, binaural	V5160	_____
☐	Hearing Aid, CROS, ITE	V5170	_____
☐	Hearing Aid, CROS, BTE	V5180	_____
☐	Hearing Aid, CROS, glasses	V5190	_____
☐	Dispensing fee, CROS	V5200	_____
☐	Hearing Aid, BICROS, ITE	V5210	_____
☐	Hearing Aid, BICROS, BTE	V5220	_____
☐	Hearing Aid, BICROS, glasses	V5230	_____
☐	Dispensing Fee, BICROS	V5240	_____
☐	Dispensing Fee, Monaural Hearing Aid	V5241	_____
☐	Hearing Aid, Analog, monaural, completely in the ear canal (CIC)	V5242	_____
☐	Hearing aid, analog, monaural, in the canal (ITC)	V5243	_____
☐	Hearing aid, digitally programmable analog, monaural, CIC	V5244	_____
☐	Hearing aid, digitally programmable analog, monaural, ITC	V5245	_____
☐	Hearing aid, digitally programmable analog, monaural, ITE	V5246	_____
☐	Hearing aid, digitally programmable analog, monaural, BTE	V5247	_____
☐	Hearing aid, analog, binaural, CIC	V5248	_____
☐	Hearing aid, analog, binaural, ITC	V5249	_____
☐	Hearing aid, digitally programmable analog, binaural, CIC	V5250	_____
☐	Hearing aid, digitally programmable analog, binaural, ITC	V5251	_____
☐	Hearing aid, digitally programmable, binaural, ITE	V5252	_____
☐	Hearing aid, digitally programmable, binaural, BTE	V5253	_____
☐	Hearing aid, digital, monaural, CIC	V5254	_____
☐	Hearing aid, digital, monaural, ITC	V5255	_____
☐	Hearing aid, digital, monaural, ITE	V5256	_____
☐	Hearing aid, digital, monaural, BTE	V5257	_____

369

☑	PROCEDURE	CPT	CHARGE
☐	Hearing aid, digital, binaural, CIC	V5258	_____
☐	Hearing aid, digital, binaural, ITC	V5259	_____
☐	Hearing aid, digital, binaural, ITE	V5260	_____
☐	Hearing aid, digital, binaural, BTE	V5261	_____
☐	Hearing aid, disposable, any type, monaural	V5262	_____
☐	Hearing aid, disposable, any type, binaural	V5263	_____
☐	Earmold/insert, not disposable, any type	V5264	_____
☐	Earmold/insert, disposable, any type	V5265	_____
☐	Battery for use in hearing device	V5266	_____
☐	Hearing aid supplies/accessories	V5267	_____
☐	Assistive listening device, telephone amplifier, any type	V5268	_____
☐	Assistive listening device, alerting, any type	V5269	_____
☐	Assistive listening device, television amplifier, any type	V5270	_____
☐	Assistive listening device, television caption decoder	V5271	_____
☐	Assistive listening device, TDD	V5272	_____
☐	Assistive listening device, for use with cochlear implant	V5273	_____
☐	Assistive learning device not otherwise specified	V5274	_____
☐	Ear impression, each	V5275	_____
☐	Hearing Service, Miscellaneous	V5299	_____

Other Procedures

☑	PROCEDURE	CPT	CHARGE
☐	Otorhinolaryngological service or procedure	92700	_____

☑	PROCEDURE	CPT	CHARGE
☐	Telephone assessment and management service provided by a qualified nonphysician health care professional to an established patient, parent, or guardian not originating from a related assessment and management service provided within the previous seven days nor leading to an assessment and management service or procedure with the next 24 hours or soonest available appointment; 5-10 minutes of medical discussion	98966	_____
☐	11-20 minutes of medical discussion	98967	_____
☐	21-30 minutes of medical discussion	98968	_____
☐	Online assessment & management service provided by a qualified nonphysician health care professional to an established patient, guardian, or health care provider not originating from a related assessment & management service provided within the previous 7 days, using the Internet or similar electronic communications network.	98969	_____
☐	Medical team conference with interdisciplinary team of health care professionals, face-to-face with patient and/or family, 30 minutes or more; participation by nonphysician qualified health care professional	99366	_____
☐	Medical team conference with interdisciplinary team of health care professionals, patient and/or family not present, 30 minutes or more; participation by nonphysician qualified health care professional	99368	_____

Total Charges: $ _____

BILLING INFORMATION

PREVIOUS BALANCE:	$
TODAY'S CHARGES:	$
TOTAL DUE:	$
PAID TODAY:	$

PAID BY: ☐ CASH   ☐ CREDIT   ☐ CHECK
O VISA O MC O OTHER

BALANCE:	$

AUTHORIZATIONS

I hereby authorize direct payment of benefits to Audiology & Hearing Center, Inc.

SIGNATURE: _____

DATE: _____

I hereby authorize Steven Smith, AuD, CCC-A to release any information acquired in the course of treatment.

SIGNATURE: _____

DATE: _____

Steven Smith, AuD, CCC-A
Audiology & Hearing Center, Inc.
999 Anywhere Street
Rockville, MD 00000
(999) 999-9999 PHONE
(888) 888-8888 FAX

NPI # 1234567890 ♦ TAX ID # 22-22222 ♦ MARYLAND LICENSE # 3333

White Copy: Office   Canary Copy: Insurance   Pink Copy: Patient

Appendix F

AAA Code of Ethics

Highlighted Changes Effective April 2011

Preamble

The Code of Ethics of the American Academy of Audiology specifies professional standards that allow for the proper discharge of audiologists' responsibilities to those served, and that protect the integrity of the profession. The Code of Ethics consists of two parts. The first part, the Statement of Principles and Rules, presents precepts that members (all categories of members, including Student Members) effective January 1, 2009 of the Academy agree to uphold. The second part, the Procedures, provides the process that enables enforcement of the Principles and Rules.

PART I. Statement of Principles and Rules

PRINCIPLE 1: Members shall provide professional services and conduct research with honesty and compassion, and shall respect the dignity, worth, and rights of those served.

Rule la: Individuals shall not limit the delivery of professional services on any basis that is unjustifiable or irrelevant to the need for the potential benefit from such services.

Rule 1b: Individuals shall not provide services except in a professional relationship, and shall not discriminate in the provision of services to individuals on the basis of sex, race, religion, national origin, sexual orientation, or general health.

PRINCIPLE 2: Members shall maintain high standards of professional competence in rendering services.

Rule 2a: Members shall provide only those professional services for which they are qualified by education and experience.

Rule 2b: Individuals shall use available resources, including referrals to other specialists, and shall not give or accept benefits or items of value for receiving or making referrals.

Rule 2c: Individuals shall exercise all reasonable precautions to avoid injury to persons in the delivery of professional services or execution of research.

Rule 2d: Individuals shall provide appropriate supervision and assume full responsibility for services delegated to supportive personnel. Individuals shall not delegate any service requiring professional competence to unqualified persons.

Rule 2e: Individuals shall not knowingly permit personnel under their direct or indirect supervision to engage in any practice that is a violation of the Code of Ethics.

Rule 2f: Individuals shall maintain professional competence, including participation in continuing education.

PRINCIPLE 3: Members shall maintain the confidentiality of the information and records of those receiving services or involved in research.

Rule 3a: Individuals shall not reveal to unauthorized persons any professional or personal information obtained from the person served professionally, unless required by law.

PRINCIPLE 4: Members shall provide only services and products that are in the best interest of those served.

Rule 4a: Individuals shall not exploit persons in the delivery of professional services.

Rule 4b: Individuals shall not charge for services not rendered.

Rule 4c: Individuals shall not participate in activities that constitute a conflict of professional interest.

Rule 4d: Individuals using investigational procedures with human participants or prospectively collecting research data from human participants shall obtain full informed consent from the participants or legal representatives. Members conducting research with human participants or animals shall follow accepted standards, such as those promulgated in the current Responsible Conduct of Research (current edition, 2009) by the U.S. Office of Research Integrity.

PRINCIPLE 5: Members shall provide accurate information about the nature and management of communicative disorders and about the services and products offered.

Rule 5a: Individuals shall provide persons served with the information a reasonable person would want to know about the nature and possible effects of services rendered, or products provided or research being conducted.

Rule 5b: Individuals may make a statement of prognosis, but shall not guarantee results, mislead, or misinform persons served or studied.

Rule 5c: Individuals shall conduct and report product-related research only according to accepted standards of research practice.

Rule 5d: Individuals shall not carry out teaching or research activities in a manner that constitutes an invasion of privacy, or that fails to inform persons fully about the nature and possible effects of these activities, affording all persons informed free choice of participation.

Rule 5e: Individuals shall maintain accurate documentation of services rendered according to accepted medical, legal, and professional standards and requirements.

PRINCIPLE 6: Members shall comply with the ethical standards of the Academy with regard to public statements or publication.

Rule 6a: Individuals shall not misrepresent their educational degrees, training, credentials, or competence. Only degrees earned from regionally accredited institutions in which training was obtained in audiology, or a directly related discipline, may be used in public statements concerning professional services.

Rule 6b: Individuals' public statements about professional services, products, or research results shall not contain representations or claims that are false, misleading, or deceptive.

PRINCIPLE 7: Members shall honor their responsibilities to the public and to professional colleagues.

Rule 7a: Individuals shall not use professional or commercial affiliations in any way that would limit services to or mislead patients or colleagues.

Rule 7b: Individuals shall inform colleagues and the public in an objective manner consistent with professional standards about products and services they have developed or research they have conducted.

PRINCIPLE 8: Members shall uphold the dignity of the profession and freely accept the Academy's self-imposed standards.

Rule 8a: Individuals shall not violate these Principles and Rules, nor attempt to circumvent them.

Rule 8b: Individuals shall not engage in dishonesty or illegal conduct that adversely reflects on the profession.

Rule 8c: Individuals shall inform the Ethical Practices Committee when there are reasons to believe that a member of the Academy may have violated the Code of Ethics.

Rule 8d: Individuals shall fully cooperate with reviews being conducted by the Ethical Practices Committee in any matter related to the Code of Ethics.

PART II. Procedures for the Management of Alleged Violations

Introduction

Members of the American Academy of Audiology are obligated to uphold the Code of Ethics of the Academy in their personal conduct and in the performance of their professional duties. To this end it is the responsibility of each Academy member to inform the Ethical Practices Committee of possible Ethics Code violations. The processing of alleged violations of the Code of Ethics will follow the procedures specified below in an expeditious manner to ensure that violations of ethical conduct by members of the Academy are halted in the shortest time possible.

Procedures

1. Suspected violations of the Code of Ethics shall be reported in letter format giving documentation sufficient to support the alleged violation. Letters must be addressed to:

   Chair, Ethical Practices Committee
   c/o Executive Director
   American Academy of Audiology
   11730 Plaza America Dr., Suite 300
   Reston, VA 20190

2. Following receipt of a report of a suspected violation, at the discretion of the Chair, the Ethical Practices Committee will request a signed Waiver of Confidentiality from the complainant indicating that the complainant will allow the Ethical Practices Committee to disclose his/her name should this become necessary during investigation of the allegation.

   a. The Ethical Practices Committee may, under special circumstances, act in the absence of a signed Waiver of Confidentiality. For example, in cases where the Ethical Practices Committee has received information from a state licensure or registration board of a member having his or her license or registration suspended or revoked, then the Ethical Practices Committee will proceed without a complainant.

   b. The Chair may communicate with other individuals, agencies, and/or programs for additional information as may be required for review at any time during the deliberation.

3. The Ethical Practices Committee will convene to review the merit of the alleged violation as it relates to the Code of Ethics

   a. The Ethical Practices Committee shall meet to discuss the case, either in person, by electronic means or by teleconference. The meeting will occur within 60 days of receipt of the waiver of confidentiality, or of notification by the complainant of refusal to sign the waiver. In cases where another form of notification brings the complaint to the attention of the Ethical Practices Committee, the Committee will convene within 60 days of notification.

   b. If the alleged violation has a high probability of being legally actionable, the case may be referred to the appropriate agency. The Ethical Practices Committee may postpone member notification and further deliberation until the legal process has been completed.

4. If there is sufficient evidence that indicates a violation of the Code of Ethics has occurred, upon majority vote, the member will be forwarded a Notification of Potential Ethics Concern.

   a. The circumstances of the alleged violation will be described.

   b. The member will be informed of the specific Code of Ethics rule that may conflict with member behavior.

   c. Supporting Academy documents that may serve to further educate the member about the ethical implications will be included, as appropriate.

   d. The member will be asked to respond fully to the allegation and submit all supporting evidence within 30 calendar days.

5. The Ethical Practices Committee will meet either in person or by teleconference:

   a. within 60 calendar days of receiving a response from the member to the Notification of Potential Ethics Concern to review the response and all information pertaining to the alleged violation, or

   b. within sixty (60) calendar days of notification to member if no response is received from the member to review the information received from the complainant.

6. If the Ethical Practices Committee determines that the evidence supports the allegation of an ethical violation, then the member will be provided written notice containing the following information:

   a. The right to a hearing in person or by teleconference before the Ethical Practices Committee;

   b. The date, time and place of the hearing;

   c. The ethical violation being charged and the potential sanction

   d. The right to present a defense to the charges.

   At this time the member should provide any additional relevant information. As this is the final opportunity for a member to provide new information, the member should carefully prepare all documentation.

7. Potential Rulings.

   a. When the Ethical Practices Committee determines there is insufficient evidence of an ethical violation, the parties to the complaint will be notified that the case will be closed.

   b. If the evidence supports the allegation of a Code violation, the rules(s) of the Code violated will be cited and sanction(s) will be specified.

8. The Committee shall sanction members based on the severity of the violation and history of prior ethical violations. A simple majority of voting members is required to institute a sanction unless otherwise noted. Sanctions may include one or more of the following:

   a. Educative Letter. This sanction alone is appropriate when:

(1) The ethics violation appears to have been inadvertent.

(2) The member's response to Notification of Potential Ethics Concern indicates a new awareness of the problem and the member resolves to refrain from future ethical violations.

b. Cease and Desist Order. The member signs a consent agreement to immediately halt the practice(s) which were found to be in violation of the Code of Ethics.

c. Reprimand. The member will be formally reprimanded for the violation of the Code of Ethics.

d. Mandatory continuing education.

(1) The EPC will determine the type of education needed to reduce chances of recurrence of violations.

(2) The member will be responsible for submitting documentation of continuing education within the period of time designated by the Ethical Practices Committee.

(3) All costs associated with compliance will be borne by the member.

e. Probation of Suspension. The member signs a consent agreement in acknowledgement of the Ethical Practices Committee decision and is allowed to retain membership benefits during a defined probationary period.

(1) The duration of probation and the terms for avoiding suspension will be determined by the Ethical Practices Committee.

(2) Failure of the member to meet the terms for probation will result in the suspension of membership.

f. Suspension of Membership.

(1) The duration of suspension will be determined by the Ethical Practices Committee.

(2) The member may not receive membership benefits during the period of suspension.

(3) Members suspended are not entitled to a refund of dues or fees.

g. Revocation of Membership. Revocation of membership is considered the maximum punishment for a violation of the Code of Ethics.

(1) Revocation requires a two-thirds majority of the voting members of the EPC.

(2) Individuals whose memberships are revoked are not entitled to a refund of dues or fees.

(3) One year following the date of membership revocation the individual may reapply for, but is not guaranteed, membership through normal channels and must meet the membership qualifications in effect at the time of application.

9. The member may appeal the Final Finding and Decision of the Ethical Practices Committee to the Academy Board of Directors. The route of Appeal is by letter format through the Ethical Practices Committee to the Board of Directors of the Academy. Requests for Appeal must:

a. be received by the Chair, Ethical Practices Committee, within 30 days of the Ethical Practices Committee's notification of the Final Finding and Decision,

b. state the basis for the appeal, and the reason(s) that the Final Finding and Decision of the Ethical Practices Committee should be changed,

c. not offer new documentation.

The EPC chair will communicate with the Executive Director of the Association to schedule the appeal at the earliest feasible Board of Director's meeting.

The Board of Directors will review the documents and written summaries, and deliberate the case.

The decision of the Board of Directors regarding the member's appeal shall be final.

10. In order to educate the membership, upon majority vote the Ethical Practices Committee, the circumstances and nature of cases shall be presented in *Audiology Today* and in the Professional Resource area of the Academy website. The member's identity will not be made public.

11. No Ethical Practices Committee member shall give access to records, act or speak independently, or on behalf of the Ethical Practices Committee, without the expressed permission of the members then active. No member may impose the sanction of the Ethical Practices Committee, or to interpret the findings of the EPC in any manner which may place members of the Ethical Practices Committee or Board of Directors, collectively or singly, at financial, professional, or personal risk.

12. The Ethical Practices Committee Chair shall maintain a Book of Precedents that shall form the basis for future findings of the Committee.

Confidentiality and Records

Confidentiality shall be maintained in all Ethical Practices Committee discussion, correspondence, communication, deliberation, and records pertaining to members reviewed by the Ethical Practices Committee.

1. Complaints and suspected violations are assigned a case number.
2. Identity of members involved in complaints and suspected violations and access to EPC files is restricted to the following:
   a. EPC Chair
   b. EPC member designated by EPC Chair when the chair recuses him or herself from a case.
   c. Executive Director
   d. Agent/s of the Executive Director
   e. Other/s, following majority vote of EPC
3. Original records shall be maintained at the Central Records Repository at the Academy office in a locked cabinet.
   a. One copy will be sent to the Ethical Practices Committee chair or member designated by the Chair.
   b. Copies will be sent to members.
4. Communications shall be sent to the members involved in complaints by the Academy office via certified or registered mail, after review by Legal Counsel.
5. When a case is closed,
   a. The chair will forward all documentation to the Academy Central Records Repository.
   b. Members shall destroy all material pertaining to the case.
6. Complete records generally shall be maintained at the Academy Central Records Repository for a period of five years.
   a. Records will be destroyed five years after a member receives a sanction less than suspension, or five years after the end of a suspension, or after membership is reinstated.
   b. Records of membership revocations for persons who have not returned to membership status will be maintained indefinitely.

http://www.audiology.org/resources/documentlibrary/Pages/codeofethics.aspx

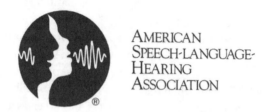

AMERICAN
SPEECH-LANGUAGE-
HEARING
ASSOCIATION

Code of Ethics

Reference this material as: American Speech-Language-Hearing Association. (2010). *Code of Ethics* [Ethics].
Available from www.asha.org/policy.

Index terms: ethics

doi:10.1044/policy.ET2010-00309

Preamble

The preservation of the highest standards of integrity and ethical principles is vital to the responsible discharge of obligations by speech-language pathologists, audiologists, and speech, language, and hearing scientists. This Code of Ethics sets forth the fundamental principles and rules considered essential to this purpose.

Every individual who is (a) a member of the American Speech-Language-Hearing Association, whether certified or not, (b) a nonmember holding the Certificate of Clinical Competence from the Association, (c) an applicant for membership or certification, or (d) a Clinical Fellow seeking to fulfill standards for certification shall abide by this Code of Ethics.

Any violation of the spirit and purpose of this Code shall be considered unethical. Failure to specify any particular responsibility or practice in this Code of Ethics shall not be construed as denial of the existence of such responsibilities or practices.

The fundamentals of ethical conduct are described by Principles of Ethics and by Rules of Ethics as they relate to the responsibility to persons served, the public, speech-language pathologists, audiologists, and speech, language, and hearing scientists, and to the conduct of research and scholarly activities.

Principles of Ethics, aspirational and inspirational in nature, form the underlying moral basis for the Code of Ethics. Individuals shall observe these principles as affirmative obligations under all conditions of professional activity.

Rules of Ethics are specific statements of minimally acceptable professional conduct or of prohibitions and are applicable to all individuals.

Principle of Ethics I

Individuals shall honor their responsibility to hold paramount the welfare of persons they serve professionally or who are participants in research and scholarly activities, and they shall treat animals involved in research in a humane manner.

Rules of Ethics

A. Individuals shall provide all services competently.
B. Individuals shall use every resource, including referral when appropriate, to ensure that high-quality service is provided.
C. Individuals shall not discriminate in the delivery of professional services or the conduct of research and scholarly activities on the basis of race or ethnicity, gender, gender identity/gender expression, age, religion, national origin, sexual orientation, or disability.
D. Individuals shall not misrepresent the credentials of assistants, technicians, support personnel, students, Clinical Fellows, or any others under their supervision, and they shall inform those they serve professionally of the name and professional credentials of persons providing services.
E. Individuals who hold the Certificate of Clinical Competence shall not delegate tasks that require the unique skills, knowledge, and judgment that are within the scope of their profession to assistants, technicians, support personnel, or any nonprofessionals over whom they have supervisory responsibility.

F. Individuals who hold the Certificate of Clinical Competence may delegate tasks related to provision of clinical services to assistants, technicians, support personnel, or any other persons only if those services are appropriately supervised, realizing that the responsibility for client welfare remains with the certified individual.

G. Individuals who hold the Certificate of Clinical Competence may delegate tasks related to provision of clinical services that require the unique skills, knowledge, and judgment that are within the scope of practice of their profession to students only if those services are appropriately supervised. The responsibility for client welfare remains with the certified individual.

H. Individuals shall fully inform the persons they serve of the nature and possible effects of services rendered and products dispensed, and they shall inform participants in research about the possible effects of their participation in research conducted.

I. Individuals shall evaluate the effectiveness of services rendered and of products dispensed, and they shall provide services or dispense products only when benefit can reasonably be expected.

J. Individuals shall not guarantee the results of any treatment or procedure, directly or by implication; however, they may make a reasonable statement of prognosis.

K. Individuals shall not provide clinical services solely by correspondence.

L. Individuals may practice by telecommunication (e.g., telehealth/e-health), where not prohibited by law.

M. Individuals shall adequately maintain and appropriately secure records of professional services rendered, research and scholarly activities conducted, and products dispensed, and they shall allow access to these records only when authorized or when required by law.

N. Individuals shall not reveal, without authorization, any professional or personal information about identified persons served professionally or identified participants involved in research and scholarly activities unless doing so is necessary to protect the welfare of the person or of the community or is otherwise required by law.

O. Individuals shall not charge for services not rendered, nor shall they misrepresent services rendered, products dispensed, or research and scholarly activities conducted.

P. Individuals shall enroll and include persons as participants in research or teaching demonstrations only if their participation is voluntary, without coercion, and with their informed consent.

Q. Individuals whose professional services are adversely affected by substance abuse or other health-related conditions shall seek professional assistance and, where appropriate, withdraw from the affected areas of practice.

R. Individuals shall not discontinue service to those they are serving without providing reasonable notice.

Principle of Ethics II   Individuals shall honor their responsibility to achieve and maintain the highest level of professional competence and performance.

Rules of Ethics	A. Individuals shall engage in the provision of clinical services only when they hold the appropriate Certificate of Clinical Competence or when they are in the certification process and are supervised by an individual who holds the appropriate Certificate of Clinical Competence.
	B. Individuals shall engage in only those aspects of the professions that are within the scope of their professional practice and competence, considering their level of education, training, and experience.
	C. Individuals shall engage in lifelong learning to maintain and enhance professional competence and performance.
	D. Individuals shall not require or permit their professional staff to provide services or conduct research activities that exceed the staff member's competence, level of education, training, and experience.
	E. Individuals shall ensure that all equipment used to provide services or to conduct research and scholarly activities is in proper working order and is properly calibrated.

Principle of Ethics III

Individuals shall honor their responsibility to the public by promoting public understanding of the professions, by supporting the development of services designed to fulfill the unmet needs of the public, and by providing accurate information in all communications involving any aspect of the professions, including the dissemination of research findings and scholarly activities, and the promotion, marketing, and advertising of products and services.

Rules of Ethics

A. Individuals shall not misrepresent their credentials, competence, education, training, experience, or scholarly or research contributions.

B. Individuals shall not participate in professional activities that constitute a conflict of interest.

C. Individuals shall refer those served professionally solely on the basis of the interest of those being referred and not on any personal interest, financial or otherwise.

D. Individuals shall not misrepresent research, diagnostic information, services rendered, results of services rendered, products dispensed, or the effects of products dispensed.

E. Individuals shall not defraud or engage in any scheme to defraud in connection with obtaining payment, reimbursement, or grants for services rendered, research conducted, or products dispensed.

F. Individuals' statements to the public shall provide accurate information about the nature and management of communication disorders, about the professions, about professional services, about products for sale, and about research and scholarly activities.

G. Individuals' statements to the public when advertising, announcing, and marketing their professional services; reporting research results; and promoting products shall adhere to professional standards and shall not contain misrepresentations.

Principle of Ethics IV

Individuals shall honor their responsibilities to the professions and their relationships with colleagues, students, and members of other professions and disciplines.

Rules of Ethics

A. Individuals shall uphold the dignity and autonomy of the professions, maintain harmonious interprofessional and intraprofessional relationships, and accept the professions' self-imposed standards.

B. Individuals shall prohibit anyone under their supervision from engaging in any practice that violates the Code of Ethics.

C. Individuals shall not engage in dishonesty, fraud, deceit, or misrepresentation.

D. Individuals shall not engage in any form of unlawful harassment, including sexual harassment or power abuse.

E. Individuals shall not engage in any other form of conduct that adversely reflects on the professions or on the individual's fitness to serve persons professionally.

F. Individuals shall not engage in sexual activities with clients, students, or research participants over whom they exercise professional authority or power.

G. Individuals shall assign credit only to those who have contributed to a publication, presentation, or product. Credit shall be assigned in proportion to the contribution and only with the contributor's consent.

H. Individuals shall reference the source when using other persons' ideas, research, presentations, or products in written, oral, or any other media presentation or summary.

I. Individuals' statements to colleagues about professional services, research results, and products shall adhere to prevailing professional standards and shall contain no misrepresentations.

J. Individuals shall not provide professional services without exercising independent professional judgment, regardless of referral source or prescription.

K. Individuals shall not discriminate in their relationships with colleagues, students, and members of other professions and disciplines on the basis of race or ethnicity, gender, gender identity/gender expression, age, religion, national origin, sexual orientation, or disability.

L. Individuals shall not file or encourage others to file complaints that disregard or ignore facts that would disprove the allegation, nor should the Code of Ethics be used for personal reprisal, as a means of addressing personal animosity, or as a vehicle for retaliation.

M. Individuals who have reason to believe that the Code of Ethics has been violated shall inform the Board of Ethics.

N. Individuals shall comply fully with the policies of the Board of Ethics in its consideration and adjudication of complaints of violations of the Code of Ethics.

Appendix H

Audiometry Time Line

Adapted from Vogel et al., 2007

Events Relevant to Audiology	Audiometric-Related Events
550 BC—Pythagoras explained that sound is caused by vibration	**337 BC**—Hippocrates reported a clinical case of hearing loss, the history involved deafness from skull trauma
	50 AD—Celsus reported clearly different etiologies for hearing disorders, especially those involving the outer and middle ears
	600 AD—Alexander of Tralles reported physicians making noises with bells for the purpose of investigating the auditory system
1543—Vasalius described middle ear anatomy	
1543—Fallopio discovered the cochlea	**1550**—Cardano described method of transmitting sound to the ears by placing a hard object between one's teeth
	1578—Capivacci differentiated between conductive hearing loss and a nerve loss by use of zither string attached to the patient's teeth
	1711—Shore invented the tuning fork
	1804—Psfingsten classified speech sounds into vowels, voiced consonants, and voiceless consonants
	1821—Itarod first used a tuning ring of copper to scientifically test hearing
	1820—Wallaston reported the upper and lower frequency limits of hearing (30–18,000 Hz)
	1834—Weber described cochlear anatomy and his Weber Test
	1855—Rinne reported the findings of differentiating tuning fork sounds to the ear from bone conduction versus air conduction
	1875—Bing introduced an "acumeter" with built-in tape measure for measuring distance between patient and sound source
	1877—Politaer invented an "acumeter" to assist in bone conduction testing
Telephone invented; commercial development and widespread use of electricity	**1879**—Richardson coined the term "audiometer"
	1885—Hartmann created the "Auditory Chart"
	1899—Seashore used induction coils to create an electric "acumeter" with logarithmic intensity regulation
	1903—Wien created graphs that showed sensitivity curves in relation to hearing threshold
	1907—Zwaardemaker described construction of a "noise-proof" test room
First commercially manufactured hearing aid	**1909**—Congress of Otology adopted the Politzer et al. proposal to standardize nomenclature and record forms for hearing testing
	1910—Bárány attempted to test one speech sound per test word

Events Relevant to Audiology	Audiometric-Related Events
1918— American Standards Associate (ASA) later to be called American National Standards Institute (ANSI) was founded	**1919**—Schwarz presented an electronic audiometer – "Otaudion." This included the "Otosklerometer" which attempted to involve the Wheatstone-Gelle phenomenon (occlusion effect)
	1922—Fletcher et al. initiated the convention of recording hearing with frequency shown along the abscissa and intensity downward on the ordinate
	1923—Fowler and Wegel reported the use of the Western Electric 1A Audiometer—the first commercially available hearing testing instrument and use of a "sound-proof" room for testing was first employed
	1924—Jones and Knudsen included speech transmission through their instrument, the "audio-amplified"
Penicillin was discovered	**1928**—Fowler employed the use of binaural loudness balance testing to test the perception of intensity, later, recruitment; Western Electric audiometers were routinely equipped with bone conduction vibrators; otologic journals included instructions for building audiometers
	1937—manufacturer Western Electric introduced D-5 audiometer enabling the selection of "0" for each frequency, and dispensed with the need for calculating hearing loss via calibration curve
	1938—ASA (Later, ANSI), AMA, and manufacturers of audiometers—initiated standards for hearing instruments
WWII: Military showed interest in rehabilitation of hearing	**1939**—Davis reported on human brain activity after acoustic stimulation
1946—International Standards Organization (ISO) was founded	**1946**—Hudgins et al. developed spondee word lists in English. Word lists in other languages were concurrently under development during the same period
	1947—Békésy introduced the semiautomatic self-testing audiometer which enabled the graphing of a diagram of hearing
	1949—International Congress of Audiology—accepted proposals for standardization of audiogram charts
	1951—ASA introduced the standard for audiometric "0"
Introduction of transistorized Behind The Ear hearing aids	**1956**—Zwislocki initiated use of narrow-band noise for purposes of masking
	1958—Matzker used a "central synthesis" of signals to be received binaurally in order to judge central auditory function
	1960—Madsen presented the first commercially available electroacoustic bridge for impedance audiometry
	1963—Zwislocki introduced the first commercial use of the acoustic impedance bridge
	1964—International Standards Association introduced its standard for audiometric zero
	1969—ANSI released its standard for audiometric zero
	1970—Jerger introduced tympanogram classification
	1974—ASHA published "Guidelines for Audiometric Symbols"

Events Relevant to Audiology	Audiometric-Related Events
First Cochlear implant	**1978**—ANSI published "Methods for Manual Pure-Tone Threshold Audiometry"—included audiogram specifications; Kemp reported on acoustic emissions from within the human auditory system
	1979—Fausti et al. indicated the need for ultrahigh-frequency testing to monitor ototoxic medication exposure
Widespread availability of desktop computers	**1990s**—Manufacturers marketed instruments capable of producing audiograms directly from their audiometers; hospitals began using paperless charts; Universal newborn hearing screening programs became
Health Insurance Portability and Accountability Act of 1996 (HIPPAA)	widespread initiating the delivery of economical hand-held OAE screeners
	2010—ANSI published most recent audiometric standards (ANSI, 2010)
	2013—James Jerger publishes article explaining why the audiogram is upside-down

American National Standards Institute. (2010). *Specification for audiometers* (S3. 6-2010). New York, NY.

Jerger, J. (2013). Why the audiogram is upside-down. *International Journal of Audiology, 52*(3), 146–150.

Vogel, D. A., McCarthy, P. A., Bratt, G. W., & Brewer, C. (2007). The clinical audiogram: Its history and current use. *Communication Disorders Review, 1*(2), 81-94.

SII 2010 Revision of the 1990 Mueller and Killion Count-The-Dots Audiogram

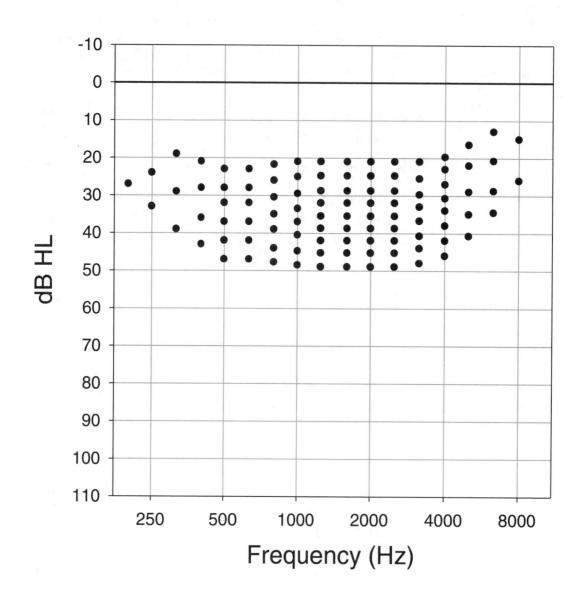

LDL Instructions

The purpose of this test is to find your judgments of the loudness of different sounds.

You will hear sounds that increase and decrease in volume. You must make a judgment about how loud the sounds are. Pretend you are listening to the radio at that volume. How loud would it be?

After each sound, tell me which of these categories best describes the loudness. It is okay to repeat a loudness category, and it is okay to skip a category.

Keep in mind that an uncomfortably loud sound is louder than you would ever choose on your radio no matter what mood you are in.

LDL Instructions

#7. Uncomfortably Loud

#6. Loud, But Okay

#5. Comfortable, But Slightly Loud

#4. Comfortable

#3. Comfortable, But Slightly Soft

#2. Soft

#1. Very Soft

Appendix L

NU Auditory Test #6

LIST 1A	LIST 2A	LIST 3A	LIST 4A
1. laud	1. pick	1. base	1. pass
2. boat	2. room	2. mess	2. doll
3. pool	3. nice	3. cause	3. back
4. nag	4. said	4. mop	4. red
5. limb	5. fail	5. good	5. wash
6. shout	6. south	6. luck	6. sour
7. sub	7. white	7. walk	7. bone
8. vine	8. keep	8. youth	8. get
9. dime	9. dead	9. pain	9. wheat
10. goose	10. loaf	10. date	10. thumb
11. whip	11. dab	11. pearl	11. sail
12. tough	12. numb	12. search	12. yearn
13. puff	13. juice	13. ditch	13. wife
14. keen	14. chief	14. talk	14. such
15. death	15. merge	15. ring	15. neat
16. sell	16. wag	16. germ	16. peg
17. take	17. rain	17. life	17. mob
18. fall	18. witch	18. team	18. gas
19. raise	19. soap	19. lid	19. check
20. third	20. young	20. pole	20. join
21. gap	21. ton	21. road	21. lease
22. fat	22. keg	22. shall	22. long
23. met	23. calm	23. late	23. chain
24. jar	24. tool	24. cheek	24. kill
25. door	25. pike	25. beg	25. hole
26. love	26. mill	26. gun	26. lean
27. sure	27. hush	27. jug	27. tape
28. knock	28. shack	28. sheep	28. tire
29. choice	29. read	29. five	29. dip
30. hash	30. rot	30. rush	30. rose
31. lot	31. hate	31. rat	31. came
32. raid	32. live	32. void	32. fit
33. hurl	33. book	33. wire	33. make
34. moon	34. voice	34. half	34. vote
35. page	35. gaze	35. note	35. judge
36. yes	36. pad	36. when	36. food
37. reach	37. thought	37. name	37. ripe
38. king	38. bought	38. thin	38. have
39. home	39. turn	39. tell	39. rough
40. rag	40. chair	40. bar	40. kick
41. which	41. lore	41. mouse	41. lose
42. week	42. bite	42. hire	42. near
43. size	43. haze	43. cab	43. perch
44. mode	44. match	44. hit	44. shirt
45. bean	45. learn	45. chat	45. bath
46. tip	46. shawl	46. phone	46. time
47. chalk	47. deep	47. soup	47. hall
48. jail	48. gin	48. dodge	48. mood
49. burn	49. goal	49. seize	49. dog
50. kite	50. far	50. cool	50. should

Appendix M

AUDITEC
Northwestern University Auditory Test #6 NU-6
Ordered by Difficulty Version II

LIST 1	LIST 2	LIST 3	LIST 4
1. Death	1. Gin	1. Chat	1. Yearn
2. Knock	2. Pike	2. Thin	2. Perch
3. Laud	3. Keg	3. Mouse	3. Fit
4. Puff	4. Pick	4. Mess	4. Pass
5. Keen	5. Keep	5. Pearl	5. Shirt
6. Burn	6. Turn	6. Germ	6. Ripe
7. Take	7. Dab	7. Ditch	7. Came
8. Third	8. Gaze	8. Dodge	8. Peg
9. Met	9. Learn	9. Cheek	9. Tape
10. Pool	10. Ton	10. Tell	10. Kick
11. Kite	11. Shack	11. Beg	11. Neat
12. Hurl	12. Pad	12. Pain	12. Lease
13. Jar	13. Mill	13. Team	13. Bath
14. Fat	14. Thought	14. Ring	14. Back
15. Sell	15. Nice	15. Mop	15. Gas
16. Tip	16. Wag	16. Hit	16. Check
17. Lot	17. Rot	17. Talk	17. Thumb
18. Chalk	18. Match	18. Youth	18. Wash
19. Week	19. Said	19. Cause	19. Join
20. Which	20. Chief	20. Pole	20. Judge
21. Page	21. Lore	21. Search	21. Should
22. Gap	22. Bought	22. Sheep	22. Make
23. Shout	23. Dead	23. Shall	23. Long
24. Dime	24. Shawl	24. Jug	24. Such
25. Hash	25. Calm	25. Lid	25. Wife
26. Nag	26. Goal	26. Seize	26. Sour
27. Mode	27. Witch	27. Half	27. Kill
28. Tough	28. Merge	28. Cab	28. Get
29. Sub	29. Far	29. Rat	29. Chain
30. Raise	30. Tool	30. Phone	30. Bone
31. Yes	31. Fail	31. Date	31. Doll
32. Size	32. Chair	32. Five	32. Dip
33. Whip	33. Hush	33. Rush	33. Time
34. King	34. Live	34. Hire	34. Wheat
35. Fall	35. Haze	35. Life	35. Tire
36. Choice	36. Bite	36. Void	36. Hole
37. Bean	37. Soap	37. Base	37. Red
38. Limb	38. South	38. Road	38. Mob
39. Moon	39. Loaf	39. Wire	39. Mood
40. Vine	40. Voice	40. Bar	40. Rough
41. Rag	41. Deep	41. When	41. Sail
42. Goose	42. Young	42. Name	42. Near
43. Door	43. Juice	43. Luck	43. Dog
44. Sure	44. Numb	44. Gun	44. Vote
45. Reach	45. Read	45. Late	45. Rose
46. Jail	46. Book	46. Note	46. Food
47. Raid	47. Hate	47. Walk	47. Hall
48. Boat	48. White	48. Cool	48. Have
49. Home	49. Rain	49. Soup	49. Lose
50. Love	50. Room	50. Good	50. Lean

Hurley, R. M., & Sells, J. P. "An Abbreviated Word Recognition Protocol Based on Item Difficulty" *Ear and Hearing, 24,* 2003 (111–118).

SPRINT CHART for 25-WORD LISTS

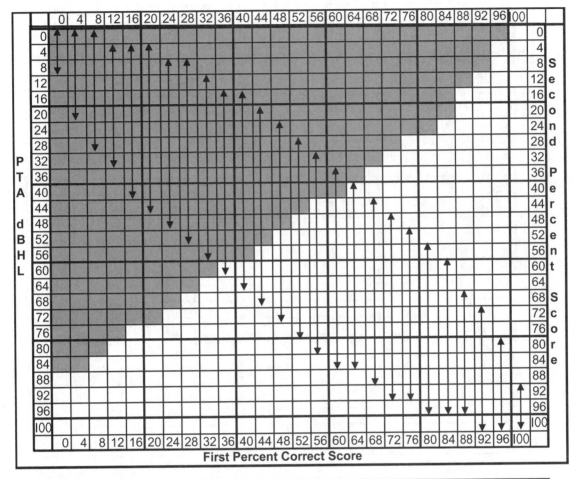

95% Confidence Limit for PBmax on NU6 25-word list. Plot score according to PTA on left ordinate and percent correct score on the abscissa. If it falls in the shaded area, it is considered disproportionately low. (Adapted from Dubno et al.,1995)

95% Critical differences for 25-word list. Plot first and second score according to the abscissa and right ordinate. If it falls within the arrow, the two scores are not significantly different (Adapted from Thornton & Raffin, 1978)

SPRINT CHART for 50-WORD LISTS

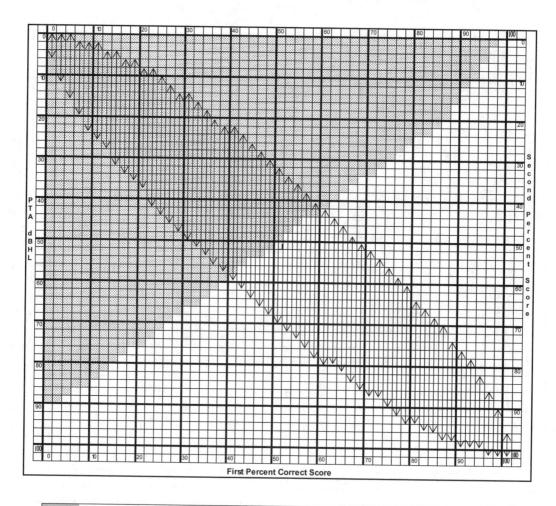

95% Confidence Limit for PBmax on NU6 50-word list. Plot score according
to PTA on left ordinate and percent correct score on the abscissa.
If it falls in the shaded area, it is considered disproportionately low.
(Adapted from Dubno et al.,1995)

95% Critical differences for 50-word list. Plot first and second score
according to the abscissa and right ordinate. If it falls within the arrow, the two
scores are not significantly different. (Adapted from Thornton & Raffin, 1978)

© Linda M. Thibodeau

Maryland CNC Word List
Left Channel

TRACK 3 LIST 1		TRACK 5 LIST 3		TRACK 7 LIST 6		TRACK 9 LIST 7	
1.	JAR	1.	JAIL	1.	WHIP	1.	NOTE
2.	BOIL	2.	RAT	2.	BUD	2.	DOOM
3.	TOUGH	3.	TOSS	3.	SHONE	3.	COKE
4.	TOOTH	4.	SOON	4.	RUG	4.	HOLE
5.	GOOSE	5.	FAITH	5.	CHEESE	5.	JOIN
6.	TOAD	6.	SUNG	6.	CHAIN	6.	THRID
7.	ROUTE	7.	KEG	7.	LOOK	7.	MOUTH
8.	MESS	8.	VOT	8.	DULL	8.	SURE
9.	KITE	9.	SIZE	9.	POPE	9.	VAGUE
10.	JUG	10.	NUMB	10.	CALF	10.	BIG
11.	PAD	11.	DAB	11.	FIRE	11.	FAR
12.	SALVE	12.	WHAT	12.	TURN	12.	GUN
13.	VAN	13.	ROOM	13.	RAISE	13.	PEARL
14.	HOME	14.	KID	14.	SOUR	14.	LOOT
15.	CAPE	15.	DIKE	15.	BED	15.	SAVE
16.	SHORE	16.	MATE	16.	LAWN	16.	SIDE
17.	WRECK	17.	WELL	17.	SIT	17.	HEAT
18.	SHIRT	18.	RIG	18.	TUBE	18.	BUN
19.	KNIFE	19.	FOUR	19.	VEAL	19.	FISH
20.	HULL	20.	BUSH	20.	GET	20.	HAVE
21.	YEARN	21.	DIP	21.	PACE	21.	MOLE
22.	SUN	22.	GAP	22.	NIGHT	22.	PINE
23.	WHEEL	23.	PERCH	23.	HISS	23.	NAP
24.	FIT	24.	SHEEP	24.	SHOCK	24.	MINE
25.	PATCH	25.	HOUSE	25.	WING	25.	WAS

TRACK 4 LIST 1		TRACK 6 LIST 3		TRACK 8 LIST 6		TRACK 10 LIST 7	
26.	MAKE	26.	FADE	26.	DOOR	26.	REACH
27.	DIME	27,	LAKE	27.	NIECE	27.	FACE
28.	BEAN	28.	GULL	28.	CAT	28.	BET
29.	THIN	29.	ROUGE	29.	MOVE	29.	CAUGHT
30.	SEIZE	30.	BAR	30.	COOL	30.	LAUGH
31.	HATE	31.	TONE	31.	WEB	31.	SHALL
32.	WOOD	32.	CHIN	32.	KNOCK	32.	GEESE
33.	CHECK	33.	PIECE	33.	JOT	33.	TAPE
34.	DITCH	34.	PURGE	34.	CAGE	34.	SLACK
35.	ROSE	35.	BELL	35.	MODE	35.	RIDGE
36.	MERGE	36.	WORK	36.	SEARCH	36.	CHEEK
37.	LEASE	37.	LIFE	37.	GONE	37.	DUMB
38.	LOOP	38.	POD	38.	RUSH	38.	TOP
39.	KING	39.	SHINE	39.	POLE	39.	YOUNG
40.	DEAD	40.	TOLL	40.	DIG	40.	LED
41.	CHORE	41.	JOKE	41.	BAD	41.	RIB
42.	BOAT	42.	HEAD	42.	LIVE	42.	PASS
43.	WISH	43.	WITH	43.	MAP	43.	WIT
44.	NAME	44.	KEEN	44.	WIFE	44.	DID
45.	PICK	45.	MORE	45.	FAN	45.	CALL
46.	RIPE	46.	LEAVE	46.	BIRTH	46.	NECK
47.	FALL	47.	HUT	47.	TEAM	47.	SUCH
48.	LAG	48.	NOISE	48.	HOWL	48.	LOSE
49.	GALE	49.	MAN	49.	HIKE	49.	GEM
50.	SOB	50.	YAM	50.	JAM	50.	TAR

Maryland CNC Word List
Left Channel

TRACK 11
LIST 9

1.	LACK
2.	WATCH
3.	POWER
4.	MIRE
5.	NAIL
6.	THINE
7.	WORD
8.	TOOL
9.	MOB
10.	HEN
11.	GOT
12.	SANE
13.	SHOUT
14.	PILL
15.	BOTH
16.	SHADE
17.	JAZZ
18.	LATHE
19.	CATCH
20.	WHITE
21.	CHAIR
22.	LOAF
23.	PUN
24.	HAM
25.	LIP

TRACK 13
LIST 10

1.	SUB
2.	LOT
3.	DIN
4.	DEATH
5.	CHILL
6.	COIN
7.	CAUSE
8.	BURN
9.	LOOSE
10.	PALM
11.	JUDGE
12.	WASH
13.	ROB
14.	FINE
15.	WHILE
16.	CHAT
17.	BIT
18.	NICK
19.	NEAT
20.	HAIR
21.	SAFE
22.	HIT
23.	JADE
24.	HURT
25.	PILE

TRACK 12
LIST 9

26.	WRONG
27.	YES
28.	SIN
29.	CURVE
30.	HAZE
31.	GIRL
32.	TIME
33.	BOOK
34.	REAP
35.	FUDGE
36.	VOICE
37.	RAG
38.	MUD
39.	BALL
40.	DECK
41.	CUT
42.	NEED
43.	CHEER
44.	SOAP
45.	FEET
46.	TICK
47.	ROOF
48.	DOG
49.	BEAT
50.	DISH

TRACK 14
LIST 10

26.	SHACK
27.	CONE
28.	SELL
29.	YOUR
30.	TERM
31.	MOOD
32.	DEEP
33.	MEEK
34.	ROPE
35.	WITCH
36.	RIDE
37.	BAKE
38.	GORE
39.	FOOL
40.	GUESS
41.	MOUSE
42.	LUNG
43.	LOAD
44.	PATH
45.	PEAK
46.	RUN
47.	SAG
48.	CAVE
49.	THATCH
50.	TOWEL

Appendix Q

Revised SPIN Test

List 1

1. His plans meant taking a big <u>RISK</u>.   H
2. Stir your coffee with a <u>SPOON</u>.   H
3. Miss White won't think about the <u>CRACK</u>.   L
4. He would think about the <u>RAG</u>.   L
5. The plow was pulled by an <u>OX</u>.   H
6. The old train was powered by <u>STEAM</u>.   H
7. The old man was talking about the <u>LUNGS</u>.   L
8. I was considering the <u>CROOK</u>.   L
9. Let's decide by tossing a <u>COIN</u>.   H
10. The doctor prescribed the <u>DRUG</u>.   H
11. Bill might discuss the <u>FOAM</u>.   L
12. Nancy didn't discuss the <u>SKIRT</u>.   L
13. Hold the baby on your <u>LAP</u>.   H
14. Bob has discussed the <u>SPLASH</u>.   L
15. The dog chewed on a <u>BONE</u>.   H
16. Ruth hopes he heard about the <u>HIPS</u>.   L
17. The war was fought with armored <u>TANKS</u>. H
18. She wants to talk about the <u>CREW</u>.   L
19. They had a problem with the <u>CLIFF</u>.   L
20. They drank a whole bottle of <u>GIN</u>.   H
21. You heard Jane called about the <u>VAN</u>.   L
22. The witness took a solemn <u>OATH</u>.   H
23. We could consider the <u>FEAST</u>.   L
24. Bill heard we asked about the <u>HOST</u>.   L
25. They tracked the lion to his <u>DEN</u>.   H
26. The cow gave birth to a <u>CALF</u>.   H
27. I had not thought about the <u>GROWL</u>.   L
28. The scarf was made of shiny <u>SILK</u>.   H
29. The super highway has six <u>LANES</u>,   H
30. He should know about the <u>HUT</u>.   L
31. For dessert he had apple <u>PIE</u>.   H
32. The beer drinkers raised their <u>MUGS</u>.   H
33. I'm glad you heard about the <u>BEND</u>.   L
34. You're talking about the <u>POND</u>.   L
35. The rude remark made her <u>BLUSH</u>.   H
36. Nancy had considered the <u>SLEEVES</u>.   L
37. We heard the ticking of the <u>CLOCK</u>.   H
38. He can't consider the <u>CRIB</u>.   L
39. He killed the dragon with his <u>SWORD</u>.   H
40. Tom discussed the <u>HAY</u>.   L
41. Mary wore her hair in <u>BRAIDS</u>.   H
42. She's glad Jane asked about the <u>DRAIN</u>.   L
43. Bill hopes Paul heard about the <u>MIST</u>.   L
44. We're lost so let's look at the <u>MAP</u>.   H
45. No one was injured in the <u>CRASH</u>.   H
46. We're speaking about the <u>TOLL</u>.   L
47. My son has a dog for a <u>PET</u>.   H
48. He was scared out of his <u>WITS</u>.   H
49. We spoke about the <u>KNOB</u>.   L
50. I've spoken about the <u>PILE</u>.   L

List 2

1. Miss Black thought about the <u>LAP</u>.   L
2. The baby slept in his <u>CRIB</u>.   H
3. The watchdog gave a warning <u>GROWL</u>.   H
4. Miss Black would consider the <u>BONE</u>.   L
5. The natives built a wooden <u>HUT</u>.   H
6. Bob could have known about the <u>SPOON</u>.   L
7. Unlock the door and turn the <u>KNOB</u>.   H
8. He wants to talk about the <u>RISK</u>.   L
9. He heard they called about the <u>LANES</u>.   L
10. Wipe your greasy hands on the <u>RAG</u>.   H
11. She has known about the <u>DRUG</u>.   L
12. I want to speak about the <u>CRASH</u>.   L
13. The wedding banquet was a <u>FEAST</u>.   H
14. I should have considered the <u>MAP</u>.   L
15. Paul hit the water with a <u>SPLASH</u>.   H
16. The ducks swam around on the <u>POND</u>.   H
17. Ruth must have known about the <u>PIE</u>.   L
18. The man should discuss the <u>OX</u>.   L
19. Bob stood with his hands on his <u>HIPS</u>.   H
20. The cigarette smoke filled his <u>LUNGS</u>.   H
21. They heard I called about the <u>PET</u>.   L
22. The cushion was filled with <u>FOAM</u>.   H
23. Ruth poured the water down the <u>DRAIN</u>.   H
24. Bill cannot consider the <u>DEN</u>.   L
25. This nozzle sprays a fine <u>MIST</u>.   H
26. The sport shirt has short <u>SLEEVES</u>.   H
27. She hopes Jane called about the <u>CALF</u>.   L
28. Jane has a problem with the <u>COIN</u>.   L
29. She shortened the hem of her <u>SKIRT</u>.   H
30. Paul hopes she called about the <u>TANKS</u>.   L
31. The girl talked about the <u>GIN</u>.   L
32. The guests were welcomed by the <u>HOST</u>. H
33. Mary should think about the <u>SWORD</u>.   L
34. Ruth could have discussed the <u>WITS</u>.   L
35. The ship's Captain summoned his <u>CREW</u>. H
36. You had a problem with a <u>BLUSH</u>.   L
37. The flood took a heavy <u>TOLL</u>.   H
38. The car drove off the steep <u>CLIFF</u>.   H
39. We have discussed the <u>STEAM</u>.   L
40. The policemen captured the <u>CROOK</u>.   H
41. The door was opened just a <u>CRACK</u>.   H
42. Tom is considering the <u>CLOCK</u>.   L
43. The sand was heaped in a <u>PILE</u>.   H
44. You should not speak about the <u>BRAIDS</u>.   L
45. Peter should speak about the <u>MUGS</u>.   L
46. Household goods are moved in a <u>VAN</u>.   H
47. He has a problem with the <u>OATH</u>.   L
48. Follow this road around the <u>BEND</u>.   H
49. Tom won't consider the <u>SILK</u>.   L
50. The farmer baled the <u>HAY</u>.   H

Revised SPIN Test

List 3

1.	Kill the bugs with this <u>SPRAY</u>.	H	
2.	Mr. White discussed the <u>CRUISE</u>.		L
3.	How much can I buy for a <u>DIME</u>?	H	
4.	Miss White thinks about the <u>TEA</u>.		L
5.	We shipped the furniture by <u>TRUCK</u>.	H	
6.	He is thinking about the <u>ROAR</u>.		L
7.	She's spoken about the <u>BOMB</u>.		L
8.	My T. V. has a twelve-inch <u>SCREEN</u>.	H	
9.	That accident gave me a <u>SCARE</u>.	H	
10.	You want to talk about the <u>DITCH</u>.		L
11.	The king wore a golden <u>CROWN</u>.	H	
12.	The girls swept the floor with a <u>BROOM</u>.	H	
13.	We're discussing the <u>SHEETS</u>.		L
14.	The nurse gave him first <u>AID</u>.	H	
15.	She faced them with a foolish <u>GRIN</u>.	H	
16.	Betsy has considered the <u>BARK</u>.		L
17.	Watermelons have lots of <u>SEEDS</u>.	H	
18.	Use this spray to kill the <u>BUGS</u>.	H	
19.	Tom will discuss the <u>SWAN</u>.		L
20.	The teacher sat on a sharp <u>TACK</u>.	H	
21.	You'd been considering the <u>GEESE</u>.		L
22.	The sailor swabbed the <u>DECK</u>.	H	
23.	They were interested in the <u>STRAP</u>.		L
24.	He could discuss the <u>BREAD</u>.		L
25.	He tossed the drowning man a <u>ROPE</u>.	H	
26.	Jane hopes Ruth asked about the <u>STRIPES</u>.		L
27.	Paul spoke about the <u>PORK</u>.		L
28.	The boy gave the football a <u>KICK</u>.	H	
29.	The storm broke the sailboat's <u>MAST</u>.	H	
30.	Mr. Smith thinks about the <u>CAP</u>.		L
31.	We are speaking about the <u>PRIZE</u>.		L
32.	Mr. Brown carved the roast <u>BEEF</u>.	H	
33.	The glass had a chip on the <u>RIM</u>.	H	
34.	Harry had thought about the <u>LOGS</u>.		L
35.	Bob could consider the <u>POLE</u>.		L
36.	Her cigarette had a long <u>ASH</u>.	H	
37.	Ruth has a problem with the <u>JOINTS</u>.		L
38.	He is considering the <u>THROAT</u>.		L
39.	The soup was served in a <u>BOWL</u>.	H	
40.	We can't consider the <u>WHEAT</u>.		L
41.	The man spoke about the <u>CLUE</u>.		L
42.	The lonely bird search for its <u>MATE</u>.	H	
43.	Please wipe your feet on the <u>MAT</u>.	H	
44.	David has discussed the <u>DENT</u>.		L
45.	The pond was full of croaking <u>FROGS</u>.	H	
46.	He hit me with a clenched <u>FIST</u>.	H	
47.	Bill heard Tom called about the <u>COACH</u>.		L
48.	A bicycle has two <u>WHEELS</u>.	H	
49.	Jane has spoken about the <u>CHEST</u>.		L
50.	Mr. White spoke about the <u>FIRM</u>.		L

List 4

1.	The doctor X-rayed his <u>CHEST</u>.	H	
2.	Mary had considered the <u>SPRAY</u>.		L
3.	The woman talked about the <u>FROGS</u>.		L
4.	The workers are digging a <u>DITCH</u>.	H	
5.	Miss Brown will speak about the <u>GRIN</u>.		L
6.	Bill can't have considered the <u>WHEELS</u>.		L
7.	The duck swam with the white <u>SWAN</u>.	H	
8.	Your knees and elbows are <u>JOINTS</u>.	H	
9.	Mr. Smith spoke about the <u>AID</u>.		L
10.	He hears she asked about the <u>DECK</u>.		L
11.	Raise the flag up the <u>POLE</u>.	H	
12.	You want to think about the <u>DIME</u>.		L
13.	You've considered the <u>SEEDS</u>.		L
14.	The detectives searched for a <u>CLUE</u>.	H	
15.	Ruth's Grandmother discussed the <u>BROOM</u>.		L
16.	The steamship left on a <u>CRUISE</u>.	H	
17.	Miss Smith considered the <u>SCARE</u>.		L
18.	Peter has considered the <u>MAT</u>.		L
19.	Tree trunks are covered with <u>BARK</u>.	H	
20.	The meat from a pig is called <u>PORK</u>.	H	
21.	The old man considered the <u>KICK</u>.		L
22.	Ruth poured herself a cup of <u>TEA</u>.	H	
23.	We saw a flock of wild <u>GEESE</u>.	H	
24.	Paul could not consider the <u>RIM</u>.		L
25.	How did your car get that <u>DENT</u>?	H	
26.	She made the bed with clean <u>SHEETS</u>.	H	
27.	I've been considering the <u>CROWN</u>.		L
28.	The team was trained by their <u>COACH</u>.	H	
29.	I've got a cold and a sore <u>THROAT</u>.	H	
30.	We've spoken about the <u>TRUCK</u>.		L
31.	She wore a feather in her <u>CAP</u>.	H	
32.	The bread was made from whole <u>WHEAT</u>.	H	
33.	Mary could not discuss the <u>TACK</u>.		L
34.	Spread some butter on your <u>BREAD</u>.	H	
35.	The cabin was made of <u>LOGS</u>.	H	
36.	Harry might consider the <u>BEEF</u>.		L
37.	We're glad Bill heard about the <u>ASH</u>.		L
38.	The lion gave an angry <u>ROAR</u>.	H	
39.	The sandal has broken a <u>STRAP</u>.	H	
40.	Nancy should consider the <u>FIST</u>.		L
41.	He's employed by a large <u>FIRM</u>.	H	
42.	They did not discuss the <u>SREEN</u>.		L
43.	Her entry should win first <u>PRIZE</u>.	H	
44.	The old man thinks about the <u>MAST</u>,		L
45.	Paul wants to speak about the <u>BUGS</u>.		L
46.	The airplane dropped a <u>BOMB</u>.	H	
47.	You're glad she called about the <u>BOWL</u>.		L
48.	A zebra has black and white <u>STRIPES</u>.	H	
49.	Miss Black could have discussed the <u>ROPE</u>.		L
50.	I hope Paul asked about the <u>MATE</u>.		L

Revised SPIN Test

List 5

1.	Betty knew about the NAP.	L
2.	The girl should consider the FLAME.	L
3.	It's getting dark, so light the LAMP.	H
4.	To store his wood he built a SHED.	H
5.	They heard I asked about the BET.	L
6.	The mouse was caught in the TRAP.	H
7.	Mary knows about the RUG.	L
8.	The airplane went into a DIVE.	H
9.	The fireman heard her frightened SCREAM.	H
10.	He was interested in the HEDGE.	L
11.	He wiped the sink down with a SPONGE.	H
12.	Jane did not speak about the SLICE.	L
13.	Mr. Brown can't discuss the SLOT.	L
14.	The papers were held by a CLIP.	H
15.	Paul can't discuss the WAX.	L
16.	Miss Brown shouldn't discuss the SAND.	L
17.	The chicks followed the mother HEN.	H
18.	David might consider the FUN.	L
19.	She wants to speak about the ANT.	L
20.	The fur coat was made of MINK.	H
21.	The boy took shelter in a CAVE.	H
22.	He hasn't considered the DART.	L
23.	Eve was made from Adam's RIB.	H
24.	The boat sailed along the COAST.	H
25.	We've been discussing the CRATES.	L
26.	The judge is sitting on the BENCH.	H
27.	We've been thinking about the FAN.	L
28.	Jane didn't think about the BROOK.	L
29.	Cut a piece of meat from the ROAST.	H
30.	Betty can't consider the GRIEF.	L
31.	The heavy rains caused a FLOOD.	H
32.	The swimmer dove into the POOL.	H
33.	Harry will consider the TRAIL.	L
34.	Let's invite the whole GANG.	H
35.	The house was robbed by a THIEF.	H
36.	Tom is talking about the FEE.	L
37.	Bob wore a watch on his WRIST.	H
38.	Tom had spoken about the PILL.	L
39.	Tom has been discussing the BEADS.	L
40.	The secret agent was a SPY.	H
41.	The rancher rounded up his HERD.	H
42.	Tom could have thought about the SPORT.	L
43.	Mary can't consider the TIDE.	L
44.	Ann works in the bank as a CLERK.	H
45.	A chimpanzee is an APE.	H
46.	He hopes Tom asked about the BAR.	L
47.	We could discuss the DUST.	L
48.	The bandits escaped from JAIL.	H
49.	Paul hopes we heard about the LOOT.	L
50.	The landlord raised the RENT.	H

List 6

1.	You were considering the GANG.	L
2.	The boy considered the MINK.	L
3.	Playing checkers can be FUN.	H
4.	The doctor charged a low FEE.	H
5.	He wants to know about the RIB.	L
6.	The gambler lost the BET.	H
7.	Get the bread and cut me a SLICE.	H
8.	She might have discussed the APE.	L
9.	The sleepy child took a NAP.	H
10.	Instead of a fence, plant a HEDGE.	H
11.	The old woman discussed the THIEF.	L
12.	Drop the coin through the SLOT,	H
13.	They fished in the babbling BROOK.	H
14.	You were interested in the SCREAM.	L
15.	We hear they asked about the SHED.	L
16.	The widow's sob expressed her GRIEF.	H
17.	The candle flame melted the WAX.	H
18.	I haven't discussed the SPONGE.	L
19.	He was hit by a poisoned DART.	H
20.	Ruth had a necklace of glass BEADS.	H
21.	Ruth will consider the HERD.	L
22.	The singer was mobbed by her FANS.	H
23.	The old man discussed the DIVE.	L
24.	The class should consider the FLOOD.	L
25.	The fruit was shipped in wooden CRATES.	H
26.	I'm talking about the BENCH.	L
27.	Paul has discussed the LAMP.	L
28.	The candle burned with a bright FLAME.	H
29.	You knew about the CLIP.	L
30.	She might consider the POOL.	L
31.	We swam at the beach at high TIDE.	H
32.	Bob was considering the CLERK.	L
33.	We got drunk in the local BAR.	H
34.	A termite looks like an ANT.	H
35.	The man knew about the SPY.	L
36.	The sick child swallowed the PILL.	H
37.	The class is discussing the WRIST.	L
38.	The burglar escaped with the LOOT.	H
39.	They hoped he heard about the RENT.	L
40.	Mr. White spoke about the JAIL.	L
41.	He rode off in a cloud of DUST.	H
42.	Miss Brown might consider the COAST.	L
43.	Bill didn't discuss the HEN.	L
44.	The bloodhound followed the TRAIL.	H
45.	The boy might consider the TRAP.	L
46.	On the beach we played in the SAND.	H
47.	He should consider the ROAST.	L
48.	Miss Brown spoke about the CAVE.	L
49.	She hated to vacuum the RUG.	H
50.	Football is a dangerous SPORT.	H

Revised SPIN Test

List 7

1.	We're considering the BROW.	L
2.	You cut the wood against the GRAIN.	H
3.	I am thinking about the KNIFE.	L
4.	They've considered the SHEEP.	L
5.	The cop wore a bullet-proof VEST.	H
6.	He's glad we heard about the SKUNK.	L
7.	His pants were held up by a BELT.	H
8.	Paul took a bath in the TUB.	H
9.	The girl should not discuss the GOWN.	L
10.	Maple syrup is made from SAP.	H
11.	Mr. Smith knew about the BAY.	L
12.	They played a game of cat and MOUSE.	H
13.	The thread was wound on a SPOOL.	H
14.	We did not discuss the SHOCK.	L
15.	The crook entered a guilty PLEA.	H
16.	Mr. Black has discussed the CARDS.	L
17.	A bear has a thick coat of FUR.	H
18.	Mr. Black considered the FLEET.	L
19.	To open the jar, twist the LID.	H
20.	We are considering the CHEERS.	L
21.	Sue was interested in the BRUISE.	L
22.	Tighten the belt by a NOTCH.	H
23.	The cookies were kept in a JAR.	H
24.	Miss Smith couldn't discuss the ROW.	L
25.	I am discussing the TASK.	L
26.	The marksman took careful AIM.	H
27.	I ate a piece of chocolate FUDGE.	H
28.	Paul should know about the NET.	L
29.	Miss Smith might consider the SHELL.	L
30.	John's front tooth had a CHIP.	H
31.	At breakfast he drank some JUICE.	H
32.	You cannot have discussed the GREASE.	L
33.	I did not know about the CHUNKS.	L
34.	Our cat is good at catching MICE.	H
35.	I should have known about the GUM.	L
36.	Mary hasn't discussed the BLADE.	L
37.	The stale bread was covered with MOLD.	H
38.	Ruth has discussed the PEG.	L
39.	How long can you hold your BREATH?	H
40.	His boss made him work like a SLAVE.	H
41.	We have not thought about the HINT.	L
42.	Air mail requires a special STAMP.	H
43.	The bottle was sealed with a CORK.	H
44.	The old man discussed the YELL.	L
45.	They're glad we heard about the TRACK.	L
46.	Cut the bacon into STRIPS.	H
47.	Throw out all this useless JUNK.	H
48.	The boy can't talk about the THORNS.	L
49.	Bill won't consider the BRAT.	L
50.	The shipwrecked sailors built a RAFT.	H

List 8

1.	Bob heard Paul called about the STRIPS.	L
2.	My turtle went into its SHELL.	H
3.	Paul has a problem with the BELT.	L
4.	I cut my finger with a KNIFE.	H
5.	They knew about the FUR.	L
6.	We're glad Ann asked about the FUDGE.	L
7.	Greet the heroes with loud CHEERS.	H
8.	Jane was interested in the STAMP.	L
9.	That animal stinks like a SKUNK.	L
10.	A round hole won't take a square PEG.	H
11.	Miss White would consider the MOLD.	L
12.	They want to know about the AIM.	L
13.	The Admiral commands the FLEET.	H
14.	The bride wore a white GOWN.	H
15.	The woman discussed the GRAIN.	L
16.	You hope they asked about the VEST.	L
17.	I can't guess so give me a HINT.	H
18.	Our seats were in the second ROW.	H
19.	We should have considered the JUICE.	L
20.	The boat sailed across the BAY.	H
21.	The woman considered the NOTCH.	L
22.	That job was an easy TASK.	H
23.	The woman knew about the LID.	L
24.	Jane wants to speak about the CHIP.	L
25.	The shepherd watched his flock of SHEEP.	H
26.	Bob should not consider the MICE.	L
27.	David wiped the sweat from his BROW.	H
28.	Ruth hopes she called about the JUNK.	L
29.	I can't consider the PLEA.	L
30.	The bad news came as a SHOCK.	H
31.	A spoiled child is a BRAT.	H
32.	Paul has interest in the SAP.	L
33.	The drowning man let out a YELL.	H
34.	A rose bush has prickly THORNS.	H
35.	He's glad you called about the JAR.	L
36.	The dealer shuffled the CARDS.	H
37.	Miss Smith knows about the TUB.	L
38.	The man would not discuss the MOUSE.	L
39.	The railroad train ran off the TRACK.	H
40.	My jaws ache when I chew GUM.	H
41.	Ann was interested in the BREATH.	L
42.	You're glad they heard about the SLAVE.	L
43.	He caught the fish in his NET.	H
44.	Bob was cut by the jackknife's BLADE.	H
45.	The man could consider the SPOOL.	L
46.	Tom fell down and got a bad BRUISE.	H
47.	Lubricate the car with GREASE.	H
48.	Peter knows about the RAFT.	L
49.	Cut the meat into small CHUNKS.	H
50.	She hears Bob asked about the CORK.	L

Appendix R

CST Passages

Test Passage Pair 1 (Window/Glove)
Psg: 1 WINDOW
Windows **PROVIDE LIGHT** and air to **ROOMS.**
Windows were **ONCE COVERED** with **CRUDE SHUTTERS.**
Later, oiled **PAPER** was **USED** for windowpanes.
GLASS windows **FIRST** appeared in ancient Rome.
COLORED glass was used in European **WINDOWS.**
SOME CHURCHES were **FAMOUS** for their **BEAUTIFUL** windows.
These windows **DISPLAYED PICTURES** from the **BIBLE**
PIECES of glass were **HELD** together by lead.
SUCH windows **MAY** be seen in French cathedrals.
English churches also contain **STAINED** glass windows.

Psg: 2 GLOVE ___/50
Gloves are **CLOTHING WORN ON** the **HANDS.**
The **WORD "GLOVE" MEANS** "palm of the hand."
CRUDE GLOVES were **WORN** by **PRIMITIVE MAN.**
Greeks wore **WORKING** gloves to **PROTECT** their hands.
The **ROMANS USED** gloves as a sign of **RANK.**
Knights used to fasten gloves to their helmets.
The gloves **SHOWED** their **DEVOTION** to their **LADIES.**
A glove thrown on the **GROUND SIGNALED** a challenge.
Knights threw them at their enemy's feet.
FIGHTING STARTED WHEN the enemy picked up the glove.

Test Passage Pair 2 (Umbrella/Giraffe)
Psg: 3 UMBRELLA
The **NAME** "umbrella means small shadow.
Umbrellas **WERE** first used in **ANCIENT** Egypt.
THEY GAVE protection **FROM** the fierce **SUNSHINE.**
SLAVES held **UMBRELLAS** over their **MASTERS.**
In Egypt today, many people **CARRY** umbrellas.
In **EARLY** Rome, **ONLY WOMEN** used umbrellas.
IF a **MAN** did, he **WAS CONSIDERED** a sissy.
Umbrellas were **USED** by both **SEXES** in **ENGLAND.**
TODAY, people use umbrellas to keep **OUT** the **RAIN.**
Umbrellas **USED** as sunshades are called parasols.

Psg: 4 GIRAFFE ___/50
The giraffe is the tallest wild **ANIMAL.**
It is three time taller than a man.
A full grown giraffe is eighteen **FEET** high.
The giraffe has an extremely **LONG NECK.**
The neck **HAS ONLY** seven **NECKBONES.**
The **GIRAFFE'S BODY** is about the **SIZE** of a **HORSE'S.**
The **BODY** is **SHAPED LIKE** a triangle.
Africa is the only **COUNTRY WHERE** giraffes **LIVE WILD.**
LARGE GROUPS of them are **FOUND ON** the **PLAINS.**
They live there with **LIONS** and **ELEPHANTS.**

Test Passage Pair 3 (Lung/Dove)
Psg: 5 LUNG
The lungs are the **ORGANS** of breathing.
They **LIE** in the **CENTER** of the chest.
The heart lies **BETWEEN** the lungs.
The two lungs **ARE SURROUNDED** by the **RIBS.**
BOTH ARE JOINED together by the **WINDPIPE.**
This airway **EXTENDS FROM** the mouth and **NOSE.**
The lungs **CONTAIN SEVERAL MILLION AIR** cells.
BLOOD is pumped **THROUGH** the lungs by the **HEART.**
OXYGEN is carried to the **CELLS THIS WAY.**

Psg: 6 DOVE ___/50
A dove is a small **TRIM BIRD.**
The **BEST** known is the **MOURNING** dove.
The mourning **DOVE** lives in **NORTH** America.
Its **NAME COMES** from its **SAD MATING** call.
It is sometimes **INCORRECTLY CALLED TURTLEDOVE.**
The mourning dove is about a **FOOT LONG.**
Its **BODY** is **BROWN** with **GRAY** wings.
It **FEEDS** on **GRAINS** , grasses and **WEEDS.**
The mourning dove is a **CARELESS HOUSEKEEPER.**
Its **NEST** is just some **STICKS** tossed together.

Test Passage Pair 4 (Carrot/Grass)
Psg: 7 CARROT
A carrot is a **VEGETABLE RELATED** to parsley.
The **LONG** stem of the carrot **GROWS UNDERGROUND.**
It is **THIS STEM** that most people **EAT.**
The **LEAVES** of the **CARROT** are also eaten.
They are often used to **FLAVOR** foods.
Spring **CROPS** are **GROWN** in the western **STATES.**
The crop is **HARVESTED** in one **HUNDRED** days.
Fall crops **ARE GROWN** in the **NORTHERN STATES.**
Winter **HARVESTS** usually come from **CALIFORNIA.**
WINTER crops are also **GROWN** in **TEXAS.**

Psg: 8 GRASS ___/50
Grass **CAN GROW** in all climates.
THERE are many forms of grasses.
MANY GRASSES are important food **SOURCES.**
Some grasses **GROW** higher than a **MAN'S HEAD.**
AMONG THESE are bamboo an sugar cane.
Other types are **ONLY** a **FEW INCHES** tall.
Some grasses **ARE AS SLENDER** as threads.
Others are stiff enough to **STAND** a heavy **SNOW.**
MOST grasses are **FLOWERING PLANTS.**
These flowers bloom **MAINLY** in the **SPRING.**

Test Passage Pair 5 (Nail/Woodpecker)
Psg: 9 NAIL
Nails are use to **FASTEN WOOD TOGETHER.**
Pioneers **USED WOODEN** pegs **INSTEAD** of nails.
One **END** of a nail is quite **POINTED.**
The **POINT** creates an **OPENING** for the **NAIL.**
It also helps **KEEP** the **WOOD** from **SPLITTING.**
At the nail's **OTHER** end is a **HEAD.**
It provides a **STRIKING SURFACE** for the hammer.
It also **COVERS** the nail **HOLE** in the wood.
There is a **SPECIAL NAIL** for every **PURPOSE.**
For **MOST** purposes a **ROUND** nail will do.

Psg: 10 WOODPECKER ___/50
The woodpecker is a bird with a **STRONG BEAK.**
It bores **HOLES** in **TREES** looking for **INSECTS.**
Woodpeckers **LIVE** in all parts of the world.
The **TOES** of woodpeckers **ARE VERY UNUSUAL.**
Two **POINT FORWARD** and two face **BACKWARD.**
This allows the **BIRD** to cling to **TREES.**
The **TAIL FEATHERS** of a woodpecker are **STIFF.**
THEY can **USE** their tails as a **SUPPORT.**
They also use their tails to grasp **TREES.**
Woodpeckers **HAVE** long **TONGUES** with pointed **TIPS.**

CST Passages

Test Passage Pair 6 (Owl/Vegetable)
Psg: 11 **OWL**
Owls **HUNT** alone at **NIGHT** for food.
THESE BIRDS kill and **EAT** small **ANIMALS**.
They are **BIRDS** of prey, like **EAGLES**.
OWLS defend our **GARDENS** by eating **MICE**.
They are **CLOSELY** related to night **HAWKS**.
There are five **HUNDRED** different **KINDS** of owls.
They live throughout **COLD** and **TROPICAL** climates.
Owls **USUALLY** live **ALONE** in the **FOREST**.
SOMETIMES they exist on remote **SEA** islands.
Owls are **KNOWN FOR** their **SOLEMN** expression.

Psg: 12 **VEGETABLE**   ___/50
The **WORD** "vegetable" **HAS** several **MEANINGS**.
It is **USED** in the phrase "vegetable **KINGDOM**."
This **REFERS** to the entire plant **WORLD**.
SOME WILD vegetables can be eaten.
Vegetables **COME** from the **LEAVES** and **FLOWERS** of plants.
Some vegetables come **FROM** a plant's **ROOTS**.
Vegetables can be **EATEN** raw or **COOKED**.
The **BEST** way to **COOK** vegetables is by **STEAMING**.
THEY are **USUALLY** chopped or **MASHED** before eaten.
Vegetables are **VERY DIFFERENT FROM** fruits.

Test Passage Pair 7 (Lemon/Violin)
Psg: 13 **LEMON**
A **LEMON** is an oval, yellow citrus **FRUIT**.
It **GROWS** in Southern California and **FLORIDA**.
Lemon trees are **MEDIUM** sized, **WITH SPREADING BRANCHES**.
They have **PALE GREEN LEAVES** and large flowers.
The flowers are **WHITE**, with **PURPLE UNDERNEATH**.
The lemon **FLOWER** smells sweet.
SOME types of lemons have **NO** seeds.
OTHER types have **MANY** seeds.
Their **FRUIT** is a **SPECIAL TYPE** of **CITRUS**.
It usually has a **SOUR TASTE**.

Psg: 14 **VIOLIN**   ___/50
The violin is the best **KNOWN** stringed **INSTRUMENT**.
EARLY VIOLINS did not produce clear tones.
These violins were **VERY ROUGH SOUNDING**.
LATER violin **MAKERS** improved their craft.
Their **VIOLINS** were **EXTREMELY** well made.
The **VIOLIN BECAME** an **INSTRUMENT** for beautiful
         MUSIC.
Only **SMALL CHANGES** have occurred in violin **DESIGN**.
Violins must be **MADE** with **GREAT** care.
The **WOOD USED** greatly influences the tone.
The parts **MUST** be glued **TOGETHER** by **HAND**.

Test Passage Pair 8 (Wheat/Ice)
Psg: 15 **WHEAT**
Wheat is a **CHIEF SOURCE** of food.
MILLIONS of **PEOPLE DEPEND** on wheat **PRODUCTS**.
It is the most **WIDELY** used human **FOOD**.
Americans **PRIZE** wheat **MORE HIGHLY** than **OTHER** grains.
Wheat is **GROWN** on the **PLAINS** of the United States.
More wheat is **PRODUCED** there than **RICE**.
However, rice is **CHEAPER** to **PRODUCE**.
It **CAN** be **PLANTED** and **HARVESTED** by **HAND**.
Rice is **IMPORTANT** to **OVERPOPULAED** countries.
It is their **PRIMARY** source of nutrition.

Psg: 16 **ICE**   ___/50
Ice forms when **WATER REACHES** the freezing **POINT**.
This point **OCCURS** at thirty-two degrees.
Lower **TEMPERATURES** are needed to freeze impure **WATER**.
SNOWFLAKES and **FROST** are forms of **ICE**.
Large bodies of water **FREEZE** very **SLOWLY**.
MOVING water takes **EVEN LONGER** to freeze.
It **TAKES DAYS** for ice to form on a **LAKE**.
It **TAKES** weeks for **RIVERS** to freeze.
Ice can also **FORM** on **ROADS** and **SIDEWALKS**.
This **CAN** make **TRAVELING** very **DANGEROUS**.

Test Passage Pair 9 (Donkey/Guitar)
Psg: 17 **DONKEY**
Donkeys are **SMALLER**, sturdier relatives of **HORSES**.
The **WILD** donkey is **SHAPED** like a **ZEBRA**.
It is four **FEET** high at the **SHOULDERS**.
The donkey's **COAT** is **GRAY** and black.
It **HAS** a **DARK LINE** along its **BACK**.
This **ANIMAL** is **EXTREMELY INTELLIGENT**.
SURPRISINGLY, it is also a **SWIFT RUNNER**.
Man has **TAMED** donkeys for his personal use.
Donkeys are **OFTEN** used as **BEASTS** of burden.
All donkeys are **NOTED** for their **HUGE EARS**.

Psg: 18 **GUITAR**   ___/50
The guitar is a stringed **MUSICAL INSTRUMENT**.
Guitars are used to **ACCOMPANY SINGING**.
They are played in **GROUPS** with other **INSTRUMENTS**.
A **POPULAR** style of guitar **HAS** a flat top.
It is made of wood and **HAS** six **STRINGS**.
You **TUNE** a guitar **BY** comparing **OCTAVE NOTES**.
The **FINGERBOARD** is **HELD** with the **LEFT** hand.
The **MUSICIAN'S** right hand **PULLS** the strings.
He plays **BASS NOTES** with his **RIGHT** thumb.
OTHER notes are **PLAYED** with the first **THREE** fingers.

Test Passage Pair 10 (Envelope/Grasshopper)
Psg: 19 **ENVELOPE**
An **ENVELOPE** is a **POUCH CONTAINING** a letter.
The **ADDRESS** is **WRITTEN** on the outside.
Envelopes **MAY** be used to **PROTECT IMPORTANT** documents
EACH envelope is a **FOLDED** sheet of **PAPER**.
One flap is **COVERED** with **GLUE**.
The **ENVELOPE** is **GLUED** shut before mailing.
Self sealing envelopes use a **SPECIAL GUM**.
THEY NEED not be **MOISTENED** to stick shut.
Envelopes were **FIRST MADE** in eighteen **THIRTY** nine.
BEFORE that time, **LETTERS** were simply folded.

Psg: 20 **GRASSHOPPER**   ___/50
"**GRASSHOPPER**" refers to **TWO** types of **BUGS**.
They **HAVE** long, **THIN** back legs.
Grasshoppers leap **THROUGH** fields and meadows.
They can **JUMP** many times their own **LENGTH**.
A man could never jump **THAT FAR**.
Grasshoppers include all the **INSECTS CALLED** locusts.
The **DIFFERENCE BETWEEN** the **TWO** is **THEIR** feelers.
Locusts **HAVE** much shorter **FEELERS** than **GRASSHOPPERS**.
Grasshoppers are **MORE GREEN** in **COLOR** than **LOCUSTS**.
Locusts **ARE USUALLY** brown colored.

CST Passages

Test Passage Pair 11 (Lettuce/Dictionary)

Psg: 21 **LETTUCE**

Lettuce is a **GREEN VEGETABLE** with **CRISP** leaves.
It is used to **MAKE** healthy **SALADS**.
It **GROWS** in the northern **HALF** of the **WORLD**.
There are **LOOSE** leaf and **HEAD** lettuces.
Loose **LEAF** lettuce is **POPULAR** in home gardens.
This **VARIETY** is found **MORE** often in **EUROPE**.
Its **LEAVES CURL LOOSELY** inside one another.
Most lettuce **GROWN** in America is **HEAD** lettuce.
Its **LEAVES FOLD** tightly **OVER** one another.
The leaves form a **BALL CALLED** a head.

Psg: 22 **DICTIONARY**   ___/50

A dictionary **LISTS** the meanings of words.
IT LETS a **PERSON DEFINE** a word quickly.
A dictionary **CONTAINS** over six **HUNDRED** thousand words.
MOST educated **ADULTS** know **ABOUT TEN** thousand words.
A **FIFTH** grade child **KNOWS** two **THOUSAND** words.
Adults and children **NEED** to use dictionaries.
DICTIONARIES TELL us many **USEFUL** things about words.
Every **DICTIONARY SHOWS** the **CORRECT** spelling of a
          WORD.
It also **SHOWS** how a word is **PRONOUNCED**.
CREATIVE writing would be difficult without dictionaries.

Test Passage Pair 12 (Lawn/Cactus)

Psg: 23 **LAWN**

A lawn is an **AREA** planted **WITH** grass.
GREEN, trimmed lawns are a beautiful **SIGHT**.
People **LIKE** to plant lawns around their **HOMES**.
Hospitals **OFTEN HAVE** lawns **AROUND** them.
MOST public **BUILDINGS** have **LAWNS**.
Lawns **HELP** to keep **SOIL** from eroding.
A **GOOD** lawn is **VERY** thickly **PLANTED**.
There are **FOUR** hundred plants **PER** square **FOOT**.
EACH plant has several **BLADES** of grass.
There are several **DIFFERENT KINDS** of **GRASSES**.

Psg: 24 **CACTUS**   ___/50

The cactus is a plant with **SHARP** thorns.
Five **HUNDRED DIFFERENT** kinds grow in **MEXICO**.
NEARLY all cactus **PLANTS LIVE** in America.
Cactus **LIVE** best **WHERE** there is little **RAINFALL**.
MOST CACTUS is found in the **DESERT** southwest.
PLANTS usually make food in their **LEAVES**.
The cactus does **NOT** have any **LEAVES**.
They **HAVE DISAPPEARED** so the cactus can stay moist.
The cactus stores the **WATER IN** its **STEM**.
DESERT cactus **FLOWERS BLOOM** in the spring.

Test Passage Pair 13 (Cabbage/Gold)

Psg: 25 **CABBAGE**

Cabbage is the **MOST COMMON** garden **VEGETABLE**.
It has **THICK LEAVES** which curl inward.
They form a **ROUND HEAD** eight inches **ACROSS**.
The **WORD** cabbage is Latin for "**HEAD**."
The **CABBAGE** plant can live through **SEVERAL FREEZES**.
It also **GROWS** in the heat of **SUMMER**.
EARLY SPRING cabbage is **PLANTED** in greenhouses.
This protects the **YOUNG PLANTS FROM FROST**.
AFTER six **WEEKS** they may be moved outdoors.
TRANSPLANTING is done before the end of spring.

Psg: 26 **GOLD**   ___/50

Gold was one of the first know **METALS**.
For **MANY YEARS** gold has **SYMBOLIZED WEALTH**.
EVEN the early cave man knew **ABOUT** gold.
ANCIENT EGYPTIANS hammered gold into **LEAVES**.
They used these leaves to **DECORATE** their **TOMBS**.
A **SCIENCE** grew up around efforts to make gold.
It **STARTED DURING** the **MIDDLE** ages.
The ancient scientists **NEVER ACHIEVED** their **GOAL**.
Modern **SCIENTISTS** have made these **DREAMS** come **TRUE**.
THEY now **MAKE** gold by a **CHEMICAL** process.

Test Passage Pair 14 (Weed/Chimney)

Psg: 27 **WEED**

Weeds are considered **WORTHLESS PLANTS**.
The **DIFFERENCE BETWEEN** weeds and useful **PLANTS** is
     unclear.
WHERE a **WEED GROWS** determines its usefulness.
OATS GROWNING in a **CORNFIELD** are considered weeds.
Oats growing in an **OATFIELD** are useful **PLANTS**.
Much crop damage is **CAUSED BY** weeds.
Experts estimate it at **FIVE** dollars per person.
FARMERS SPEND THOUSANDS of **DOLLARS** for **WEED** sprays.
Chemicals used to **KILL** weeds can be harmful.
These chemicals are **SOMETIMES** found in **DRINKING WATER**.

                                                          ___/50

Psg: 28 **CHIMNEY**

A chimney **CARRIES SMOKE** from a **FIREPLACE**.
It **ALSO SUPPLIES** the fire with **OXYGEN**.
Warm air is **LIGHTER** than **COLD** air.
Warm air **ABOVE** the fire **TENDS** to rise.
As the **WARM** air **RISES**, cold air rushes in.
A draft is **CREATED** in the **CHIMNEY**.
The draft **PROVIDES** the oxygen **NEEDED** for the **FIRE**.
Chimneys must **STAND HIGHER** than the **BUILDING**.
Otherwise, the chimney **WILL** not **DRAW PROPERLY**.
CHIMNEYS can **IMPROVE** the appearance of a home.

Test Passage Pair 15 (Lead/Calendar)

Psg: 29 **LEAD**

Lead is a **SOFT**, **HEAVY**, metallic element.
It is **OFTEN** combined with other **METALS**.
MANY USEFUL OBJECTS contain some lead **MIXTURE**.
The Romans **USED LEAD** for **WATER PIPES**.
Their **PUBLIC** baths were lined **WITH** lead.
The **WORD** "plumber" means a **WORKER** in lead.
Lead is **ONE** of the **HEAVIEST KNOWN** metals.
It is **ELEVEN** times as **HEAVY** as **WATER**.
The **EXPRESSION** "as **HEAVY** as lead" is common.
It **DESCRIBES** an obiect of great weight.

Psg: 30 **CALENDAR**   ___/50

A calendar is a **SYSTEM** for **RECORDING TIME**.
All **CALENDARS INCLUDE** the day and the **YEAR**.
THESE are two **NATURAL DIVISIONS** of time.
Both are based **ON** the **EARTH** and the **SUN**.
The **MONTH** depends on the **APPEARANCE** of the **MOON**.
The week **IS** an **ARTIFICIAL** division of **TIME**.
WEEKS are not **BASED** on observable **EVENTS**.
The calendar was a **GREAT HUMAN** achievement.
THROUGH it, men learned to measure **TIME**.

CST Passages

Test Passage Pair 16 (Lion/Zebra)
Psg: 31 **LION**
The lion is a **WILD MEMBER** of the cat **FAMILY.**
IT is related to the tiger and the **BOBCAT.**
The lion and **TIGER** are the largest **CATS.**
The **TIGER** is the **FIERCEST** of all.
The lion is a strong, **WILD CREATURE.**
It **HAS** a large, **HEAVY** and powerful **BODY.**
ITS long **MANE** gives it a proud appearance.
The lion is **KNOWN** as the "**KING** of **BEASTS.**"
Lions are also **CALLED** "**LORDS** of the jungle."
HOWEVER, they are **SELDOM FOUND** in the **JUNGLE.**

Psg 32 **ZEBRA** ___/50
A zebra is an animal that **LIVES** in Africa.
It is a wild, **GRASS** eating **ANIMAL.**
It **LOOKS VERY** much like a **HORSE.**
MOST zebras **STAND** four to five **FEET** high.
The zebra has a **SURPRISINGLY** different **COLOR** pattern.
Zebras **HAVE PARALLEL** black and **WHITE STRIPES.**
The stripes are arranged in **EXACT DESIGNS.**
These stripes **RUN** all **OVER** their **BODIES.**
They even run **UP** and **DOWN THEIR** faces.
The stripes **ALSO** appear on the zebra's **EARS.**

Test Passage Pair 17 (Lizard/Wolf)
Psg: 33 **LIZARD**
The **LIZARDS ARE** the **CLOSEST RELATIVES** of **SNAKES.**
SOME lizards look **LIKE** snakes with **LEGS.**
Some **LARGE** ones look like **CROCODILES.**
They come in a **VARIETY** of **SHAPES** and **COLORS.**
Lizards have **MANY WAYS** of moving and fighting.
LIZARDS and **SALAMANDERS** are often **CONFUSED.**
They **LOOK** very much **ALIKE BUT** aren't related.
Up **NORTH** there are few lizards but **MANY** salamanders.
In the **SOUTHWEST,** just the **OPPOSITE** is true.

Psg: 34 **WOLF** ___/50
The wolf **IS** a **MEMBER** of the **DOG** family.
A wolf **LOOKS** like a **SKINNY** wild **DOG.**
It has a **WIDE HEAD** and pointed **NOSE.**
Wolves **LIVE** in North **AMERICA,** Europe, and Asia.
Wolves **USED** to **LIVE** all over the United **STATES.**
GRAY wolves are **SELDOM SEEN** nowadays.
THEY live in the Rockies and **NORTHERN** states.
Wolves **HUNT** in packs and **MATE** for **LIFE.**
The average wolf pack consists of **TEN** wolves.
A female wolf gives **BIRTH** every other **YEAR.**

Test Passage Pair 18 (Orange/Oyster)
Psg 35: **ORANGE**
The orange is the most important **CITRUS FRUIT.**
It is a **GOOD** source of **VITAMIN** C.
It **CAN BE** eaten **OR** made **INTO** juice.
Eating oranges **MAY PREVENT** the common **COLD.**
There are **TWO** different kinds of oranges.
The sweet orange is **EATEN** in the United States.
It is **THOUGHT** to have **COME FROM CHINA.**
The other **KIND** of orange is **MORE** bitter.
It **IS** used often in **COOKING.**
The **TANGERINE** is often **INCORRECTLY CALLED** an **ORANGE.**

Psg: 36 **OYSTER** ___/50
Oysters are animals that live in **SEA** shells.
The oyster lives in many **PARTS** of the **WORLD.**
It **LIVES MOSTLY** in quiet, shallow **WATERS.**
It **IS MAN'S** most **VALUABLE SEAFOOD.**
The oyster's **SHELL** forms a **SHELTER.**
The **SHELL** is divided into two halves.
They are **FASTENED TOGETHER** at **ONE END.**
The left **HALF** is larger and **THICKER.**
A **MUSCLE ATTACHES** the soft **BODY** to the **SHELL.**
This muscle **HELPS** the **OYSTER** open the shell.

Test Passage Pair 19 (Dice/Eagle)
Psg: 37 **DICE**
DICE are cubes **USED** in games of chance.
They may be **MADE** of ivory, wood, **OR PLASTIC.**
A **SINGLE** such **CUBE** is **CALLED** a die.
Each **SIDE** of a **DIE** has **ONE** to six dots.
DOTS on **OPPOSTIE SIDES** add up to **SEVEN.**
Players **TOSS** the dice on a flat **SURFACE.**
The **NUMBERS** that come up **DECIDE** the game.
The **COMBINATION** of numbers **DEPENDS** on chance.
A **GAME** of dice is **THEREFORE** a gamble.
Gambling is not legal in **MOST STATES.**

Psg: 38 **EAGLE** ___/50
The eagle is a large bird of **PREY.**
It has powerful **WINGS** and **SHARP** eyes.
The **EAGLE** is a **SYMBOL** of courage and freedom.
The **BALD** eagle is America's **NATIONAL BIRD.**
THERE are **SEVERAL** different kinds of eagles.
Each **TYPE IS** very **DIFFERENT** in **SIZE** and color.
Eagles **HAVE** strong beaks and **POWERFUL CLAWS.**
The eagle's **BEAK** is as long as its **HEAD.**
The beak's upper **HALF** hooks over the **LOWER.**
The eagle **USES** its **POWERFUL** beak to **CATCH** its **PREY**

Test Passage Pair 20 (Ear/Liver)
Psg: 39 **EAR**
The ear is an important **SENSE ORGAN.**
The ear **HAS** two main **PURPOSES.**
It lets **MAN HEAR** and **MAINTAIN** his balance.
GOOD hearing permits **PEOPLE** to understand **SPEECH.**
Through speech, we **EXCHANGE** ideas and **OPINIONS.**
HEARING ALSO makes man **AWARE** of **DANGER.**
The ear's **BALANCE** mechanism helps us walk **UPRIGHT.**
DAMAGE to this section causes **STAGGERING.**
The **PERSON** also **GETS** disoriented and **DIZZY.**
This kind of dizziness is **CALLED VERTIGO.**

Psg: 40 **LIVER** ___/50
The liver is a very important **INTERNAL** organ.
Its **MAIN FUNCTION** is to filter the **BLOOD.**
The liver is the **LARGEST** organ in **MAN.**
It can **WEIGH** three to four **POUNDS.**
The liver is **DARK RED** or **CHOCOLATE** colored.
It is **LOCATED** in the **MIDDLE SECTION** of the **BODY.**
It **FITS** closely to the intestines and kidneys.
It is **POSSIBLE** to **TRANSPLANT** a liver.
This **ADVANCED** operation is **VERY** expensive.
HOWEVER, it is **RESPONSIBLE** for **SAVING MANY LIVES.**

CST Passages

Psg: 41 LEOPARD
The leopard is a **MEMBER** of the **CAT** family.
It is the **THIRD** largest cat in the **WORLD**.
ONLY the **LION** and tiger are **LARGER**.
Leopards live in the **JUNGELS** of Africa.
They are **EXCELLENT** night time **HUNTERS**.
LEOPARDS STAND ALMOST two feet high at the **SHOULDERS**.
A big **MALE MAY MEASURE** nine **FEET LONG**.
It **CAN WEIGH** one hundred and sixty pounds.
A large **FEMALE** will weigh **ONLY** seventy pounds.
LEOPARDS have only a few **CUBS** in a litter.

Psg: 42 EYE ___/50
The eye is the most **IMPORTANT SNESE** organ.
We **USE** it to **VIEW** the **WORLD**.
ALMOST EVERY ACTIVITY INVOLVES the eyes.
EYES are **OUR** windows to the **WORLD**.
The **LENS** of the eye collects **LIGHT**.
The **LIGHT** is **FOCUSED INSIDE** the eye.
This information is sent to the **BRAIN**.
The brain the begins to **PROCESS** the **IMAGE**.
Eyes help us to enjoy **BOOKS** and **PAINTINGS**.
We **SEE** beauty in **MOUNTAINS** and **SUNSETS**.

Test Passage 22 (Zipper/Egg)
Psg: 43 ZIPPER
A zipper is any kind of **SLIDE FASTENER**.
ALL zippers **HAVE** two rows of **TEETH**.
The two **EDGES** of the zipper fasten **TOGETHER**.
The **TEETH HOLD** the zipper **TOGETHER**.
The edges **STAY** fastened **TILL** they are **RELEASED**.
They are released **BY DRAWING** the slide back.
Slide zippers are **OFTEN** used to **FASTEN CLOTHING**.
They **ARE USED** on **LUGGAGE** and briefcases.
The **FIRST** zipper was invented by an **AMERICAN**.
It **WAS** made of connected **HOOKS** and eyes.

Psg: 44 EGG ___/50
Many kinds of animals and **BIRDS PRODUCE** eggs.
The **MAIN PURPOSE** of eggs is to breed **YOUNG**.
Most young **ANIMALS BEGIN** as an **EGG**.
PEOPLE usually think of the egg as **FOOD**.
Actually, **FEW** kinds of eggs are **EATEN**.
Bird's eggs are **LARGER** than **MAMMAL'S**.
Their eggs **CONTAIN FOOD** for the young **BIRD**.
Young birds **DEVELOP OUTSIDE** the mother's **BODY**.
The ostrich **EGG** is the **LARGEST** type.
The **HUMAN EGG** is **ONE** of the smallest.

Test Passage Pair 23 (Clock/Kangaroo)
Psg: 45 CLOCK
Clocks are **INSTRUMENTS** that can **MEASURE** time.
They **DIVIDE** days into regular **INTERVALS**.
Originally, **TREE SHADOWS** were **USED** to mark time.
The **SHORTEST** shadows **OCCUR** around midday.
LONGER shadows occur in morning and **LATE AFTERNOON**.
The **FIRST** clock invented was the **SUNDIAL**.
LATER, the water clock was **DEVELOPED** in **CHINA**.
It could **MEASURE** time on **CLOUDY** days.
WATER clocks were used for several **THOUSAND YEARS**.
EARLY GREEKS and Romans **ALSO** used clocks.

Psg: 46 KANGAROO ___/50
The kangaroo **CARRIES** its **YOUNG** in a **POUCH**.
The pouch is **LOCATED** outside of the **ABDOMEN**.
ANIMALS with **POUCHES** are not found in **AMERICA**.
The kangaroo's **NATIVE COUNTRY** is **AUSTRALIA**.
There are many different kinds of **KANGAROOS**.
The **SMALLEST ARE** the same size as a **RABBIT**.
The largest **ARE NEARLY** seven feet tall.
Their back **LEGS** are larger than their **FRONT** legs.
Kangaroo fossils have **RECENTLY BEEN FOUND**.
Prehistoric kangaroos **GREW** to **BE** very **LARGE**.

Test Passage Pair 24 (Camel/Goose)
Psg: 47 CAMEL
The camel is a very **UGLY** animal.
It is also **ONE** of the most **USEFUL**.
It has **BEEN** man's **SERVANT** for **MANY CENTURIES**.
Camels were **ONCE** a measure of **WEALTH**.
In the **BIBLE,** God gave camels to **ABRAHAM**.
Camels are called the "**SHIP** of the desert."
They **CAN** endure long, **HARD** desert **JOURNEYS**.
Camels can **TRAVEL** man **MILES** without **NEEDING** water.
WITHOUT the camel, man **COULDN'T TRAVEL** the **DESERTS**.
Camel **CARAVANS** are **STILL** seen in the **SAHARA**.

Psg: 48 GOOSE ___/50
The goose is a **WEB FOOTED BIRD**.
It **IS CLOSELY RELATED TO** the **DUCK**.
A goose is larger than a **DUCK**.
Its **NECK** is slightly **LONGER** than a duck's.
There are forty different varieties of **GEESE**.
Seventeen kinds of wild **GEESE** live in **AMERICA**.
GEESE ARE KNOWN to **MOVE WITH** the seasons.
They **FLY NORTH** in the summer and south in the **WINTER**.
Some fly as far north as the **ARCTIC**.
OTHERS fly as far south as **MEXICO**.

Appendix S

HINT Sentence Lists

List 1

1. (A/the) **boy fell from** (A/the) **window**
2. (A/the) **wife helped her husband**
3. **Big dogs can be dangerous**
4. **Her shoes (are/were) very dirty**
5. (A/the) **player lost** (a/the) **shoe**
6. **Somebody stole the money**
7. (A/the) **fire (is/was) very hot**
8. **She's drinking from her own cup**
9. (A/the) **picture came from** (a/the) **book**
10. (A/the) **car (is/was) going too fast**

List 2

1. (A/the) **boy ran down** (a/the) **path**
2. **Flowers grow in** (a/the) **garden**
3. **Strawberry jam (is/was) sweet**
4. (A/the) **shop closes for lunch**
5. **The police helped** (a/the) **driver**
6. **She looked in her mirror**
7. (A/the) **match fell on** (a/the) **floor**
8. (An/the) **fruit came in** (a/the) **box**
9. **He really scared his sister**
10. (A/the) **tub faucet (is/was) leaking**

List 3

1. **They heard** (a/the) **funny noise**
2. **He found his brother hiding**
3. (A/the) **dog played with** (a/the) **stick**
4. (A/the) **book tells** (a/the) **story**
5. **The matches (are/were) on** (a/the) **shelf**
6. **The milk (is/was) by** (a/the) **front door**
7. (A/the) **broom (is/was) in** (a/the) **corner**
8. (A/the) **new road (is/was) on** (a/the) **map**
9. **She lost her credit card**
10. (A/the) **team (is/was) playing well**

List 4

1. (A/the) **little boy left home**
2. **They're going out tonight**
3. (A/the) **cat jumped over** (a/the) **fence**
4. **He wore his yellow shirt**
5. (A/the) **lady sits in her chair**
6. **He needs his vacation**
7. **She's washing her new silk dress**
8. (A/the) **cat drank from** (a/the) **saucer**
9. **Mother opened** (a/the) **drawer**
10. (A/the) **lady packed her bag**

List 5

1. (A/the) **boy did a handstand**
2. **They took some food outside**
3. **The young people (are/were) dancing**
4. **They waited for an hour**
5. **The shirts (are/were) in** (a/the) **closet**
6. **They watched** (a/the) **scary movie**
7. **The milk (is/was) in** (a/the) **pitcher**
8. (A/the) **truck drove up** (a/the) **road**
9. (A/the) **tall man tied his shoes**
10. (A/the) **letter fell on** (a/the) **floor**

List 6

1. (A/the) **silly boy (is/was) hiding**
2. (A/the) **dog growled at the neighbors**
3. (A/the) **tree fell on** (a/the) **house**
4. **Her husband brought some flowers**
5. **The children washed the plates**
6. **They went on vacation**
7. **Mother tied** (a/the) **string too tight**
8. (A/the) **mailman shut** (a/the) **gate**
9. (A/the) **grocer sells butter**
10. (A/the) **baby broke his cup**

List 7

1. **The cows (are/were) in** (a/the) **pasture**
2. (A/the) **dishcloth (is/was) soaking wet**
3. **They (have/had) some chocolate pudding**
4. **She spoke to her eldest son**
5. (An/the) **oven door (is/was) open**
6. **She's paying for her bread**
7. **My mother stirred her tea**
8. **He broke his leg again**
9. (A/the) **lady wore** (a/the) **coat**
10. **The cups (are/were) on** (a/the) **table**

List 8

1. (A/the) **ball bounced very high**
2. **Mother cut** (a/the) **birthday cake**
3. (A/the) **football game (is/was) over**
4. **She stood near** (a/the) **window**
5. (A/the) **kitchen clock (is/was) wrong**
6. **The children helped their teacher**
7. **They carried some shopping bags**
8. **Someone (is/was) crossing** (a/the) **road**
9. **She uses her spoon to eat**
10. (A/the) **cat lay on** (a/the) **bed**

List 9

1. **School got out early today**
2. (A/the) **football hit the goalpost**
3. (A/the) **boy ran away from school**
4. **Sugar (is/was) very sweet**
5. **The two children (are/were) laughing**
6. (A/the) **fire truck (is/was) coming**
7. **Mother got** (a/the) **sauce pan**
8. (A/the) **baby wants his bottle**
9. (A/the) **ball broke** (a/the) **window**
10. **There (is/was) a bad train wreck**

List 10

1. (A/the) **boy broke** (A/the) **wooden fence**
2. (An/the) **angry man shouted**
3. **Yesterday he lost his hat**
4. (A/the) **nervous driver got lost**
5. (A/the) **cook (is/was) baking** (a/the) **cake**
6. (A/the) **chicken laid some eggs**
7. (A/the) **fish swam in** (a/the) **pond**
8. **They met some friends at dinner**
9. (A/the) **man called the police**
10. (A/the) **truck made it up** (a/the) **hill**

List 11

1. (A/the) **neighbor's boy (has/had) black hair**
2. **The rain came pouring down**
3. (A/the) **orange (is/was) very sweet**
4. **He took the dogs for a walk**
5. **Children like strawberries**
6. **Her sister stayed for lunch**
7. (A/the) **train (is/was) moving fast**
8. **Mother shut** (a/the) **window**
9. (A/the) **bakery (is/was) open**
10. **Snow falls in the winter**

List 12

1. (A/the) **boy went to bed early**
2. (A/the) **woman cleaned her house**
3. (A/the) **sharp knife (is/was) dangerous**
4. (A/the) **child ripped open** (a/the) **bag**
5. **They had some cold cuts for lunch**
6. **She's helping her friend move**
7. **They ate** (a/the) **lemon pie**
8. **They (are/were) crossing** (a/the) **street**
9. **The sun melted the snow**
10. (A/the) **little girl (is/was) happy**

HINT Sentence Lists

List 13

1. **She found her purse in** (a/the) **trash**
2. (A/the) **table** (has/had) **three legs**
3. The **children waved at** (a/the) **train**
4. **Her coat** (is/was) **on** (a/the) **chair**
5. (A/the) **girl** (is/was) **fixing her dress**
6. **It's time to go to bed**
7. **Mother read** the **instructions**
8. (A/the) **dog** (is/was) **eating some meat**
9. **Father forgot** the **bread**
10. (A/the) **road goes up** (a/the) **hill**

List 14

1. The **fruit** (is/was) **on** the **ground**
2. **They followed** (a/the) **garden path**
3. **They like orange marmalade**
4. **There** (are/were) **branches everywhere**
5. (A/the) **kitchen sink** (is/was) **empty**
6. The **old gloves** (are/were) **dirty**
7. The **scissors** (are/were) **very sharp**
8. (A/the) **man cleaned his suede shoes**
9. (A/the) **raincoat** (is/was) **dripping wet**
10. **It's getting cold in here**

List 15

1. (A/the) **house** (has/had) **nine bedrooms**
2. **They're shopping for school clothes**
3. **They're playing in** (a/the) **park**
4. **Rain** (is/was) **good for** the **trees**
5. **They sat on** (a/the) **wooden bench**
6. (A/the) **child drank some fresh milk**
7. (A/the) **baby slept all night**
8. (A/the) **salt shaker** (is/was) **empty**
9. (A/the) **policeman knows** the **way**
10. The **buckets fill up quickly**

List 16

1. **He played with his toy train**
2. **They're watching** (a/the) **cuckoo clock**
3. **Potatoes grow in** the **ground**
4. (A/the) **girl ran along** (a/the) **fence**
5. (A/the) **dog jumped on** (a/the) **chair**
6. **They finished dinner on time**
7. **He got mud on his shoes**
8. **They're clearing** (a/the) **table**
9. **Some animals sleep on straw**
10. The **police cleared** (a/the) **road**

List 17

1. **Mother picked some flowers**
2. (A/the) **puppy played with** (a/the) **ball**
3. (An/the) **engine** (is/was) **running**
4. (An/the) **old woman** (is/was) **at home**
5. **They're watching** (a/the) **train go by**
6. (An/the) **oven** (is/was) **too hot**
7. **They rode their bicycles**
8. (A/the) **big fish got away**
9. **They laughed at his story**
10. **They walked across** the **grass**

List 18

1. (A/the) **boy** (is/was) **running away**
2. (A/the) **towel** (is/was) **near** (a/the) **sink**
3. **Flowers can grow in** (a/the) **pot**
4. **He's skating with his friend**
5. (A/the) **janitor swept** (a/the) **floor**
6. (A/the) **lady washed** (a/the) **shirt**
7. **She took off her fur coat**
8. The **match boxes** (are/were) **empty**
9. (A/the) **man** (is/was) **painting** (a/the) **sign**
10. (A/the) **dog came home at last**

List 19

1. (A/the) **painter uses** (a/the) **brush**
2. (A/the) **family bought** (a/the) **house**
3. **Swimmers can hold their breath**
4. **She cut** (a/the) **steak with her knife**
5. **They're pushing** an **old car**
6. The **food** (is/was) **expensive**
7. The **children** (are/were) **walking home**
8. **They** (have/had) **two empty bottles**
9. **Milk comes in** (a/the) **carton**
10. (A/the) **dog sleeps in** (a/the) **basket**

List 20

1. (A/the) **clown** (has/had) (a/the) **funny face**
2. The **bath water** (is/was) **warm**
3. **She injured four of her fingers**
4. **He paid his bill in full**
5. **They stared at** (a/the) **picture**
6. (A/the) **driver started** (a/the) **car**
7. (A/the) **truck carries fresh fruit**
8. (A/the) **bottle** (is/was) **on** (a/the) **shelf**
9. The **small tomatoes** (are/were) **green**
10. (A/the) **dinner plate** (is/was) **hot**

List 21

1. **They're running past** (a/the) **house**
2. **He's washing his face with soap**
3. (A/the) **dog's chasing** (a/the) **cat**
4. (A/the) **milkman drives** (a/the) **small truck**
5. (A/the) **bus leaves before** (a/the) **train**
6. (A/the) **baby** (has/had) **blue eyes**
7. (A/the) **bag fell off** (a/the) **shelf**
8. **They** (are/were) **coming for dinner**
9. **They wanted some potatoes**
10. **They knocked on** (a/the) **window**

List 22

1. (A/the) **girl came into** (a/the) **room**
2. (A/the) **field mouse found** (a/the) **cheese**
3. **They're buying some fresh bread**
4. (A/the) **machine** (is/was) **noisy**
5. The **rice pudding** (is/was) **ready**
6. **They had** a **wonderful day**
7. (An/the) **exit** (is/was) **well lit**
8. (A/the) **train stops at** (a/the) **station**
9. **He** (is/was) **sucking his thumb**
10. (A/the) **big boy kicked** the **ball**

List 23

1. The **paint dripped on** the **ground**
2. (A/the) **towel fell on** (a/the) **floor**
3. (A/the) **family likes fish**
4. The **bananas** (are/were) **too ripe**
5. **He grew lots of vegetables**
6. **She argues with her sister**
7. (A/the) **kitchen window** (is/was) **clean**
8. **He hung up his raincoat**
9. (A/the) **mailman brought** (a/the) **letter**
10. (A/the) **mother heard** (a/the) **baby**

List 24

1. (A/the) **waiter brought** (a/the) **cream**
2. (A/the) **teapot** (is/was) **very hot**
3. (A/the) **apple pie** (is/was) **good**
4. (A/the) **jelly jar** (is/was) **full**
5. (A/the) **girl** (is/was) **washing her hair**
6. (A/the) **girl played with** (a/the) **baby**
7. (A/the) **cow** (is/was) **milked every day**
8. **They called an ambulance**
9. **They** (are/were) **drinking coffee**
10. **He climbed up** (a/the) **ladder**

HINT Sentence Lists

List 25

1. (A/the) **boy slipped on** the **stairs**
2. **New neighbors (are/were) moving in**
3. (A/the) **girl caught** (a/the) **head cold**
4. **His father will come home soon**
5. (A/the) **bus stopped suddenly**
6. **He (is/was) washing his car**
7. (A/the) **cat caught** (a/the) **little mouse**
8. **They broke all** the **brown eggs**
9. (A/the) **candy shop (is/was) empty**
10. (A/the) **lady went to** (a/the) **store**

Appendix T

Quick SIN Score Sheet

List 1

Tracks 3, 24, 36, 52	**Score**
1. A white silk jacket goes with any shoes.	S/N 25____
2. The child crawled into the dense grass.	S/N 20____
3. Footprints showed the path he took up the beach.	S/N 15____
4. A vent near the edge brought in fresh air.	S/N 10 ____
5. It is a band of steel three inches wide.	S/N 5 ____
6. The weight of the package was seen on the high scale.	S/N 0 ____

25.5 – TOTAL=____ SNR loss   **TOTAL** _____

List 2

Tracks 4, 25, 37, 53	**Score**
1. Tear a thin sheet from the yellow pad.	S/N 25____
2. A cruise in warm waters in a sleek yacht is fun.	S/N 20____
3. A streak of color ran down the left edge.	S/N 15____
4. It was done before the boy could see it.	S/N 10 ____
5. Crouch before you jump or miss the mark.	S/N 5 ____
6. The square peg will settle in the round hole.	S/N 0 ____

25.5 – TOTAL=____ SNR loss   **TOTAL** _____

List 6

Tracks 8, 29, 41, 57	**Score**
1. The leaf drifts along with a slow spin.	S/N 25____
2. The pencil was cut to be sharp at both ends.	S/N 20____
3. Down that road is the way to the grain farmer.	S/N 15____
4. The best method is to fix it in place with clips.	S/N 10 ____
5. If you mumble your speech will be lost.	S/N 5 ____
6. A toad and a frog are hard to tell apart.	S/N 0 ____

25.5 – TOTAL=____ SNR loss   **TOTAL** _____

List 8

Tracks 10, 31, 43, 59	**Score**
1. The sun came up to light the eastern sky.	S/N 25____
2. The stale smell of old beer lingers.	S/N 20____
3. The desk was firm on the shaky floor.	S/N 15____
4. A list of names is carved around the base.	S/N 10 ____
5. The news struck doubt into restless minds.	S/N 5 ____
6. The sand drifts over the sill of the old house.	S/N 0 ____

25.5 – TOTAL=____ SNR loss   **TOTAL** _____

List 10

Tracks 12, 33, 45, 61	**Score**
1. Dots of light betrayed the black cat.	S/N 25____
2. Put the chart on the mantel and tack it down.	S/N 20____
3. The steady drip is worse than a drenching rain.	S/N 15____
4. A flat pack takes less luggage space.	S/N 10 ____
5. The gloss on top made it unfit to read.	S/N 5 ____
6. Seven seals were stamped on great sheets.	S/N 0 ____

25.5 – TOTAL= ____ SNR loss   **TOTAL** _____

List 12

Tracks 14, 35, 47, 63	**Score**
1. The hinge on the door creaked with old age.	S/N 25____
2. The bright lanterns were gay on the dark lawn.	S/N 20____
3. He offered proof in the form of a large chart.	S/N 15____
4. Their eyelids droop for want of sleep.	S/N 10 ____
5. There are many ways to do these things.	S/N 5 ____
6. We like to see clear weather.	S/N 0 ____

25.5 – TOTAL= ____ SNR loss   **TOTAL** _____

List 15

Tracks 17, 50, 66	**Score**
1. Poached eggs and tea must suffice.	S/N 25____
2. They sang the same tunes at each party	S/N 20____
3. A gold vase is both rare and costly	S/N 15____
4. Cod is the main business of the north shore.	S/N 10 ____
5. A round mat will cover the dull spot.	S/N 5 ____
6. A good book informs of what we ought to know.	S/N 0 ____

25.5 – TOTAL= ____ SNR loss   **TOTAL** _____

List 17

Track 19	**Score**
1. The point of the steel pen was bent and twisted.	S/N 25____
2. There is a lag between thought and act.	S/N 20____
3. Seed is needed to plant the spring corn.	S/N 15____
4. This horse will nose his way to the finish.	S/N 10 ____
5. The dry wax protects the deep scratch.	S/N 5 ____
6. Twist the valve and release hot steam.	S/N 0 ____

25.5 – TOTAL= ____ SNR loss   **TOTAL** _____

Appendix U

BKB SIN Sentences

List Pair 1

List 1A	Key Words	#Correct	SNR
1. They are looking at the clock.	4	_____	+21 dB
2. The car engine is running.	3	_____	+18 dB
3. Children like strawberries.	3	_____	+15 dB
4. They are buying some bread.	3	_____	+12 dB
5. The green tomatoes are small.	3	_____	+9 dB
6. He played with his train.	3	_____	+6 dB
7. The bag fell to the ground.	3	_____	+3 dB
8. The boy did a handstand.	3	_____	+0 dB
9. The water boiled quickly.	3	_____	-3 dB
10. The man is painting a sign.	3	_____	-6 dB

Total Key Word Correct_____

SNR-50= (23.5)-(# Correct)=_____dB

List 1B	Key Words	#Correct	SNR
1. The dog made an angry noise.	4	_____	+21 dB
2. They followed the path.	3	_____	+18 dB
3. Someone is crossing the road.	3	_____	+15 dB
4. The mailman brought a letter.	3	_____	+12 dB
5. The milk was by the front door.	3	_____	+9 dB
6. The candy shop was empty.	3	_____	+6 dB
7. The lady stayed for lunch.	3	_____	+3 dB
8. The policeman knows the way.	3	_____	+0 dB
9. The little girl was happy.	3	_____	-3 dB
10. They are coming for Christmas.	3	_____	-6 dB

Total Key Word Correct_____

SNR-50= (23.5)-(# Correct)= _____dB

Average SNR-50, Lists 1A and 1B= _____dB

List Pair 2

List 2A	Key Words	#Correct	SNR
1. The cat is sitting on the bed.	4	_____	+21 dB
2. They had a lovely day.	3	_____	+18 dB
3. The thin dog was hungry.	3	_____	+15 dB
4. They are watching the train.	3	_____	+12 dB
5. The dog played with a stick.	3	_____	+9 dB
6. The farmer keeps a bull.	3	_____	+6 dB
7. The lady wore a coat.	3	_____	+3 dB
8. The boy is running away.	3	_____	+0 dB
9. The room is getting cold.	3	_____	-3 dB
10. The wife helped her husband.	3	_____	-6 dB

Total Key Word Correct_____

SNR-50= (23.5)-(# Correct)=_____dB

List 2B	Key Words	#Correct	SNR
1. The lady went to the store.	4	_____	+21 dB
2. A tree fell on the house.	3	_____	+18 dB
3. The fruit came in a box.	3	_____	+15 dB
4. The husband brought some flowers.	3	_____	+12 dB
5. A man told the police.	3	_____	+9 dB
6. Potatoes grow in the ground.	3	_____	+6 dB
7. The big dog was dangerous.	3	_____	+3 dB
8. The strawberry jam was sweet.	3	_____	+0 dB
9. The boy has black hair/ tie.	3	_____	-3 dB
10. The mother heard the baby.	3	_____	-6 dB

Total Key Word Correct_____

SNR-50= (23.5)-(# Correct)= _____dB

Average SNR-50, Lists 2A and 2B= _____dB

List Pair 3

List 3A	Key Words	#Correct	SNR
1. The ball went into the goal.	4	_____	+21 dB
2. The house had a nice garden.	3	_____	+18 dB
3. He found his brother.	3	_____	+15 dB
4. Some animals sleep on straw.	3	_____	+12 dB
5. The jelly jar was full.	3	_____	+9 dB
6. They are kneeling down.	3	_____	+6 dB
7. The cook is making a cake.	3	_____	+3 dB
8. The child grabbed the toy.	3	_____	+0 dB
9. A boy fell from the window.	3	_____	-3 dB
10. She used her spoon.	3	_____	-6 dB

Total Key Word Correct_____

SNR-50= (23.5)-(# Correct)= _____dB

List 3B	Key Words	#Correct	SNR
1. Mother cut the birthday cake.	4	_____	+21 dB
2. The mailman comes early.	3	_____	+18 dB
3. The sign showed the way.	3	_____	+15 dB
4. The grass is getting long.	3	_____	+12 dB
5. A man is turning the faucet.	3	_____	+9 dB
6. The fire was very hot.	3	_____	+6 dB
7. He is sucking his thumb.	3	_____	+3 dB
8. The driver started the engine.	3	_____	+0 dB
9. The janitor swept the floor.	3	_____	-3 dB
10. A grocer sells butter.	3	_____	-6 dB

Total Key Word Correct_____

SNR-50= (23.5)-(# Correct)=_____dB

Average SNR-50, Lists 3A and 3B= _____dB

List Pair 4

List 4A	Key Words	#Correct	SNR
1. A mouse ran down the hole.	4	_____	+21 dB
2. The light went out.	3	_____	+18 dB
3. They wanted some potatoes.	3	_____	+15 dB
4. The little girl is shouting.	3	_____	+12 dB
5. The cold milk is in a pitcher.	3	_____	+9 dB
6. The paint dripped on the ground.	3	_____	+6 dB
7. Mother stirred her tea.	3	_____	+3 dB
8. The father is coming home.	3	_____	+0 dB
9. They painted the wall.	3	_____	-3 dB
10. The towel dropped on the floor.	3	_____	-6 dB

Total Key Word Correct_____

SNR-50= (23.5)-(# Correct)= _____dB

List 4B	Key Words	#Correct	SNR
1. The boy got into bed.	4	_____	+21 dB
2. He is reaching for his spoon.	3	_____	+18 dB
3. They are staying for supper.	3	_____	+15 dB
4. The girl held a mirror.	3	_____	+12 dB
5. The cows are in the pasture.	3	_____	+9 dB
6. He paid his bill.	3	_____	+6 dB
7. Mother made some curtains.	3	_____	+3 dB
8. The oven is too hot.	3	_____	+0 dB
9. The two children are laughing.	3	_____	-3 dB
10. The pepper shaker was empty.	3	_____	-6 dB

Total Key Word Correct_____

SNR-50= (23.5)-(# Correct)=_____dB

Average SNR-50, Lists 4A and 4B= _____dB

List Pair 5

List 5A	Key Words	#Correct	SNR
1. They ate the lemon pie.	4	_____	+21 dB
2. A sharp knife is dangerous.	3	_____	+18 dB
3. The smart girls are reading.	3	_____	+15 dB
4. The broom stood in the corner.	3	_____	+12 dB
5. The woman cleaned her house.	3	_____	+9 dB
6. Mother got a saucepan.	3	_____	+6 dB
7. The young people are dancing.	3	_____	+3 dB
8. The bus left early.	3	_____	+0 dB
9. The ball is bouncing very high.	3	_____	-3 dB
10. Father forgot the bread.	3	_____	-6 dB

Total Key Word Correct_____

SNR-50= (23.5)-(# Correct)= _____dB

List 5B	Key Words	#Correct	SNR
1. They had two empty bottles.	4	_____	+21 dB
2. He closed his eyes.	3	_____	+18 dB
3. The lady bought some butter.	3	_____	+15 dB
4. They called an ambulance.	3	_____	+12 dB
5. The policeman found a dog.	3	_____	+9 dB
6. The driver lost his way.	3	_____	+6 dB
7. They stared at the picture.	3	_____	+3 dB
8. The cat drank from the saucer.	3	_____	+0 dB
9. The oven door was open.	3	_____	-3 dB
10. The silly boy is hiding.	3	_____	-6 dB

Total Key Word Correct_____

SNR-50= (23.5)-(# Correct)=_____dB

Average SNR-50, Lists 5A and 5B=   _____dB

List Pair 6

List 6A	Key Words	#Correct	SNR
1. A boy ran down the path.	4	_____	+21 dB
2. The orange was very sweet.	3	_____	+18 dB
3. He is holding his nose.	3	_____	+15 dB
4. The new road is on the map.	3	_____	+12 dB
5. The boy forgot his book.	3	_____	+9 dB
6. A friend came for lunch.	3	_____	+6 dB
7. The match boxes are empty.	3	_____	+3 dB
8. The family bought a house.	3	_____	+0 dB
9. The ball broke the window.	3	_____	-3 dB
10. The pond water is dirty.	3	_____	-6 dB

Total Key Word Correct_____

SNR-50= (23.5)-(# Correct)=_____dB

List 6B	Key Words	#Correct	SNR
1. They are running past the house.	4	_____	+21 dB
2. The police are clearing the road.	3	_____	+18 dB
3. She writes to her brother.	3	_____	+15 dB
4. The book tells a story.	3	_____	+12 dB
5. They are climbing the tree.	3	_____	+9 dB
6. She stood near her window.	3	_____	+6 dB
7. The baby broke his cup.	3	_____	+3 dB
8. The dinner plate is hot.	3	_____	+0 dB
9. A dish towel is by the sink.	3	_____	-3 dB
10. The good boy is helping.	3	_____	-6 dB

Total Key Word Correct_____

SNR-50= (23.5)-(# Correct)=_____dB

Average SNR-50, Lists 6A and 6B=   _____dB

List Pair 7

List 7A	Key Words	#Correct	SNR
1. Men wear long pants.	4	_____	+21 dB
2. The two farmers are talking.	3	_____	+18 dB
3. Father wrote a letter.	3	_____	+15 dB
4. The food cost a lot.	3	_____	+12 dB
5. The girl is washing her hair.	3	_____	+9 dB
6. He lost his hat.	3	_____	+6 dB
7. The faucets are above the sink.	3	_____	+3 dB
8. They had some cold meat.	3	_____	+0 dB
9. The children helped the milkman.	3	_____	-3 dB
10. The rice pudding was ready.	3	_____	-6 dB

Total Key Word Correct_____

SNR-50= (23.5)-(# Correct)=_____dB

List 7B	Key Words	#Correct	SNR
1. The boy slipped on the stairs.	4	_____	+21 dB
2. The snow is on the roof.	3	_____	+18 dB
3. Sugar is very sweet.	3	_____	+15 dB
4. The washing machine broke.	3	_____	+12 dB
5. They are clearing the table.	3	_____	+9 dB
6. She hurt her hand.	3	_____	+6 dB
7. The cup is on the saucer.	3	_____	+3 dB
8. The boy got into trouble.	3	_____	+0 dB
9. The truck carried fruit.	3	_____	-3 dB
10. The ice cream was pink.	3	_____	-6 dB

Total Key Word Correct_____

SNR-50= (23.5)-(# Correct)= _____dB

Average SNR-50, Lists 7A and 7B=   _____dB

List Pair 8

List 8A	Key Words	#Correct	SNR
1. They washed in cold water.	4	_____	+21 dB
2. The dog sleeps in a basket.	3	_____	+18 dB
3. An old woman was at home.	3	_____	+15 dB
4. The girl played with the baby.	3	_____	+12 dB
5. The children washed the plate/plates.	3	_____	+9 dB
6. The match fell on the floor.	3	_____	+6 dB
7. The shop closed for lunch.	3	_____	+3 dB
8. The boy hurried to school.	3	_____	+0 dB
9. Flowers grow in the garden.	3	_____	-3 dB
10. The children waved at the train.	3	_____	-6 dB

Total Key Word Correct_____

SNR-50= (23.5)-(# Correct)= _____dB

List 8B	Key Words	#Correct	SNR
1. They broke all the eggs.	4	_____	+21 dB
2. The car hit a wall.	3	_____	+18 dB
3. They are riding their bicycles.	3	_____	+15 dB
4. He broke his leg.	3	_____	+12 dB
5. The shirts are hanging in the closet.	3	_____	+9 dB
6. The ground was very hard.	3	_____	+6 dB
7. The buckets hold water.	3	_____	+3 dB
8. The chicken laid some eggs.	3	_____	+0 dB
9. He/ She had her spending money.	3	_____	-3 dB
10. He is bringing his raincoat.	3	_____	-6 dB

Total Key Word Correct_____

SNR-50= (23.5)-(# Correct)=_____dB

Average SNR-50, Lists 8A and 8B=   _____dB

List Pair 9

List 9A	Key Words	#Correct	SNR
1. The <u>football</u> <u>player</u> <u>lost</u> a <u>shoe</u>.	4	_____	+21 dB
2. The <u>painter</u> <u>used</u> a <u>brush</u>.	3	_____	+18 dB
3. The <u>lady</u> <u>sat</u> on her <u>chair</u>.	3	_____	+15 dB
4. The <u>milkman</u> <u>brought</u> the <u>cream</u>.	3	_____	+12 dB
5. The <u>dog</u> <u>chased</u> the <u>cat</u>.	3	_____	+9 dB
6. <u>Mother</u> <u>shut</u> the <u>window</u>.	3	_____	+6 dB
7. The <u>apple</u> <u>pie</u> was <u>good</u>.	3	_____	+3 dB
8. <u>Rain</u> <u>falls</u> from the <u>clouds</u>.	3	_____	+0 dB

Total Key Word Correct_____
SNR-50=(23.5)-(# Correct)= _____dB

List 9B	Key Words	#Correct	SNR
1. <u>They</u> <u>carried</u> some <u>shopping</u> <u>bags</u>.	4	_____	+21 dB
2. <u>They</u> <u>laughed</u> at his <u>story</u>.	3	_____	+18 dB
3. The <u>small</u> <u>boy</u> was <u>asleep</u>.	3	_____	+15 dB
4. The <u>sun</u> <u>melted</u> the <u>snow</u>.	3	_____	+12 dB
5. The <u>truck</u> <u>drove</u> up the <u>road</u>.	3	_____	+9 dB
6. The <u>children</u> <u>dropped</u> the <u>bag</u>.	3	_____	+6 dB
7. The <u>dog</u> <u>came</u> <u>back</u>.	3	_____	+3 dB
8. She <u>found</u> her <u>purse</u>.	3	_____	+0 dB

Total Key Word Correct_____
SNR-50= (23.5)-(# Correct)= _____dB
Average SNR-50, Lists 9A and 9B=   _____dB

List Pair 10

List 10A	Key Words	#Correct	SNR
1. <u>She</u> <u>looked</u> <u>in</u> her <u>mirror</u>.	4	_____	+21 dB
2. The <u>dog</u> is <u>eating</u> some <u>meat</u>.	3	_____	+18 dB
3. A <u>boy</u> <u>broke</u> the <u>fence</u>.	3	_____	+15 dB
4. The <u>yellow</u> <u>pears</u> tasted <u>good</u>.	3	_____	+12 dB
5. The <u>lady</u> <u>washed</u> the <u>shirt</u>.	3	_____	+9 dB
6. The <u>cup</u> is <u>hanging</u> on a <u>hook</u>.	3	_____	+6 dB
7. The <u>family</u> <u>likes</u> <u>fish</u>.	3	_____	+3 dB
8. The <u>baby</u> <u>is</u> on the <u>rug</u>.	3	_____	+0 dB

Total Key Word Correct_____
SNR-50= (23.5)-(# Correct)= _____dB

List 10B	Key Words	#Correct	SNR
1. <u>They</u> <u>waited</u> for <u>one</u> <u>hour</u>.	4	_____	+21 dB
2. The <u>fruit</u> <u>is</u> on the <u>ground</u>.	3	_____	+18 dB
3. The <u>girl</u> has a <u>picture</u> <u>book</u>.	3	_____	+15 dB
4. The <u>jug</u> <u>is</u> on the <u>shelf</u>.	3	_____	+12 dB
5. <u>They</u> are <u>shopping</u> for <u>cheese</u>.	3	_____	+9 dB
6. The <u>bus</u> <u>stopped</u> <u>suddenly</u>.	3	_____	+6 dB
7. The <u>three</u> <u>girls</u> are <u>listening</u>.	3	_____	+3 dB
8. The <u>coat</u> <u>is</u> on the <u>chair</u>.	3	_____	+0 dB

Total Key Word Correct_____
SNR-50= (23.5)-(# Correct)= _____dB
Average SNR-50, Lists 10A and 10B=   dB

List Pair 11

List 11A	Key Words	#Correct	SNR
1. <u>Father</u> <u>paid</u> <u>at</u> the <u>gate</u>.	4	_____	+21 dB
2. A <u>girl</u> <u>came</u> into the <u>room</u>.	3	_____	+18 dB
3. The <u>cat</u> <u>caught</u> a <u>mouse</u>.	3	_____	+15 dB
4. <u>She</u> <u>made</u> her <u>bed</u>.	3	_____	+12 dB
5. <u>Bananas</u> are <u>yellow</u> <u>fruit</u>.	3	_____	+9 dB
6. The <u>coffee</u> <u>cups</u> are on the <u>table</u>.	3	_____	+6 dB
7. The <u>basketball</u> <u>team</u> is <u>playing</u>.	3	_____	+3 dB
8. <u>Father</u> <u>picked</u> some <u>pears</u>.	3	_____	+0 dB

Total Key Word Correct_____
SNR-50= (23.5)-(# Correct)= _____dB

List 11B	Key Words	#Correct	SNR
1. <u>She</u> <u>spoke</u> to <u>her</u> <u>son</u>.	4	_____	+21 dB
2. The <u>clown</u> had a <u>funny</u> <u>face</u>.	3	_____	+18 dB
3. <u>She</u> <u>cut</u> with her <u>knife</u>.	3	_____	+15 dB
4. The <u>house</u> had <u>nine</u> <u>rooms</u>.	3	_____	+12 dB
5. The <u>mailman</u> <u>shut</u> the <u>gate</u>.	3	_____	+9 dB
6. The <u>rain</u> <u>came</u> <u>down</u>.	3	_____	+6 dB
7. The <u>old</u> <u>gloves</u> are <u>dirty</u>.	3	_____	+3 dB
8. The <u>boy</u> <u>knew</u> the <u>game</u>.	3	_____	+0 dB

Total Key Word Correct_____
SNR-50= (23.5)-(# Correct)= _____dB
Average SNR-50, Lists 11A and 11B=   dB

List Pair 12

List 12A	Key Words	#Correct	SNR
1. <u>They</u> <u>heard</u> a <u>funny</u> <u>noise</u>.	4	_____	+21 dB
2. <u>Snow</u> <u>falls</u> at <u>Christmas</u>.	3	_____	+18 dB
3. <u>She</u> is <u>taking</u> her <u>coat</u>.	3	_____	+15 dB
4. The <u>police</u> <u>chased</u> the <u>car</u>.	3	_____	+12 dB
5. The <u>lady</u> is <u>making</u> a <u>toy</u>.	3	_____	+9 dB
6. Some <u>sticks</u> were <u>under</u> the <u>tree</u>.	3	_____	+6 dB
7. The <u>little</u> <u>baby</u> is <u>sleeping</u>.	3	_____	+3 dB
8. <u>School</u> <u>finished</u> <u>early</u> today.	3	_____	+0 dB

Total Key Word Correct_____
SNR-50= (23.5)-(# Correct)= _____dB
SNR-50= (23.5)-(# Correct)= _____dB

List 12B	Key Words	#Correct	SNR
1. <u>They</u> <u>walked</u> <u>across</u> the <u>grass</u>.	4	_____	+21 dB
2. The <u>children</u> are <u>all</u> <u>eating</u>.	3	_____	+18 dB
3. The <u>angry</u> <u>man</u> <u>shouted</u>.	3	_____	+15 dB
4. <u>They</u> are <u>drinking</u> <u>tea</u>.	3	_____	+12 dB
5. <u>Mother</u> <u>opened</u> the <u>drawer</u>.	3	_____	+9 dB
6. <u>He</u> <u>dropped</u> his <u>money</u>.	3	_____	+6 dB
7. The <u>kitchen</u> <u>window</u> was <u>clean</u>.	3	_____	+3 dB
8. <u>She</u> is <u>helping</u> her <u>friend</u>.	3	_____	+0 dB

Total Key Word Correct_____
SNR-50= (23.5)-(# Correct)= _____dB
Average SNR-50, Lists 12A and 12B=   dB

List Pair 13

List 13A	Key Words	#Correct	SNR
1. The <u>young</u> <u>boy</u> <u>left</u> <u>home</u>.	4	_____	+21 dB
2. The <u>glass</u> <u>bowl</u> <u>broke</u>.	3	_____	+18 dB
3. The <u>teapot</u> is <u>very</u> <u>hot</u>.	3	_____	+15 dB
4. The <u>children</u> are <u>walking</u> <u>home</u>.	3	_____	+12 dB
5. The <u>man</u> <u>cleaned</u> his <u>shoes</u>.	3	_____	+9 dB
6. <u>Father</u> <u>looked</u> at the <u>book</u>.	3	_____	+6 dB
7. <u>She</u> <u>drinks</u> from her <u>cup</u>.	3	_____	+3 dB
8. A <u>girl</u> <u>kicked</u> the <u>table</u>.	3	_____	+0 dB

Total Key Word Correct_____
SNR-50= (23.5)-(# Correct)= _____dB
SNR-50= (23.5)-(# Correct)= _____dB

List 13B	Key Words	#Correct	SNR
1. The <u>plant</u> is <u>hanging</u> <u>above</u> the <u>door</u>.	4	_____	+21 dB
2. The <u>table</u> has <u>three</u> <u>legs</u>.	3	_____	+18 dB
3. A <u>letter</u> <u>fell</u> on the <u>floor</u>.	3	_____	+15 dB
4. The <u>five</u> <u>men</u> are <u>working</u>.	3	_____	+12 dB
5. The <u>shoes</u> were <u>very</u> <u>dirty</u>.	3	_____	+9 dB
6. <u>They</u> <u>went</u> on a <u>vacation</u>.	3	_____	+6 dB
7. The <u>lady</u> <u>packed</u> her <u>bag</u>.	3	_____	+3 dB
8. The <u>child</u> <u>drank</u> some <u>milk</u>.	3	_____	+0 dB

Total Key Word Correct_____
SNR-50= (23.5)-(# Correct)= _____dB
Average SNR-50, Lists 13A and 13B=   _____dB

List Pair 14

List 14A	Key Words	#Correct	SNR
1. He <u>listened</u> <u>to</u> his <u>father</u>.	4	_____	+21 dB
2. The <u>machine</u> was <u>very</u> <u>noisy</u>.	3	_____	+18 dB
3. The <u>old</u> <u>man</u> is <u>worried</u>.	3	_____	+15 dB
4. <u>They</u> are <u>crossing</u> the <u>street</u>.	3	_____	+12 dB
5. <u>Lemons</u> <u>grow</u> on <u>trees</u>.	3	_____	+9 dB
6. The <u>girl</u> <u>lost</u> her <u>doll</u>.	3	_____	+6 dB
7. The <u>mud</u> <u>stuck</u> on his <u>shoe</u>.	3	_____	+3 dB
8. The <u>bath</u> <u>towel</u> was <u>wet</u>.	3	_____	+0 dB

Total Key Word Correct_____
SNR-50= (23.5)-(# Correct)= _____dB
SNR-50= (23.5)-(# Correct)= _____dB

List 14B	Key Words	#Correct	SNR
1. The <u>big</u> <u>boy</u> <u>kicked</u> the <u>ball</u>.	4	_____	+21 dB
2. Some <u>nice</u> <u>people</u> are <u>coming</u>.	3	_____	+18 dB
3. <u>She</u> <u>bumped</u> her <u>head</u>.	3	_____	+15 dB
4. The <u>tiny</u> <u>baby</u> was <u>pretty</u>.	3	_____	+12 dB
5. The <u>daughter</u> <u>set</u> the <u>table</u>.	3	_____	+9 dB
6. <u>Mother</u> <u>tied</u> the <u>string</u>.	3	_____	+6 dB
7. The <u>train</u> <u>stops</u> at the <u>station</u>.	3	_____	+3 dB
8. The <u>puppy</u> <u>plays</u> with the <u>ball</u>.	3	_____	+0 dB

Total Key Word Correct_____
SNR-50= (23.5)-(# Correct)= _____dB
Average SNR-50, Lists 14A and 14B=   _____dB

List Pair 15

List 15A	Key Words	#Correct	SNR
1. He <u>wore</u> his <u>yellow</u> <u>shirt</u>.	4	_____	+21 dB
2. The <u>matches</u> <u>are</u> on the <u>shelf</u>.	3	_____	+18 dB
3. The <u>train</u> had a <u>bad</u> <u>accident</u>.	3	_____	+15 dB
4. The <u>kitchen</u> <u>sink</u> is <u>empty</u>.	3	_____	+12 dB
5. The <u>park</u> is <u>near</u> the <u>road</u>.	3	_____	+9 dB
6. The <u>cook</u> <u>cut</u> up some <u>onions</u>.	3	_____	+6 dB
7. <u>He</u> is <u>washing</u> his <u>face</u>.	3	_____	+3 dB
8. <u>Somebody</u> <u>took</u> the <u>money</u>.	3	_____	+0 dB

Total Key Word Correct_____
SNR-50= (23.5)-(# Correct)= _____dB
SNR-50= (23.5)-(# Correct)= _____dB

List 15B	Key Words	#Correct	SNR
1. <u>They</u> <u>sat</u> on a <u>wooden</u> <u>bench</u>.	4	_____	+21 dB
2. The <u>man</u> <u>tied</u> his <u>shoes</u>.	3	_____	+18 dB
3. The <u>flowers</u> <u>grow</u> in a <u>pot</u>.	3	_____	+15 dB
4. The <u>dog</u> <u>drank</u> from a <u>bowl</u>.	3	_____	+12 dB
5. The <u>cow</u> <u>is/was</u> on the <u>grass</u>.	3	_____	+9 dB
6. <u>He</u> <u>frightened</u> his <u>sister</u>.	3	_____	+6 dB
7. The <u>ladder</u> is <u>near</u> the <u>door</u>.	3	_____	+3 dB
8. The <u>janitor</u> <u>used</u> a <u>broom</u>.	3	_____	+0 dB

Total Key Word Correct_____
SNR-50= (23.5)-(# Correct)= _____dB
Average SNR-50, Lists 15A and 15B=   _____dB

List Pair 16

List 16A	Key Words	#Correct	SNR
1. The <u>big</u> <u>fish</u> got <u>away</u>.	4	_____	+21 dB
2. The <u>dogs</u> <u>went</u> for a <u>walk</u>.	3	_____	+18 dB
3. The <u>driver</u> <u>waited</u> by the <u>corner</u>.	3	_____	+15 dB
4. <u>They</u> <u>finished</u> the <u>dinner</u>.	3	_____	+12 dB
5. <u>Mother</u> <u>picked</u> some <u>flowers</u>.	3	_____	+9 dB
6. A <u>fish</u> <u>swam</u> in the <u>pond</u>.	3	_____	+6 dB
7. The <u>front</u> <u>garden</u> was <u>pretty</u>.	3	_____	+3 dB
8. <u>She</u> is <u>waiting</u> for her <u>bus</u>.	3	_____	+0 dB

Total Key Word Correct_____
SNR-50= (23.5)-(# Correct)= _____dB
SNR-50= (23.5)-(# Correct)= _____dB

List 16B	Key Words	#Correct	SNR
1. A <u>cat</u> <u>jumped</u> <u>off</u> the <u>fence</u>.	4	_____	+21 dB
2. <u>They</u> are <u>going</u> <u>out</u>.	3	_____	+18 dB
3. The <u>football</u> <u>hit</u> the <u>goalpost</u>.	3	_____	+15 dB
4. The <u>dishcloth</u> is <u>very</u> <u>wet</u>.	3	_____	+12 dB
5. The <u>baby</u> has <u>blue</u> <u>eyes</u>.	3	_____	+9 dB
6. The <u>girl</u> <u>caught</u> a <u>cold</u>.	3	_____	+6 dB
7. The <u>raincoat</u> is <u>hanging</u> <u>up</u>.	3	_____	+3 dB
8. <u>She</u> <u>brushed</u> her <u>hair</u>.	3	_____	+0 dB

Total Key Word Correct_____
SNR-50= (23.5)-(# Correct)= _____dB
Average SNR-50, Lists 16A and 16B=   _____dB

List Pair 17

List 17A	Key Words	#Correct	SNR
1. They met some friends.	4	_____	+21 dB
2. The bread truck is coming.	3	_____	+18 dB
3. The picture came from a book.	3	_____	+15 dB
4. The boy had a toy dragon.	3	_____	+12 dB
5. They are playing in the park.	3	_____	+9 dB
6. She argued with her sister.	3	_____	+6 dB
7. He is cleaning his car.	3	_____	+3 dB
8. The mouse found the cheese.	3	_____	+0 dB

Total Key Word Correct_____

SNR-50= (23.5)-(# Correct)= _____dB

SNR-50= (23.5)-(# Correct)= _____dB

List 17B	Key Words	#Correct	SNR
1. They like orange marmalade.	4	_____	+21 dB
2. The apple pie is baking.	3	_____	+18 dB
3. He drinks from his mug.	3	_____	+15 dB
4. The sky was very blue.	3	_____	+12 dB
5. They knocked on the window.	3	_____	+9 dB
6. People are going home.	3	_____	+6 dB
7. The baby wants his bottle.	3	_____	+3 dB
8. They had some chocolate pudding.	3	_____	+0 dB

Total Key Word Correct_____

SNR-50= (23.5)-(# Correct)= _____dB

Average SNR-50, Lists 17A and 17B= _____dB

List Pair 18

List 18A	Key Words	#Correct	SNR
1. The milkman drives a small truck.	4	_____	+21 dB
2. The scissors are very sharp.	3	_____	+18 dB
3. She is calling her daughter.	3	_____	+15 dB
4. The girl ran along.	3	_____	+12 dB
5. Mother read the paper.	3	_____	+9 dB
6. The bakery is open.	3	_____	+6 dB
7. She talks/talked to her doll.	3	_____	+3 dB
8. The police helped the driver.	3	_____	+0 dB

Total Key Word Correct_____

SNR-50= (23.5)-(# Correct)= _____dB

SNR-50= (23.5)-(# Correct)= _____dB

List 18B	Key Words	#Correct	SNR
1. They are pushing an old car.	4	_____	+21 dB
2. He needed his vacation.	3	_____	+18 dB
3. She is washing her dress.	3	_____	+15 dB
4. The cow gave some milk.	3	_____	+12 dB
5. The football game is over.	3	_____	+9 dB
6. The bath water was warm.	3	_____	+6 dB
7. The floor looked clean.	3	_____	+3 dB
8. Some men shave in the morning.	3	_____	+0 dB

Total Key Word Correct_____

SNR-50= (23.5)-(# Correct)= _____dB

Average SNR-50, Lists 18A and 18B= _____dB

Appendix V

Az Bio Sentence Test Score Sheet

Name:_____

Date: _____

List 1

Sentence	Text	Poss	Score
1	The pool was filled with dirt and leaves.	8	
2	He ducked under the counter to avoid eye contact.	9	
3	What are you feeding this dog?	6	
4	Do you think this is easy?	6	
5	Today we honor a legend.	5	
6	Traffic school was not where I wanted to be.	9	
7	She struggled with a significant weight problem.	7	
8	You are welcome, regardless of your age.	7	
9	I have a sneaking suspicion history will repeat itself.	9	
10	There is no need to be cruel.	7	
11	They cleaned the office for the new faculty member.	9	
12	He cried when the pet goat was sent to market.	10	
13	He did not have an original thought in his head.	10	
14	Do you believe in miracles?	5	
15	How does a lizard's tail grow back?	7	
16	The dog ate the snow.	5	
17	Try to stay focused on the task at hand.	9	
18	The bone structure of her face was striking.	8	
19	She directly said no to the family's plea.	8	
20	It was the first time she ever offered to pay.	10	

Words Correct _____

Words Possible   **154**

Percent Correct   ☐

Appendix W

BEST Sentences

BEST- Test List 1
Track 4   Score= Noise =

He	lock	ed	the	car	door			/6	_____
She	is	eat	ing	a	meat	pie		/7	_____
They	are	paint	ing	the	house			/6	_____
The	teach	er	is	mark	ing	home	work	/8	_____
A	lamb	is	drink	ing	milk			/6	_____
A	naughtyboy	climb	ed	the	fence			/7	_____
A	girl	twist	ed	her	ankle			/6	_____
Child	ren	play	on	the	park	swing	s	/8	_____
The	boss	wait	ed	for	the	lift		/7	_____
A	cat	crept	up	the	stair	s		/7	_____
The	run	ner	is	go	ing	fast		/7	_____
He	is	rid	ing	on	the	foot	path	/8	_____
The	whole	class	went	out	side			/6	_____
The	old	lady	was	tired				/5	_____
Lollie	s	taste	very	sweet				/5	_____
The	fresh	bread	is	bak	ing			/6	_____

1) Average of midpoint of reversals (dB SPL) _____
2) S/N ratio at SRT _____

BEST- Test List 2
Track 5   Score= Noise =

A	lady	drink	s	white	wine			/6	_____
She	wrote	a	long	story				/5	_____
The	child	ren	ate	all	the	grape	s	/8	_____
Grand	pa	is	sweep	ing	the	path		/7	_____
A	man	is	play	ing	the	drum	s	/8	_____
The	cat	chas	ed	a	butter	fly		/7	_____
Those	girl	s	are	play	ing	net	ball	/8	_____
She	walk	s	past	the	shop	s		/7	_____
The	apple	fell	on	the	floor			/6	_____
Boat	s	float	on	water				/5	_____
This	coat	is	very	warm				/5	_____
The	back	pack	was	quite	heavy			/6	_____
My	old	er	sister	is	sing	ing		/7	_____

1) Average of midpoint of reversals (dB SPL) _____
2) S/N ratio at SRT _____

BEST- Test List 3
Track 6   Score= Noise =

Doctor	s	help	sick	people				/5	_____
The	dog	dig	s	a	deep	hole		/7	_____
A	clean	er	dust	ed	the	shelf		/7	_____
He	rode	the	small	horse				/5	_____
The	student	s	are	play	ing	game	s	/8	_____
He	is	clear	ing	the	back	yard		/7	_____
Grand	ma	is	hid	ing	the	present		/7	_____
She	crawl	s	under	the	table			/6	_____
The	child	is	drink	ing	slow	ly		/7	_____
The	lady	pay	s	by	credit	card		/7	_____
The	girl	is	read	ing	in	bed		/7	_____
They	ran	to	the	bus	stop			/6	_____
A	baby	slept	in	the	car			/6	_____
A	jewelry	box	was	lost				/5	_____
That	old	picture	is	beauti	ful			/6	_____
A	little	boy	is	swim	ming			/6	_____

1) Average of midpoint of reversals (dB SPL) _____
2) S/N ratio at SRT _____

BEST- Test List 4

Track 7   **Score= Noise =**

He	carrie	s	the	rubbish	bin			/6	_____
Mum	is	sweep	ing	the	floor			/6	_____
The	man	forgot	his	rain	coat			/6	_____
The	girl	play	ed	the	guitar			/6	_____
She	drove	a	red	car				/5	_____
He	is	climb	ing	the	lemon	tree		/7	_____
They	are	sing	ing	a	new	song		/7	_____
A	boy	stepp	ed	on	a	nail		/7	_____
The	mail	came	early					/4	_____
The	snow	man	melt	ed	in	the	sun	/8	_____
A	door	open	ed	quiet	ly			/6	_____
A	ball	bounc	ed	over	the	fence		/7	_____
A	police	man	shout	s	angri	ly		/7	_____
The	little	bug	s	are	yellow			/6	_____
Fresh	fruit	salad	is	good				/5	_____
A	foot	ball	team	is	train	ing		/7	_____

1) Average of midpoint of reversals (dB SPL) _____

2) S/N ratio at SRT _____

BEST- Test List 5

Track 8   **Score= Noise =**

My	sister	clean	ed	the	bath	room	/7	_____
He	won	a	lot	of	money		/6	_____
The	girl	is	blow	ing	her	nose	/7	_____
Some	one	lost	a	pencil	case		/6	_____
A	horse	ate	the	apple	s		/6	_____
The	boy	ask	ed	a	question		/6	_____
Dad	is	wear	ing	new	shoe	s	/7	_____
He	went	for	a	long	drive		/6	_____
The	student	s	travel	by	train		/6	_____
A	ball	roll	s	down	the	hill	/7	_____
A	spider	climb	ed	up	the	wall	/7	_____
The	turtle	walk	ed	slow	ly		/6	_____
They	ran	away	from	the	house		/6	_____
That	baby	sitter	is	nice			/5	_____
The	orange	was	very	juicy			/5	_____
A	little	dog	is	bark	ing		/6	_____

1) Average of midpoint of reversals (dB SPL) _____

2) S/N ratio at SRT _____

BEST- Test List 6

Track 9   **Score= Noise =**

The	doctor	wrote	a	letter				/5	_____
They	are	eat	ing	straw	berries			/6	_____
The	family	had	a	picnic	lunch			/6	_____
We	had	pop	corn	with	butter			/6	_____
My	friend	wear	s	hearing	aid	s		/7	_____
They	built	a	big	house				/5	_____
Most	people	like	chocolate					/4	_____
Two	lollie	s	were	in	the	bag		/7	_____
A	boy	sang	soft	ly				/5	_____
A	bird	flew	across	the	lake			/6	_____
Mum	is	run	ning	in	a	race		/7	_____
The	girl	s	dance	beauti	ful	ly		/7	_____
Monkey	s	sleep	in	tree	s			/6	_____
These	new	shoe	s	are	red			/6	_____
The	school	book	s	are	expensive			/6	_____
A	search	party	is	com	ing			/6	_____

1) Average of midpoint of reversals (dB SPL) _____

2) S/N ratio at SRT _____

Appendix X

Hearing Handicap for the Elderly (HHIE)

Name: _____ Date: _____

The purpose of this scale is to identify the problems your hearing loss may be causing you. Check 'Yes,' 'Sometimes,' or 'No' for each question. Do not skip any questions. If you use a hearing aid, please answer the way you hear without a hearing aid.

	Yes	Sometimes	No
1. Does a hearing problem cause you to use the phone less often than you would like? (S)			
2. Does a hearing problem cause you to feel embarrassed when meeting new people? (E)			
3. Does a hearing problem cause you to avoid groups of people? (S)			
4. Does a hearing problem make you irritable? (E)			
5. Does a hearing problem cause you to feel frustrated when talking to members of your family? (E)			
6. Does a hearing problem cause you difficulty when attending a party? (S)			
7. Does a hearing problem cause you to feel "stupid" or "dumb?" (E)			
8. Do you have difficulty hearing when someone speaks in a whisper? (S)			
9. Do you feel handicapped by a hearing problem? (E)			
10. Does a hearing problem cause you difficulty when visiting friends, relatives, or neighbors? (S)			
11. Does a hearing problem cause you to attend religious services less often than you would like? (S)			
12. Does a hearing problem cause you to be nervous? (E)			
13. Does a hearing problem cause you to visit friends, relatives, or neighbors less often than you would like? (S)			

	Yes	Sometimes	No
14. Does a hearing problem cause you to have arguments with family members? (E)			
15. Does a hearing problem cause you difficulty when listening to TV or radio? (S)			
16. Does a hearing problem cause you to go shopping less often than you would like? (S)			
17. Does any problem or difficulty with your hearing upset you at all? (E)			
18. Does a hearing problem cause you to want to be by yourself? (E)			
19. Does a hearing problem cause you to talk to family members less often than you would like? (S)			
20. Do you feel that any difficulty with your hearing limits or hampers your personal or social life? (E)			
21. Does a hearing problem cause you difficulty when in a restaurant with relatives or friends? (S)			
22. Does a hearing problem cause you to feel depressed? (E)			
23. Does a hearing problem cause you to listen to TV or radio less often than you would like? (S)			
24. Does a hearing problem cause you to feel uncomfortable when talking to friends? (E)			
25. Does a hearing problem cause you to feel left out when you are with a group of people? (E)			

Ventry, I. M., & Weinstein, B. E. (1982). The Hearing Handicap Inventory for the Elderly: A new tool. *Ear and Hearing, 3*, 128-134.

For clinician use only:

Fill in the number of points for each question, 'Yes' = 4, 'Sometimes'= 2, 'No' = 0

Emotional (E) questions:

2 _____
4 _____
5 _____
7 _____
9 _____
12 _____
14 _____
17 _____
18 _____
20 _____
22 _____
24 _____
25 _____

Subtotal E: _____
(52 maximum)

Situational (S) questions:

1 _____
3 _____
6 _____
8 _____
10 _____
11 _____
13 _____
15 _____
16 _____
19 _____
21 _____
23 _____

Subtotal S: _____
(48 Maximum)

Determine presence of perceived emotional and situational hearing handicaps based on E and S scores.

0–16: No Handicap
17– 42: Mild to Moderate Handicap
> or = 43: Significant Handicap

Appendix Y

Hearing Handicap for the Elderly (HHIE)—Screening

Name: _____   Date: _____

The purpose of this scale is to identify the problems your hearing loss may be causing you. Check 'Yes,' 'Sometimes,' or 'No' for each question. Do not skip any questions. If you use a hearing aid, please answer the way you hear without a hearing aid.

	Yes	Sometimes	No
1. Does a hearing problem cause you to feel embarrassed when meeting new people?			
2. Does a hearing problem cause you to feel frustrated when talking to members of your family?			
3. Do you have difficulty hearing when someone speaks in a whisper?			
4. Do you feel handicapped by a hearing problem?			
5. Does a hearing problem cause you difficulty when visiting friends, relatives, or neighbors?			
6. Does a hearing problem cause you to attend religious services less often than you would like?			
7. Does a hearing problem cause you to have arguments with family members?			
8. Does a hearing problem cause you difficulty when listening to TV or radio?			
9. Do you feel that any difficulty with your hearing limits or hampers your personal or social life?			
10. Does a hearing problem cause you difficulty when in a restaurant with relatives or friends?			

Appendix Z

Hearing Handicap for Adults (HHIA)

Name: _____ Date: _____

The purpose of this scale is to identify the problems your hearing loss may be causing you. Check 'Yes,' 'Sometimes,' or 'No' for each question. Do not skip any questions. If you use a hearing aid, please answer the way you hear without a hearing aid.

	Yes	Sometimes	No
1. Does a hearing problem cause you to use the phone less often than you would like? (S)			
2. Does a hearing problem cause you to feel embarrassed when meeting new people? (E)			
3. Does a hearing problem cause you to avoid groups of people? (S)			
4. Does a hearing problem make you irritable? (E)			
5. Does a hearing problem cause you to feel frustrated when talking to members of your family? (E)			
6. Does a hearing problem cause you difficulty when attending a party? (S)			
7. Does a hearing problem cause you difficulty hearing/understanding co-workers, clients or customers? (S)			
8. Do you feel handicapped by a hearing problem? (E)			
9. Does a hearing problem cause you difficulty when visiting friends, relatives, or neighbors? (S)			
10. Does a hearing problem cause you to feel frustrated when talking co-workers, clients or customers? (E)			
11. Does a hearing problem cause you difficulty in the movies or theater? (S)			
12. Dose a hearing problem cause you to be nervous? (E)			
13. Does a hearing problem cause you to visit friends, relatives, or neighbors less often than you would like? (S)			

	Yes	Sometimes	No
14. Does a hearing problem cause you to have arguments with family members? (E)			
15. Does a hearing problem cause you difficulty when listening to TV or radio? (S)			
16. Does a hearing problem cause you to go shopping less often than you would like? (S)			
17. Does any problem or difficulty with your hearing upset you at all? (E)			
18. Does a hearing problem cause you to want to be by yourself? (E)			
19. Does a hearing problem cause you to talk to family members less often than you would like? (S)			
20. Do you feel that any difficulty with your hearing limits or hampers your personal or social life? (E)			
21. Does a hearing problem cause you difficulty when in a restaurant with relatives or friends? (S)			
22. Does a hearing problem cause you to feel depressed? (E)			
23. Does a hearing problem cause you to listen to TV or radio less often than you would like? (S)			
24. Does a hearing problem cause you to feel uncomfortable when talking to friends? (E)			
25. Does a hearing problem cause you to feel left out when you are with a group of people? (E)			

For clinician use only:

Fill in the number of points for each question, 'Yes' = 4, 'Sometimes'= 2, 'No' = 0

Emotional (E) questions:	Situational (S) questions:
2 _____	1 _____
4 _____	3 _____
5 _____	6 _____
8 _____	7 _____
10 _____	9 _____
12 _____	11 _____
14 _____	13 _____
17 _____	15 _____
18 _____	16 _____
20 _____	19 _____
22 _____	21 _____
24 _____	23 _____
25 _____	

Subtotal E: _____   Subtotal S: _____
(52 maximum)   (48 Maximum)

Determine presence of perceived emotional and situational hearing handicaps based on E and S scores.

> 0–16: No Handicap
> 17– 42: Mild to Moderate Handicap
> > or = 43: Significant Handicap

Appendix AA

Hearing Handicap for Adults (HHIA)—Screening

Name: _____ Date: _____

The purpose of this scale is to identify the problems your hearing loss may be causing you. Check 'Yes,' 'Sometimes,' or 'No' for each question. Do not skip any questions. If you use a hearing aid, please answer the way you hear without a hearing aid.

	Yes	Sometimes	No
1. Does a hearing problem cause you to feel embarrassed when meeting new people?			
2. Does a hearing problem cause you to feel frustrated when talking to members of your family?			
3. Does a hearing problem cause you difficulty hearing/understanding co-workers, clients or customers?			
4. Do you feel handicapped by a hearing problem?			
5. Does a hearing problem cause you difficulty when visiting friends, relatives, or neighbors?			
6. Does a hearing problem cause you difficulty in the movies or theater?			
7. Does a hearing problem cause you to have arguments with family members?			
8. Does a hearing problem cause you difficulty when listening to TV or radio?			
9. Do you feel that any difficulty with your hearing limits or hampers your personal or social life?			
10. Does a hearing problem cause you difficulty when in a restaurant with relatives or friends?			

Appendix AB

Abbreviated Profile of Hearing Aid Benefit

NAME: _____ ☐ Male ☐ Female TODAY'S DATE: ___/___/___
Last   First

INSTRUCTIONS: Please circle the answers that come closest to your everyday experience. Notice that each choice includes a percentage. You can use this to help you decide on your answer. For example, if a statement is true about 75% of the time, circle "C" for that item. If you have not experienced the situation we describe, try to think of a similar situation that you have been in and respond for that situation. If you have no idea, leave that item blank.

A Always (99%)
B Almost Always (87%)
C Generally (75%)
D Half-the-time (50%)
E Occasionally (25%)
F Seldom (12%)
G Never (1%)

	Without Hearing Aid	With Hearing Aid
1. When I am in a crowded grocery store, talking with the cashier, I can follow the conversation.	A B C D E F G	A B C D E F G
2. I miss a lot of information when I'm listening to a lecture.	A B C D E F G	A B C D E F G
3. Unexpected sounds, like a smoke detector or alarm bell are uncomfortable.	A B C D E F G	A B C D E F G
4. I have difficulty hearing a conversation when I'm with one of my family at home.	A B C D E F G	A B C D E F G
5. I have trouble understanding the dialogue in a movie or at the theater.	A B C D E F G	A B C D E F G
6. When I am listening to the news on the car radio, and family members are talking, I have trouble hearing the news.	A B C D E F G	A B C D E F G
7. When I'm at the dinner table with several people, and am trying to have a conversation with one person, understanding speech is difficult.	A B C D E F G	A B C D E F G
8. Traffic noises are too loud.	A B C D E F G	A B C D E F G
9. When I am talking with someone across a large empty room, I understand the words.	A B C D E F G	A B C D E F G
10. When I am in a small office, interviewing or answering questions, I have difficulty following the conversation.	A B C D E F G	A B C D E F G
11. When I am in a theater watching a movie or play, and the people around me are whispering and rustling paper wrappers, I can still make out the dialogue.	A B C D E F G	A B C D E F G
12. When I am having a quiet conversation with a friend, I have difficulty understanding.	A B C D E F G	A B C D E F G

A	Always (99%)
B	Almost Always (87%)
C	Generally (75%)
D	Half-the-time (50%)
E	Occasionally (25%)
F	Seldom (12%)
G	Never (1%)

	Without Hearing Aids	With Hearing Aids
13. The sounds of running water, such as a toilet or shower, are uncomfortably loud.	A B C D E F G	A B C D E F G
14. When a speaker is addressing a small group, and everyone is listening quietly, I have to strain to understand.	A B C D E F G	A B C D E F G
15. When I'm in a quiet conversation with my doctor in an examination room, it is hard to follow the conversation.	A B C D E F G	A B C D E F G
16. I can understand conversations even when several people are talking.	A B C D E F G	A B C D E F G
17. The sounds of construction work are uncomfortably loud.	A B C D E F G	A B C D E F G
18. It's hard for me to understand what is being said at lectures or church services.	A B C D E F G	A B C D E F G
19. I can communicate with others when we are in a crowd.	A B C D E F G	A B C D E F G
20. The sound of a fire engine siren close by is so loud that I need to cover my ears.	A B C D E F G	A B C D E F G
21. I can follow the words of a sermon when listening to a religious service.	A B C D E F G	A B C D E F G
22. The sound of screeching tires is uncomfortably loud.	A B C D E F G	A B C D E F G
23. I have to ask people to repeat themselves in one-on-one conversation in a quiet room.	A B C D E F G	A B C D E F G
24. I have trouble understanding others when an air conditioner or fan is on.	A B C D E F G	A B C D E F G

Please fill out these additional items.

HEARING AID EXPERIENCE:	DAILY HEARING AID USE	DEGREE OF HEARING DIFFICULTY (without wearing a hearing aid):
☐ None	☐ None	☐ None
☐ Less than 6 weeks	☐ Less than 1 hour per day	☐ Mild
☐ 6 weeks to 11 months	☐ 1 to 4 hours per day	☐ Moderate
☐ 1 to 10 years	☐ 4 to 8 hours per day	☐ Moderately-Severe
☐ Over 10 years	☐ 8 to 16 hours per day	☐ Severe

© University of Memphis, 1994

Appendix AC

APHAB: Items & Subscales

Form A

Ease of Communication (EC scale)

4. I have difficulty hearing a conversation when I'm with one of my family at home.

10. When I am in a small office, interviewing or answering questions, I have difficulty following the conversation.

12. When I am having a quiet conversation with a friend, I have difficulty understanding.

14. When a speaker is addressing a small group, and everyone is listening quietly, I have to strain to understand.

15. When I'm in a quiet conversation with my doctor in an examination room, it is hard to follow the conversation.

23. I have to ask people to repeat themselves in one-on-one conversation in a quiet room.

Background Noise (BN scale)

1. *(reversed)* When I am in a crowded grocery store, talking with the cashier, I can follow the conversation.

6. When I am listening to the news on the car radio, and family members are talking, I have trouble hearing the news.

7. When I am at the dinner table with several people, and am trying to have a conversation with one person, understanding speech is difficult.

16. *(reversed)* I can understand conversations even when several people are talking.

19. *(reversed)* I can communicate with others when we are in a crowd.

24. I have trouble understanding others when an air conditioner or fan is on.

Reverberation (RV scale)

2. I miss a lot of information when I'm listening to a lecture.

5. I have trouble understanding dialogue in a movie or at the theater.

9. *(reversed)* When I am talking with someone across a large empty room, I understand the words.

11. *(reversed)* When I am in a theater watching a movie or play, and the people around me are whispering and rustling paper wrappers, I can still make out the dialogue.

18. It's hard for me to understand what is being said at lectures or church services.

21. *(reversed)* I can follow the words of a sermon when listening to a religious service.

Aversiveness (AV scale)

3. Unexpected sounds, like a smoke detector or alarm bell are uncomfortable.

8. Traffic noises are too loud.

13. The sounds of running water, such as a toilet or shower, are uncomfortably loud.

17. The sounds of construction work are uncomfortably loud.

20. The sounds of a fire engine siren close by is so loud that I need to cover my ears.

22. The sound of screeching tires is uncomfortably loud.

APHAB: Items & Subscales

Form B

Ease of Communication (EC scale)

2. When a speaker is addressing a small group, and everyone is listening quietly, I have to strain to understand.

6. When I'm in a quiet conversation with my doctor in an examination room, it is hard to follow the conversation.

9. When I am having a quiet conversation with a friend, I have difficulty understanding.

15. When I am in a small office, interviewing or answering questions, I have difficulty following the conversation.

17. I have to ask people to repeat themselves in one-on-one conversation in a quiet room.

23. I have difficulty hearing a conversation when I'm with one of my family at home.

Background Noise (BN scale)

4. When I am at the dinner table with several people, and am trying to have a conversation with one person, understanding speech is difficult.

7. When I am listening to the news on the car radio, and family members are talking, I have trouble hearing the news.

10. (reversed) I can understand conversations even when several people are talking.

12. I have trouble understanding others when an air conditioner or fan is on.

20. (reversed) When I am in a crowded grocery store, talking with the cashier, I can follow the conversation.

21. (reversed) I can communicate with others when we are in a crowd.

Reverberation (RV scale)

3. It's hard for me to understand what is being said at lectures or church services.

5. (reversed) When I am in a theater watching a movie or play, and the people around me are whispering and rustling paper wrappers, I can still make out the dialogue.

13. I have trouble understanding dialogue in a movie or at the theater.

16. I miss a lot of information when I'm listening to a lecture.

19. (reversed) I can follow the words of a sermon when listening to a religious service.

24. (reversed) When I am talking with someone across a large empty room, I understand the words.

Aversiveness (AV scale)

1. The sounds of a fire engine siren close by is so loud that I need to cover my ears.

8. The sounds of running water, such as a toilet or shower, are uncomfortably loud.

11. The sounds of construction work are uncomfortably loud.

14. Traffic noises are too loud.

18. Unexpected sounds, like a smoke detector or alarm bell are uncomfortable.

22. The sound of screeching tires is uncomfortably loud.

Instructions for Manual Scoring of the APHAB

1)   Assign a value for each answer from the table below

Response	Not a Reversed Item	Reversed Item
A Always	99%	1%
B Almost always	87%	12%
C Generally	75%	25%
D Half-the-time	50%	50%
E Occasionally	25%	75%
F Seldom	12%	87%
G Never	1%	99%

2)   Calculate the average unaided score and average aided score for each subscale.

3)   The Global Score is the mean of the scores for all the items in the EC, RV and BN subscales.

4)   Benefit is calculated by subtracting the aided average from the unaided average. Make sure that you have responses for both unaided and aided on each item used for benefit calculation.

5)   Keep in mind that these scores show how frequently clients experience performance problems.

APHAB Norms

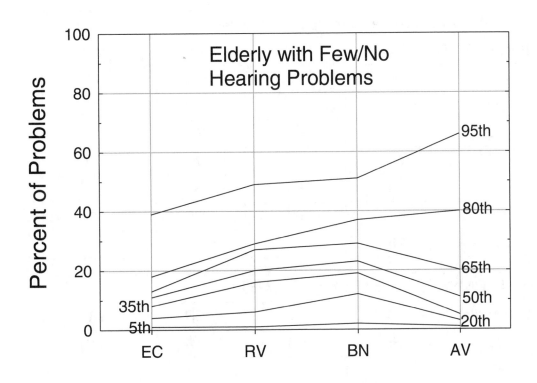

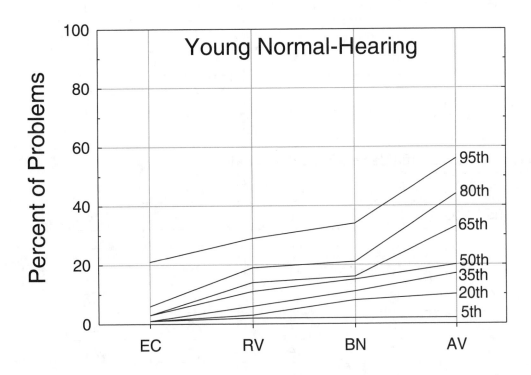

2005 APHAB Norms for WDRC-Capable Hearing Aids

Users of WDRC capable hearing aids- Unaided

Percentile	EC	RV	BN	AV
95	99	99	99	70
80	83	87	89	35
65	75	81	81	21
50	63	71	75	14
35	56	65	67	9
20	46	58	58	3
5	26	47	41	1

Users of WDRC capable hearing aids- Aided

Percentile	EC	RV	BN	AV
95	86	79	82	82
80	39	57	58	64
65	29	46	49	53
50	23	37	40	38
35	17	29	32	23
20	12	21	22	14
5	5	12	14	2

Users of WDRC capable hearing aids- Benefit

Percentile	EC	RV	BN	AV
95	76	70	56	16
80	52	52	47	0
65	46	41	39	-8
50	38	34	33	-13
35	29	27	23	-25
20	19	16	12	-41
5	-10	-3	-1	-61

Appendix AF

ECHO Questionnaire

NAME _____ GENDER M   F   DATE OF BIRTH ___/___/___   TODAY'S DATE ___/___/___

> **INSTRUCTIONS**
> *Listed below are statements about hearing aids. Please circle the letter that indicates the extent to which you agree with each statement. Use the list of words on the right to determine your answer.*

A   Not At All
B   A Little
C   Somewhat
D   Medium
E   Considerably
F   Greatly
G   Tremendously

How much do you agree with each statement?

1. My hearing aids will help me understand the people I speak with most frequently.	A B C D E F G
2. I will be frustrated when my hearing aids pick up sounds that keep me from hearing what I want to hear.	A B C D E F G
3. Getting hearing aids is in my best interest.	A B C D E F G
4. People will notice my hearing loss more when I wear my hearing aids.	A B C D E F G
5. My hearing aids will reduce the number of times I have to ask people to repeat.	A B C D E F G
6. My hearing aids will be worth the trouble.	A B C D E F G
7. Sometimes I will be bothered by an inability to get enough loudness from my hearing aids without feedback (whistling).	A B C D E F G
8. I will be content with the appearance of my hearing aids.	A B C D E F G
9. Using hearing aids will improve my self-confidence.	A B C D E F G

(Continued on next page)

A Not At All
B A Little
C Somewhat
D Medium
E Considerably
F Greatly
G Tremendously

How much do you agree with each statement?

10. My hearing aids will have a natural sound.	A B C D E F G
11. My hearing aids will be helpful on most telephones without amplifiers or loudspeakers. (If you hear well on the telephone *without* hearing aids, check here ☐)	A B C D E F G
12. The person who provides me with my hearing aids will be competent.	A B C D E F G
13. Wearing my hearing aids will make me seem less capable.	A B C D E F G
14. The cost of my hearing aids will be reasonable.	A B C D E F G
15. My hearing aids will be dependable (need few repairs).	A B C D E F G

Please respond to these additional items.

LIFETIME HEARING AID EXPERIENCE (includes all old and current hearing aids)	DAILY HEARING AID USE	DEGREE OF HEARING DIFFICULTY (without wearing a hearing aid)
☐ None ☐ Less than 6 weeks ☐ 6 weeks to 11 months ☐ 1 to 10 years ☐ Over 10 years	☐ None ☐ Less than 1 hour per day ☐ 1 to 4 hours per day ☐ 4 to 8 hours per day ☐ 8 to 16 hours per day	☐ None ☐ Mild ☐ Moderate ☐ Moderately Severe ☐ Severe

HARL
Hearing Aid Research Lab.

ECHO Scale: Items & Subscales

SCALE	ITEMS (*) = reversed item
Positive Effect	1, 3, 5, 6, 9, 10
Service & Cost	12, 14, 15
Negative Features	2*, 7*, 11
Personal Image	4*, 8, 13*

Instructions for Manual Scoring of the ECHO

1) Assign a value for each answer from the table below

Response	Not a Reversed Item	Reversed Item
A Not At All	1	7
B A Little	2	6
C Somewhat	3	5
D Medium	4	4
E Considerably	5	3
F Greatly	6	2
G Tremendously	7	1

2) Calculate the average score for each subscale, e.g., if items for the Negative Features subscale have assigned scores of 6,4,and 3, the Negative Features subscale score is (6+4+3)/3 = 4.3

3) The Global Score is the mean of the scores for all the items.

4) If the box is checked in item 11 (hears well on the telephone without hearing aids), omit this item even if an answer was also selected from the scale.

6/30/98

ECHO Reality Norms

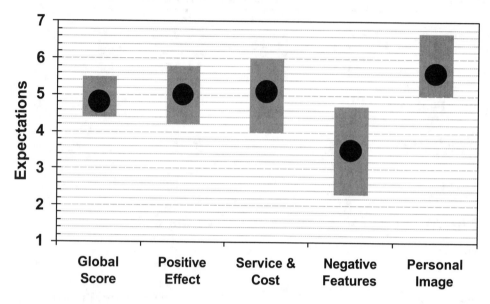

Black circle = mean score
Gray bar = 20th to 80th percentile scores

Please refer to the following article for information about the interpretation of these norms:
Cox, RM, and Alexander, GC. (2000). Expectations about hearing aids and their relationship to fitting outcome. J Am Acad Audiol 11, 368-382.

Comments:_____

_____

_____

_____

_____

_____

_____

_____

Appendix AI

NAL
CLIENT ORIENTED SCALE OF IMPROVEMENT

National Acoustic Laboratories
A division of Australian Hearing

Name : _____

Audiologist : _____

Date : _____   Category.   New _____   Return _____

1. Needs Established
2. Outcome Assessed

SPECIFIC NEEDS

Indicate Order of Significance

☐	_____
☐	_____
☐	_____
☐	_____
☐	_____

Degree of Change

	Worse	No Difference	Slightly Better	Better	Much Better

CATEGORY

CATEGORY

Final Ability (with hearing aid)

Person can hear

10% 25% 50% 75% 95%

	Hardly Ever	Occasionally	Half the Time	Most of Time	Almost Always

Categories

1. Conversation with 1 or 2 in quiet
2. Conversation with 1 or 2 in noise
3. Conversation with group in quiet
4. Conversation with group in noise
5. Television/Radio @ normal volume
6. Familiar speaker on phone
7. Unfamiliar speaker on phone
8. Hearing phone ring from another room
9. Hear front door bell or knock
10. Hear traffic
11. Increased social contact
12. Feel embarrassed or stupid
13. Feeling left out
14. Feeling upset or angry
15. Church or meeting
16. Other

433

Hearing Aid Selection Profile (HASP)

Name: _____ Age: _____ Date: _____

Instructions: Please place a √ in the box indicating how strongly you agree or disagree with each statement below. If you do not agree or disagree, place a √ in the "**Neutral**" box. Please do not skip any items. Please complete all the items regardless of whether you are going to receive one or two hearing aids.

		Strongly Agree	Agree	Neutral	Disagree	Strongly Disagree
1T.	Computers have made our lives easier and better.	☐	☐	☐	☐	☐
2A.	If I were losing my hair, I would get a transplant, wear a wig, or toupee, or take medicine to make it stop.	☐	☐	☐	☐	☐
3A.	I do not feel comfortable about leaving the house unless I look just right.	☐	☐	☐	☐	☐
4T.	I have or would like to have a cellular phone.	☐	☐	☐	☐	☐
5C.	I am not an extravagant buyer.	☐	☐	☐	☐	☐
6P.	It is easy for me to use small objects such as paper clips, coins, small buttons, and/or zippers.	☐	☐	☐	☐	☐
7CI.	It is very important for me to hear conversations with one other person.	☐	☐	☐	☐	☐
8CI.	It is very important for me to be able to hear on the telephone.	☐	☐	☐	☐	☐
9A.	There is nothing wrong with using plastic surgery to improve ones appearance.	☐	☐	☐	☐	☐
10L.	I consider myself to be an active, busy, on-the-go kind of person.	☐	☐	☐	☐	☐
11P.	I do not have arthritis in my fingers.	☐	☐	☐	☐	☐
12L.	Physical activity is an important part of my life.	☐	☐	☐	☐	☐
13E.	A hearing aid will restore my hearing to normal just as eyeglasses restore vision to normal.	☐	☐	☐	☐	☐
14E.	I expect that my hearing aid will improve my ability to understand speech in background noise.	☐	☐	☐	☐	☐
15P.	I have good sensation in my fingertips.	☐	☐	☐	☐	☐
16M.	I want to wear a hearing aid even if I still have difficulty hearing in some situations.	☐	☐	☐	☐	☐
17A.	I am self-conscious about my appearance.	☐	☐	☐	☐	☐
18E.	My hearing aid will make speech clear, distinct, and understandable in all situations.	☐	☐	☐	☐	☐

		Strongly Agree	Agree	Neutral	Disagree	Strongly Disagree
19T.	I feel that new technology has improved our lives.	☐	☐	☐	☐	☐
20M.	I know that a hearing aid will help me.	☐	☐	☐	☐	☐
21CI.	It is very important for me to hear the television and/or radio.	☐	☐	☐	☐	☐
22L.	I enjoy going to movies, lectures, parties, restaurants, and/or to the symphony.	☐	☐	☐	☐	☐
23CI.	It is very important for me to be able to hear in a place of worship, at a lecture, at a concert and/or movies.	☐	☐	☐	☐	☐
24A.	I am often concerned about how others view my appearance.	☐	☐	☐	☐	☐
25T.	I like gadgets such as remote controls and find them very useful.	☐	☐	☐	☐	☐
26C.	I don't think that I need the best that money can buy.	☐	☐	☐	☐	☐
27M.	I am prepared to do what it takes to improve my hearing.	☐	☐	☐	☐	☐
28C.	When it comes to money, I don't like to take risks.	☐	☐	☐	☐	☐
29L.	I am quite active and involved in lots of activities and social events.	☐	☐	☐	☐	☐
30L.	I consider myself to be in good physical condition.	☐	☐	☐	☐	☐
31T.	I have a microwave oven and have used one for many years.	☐	☐	☐	☐	☐
32C.	I am a price-conscious consumer.	☐	☐	☐	☐	☐
33M.	I am certain that I want a hearing aid.	☐	☐	☐	☐	☐
34M.	I am having a significant problem understanding speech.	☐	☐	☐	☐	☐
35C.	I only purchase items that I can afford.	☐	☐	☐	☐	☐
36CI.	It is very important for me to hear conversations when I am in larger groups, for example, at a party.	☐	☐	☐	☐	☐
37P.	I have no difficulty (or would have no difficulty) holding or shuffling cards.	☐	☐	☐	☐	☐
38E.	A hearing aid will make it possible for me to understand speech in all situations.	☐	☐	☐	☐	☐
39E.	My hearing aid will make speech sound natural.	☐	☐	☐	☐	☐
40P.	I can hold my hands steady, in one position, for at least 10 seconds.	☐	☐	☐	☐	☐

HASP Scoring Template

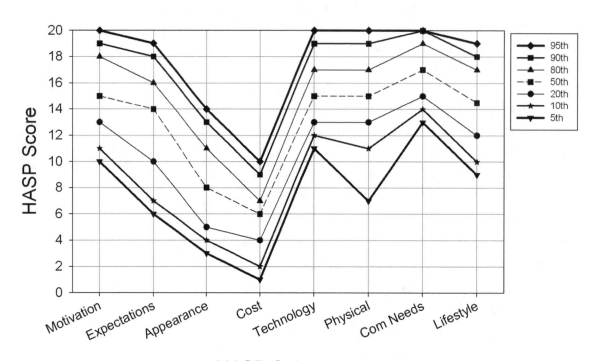

Appendix AL

Characteristics of Amplification Tool

Name: _____   Date:_____

Our goal is to maximize your ability to hear so that you can more easily communicate with others. In order to reach this goal, it is important that we understand your communication needs, your personal preferences, and your expectations. By having a better understanding of your needs, we can use our expertise to recommend the hearing aids that are most appropriate for **you**. By working together **we** will find the best solution for you.

Please complete the following questions. Be as honest as possible. Be as precise as possible. Thank you.

1. Please list the top three situations where you would most like to hear better. Be as specific as possible.

    _____

    _____

    _____

2. How important is it for you to hear better? Mark an X on the line.

    Not Very Important -- *Very Important*

3. How motivated are you to wear and use hearing aids? Mark an X on the line

    Not Very Motivated -- *Very Motivated*

4. How well do you think hearing aids will improve your hearing? Mark an X on the line.

    I expect them to:

    Not be helpful   -- *Greatly improve my*
    at all   *hearing*

5. What is your most important consideration regarding hearing aids? Rank order the following factors with **1** as the most important and **4** as the least important. Place an **X** on the line if the item has no importance to you at all.

    ____ Hearing aid size and the ability of others not to see the hearing aids

    ____ Improved ability to hear and understand speech

    ____ Improved ability to understand speech in noisy situations (e.g., restaurants, parties)

    ____ Cost of the hearing aids

Sandridge & Newman (2006)

Characteristics of Amplification Tool

6. Do you prefer hearing aids that: (check one)

    ___   are totally automatic so that you do not have to make any adjustments to them.

    ___   allow you to adjust the volume and change the listening programs as you see fit.

    ___   no preference

7. Look at the pictures of the hearing aids. Please place an X on the picture or pictures of the style you would **NOT** be willing to use. Your audiologist will discuss with you if your choices are appropriate for you—given your hearing loss and physical shape of your ear.

BTE   Full Shell   Half Shell

Mini BTE   Canal   CIC

8. How confident do you feel that you will be successful in using hearing aids?

    Not Very Confident -- *Very Confident*

9. There is a wide range in hearing aid prices. The cost of hearing aids depends on a variety of factors including the sophistication of the circuitry (for example, higher level technology is more expensive than more basic hearing aids) and size/style. The price ranges listed below are for *two* hearing aids. Please check the cost category that represents the maximum amount you are willing to spend. Please understand that you are not locked into that price range. It is just very helpful for us to know your budget so that we can provide you with the most appropriate hearing aids.

    ____   Basic digital hearing aids: Cost is between _____ to _____
    ____   Basic Plus hearing aids: Cost is between _____ to _____
    ____   Mid-level digital hearing aids: Cost is between _____ to _____
    ____   Premium digital hearing aids: Cost is between _____ to _____

Sandridge & Newman (2006)

PROFILE OF AIDED LOUDNESS

Name: _____

Date: _____

Status: __ unaided __ previous hearing aids
___ current hearing aids

Instructions: Please rate the following items by both the level of loudness of the sound and by the appropriateness of that loudness level. For example, you might rate a particular sound as "Very Soft." If "Very Soft" is your preferred level for this sound, then you would rate your loudness satisfaction as "Just Right." If, on the other hand, you think the sound should be louder than "Very Soft", then your loudness satisfaction rating might be "Not Too Good" or "Not Good At All." The Loudness Satisfaction rating is not related to how pleasing the sound is to you, but rather, the appropriateness of the loudness. Here is an example:

The hum of a refrigerator motor:

Loudness rating	Satisfaction rating
0 Do not hear	(5.) Just right
1 Very soft	4. Pretty good
(2) Soft	3. Okay
3 Comfortable, but slightly soft	2. Not too good
4 Comfortable	1. Not good at all
5 Comfortable, but slightly loud	
6 Loud, but OK	
7 Uncomfortably loud	

In this example, the hearing aid user rated the loudness level of a refrigerator motor running as "Comfortable, but slightly soft" and rated his loudness satisfaction for this sound as "Just right." This satisfaction rating indicates that the person believes that it is appropriate for a refrigerator motor to sound "Comfortable, but slightly soft."

Circle the responses that best describe your listening experiences. If you have not experienced one of the sounds listed (or a similar sound), simply leave that question blank.

1. An electric razor:

Loudness rating	Satisfaction rating
0 Do not hear	5. Just right
1 Very soft	4. Pretty good
2 Soft	3. Okay
3 Comfortable, but slightly soft	2. Not too good
4 Comfortable	1. Not good at all
5 Comfortable, but slightly loud	
6 Loud, but OK	
7 Uncomfortably loud	

2. A door slamming:

Loudness rating	Satisfaction rating
0 Do not hear	5. Just right
1 Very soft	4. Pretty good
2 Soft	3. Okay
3 Comfortable, but slightly soft	2. Not too good
4 Comfortable	1. Not good at all
5 Comfortable, but slightly loud	
6 Loud, but OK	
7 Uncomfortably loud	

3. Your own breathing:

Loudness rating	Satisfaction rating
0 Do not hear	5. Just right
1 Very soft	4. Pretty good
2 Soft	3. Okay
3 Comfortable, but slightly soft	2. Not too good
4 Comfortable	1. Not good at all
5 Comfortable, but slightly loud	
6 Loud, but OK	
7 Uncomfortably loud	

4. Water boiling on the stove:

Loudness rating	Satisfaction rating
0 Do not hear	5. Just right
1 Very soft	4. Pretty good
2 Soft	3. Okay
3 Comfortable, but slightly soft	2. Not too good
4 Comfortable	1. Not good at all
5 Comfortable, but slightly loud	
6 Loud, but OK	
7 Uncomfortably loud	

5. A car's turn signal:

Loudness rating	Satisfaction rating
0 Do not hear	5. Just right
1 Very soft	4. Pretty good
2 Soft	3. Okay
3 Comfortable, but slightly soft	2. Not too good
4 Comfortable	1. Not good at all
5 Comfortable, but slightly loud	
6 Loud, but OK	
7 Uncomfortably loud	

6. The religious leader during the sermon:

Loudness rating	Satisfaction rating
0 Do not hear	5. Just right
1 Very soft	4. Pretty good
2 Soft	3. Okay
3 Comfortable, but slightly soft	2. Not too good
4 Comfortable	1. Not good at all
5 Comfortable, but slightly loud	
6 Loud, but OK	
7 Uncomfortably loud	

7. The dryer running:

Loudness rating
0 Do not hear
1 Very soft
2 Soft
3 Comfortable, but slightly soft
4 Comfortable
5 Comfortable, but slightly loud
6 Loud, but OK
7 Uncomfortably loud

Satisfaction rating
5. Just right
4. Pretty good
3. Okay
2. Not too good
1. Not good at all

8. You chewing soft food:

Loudness rating
0 Do not hear
1 Very soft
2 Soft
3 Comfortable, but slightly soft
4 Comfortable
5 Comfortable, but slightly loud
6 Loud, but OK
7 Uncomfortably loud

Satisfaction rating
5. Just right
4. Pretty good
3. Okay
2. Not too good
1. Not good at all

9. Listening to a marching band:

Loudness rating
0 Do not hear
1 Very soft
2 Soft
3 Comfortable, but slightly soft
4 Comfortable
5 Comfortable, but slightly loud
6 Loud, but OK
7 Uncomfortably loud

Satisfaction rating
5. Just right
4. Pretty good
3. Okay
2. Not too good
1. Not good at all

10. A barking dog:

Loudness rating
0 Do not hear
1 Very soft
2 Soft
3 Comfortable, but slightly soft
4 Comfortable
5 Comfortable, but slightly loud
6 Loud, but OK
7 Uncomfortably loud

Satisfaction rating
5. Just right
4. Pretty good
3. Okay
2. Not too good
1. Not good at all

11. A lawn mower:

Loudness rating
0 Do not hear
1 Very soft
2 Soft
3 Comfortable, but slightly soft
4 Comfortable
5 Comfortable, but slightly loud
6 Loud, but OK
7 Uncomfortably loud

Satisfaction rating
5. Just right
4. Pretty good
3. Okay
2. Not too good
1. Not good at all

12. A microwave buzzer sounding:

Loudness rating
0 Do not hear
1 Very soft
2 Soft
3 Comfortable, but slightly soft
4 Comfortable
5 Comfortable, but slightly loud
6 Loud, but OK
7 Uncomfortably loud

Satisfaction rating
5. Just right
4. Pretty good
3. Okay
2. Not too good
1. Not good at all

Take an average score for soft, average, and loud sounds and compare the scores to the average scores of normally hearing individuals. The patient summary sheet is used for this type of scoring. In this manner, the clinician may compare unaided loudness perception to aided loudness perception as well as having a numeric target for the aided condition.

PATIENT SUMMARY
Profile of Aided Loudness (PAL)
Unaided Performance

Soft sounds	Q3	Q4	Q5	Q8	Category average
Loudness	__	__	__	__	____ (target = 2)
Satisfaction	__	__	__	__	____

Average sounds	Q1	Q6	Q7	Q12	Category average
Loudness	__	__	__	__	____ (target = 4)
Satisfaction	__	__	__	__	____

Loud sounds	Q2	Q9	Q10	Q11	Category average
Loudness	__	__	__	__	____ (target = 6)
Satisfaction	__	__	__	__	____

Aided Performance

Soft sounds	Q3	Q4	Q5	Q8	Category average
Loudness	__	__	__	__	____ (target = 2)
Satisfaction	__	__	__	__	____

Average sounds	Q1	Q6	Q7	Q12	Category average
Loudness	__	__	__	__	____ (target = 4)
Satisfaction	__	__	__	__	____

Loud sounds	Q2	Q9	Q10	Q11	Category average
Loudness	__	__	__	__	____ (target = 6)
Satisfaction	__	__	__	__	____

Appendix AN

Normative Data for PAL

Soft Sounds

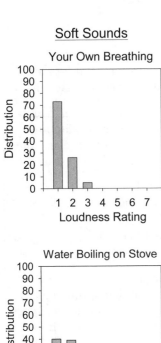

Your Own Breathing

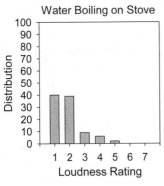

Water Boiling on Stove

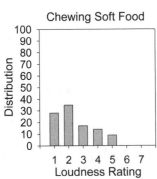

Chewing Soft Food

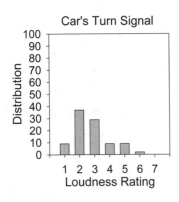

Car's Turn Signal

Average Sounds

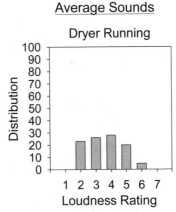

Dryer Running

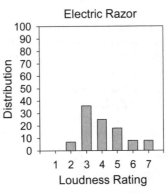

Electric Razor

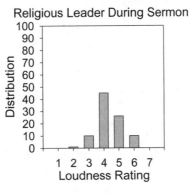

Religious Leader During Sermon

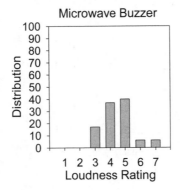

Microwave Buzzer

Loud Sounds

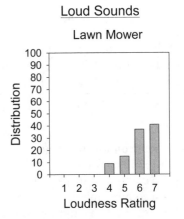

Lawn Mower

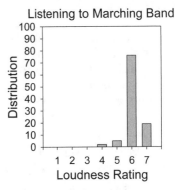

Listening to Marching Band

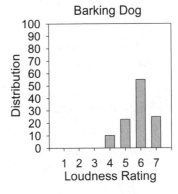

Barking Dog

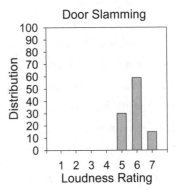

Door Slamming

Environmental Sounds Questionnaire (ESQ)

Name: _____   Date:_____

Instructions: During this week, please listen to each of the following sounds with each of your hearing aid programs. Please enter your responses to indicate the loudness of the sound and your satisfaction with that loudness level for each program.

For rating the **loudness** of the sound use the following loudness scale:		For rating your **satisfaction** with the loudness level use the following satisfaction scale:
7 = uncomfortably loud	2 = soft	5 = just right
6 = loud but okay	1 = very soft	4 = pretty good
5 = comfortable but slightly loud	0 = do not hear	3 = okay
4 = comfortable	x = don't know, e.g.,	2 = not too good
3 = comfortable but slightly soft	did not encounter that sound	1 = not good at all

For example, you might rate a particular sound as *very soft* (1). If *very soft* is your preferred level for this sound, then you would rate your loudness satisfaction as *just right* (5). If, on the other hand, you think the sound should be louder than *very soft*, then your loudness satisfaction rating might be *not too good* (2) or *not good at all* (1). The loudness satisfaction rating is not related to how pleasing or easy to hear the sound is but, rather, how satisfied you are with the loudness level perceived.

	LOUDNESS	SATISFACTION
1. Dog barking close by..	x 0 1 2 3 4 5 6 7	1 2 3 4 5
2. Travelling in a car with the windows closed.......	x 0 1 2 3 4 5 6 7	1 2 3 4 5
3. Traffic noise when standing on the curb of a busy road...	x 0 1 2 3 4 5 6 7	1 2 3 4 5
4. Your own breathing..	x 0 1 2 3 4 5 6 7	1 2 3 4 5
5. Washing machine..	x 0 1 2 3 4 5 6 7	1 2 3 4 5
6. Running water, such as a toilet or shower..........	x 0 1 2 3 4 5 6 7	1 2 3 4 5
7. Car indicator signal..	x 0 1 2 3 4 5 6 7	1 2 3 4 5
8. A motorbike passing by...	x 0 1 2 3 4 5 6 7	1 2 3 4 5
9. Chewing soft food..	x 0 1 2 3 4 5 6 7	1 2 3 4 5
10. Vacuum cleaner..	x 0 1 2 3 4 5 6 7	1 2 3 4 5
11. Water boiling on the stove..................................	x 0 1 2 3 4 5 6 7	1 2 3 4 5
12. Door slamming...	x 0 1 2 3 4 5 6 7	1 2 3 4 5
13. Telephone ringing close by................................	x 0 1 2 3 4 5 6 7	1 2 3 4 5
14. Refrigerator motor...	x 0 1 2 3 4 5 6 7	1 2 3 4 5
15. Microwave oven beeping....................................	x 0 1 2 3 4 5 6 7	1 2 3 4 5
16. Hair dryer or electric shaver.	x 0 1 2 3 4 5 6 7	1 2 3 4 5
17. Lawn mower...	x 0 1 2 3 4 5 6 7	1 2 3 4 5
18. Birds twittering..	x 0 1 2 3 4 5 6 7	1 2 3 4 5

Blamey and Martin (2009)

Appendix AP

Screening Test for Hearing Problems©

Name: _____   Date: _____

Date of Birth: _____   Gender: Male_____   Female _____
                    Month/Day/Year

Each section provides instructions and an answer key. Please circle the answer that best applies to you.

Instructions for items 1-9:

In each situation listed below, indicate how often you can
COMMUNICATE EFFECTIVELY WITH OTHERS. How often can you
give and receive information or carry on a conversation
without a great deal of effort or emotional strain?

1. Rarely, Almost Never
2. Occasionally, Sometimes
3. About Half the Time
4. Frequently, Often
5. Usually, Almost Always

---

1. You're at the dinner table with your family. 1 2 3 4 5

2. You're at a restaurant ordering food or drinks 1 2 3 4 5

3. You're talking on the telephone when you're at work or a place of business 1 2 3 4 5

4. Someone's talking to you while you're watching TV or listening to the stereo/radio..   1 2 3 4 5

5. You're talking with someone in an office. 1 2 3 4 5

6. You're at a dinner party with several other people...   1 2 3 4 5

7. You're at a meeting with several other people 1 2 3 4 5

8. You're at home and someone is talking to you from another room. 1 2 3 4 5

9. You're having a conversation at a social gathering while others are talking nearby.....   1 2 3 4 5

Please continue on the other side

Instructions for items 10-13:	1.	Rarely, Almost Never
Please indicate the experiences, feelings, and reactions that you have about hearing and communication.	2.	Occasionally, Sometimes
	3.	About Half the Time
	4.	Frequently, Often
	5.	Usually, Almost Always

10. I tend to avoid social situations where I think I'll have problems hearing 1 2 3 4 5

11. People don't speak clearly enough when they're speaking to me. 1 2 3 4 5

12. I feel foolish when I misunderstand what someone has said 1 2 3 4 5

13. People think I'm not paying attention if I don't answer them when they speak to me 1 2 3 4 5

Instructions for items 14-20:	1.	Strongly Disagree
Please indicate the level to which you agree/disagree With the following statements.	2.	Disagree
	3.	Uncertain
	4.	Agree
	5.	Strongly Agree

14. When I can't understand what's being said, I feel tense and anxious 1 2 3 4 5

15. I hate to ask others for special consideration just because I have a hearing problem 1 2 3 4 5

16. I get discouraged because of my hearing loss 1 2 3 4 5

17. I find it difficult to admit to others that I have a hearing problem 1 2 3 4 5

18. I get angry when others don't speak up 1 2 3 4 5

19. Sometimes I miss so much of what's being said that I feel left out.......................... 1 2 3 4 5

20. Others should be more understanding about my hearing problems 1 2 3 4 5

Comments:

Index

Note: Page numbers in **bold** reference non-text material.